# TOMMY DOUGLAS AND THE QUEST FOR MEDICARE IN CANADA

How and why was universal health coverage implemented so early in a poverty-stricken province in Canada? Why was its design so faithfully replicated in the national standards that ultimately shaped Medicare across the rest of Canada?

Seeking to answer these questions, *Tommy Douglas and the Quest for Medicare in Canada* explores the history of universal health care through the life of Canadian politician Tommy Douglas, identifying the pivotal moments and decisions that led to the establishment of Medicare in Canada.

The book traces the origins of Medicare back to the 1930s Depression and its devastating impact on the Prairie populations. Marchildon examines how Tommy Douglas and a new generation of reformers, radicalized by the Depression, prioritized socialized health care. The book reveals how, as the provincial party leader, Douglas leveraged support from both local and external allies to rapidly implement universal hospital insurance and lay the groundwork for a new health system.

Despite strong opposition from physician and business lobbies, Douglas continued to pressure the government for federal cost-sharing of universal health coverage. Drawing on archival sources including speeches, television broadcasts, and cabinet documents, *Tommy Douglas and the Quest for Medicare in Canada* illuminates how Douglas's vision, leadership, and coalition-building among unions were crucial to the successful establishment of Medicare in Canada.

GREGORY P. MARCHILDON is a professor emeritus at the Institute of Health Policy, Management, and Evaluation at the University of Toronto and the founding director of the North American Observatory on Health Systems and Policies.

# Tommy Douglas and the Quest for Medicare in Canada

GREGORY P. MARCHILDON

UNIVERSITY OF TORONTO PRESS
Toronto Buffalo London

© University of Toronto Press 2025
Toronto Buffalo London
utorontopress.com
Printed in Canada

ISBN 978-1-4875-6044-7 (cloth)     ISBN 978-1-4875-6046-1 (EPUB)
ISBN 978-1-4875-6043-0 (paper)     ISBN 978-1-4875-6045-4 (PDF)

Library and Archives Canada Cataloguing in Publication

Title: Tommy Douglas and the quest for medicare in Canada / Gregory P. Marchildon.
Names: Marchildon, Gregory P., 1956– author
Description: Includes bibliographical references and index.
Identifiers: Canadiana (print) 2024044857X | Canadiana (ebook) 2024044860X |
  ISBN 9781487560447 (cloth) | ISBN 9781487560430 (paper) |
  ISBN 9781487560461 (EPUB) | ISBN 9781487560454 (PDF)
Subjects: LCSH: Douglas, T. C. (Thomas Clement), 1904–1986. | LCSH: Medical care –
  Canada – History. | LCSH: Health insurance – Government policy – Canada –
  History. | LCSH: Medical policy – Canada – History.
Classification: LCC RA395.C3 M3726 2025 | DDC 362.10971 – dc23

Cover design: Sebastian Frye
Cover image: Tommy Douglas speaking at the official opening of Saskatchewan Power's natural gas system serving rural residents, 1 October 1953 (SPL B-14767)

We wish to acknowledge the land on which the University of Toronto Press operates. This land is the traditional territory of the Wendat, the Anishnaabeg, the Haudenosaunee, the Métis, and the Mississaugas of the Credit First Nation.

This book has been published with the help of a grant from the Federation for the Humanities and Social Sciences, through the Awards to Scholarly Publications Program, using funds provided by the Social Sciences and Humanities Research Council of Canada.

University of Toronto Press acknowledges the financial support of the Government of Canada, the Canada Council for the Arts, and the Ontario Arts Council, an agency of the Government of Ontario, for its publishing activities.

 Canada Council for the Arts   Conseil des Arts du Canada

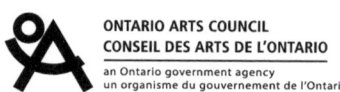 ONTARIO ARTS COUNCIL
CONSEIL DES ARTS DE L'ONTARIO
an Ontario government agency
un organisme du gouvernement de l'Ontario

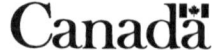 Funded by the Government of Canada   Financé par le gouvernement du Canada

*I dedicate this book to my mother who, working as a nurse's aide in City Hospital in Saskatoon during the doctors' strike of 1962, quietly disagreed with the views propounded by the hospital's medical staff and supported the Saskatchewan Medical Care Plan.*

# Contents

*Preface* ix
*Acknowledgments* xiii
*Abbreviations* xvii
*Timeline* xxi

Introduction 3
1 Medicare: The Agony and the Ecstasy 11
2 The Making of a Preacher-Politician 24
3 Federal Member of Parliament, 1935–1944 55
4 Sigerist, Sheps, and Socialism 85
5 Rise and Fall of the Green Book Proposals 124
6 Universal Hospital Insurance in Saskatchewan 143
7 National Health Grants and New Frontiers 175
8 Next-Year Country 203
9 National Influence, 1948–1958 229
10 Setting the Political Agenda Once More 267
11 The Thompson Committee and the New Party 301
12 Political Repudiation 333
13 The Doctors' Strike and the Cost of Peace 375
14 The Hall Commission and the Leftward Tilt of Canadian Politics 401

15 National Medicare    433
16 Defender of Medicare    455
Conclusion    489

*Notes*    497
*Bibliography*    639
*Index*    673

# Preface

This book is the product of a very long gestation. I have been researching the origins of universal health coverage – Medicare, as it is known in Canada – since the early 2000s. However, my fascination with Medicare, and its principal originator T.C. (Tommy) Douglas, long predates this. Growing up in Saskatchewan, I was drawn to questions of public policy in my teens. Although I moved away to complete my graduate studies in the United Kingdom and work as an academic in the United States, my interest in Canadian history, politics, and policy never abated.

In 1994, I jumped at the chance to return to Saskatchewan to work in a policy role, first as the deputy minister of intergovernmental affairs and then as cabinet secretary and deputy minister to the provincial premier, Roy Romanow. As I had had no previous experience in public administration, both jobs involved steep learning curves. To make up for my lack of experience, I spent nights and weekends studying the mechanics of Westminster-style governments, including a two-volume thesis on the structure and operations of the Douglas government. The thesis's author was A.W. (Al) Johnson, whom I soon met in South Africa as part of a Canadian project assisting the transition of that country to a multiracial democracy. This thesis and the book that grew out of it, as well as numerous conversations with Johnson, deepened my understanding of both Douglas and the establishment of universal health coverage in Saskatchewan and then Canada.

Just days after I signed an advance contract with the University of Toronto Press to write a history of Canadian Medicare, I found myself in Ottawa negotiating the mandate for what would become the Commission on the Future of Health Care in Canada (aka the Romanow Commission). This intense grappling with the question of universal health coverage, from April 2001 until November the following year, felt like drinking from a fire hose.

In the early months of the Royal Commission, I joined a confidential retreat of health system experts and practitioners, where I was confronted by a senior health official anxious about the direction of the commission. In particular, he was seeking some assurance that the commission would not be serving up what he called "that old Tommy Douglas Medicare bullshit." I immediately recognized in his statement a common enough view in the Canadian establishment: that the principles and values underpinning a strong form of universality, whatever their sentimental or popular appeal, are mere rhetoric and have nothing to do with the complex business of financing and delivering health care. The time had come, he felt, to have an "adult conversation" about Medicare, because Medicare was outdated.

In his view, T.C.'s principles and values posed a major impediment to overhauling the system. His tone and words also conveyed that, as an insider, I had too much experience with the real world, and politics and policy, to not understand this reality, as much as it was unacceptable to say so publicly because of the continuing popular support for the policy. He wanted some affirmation that I knew the time had come (finally) to ignore such high-sounding bromides and get on with recommending changes – private finance and private delivery – that could finally deliver the goods, irrespective of how such changes conflicted with the original principles and values of Medicare as expressed by Douglas. I suspect my response was less than satisfying when I said the commission would examine the strengths and weaknesses of the current system in terms of quality, timeliness, and responsiveness in serving Canada, including how Canadians were being served by existing federal-provincial arrangements. However, his words stuck, and the commission, in a partnership with the Canadian Policy Research Networks, organized twelve deliberative dialogues involving close to 500 randomly selected Canadians to interrogate the relevance of the original values and principles of Medicare as part of working through alternative reform scenarios.[1]

Once the Romanow Commission completed its work, I returned to academic life, with the idea that I would finally have the time and peace to do the historical excavation necessary to understand the polarized views on both Douglas and the policy of Medicare. I thought it would take four, possibly five, years to conduct the research and write the book. In the song "Beautiful Boy (Darling Boy)," John Lennon uses an oft-repeated quote "Life is what happens to you while you're busy making other plans." Well, life happened for the next two decades, upsetting my original plans. Almost immediately upon my return to academic life, I found myself regularly abandoning my comfortable academic cocoon to provide contemporary policy advice to governments and international organizations.

In the process, I was asked by a special operating agency of the World Health Organization's Regional Office for Europe, known as the European Observatory on Health Systems and Policies, to write a book-length review of the Canadian health system. This project would take me three years to complete and got me on a different track, including two subsequently (and considerably) revised editions of the same monograph. In these editions, I provided truncated histories of Medicare in Canada, including, of course, Saskatchewan's pioneering role in implementing universal hospital coverage eighteen months before the National Health Service was introduced in the United Kingdom. Each time I wrote and edited these sections, I was reminded of my earlier ambition to write a narrative of these events, but the lure of addressing contemporary policy problems kept drawing me away from history. In other words, the urgent continually pushed out the important. Still, I always knew that one day I would research and write the book on Douglas and Medicare.

During these many years, I was not completely negligent. I researched a wrote a few journal articles and book chapters on the history of Medicare and edited books on the subject. These more specialized pieces allowed me the research time to explore the contours of Medicare, ultimately helping shape the book I finally wrote. However, it was not until I entered into a phased retirement agreement with the University of Toronto that I finally began to work on the book in earnest. I freed myself enough to be able to spend almost all my time on the book. When I completely retired in July 2022, I was able to focus exclusively on the story I really wanted to tell, the three-decade-long gestation and infancy of Medicare. While the biographical element provides a natural structure to the story, I needed to provide some analysis of the policy as it originated, and I hope this book reflects "story and understanding in equal measure."[2]

I decided from the beginning to base my account on as much original research as possible to ensure the accuracy of the story I tell here. Wherever feasible, I used this research to shed some new light on both Douglas and the history of Medicare. While my search for documentary evidence took me to numerous archives and slowed the writing of this book, I felt it was essential to understand the story of Medicare as accurately as possible, irrespective of what the secondary sources stated about episodes or individuals. Where archival evidence was lacking, I relied heavily on contemporary newspaper and magazine articles. These sources were, in fact, invaluable in providing not only detail but some colour to key events.

This primary documentation is considerably enriched by interview evidence that has been conducted by researchers in the past and deposited in archives. The most notable examples are the hundreds of transcript pages of recorded interviews conducted by Jean Larmour with Tommy Douglas. Larmour did this work in the early 1980s on behalf of her employer, the Saskatchewan Archives Board (now the Provincial Archives of Saskatchewan). While I have interpreted interview evidence very carefully in light the frailties of human memory and the potential for self-aggrandizement, these interviews provide a richness of emotion and personality not found in official correspondence and memoranda.

As for the secondary literature, so much has been written about the history of Medicare that, at many points during my research, I felt that I was drowning in a sea of sources. There was no obvious "gap in the literature" that could be addressed only through primary sources. My life would have been far simpler if I had not selected a policy on which so much attention has been lavished.

While conducting my research and writing this book, I have been acutely aware of my natural predisposition to Douglas's goals – and to the man himself. I agree with American historian and biographer Jill Lepore that, while being so "close to your subject certainly poses some dangers," it is equally dangerous – and I would say far more problematic – not to know your subject as intimately as you can, given the availability of so many primary and secondary research sources.[3] Indeed, Lepore argues that this kind of "intimacy" should, for good historical investigators, border on invasiveness. For André Maurois, writing a biography was "a way of liberating me from myself," to which Canadian historian Brian McKillop agreed but added that biography also "enlarged and enriched and emboldened."[4] Researching and writing this book has been an enlarging, enriching, emboldening, and even liberating experience for me.

While I think there is much of interest here for current students and observers of contemporary health care in Canada, I consciously did not write this account with the present and future in mind. Admittedly, I have often used history to inform current policy, especially health reform agendas, and I wanted to be as sensitive as possible to the historical context of the times in which this narrative is placed. To do this, I had to leave the twenty-first century and live for a time in the twentieth. What I discovered in my time travel is that, while some important changes had taken place since T.C.'s death in 1986, much remains the same.

# Acknowledgments

The research, thinking, and extended dialogues that have shaped this book stretch over two decades. I owe an enormous debt to numerous individuals. My early thinking on the origins of Canadian Medicare were spurred by authors including A.W. Johnson and his biography of the Douglas government, Malcolm Taylor and his indispensable policy history of Medicare, David Naylor on the history of organized medicine and Medicare, along with comparative political scientists Antonia Maioni and Carolyn Tuohy, who have compared the evolution of universal health coverage in Canada to historical developments in other high-income countries such as the United States and the United Kingdom. I owe a special thanks to Carolyn for our insightful discussions and her rigorous analysis of the historical compact between organized medicine and the state that lies at the heart of Canadian Medicare. I owe a special debt of gratitude to historian Erika Dyck who encouraged me for years to get on with my book. I want to also thank Robert Fraser for commissioning me to write the entry for T.C. Douglas for the *Dictionary of Canadian Biography*, an assignment that ultimately led to my decision to used Douglas's life as the constant thread in this narrative history of Medicare.

Usually, historians face a paucity of sources. That is not the case for the history Medicare. Ministers and officials working for the government of Canada left a ton of documentary material recording their efforts to establish a national umbrella for Medicare, most of which is now held in trust by Library and Archives Canada, the country's largest and most comprehensive repository. Every provincial government has also generated a mass of material on the introduction of both universal hospital insurance and universal medical care coverage. Although the most notable collection, as expected, was at the Provincial Archives of Saskatchewan (PAS), the voluminous documentary evidence on the history of Medicare accessible in other provincial and university archives in Canada was amazing to me. Because of the prominent individuals who were attracted to the Saskatchewan experiment, I found documents in unlikely places outside Canada, such as the archival collections held by Yale University, Johns Hopkins University, the University of Toronto, and the London School of Economics and Political Science. Through it all, I relied heavily on the expertise of knowledgeable archivists at all these institutions, and I thank them collectively for their assistance and patience.

Although I conducted the bulk of the research for this book, I was ably assisted by some very fine research assistants in the early years of this project. I must first acknowledge Roberta Lexier, now an associate professor at Mount Royal University. Roberta spent months at PAS going through Douglas's papers and those of his ministers of health, and she did some preliminary spade work on Manningcare at the Provincial Archives of Alberta in 2004–5. Jessica Benjamin conducted targeted archival research on mental health reform and innovation in Saskatchewan during the late 1950s and early 1960s, while Scott MacNeill conducted some archival research on my behalf in Manitoba. Gordon Lawson generously provided me with access to his research on the early years of the Douglas government and spent a day on my behalf at PAS. In working with me on the history of Medicare in British Columbia and New Brunswick, my sister Nicole O'Byrne conducted research at the British Columbia Archives and the British Columbia Legislative Library in Victoria.

I never met or interviewed Douglas himself. In this regard, I was dependent on the impressions of those who worked closely with him, especially the Saskatchewan Mafia – the Douglas government bureaucrats who left a major footprint on the Pearson and Trudeau governments from the 1960s to the 1980s. Among others, these individuals included A.W. (Al) Johnson, T.K. (Tommy) Shoyama, and Donald D. Tansley. I spent valuable time with Don, who recounted in detail his experiences as the chair of the Medical Care Insurance Commission, perhaps the most dangerous position ever assumed by a civil servant in Saskatchewan. I am most indebted to Al Johnson, with whom I enjoyed a close friendship until his death in 2010. We had many discussions about Douglas's time in Regina and Ottawa as well as the evolution of Medicare from 1959 on, including important details concerning the 1962 doctors' strike, the Saskatoon Agreement, the federal-provincial negotiation of a national medical care plan, and the eventual replacement of federal shared-cost financing of Medicare with block funding.

I also had the great fortune to spend time talking to, and even interviewing, Allan Blakeney and Walter Smishek. Although I foolishly misplaced the typescripts of their interviews, I never forgot their observations and used them to buttress this narrative. Blakeney revealed the fissures in cabinet before and during the doctors' strike. Smishek, the trade union representative on the provincial Advisory Planning Committee on Medical Care (the Thompson Committee), opposed Douglas's acceptance of organized medicine's insistence on fee-for-service payment, but admitted to me that, with time, he came to accept that there was no other way that universal medical care could have been introduced.

I want to thank Roy Romanow for all our conversations about Medicare over the years. While conducting an interview with him on his student days for a short biography of his premiership, I obtained a wealth of information concerning the debate over Medicare in Saskatchewan and how it turned him into the politician he became. These discussions led to a better understanding of the extreme political polarization in the province unleashed by Medicare in the early 1960s. There were other friends such as Dr. Stuart Houston, who stood with the doctors against Medicare in 1962 only to become (unlike his father, Dr. Clarence Houston) a staunch supporter. A research economist in the Hall Commission of 1961–4, Dr. Jack Boan recounted critical details concerning that landmark commission. I was also able to spend a wonderful afternoon with Meyer Brownstone, who happened to live just a few blocks from me in Toronto. His critical analysis forced me to think more carefully about the nature of the centralized management of Medicare at the provincial level and the alternatives then available to Douglas and others.

I want to thank the amazing librarians at the University of Toronto who helped me locate the hard copies of old and obscure secondary sources. I am also grateful for U of T's enormous digital collection of books, journals, newspapers, and magazines, which I regularly accessed from the comfort of my home office. I also thank the Institute of Health Policy, Management and Evaluation at the University of Toronto for allowing me a one-year sabbatical to try to finish this book. Although it took my retirement and two more years to finish, that year was critical for the transition from researching to beginning to write.

For the sections in chapter 8 on the children's dental care program and the Saskatchewan Plan for mental health treatment, I drew on previously published work. I thank the University of Toronto Press Journals for permission to re-use portions of articles previously published in the *Canadian Journal of Health History* and *Histoire sociale / Social History*.

I am lucky to have generous friends and colleagues who share a fascination with the history of Medicare. Thank you to Patrick Farrell for reviewing and providing editorial feedback on the first very rough draft. I shared a barely improved version with Owen Adams,

Tom Bossert, Gordon Lawson, Nicole O'Byrne, Don Phillipon, and Bill Tholl, who, along with two anonymous peer reviewers as well as an insightful review from the University of Toronto Press's manuscript review committee, provided excellent feedback and suggestions. I also want to thank Jim Connor for reviewing the chapter on Fred Mott and the introduction of universal hospital insurance in Saskatchewan. I owe a special debt to Gordon Lawson, who, after reading the original draft, read the revised version of the chapters with which I had lingering concerns. He also was generous in providing me with the archival material he had collected while conducting his thesis on the question of physician remuneration in the early years of the Douglas government in Saskatchewan. These readers spurred me on to rethink and, in places, restructure the manuscript, and I am forever grateful to all of them.

Len Husband of the University of Toronto Press is owed a special thanks. He sat on my advance contract for over two decades, never once confronting me about the missing manuscript, even when I published other books in the meantime. Instead, as he said once, books take the time they need, leaving the pace entirely to me. Len, you are the most patient editor I have ever known! I am also most appreciative of Barbara Tessman's superb copyediting and was so grateful that she was selected by the publisher to be the copyeditor for this book.

# Abbreviations

| | |
|---|---|
| AMA | American Medical Association |
| AM | Archives of Manitoba |
| AO | Archives of Ontario |
| APC | Advisory Planning Committee on Medical Care (Thompson Committee), Saskatchewan |
| BCA | British Columbia Archives |
| CAR | *Canadian Annual Review* |
| CBC | Canadian Broadcasting Corporation |
| CCF | Co-operative Commonwealth Federation |
| CCYM | Co-operative Commonwealth Youth Movement |
| CEC | Citizens' Emergency Committee (Regina) |
| CLC | Canadian Labour Congress |
| CMA | Canadian Medical Association |
| CMHA | Canadian Mental Health Association |
| CMHA (Sask.) | Saskatchewan Division of the Canadian Mental Health Association |
| CPC | Communist Party of Canada |
| CPS | College of Physicians and Surgeons of Saskatchewan (acting as the Saskatchewan Division of the CMA, 1936–66) |
| DCB | *Dictionary of Canadian Biography* |
| DLAS | *Debates*, Legislative Assembly of Saskatchewan |
| EPF | Established Programs Financing |
| FERA | Federal Emergency Relief Administration (United States) |
| FFS | fee-for-service |
| FSA | Farm Security Administration (United States) |
| GMS | Group Medical Services (Saskatchewan) |
| GP | general practitioner |

| | |
|---|---|
| HCD | *House of Commons Debates*, Government of Canada |
| HIDSA | Health Insurance and Diagnostic Services Act (government of Canada) |
| HSPC | Health Services Planning Commission (government of Saskatchewan) |
| ILP | Independent Labour Party |
| JHCA | Johns Hopkins Chesney Archives |
| JLAS | Journals of the Legislative Assembly of Saskatchewan |
| KOD | Keep Our Doctors |
| LAC | Library and Archives Canada |
| LP | *Regina Leader-Post* |
| LSE | London School of Economics and Political Science, Archives and Special Collections |
| LSR | League for Social Reconstruction |
| MCA | Medical Care Act (government of Canada) |
| MCIC | Medical Care Insurance Commission (government of Saskatchewan) |
| MLA | member of the Legislative Assembly |
| MP | member of Parliament |
| MSI | Medical Services Incorporated (Saskatchewan) |
| NATO | North Atlantic Treaty Organization |
| NFB | National Film Board of Canada |
| NDP | New Democratic Party |
| NHI | national health insurance |
| NHS | National Health Service (United Kingdom) |
| PAA | Provincial Archives of Alberta |
| PAS | Provincial Archives of Saskatchewan |
| PC | Progressive Conservative Party |
| PM | prime minister |
| PSB | Psychiatric Services Branch, Department of Public Health (government of Saskatchewan) |
| QUA | Queen's University Archives |
| RM | rural municipality |
| SARM | Saskatchewan Association of Rural Municipalities |
| SFL | Saskatchewan Federation of Labour |
| SHA | Saskatchewan Hospital Association |
| SHML | State Hospital and Medical League (Saskatchewan) |
| SHSP | Saskatchewan Hospital Services Plan |
| SMA | Saskatchewan Medical Association Archives |
| Socred | Social Credit Party |
| SP | *Saskatoon Star Phoenix* |

| | |
|---|---|
| SPL | Saskatoon Public Library |
| SUMA | Saskatchewan Urban Municipalities Association |
| UHC | universal health coverage |
| UHD | union hospital district (Saskatchewan) |
| URA | University of Regina Archives |
| USAS | University of Saskatchewan Archives and Special Collections |
| UTA | University of Toronto Archives |
| WILA | Weyburn Independent Labour Association |
| YUA | Yale University Library, Manuscripts and Archives |

# Timeline

1904  Birth of Thomas Clement (T.C.) Douglas in Falkirk, Scotland, on 20 October

1912  Douglas family moves from Falkirk to Winnipeg

1916  T.C. moves to Glasgow with his mother and two sisters while his father serves with the Canadian Expeditionary Force

1919  In January, T.C. along with his mother and sisters move back to Winnipeg; his father, Tom, follows months later after release from military hospital.

1930  T.C. graduates from Brandon College and is appointed as pastor of Calvary Baptist Church in Weyburn, Saskatchewan

1931  In summer, T.C. begins graduate studies, including fieldwork, at University of Chicago

1933  T.C. completes master's thesis on the "subnormal" family; release of the CCF's Regina Manifesto and party's call for socialized health services

1934  T.C. defeated as Farmer-Labour (CCF) candidate in provincial election

1935  T.C. elected to federal Parliament as CCF MP for Weyburn

1942  T.C. elected leader of the CCF in Saskatchewan

1944  CCF government elected in Saskatchewan on 15 June; T.C. establishes Sigerist Commission to survey health system and recommend next steps

1946  Failure of the Dominion-Provincial Reconstruction Conference proposals, including comprehensive health insurance

## Timeline

| | |
|---|---|
| 1947 | Saskatchewan government implements universal hospital insurance plan |
| 1948 | Beginning of National Health Grants program |
| 1950 | Alberta government under Premier Ernest Manning implements multi-payer hospital insurance plan |
| 1957 | Passage of federal Hospital Insurance and Diagnostic Services Act (HIDSA) |
| 1958 | Saskatchewan, British Columbia, Manitoba, and Newfoundland are first provinces to be eligible for federal cost sharing under HIDSA |
| 1959 | T.C.'s December radio broadcast outlining broad principles of proposed provincial medical care insurance plan |
| 1960 | Douglas government wins single-issue election on medicare on 8 June |
| 1961 | T.C. elected leader of the federal New Democratic Party in August; medical care bill passed in Saskatchewan Legislative Assembly |
| 1962 | T.C. defeated in federal election of 18 June; Saskatchewan doctors' strike in July ends with the signing of the Saskatoon Agreement |
| 1964 | Release of Hall Commission Report recommending universal coverage for medical care and other services in Canada |
| 1966 | Passage of federal Medical Care Act in December supporting provincial implementation of universal medical care coverage |
| 1968 | T.C. defeated in Trudeaumania election of 25 June |
| 1970 | Quebec doctors' strike; October Crisis and T.C.'s opposition to imposition of War Measures Act |
| 1971 | David Lewis replaces T.C. as leader of the federal NDP |
| 1977 | Federal shared-cost financing of Medicare replaced by block funding through Established Programs Financing (EPF), a change opposed by NDP |
| 1979 | T.C. retires as MP and helps spearhead SOS Medicare Conference |
| 1984 | Passage of Canada Health Act in Parliament |
| 1986 | T.C. dies on 24 February |
| 2004 | T.C. voted "greatest Canadian" by public in CBC contest |

# TOMMY DOUGLAS AND THE QUEST FOR MEDICARE IN CANADA

# Introduction

Politics is ethics done in public.

Bernard Crick, *In Defence of Politics* (1962)[1]

After their deaths, most political leaders rapidly lose the prominence they enjoyed in their lifetimes. Only a rare few grow posthumously in reputation and stature, especially within a constantly changing historical narrative. Without a doubt, T.C. (Thomas Clement) Douglas was among these rare politicians. While he was known as T.C. for a considerable portion of his political career, he became better known as Tommy in later decades. After his death in 1986, Tommy was both lovingly remembered as the thin, bespeckled leader who had transformed Canada, despite never achieving the office of prime minister. Indeed, he was voted the greatest Canadian of all time in a popular poll conducted by the Canadian Broadcasting Corporation (CBC) as part of its 2004 television series of the same name, almost two decades after his death.

T.C.'s top ranking was unusual, given the stature of other prominent Canadian celebrities, prime ministers, and hockey players (always high on popularity lists in Canada), any one of whom could easily have taken the title based on a popular vote. Some might point to Douglas's being the lucky recipient of a popular campaign, but this too reflects the continuing salience of his legacy to many individuals. What is most interesting is that Douglas would not likely have received such acclaim in his lifetime. During his career as a politician, as premier of Saskatchewan and as the leader of a national political party, Douglas's achievements were regularly challenged by those opposed to his policies.

The achievement most associated with his name is Medicare, and almost all those voting for him as the greatest Canadian likely thought of Medicare as his greatest accomplishment. In his lifetime, he was as hated by his many adversaries as he was loved by his supporters. With death, old enemies (with some exceptions, of course) began to better appreciate this one achievement, a policy that perhaps, with the passage of time, seemed less threatening to their assumptions, beliefs, policies, and interests.[2]

**Canadian Medicare and T.C Douglas**

Is the history of universal health coverage in Canada severable from T.C. Douglas? In the popular mind, it is not. Douglas was Medicare, and Medicare was Douglas to most Canadians, at least to those who were born before the twenty-first century and have some knowledge of Canadian history. Without doubt, there were many underlying forces and key individuals that ultimately produced the policy of universal health coverage (UHC) in Canada. However, when all the evidence is sifted, T.C. still emerges as the single most important individual among the cast of characters who had a role in the introduction of Medicare.

This is not to say that Medicare would never have been introduced in Canada in the absence of T.C.: some form of public health insurance would surely have been enacted. Yet, without Douglas, UHC would never have been implemented as early as it was and, more importantly, it is highly unlikely that Medicare would have taken the form it ultimately assumed. Douglas, more than any other individual or social force, is responsible for the single-payer and single-tier universality that became essential and entrenched attributes of Canadian Medicare as it evolved from 1946 until the passage of the Canada Health Act in 1984.[3] There can be little question of T.C.'s crucial role in the advent and shaping of the first phase – universal hospital coverage. He oversaw its timing, design, and implementation from the day he was elected premier of Saskatchewan in 1944, and was the principal champion for its national adoption over a decade later. As for the second phase – universal medical care coverage – the credit is more distributed, but he nonetheless played a leading role. Consequently, T.C.'s life presents a very useful entry into a narrative history of Medicare.

Although Douglas is the central figure in this book, it is essential to recognize that Medicare is a product of circumstances and key events that occurred within a particular historical context. Two critical events are unquestionably important. The first is the Great Depression of the 1930s, which upended assumptions; radicalized many farmers, workers, and intellectuals; and created new political movements. The second is the deep desire for reconstruction that came in the wake of the

Second World War, including a welfare state that would provide access to necessary health care from cradle to grave.

It is also essential to understand the role of many other individuals aside from Douglas who contributed much to the introduction of UHC in Canada. Certainly we encounter some familiar faces, including federal health ministers Paul Martin Sr. and Allan J. MacEachen, Prime Minister Lester B. Pearson, and Justice Emmett Hall, the chair of a major royal commission. However, the reader will also encounter less familiar individuals who played an important part in the pursuit of Medicare in Canada. In other words, among the protagonists in this history, T.C. is essential, but not sufficient.

**Biography as Entry Point**

There has been a long and continuing debate among professional historians concerning the utility of biography in history. By the late 1960s, "biography had not just fallen from grace" among historians but, in the eyes of many academics, had "become the stepchild of history."[4] Although the view of biography as an "inferior type of history" or the "shallow end of history" has become attenuated in recent years, it is nonetheless perceived as potentially treacherous.[5] And undoubtedly some dangers are associated with the genre. One of the most serious is the author's identification with the subject's objectives in life, which can impair the writer's critical and impartial assessment of the individual's motives, behaviours, actions, and impacts. To be blunt, this danger was particularly real for me, given my personal identification with T.C.'s lifelong struggle to ensure that all Canadians received the benefits of comprehensive health coverage based on need rather than ability to pay. To counter this tendency, I had to interrogate throughout the very nature of this identification.

As for understanding Douglas, I had distinct disadvantages. Not only had I never met him, but even after reading previous biographies and poring over mounds of his own correspondence and a plethora of interviews with other researchers and authors, I felt I still did not have deep grasp of the inner person. My only consolation was the fact that his closest colleagues often remarked that they never truly knew the man, despite working with him for decades.[6]

Lawrence Goldman said that his biography of economic historian and Labour Party activist R.H. Tawney was "as good a way as any of presenting the history" of the welfare state in Britain.[7] In the case of Tommy Douglas, I would go further. Using his life as the narrative arc to explore the history of Canadian Medicare gives both author and reader a ring-side seat in the birth and early development of universal health coverage in Canada. Of course, we can't expect to occupy the best seat in the house forever, and, after 1962, we find that Douglas, although he remains important to the story, becomes far less central in the ongoing development of Medicare. We get moved back a few rows, although still close enough to the stage to see the actors and their more subtle expressions and even startled looks when things go off script.

The largest challenge I faced when researching this book was the fact that so much has already been written about Douglas. I could relate to British historian Robert Rotberg's predicament when he wrote his biography of imperialist Cecil Rhodes: "I was the fourteenth or so biographer of Rhodes. All but two of my counterparts passed on false rumors obtained from the writings of their predecessors. Like the 'telephone' game, one biographer after another had taken as gospel the telling (which proved not so telling) anecdotes embedded in those earlier volumes."[8] I faced almost as many biographies of Douglas, with stories that were told and retold to the point of mythmaking. The fact that many (though not all) of the existing Douglas biographies are hagiographies presents its own challenges. Like Jonathan Eig in his superb biography of Baptist preacher Martin Luther King Jr., I too felt compelled "to recover the real man from the gray mist of hagiography."[9] What emerges is, I think, a far more interesting story.

It should be obvious that my focus on T.C.'s life as it relates to Medicare means that this cannot be a comprehensive biography of the man. He already had at least a dozen biographies as well as my own short biography of him for the *Dictionary of Canadian Biography*. Of course, I have drawn on these works when helpful, but wherever possible I have used original sources to shed light on largely unexplored aspects of his life and times in the context of his continual quest for comprehensive health coverage.[10] While I use T.C.'s life mainly as an point of entry to the larger history of universal health coverage in Canada, I also try to provide a fairly rounded portrait of the man himself. In this pursuit, I was obliged to explore – and speculate on – his motives, emotions, and theology in order to understand his actions as a politician and government leader.

**Medicare and the Pragmatic Idealist**

T.C. can best be described as a pragmatic idealist.[11] Although such a phrase may seem a contradiction in terms, an equal dose of pragmatism and idealism is required for leaders highly motivated by a core set of ideals yet focused on initiating and sustaining concrete change. Such leaders must understand the societies they are trying to change in a democratic manner – in other words, what can be done and when. They must also have the wisdom to decide which compromises with the status quo are necessary in any given political term of office. For T.C., this meant finding the appropriate balance between what was ideal and what could be achieved. Pragmatism combined with idealism also defined his cabinet ministers and the senior corps of civil servants in Saskatchewan.

While you expect political parties to draw like-minded people, what was truly exceptional was the way in which T.C. attracted like-minded individuals throughout Canada and from other countries to work as civil servants in the country's first social democratic government. They came to Regina to join his government out of idealism, but they too were pragmatists who wanted to make appreciable improvements in the present, even if they had to work within certain institutional constraints and compromise with societal interests holding quite different views and objectives. The health reforms initiated and secured by the Douglas government, as well as the occasional failures or shortcomings, reflected the enormous challenges involved in finding the right balance between pragmatism and idealism.

T.C. joined the Baptist ministry to make a difference to those who lived in his community, and beyond, in the here and now, as opposed to in some presumed future after death. He entered politics in the depths of the Great Depression to try to alleviate the hardship the unemployed and destitute confronted and to give them hope that, together, they could build a better future. The socialism to which he adhered was a Christian social gospel combined with a commitment to reform within the structure of a Parliamentary democracy.

In politics, T.C. was a social democrat who stood in the tradition of the labour parties in English-speaking parliamentary democracies and in continental Europe – that is, reforming social democratic parties rather than revolutionary "socialist" parties that were Marxist in orientation.[12] Still, the terms "social democratic" and "socialist" were, and continue to be, used interchangeably. In this book, the term "social democratic" is used more often to describe the politics of Douglas and his party, the Co-operative Commonwealth Federation (CCF) and its successor, the New Democratic Party (NDP), even if "socialist" was the term more often applied to Douglas's party from the 1930s until the 1960s.

## Organization of This Book

The first chapter begins with a single day in the life of T.C., 13 October 1961, when his medical care bill was introduced in the Saskatchewan

Legislative Assembly. This was the pivotal moment in his political career – hence, my justification for beginning the narrative at this point. Before that day, Douglas had been able to use his position in government to build the programs, policies, and reputation that would allow him to introduce medical care insurance. Later, when he was no longer running a government, T.C.'s influence was more limited and indirect. Still, he used what levers were available, as well as the bully pulpit, to push for comprehensive health coverage in Canada.

The subsequent chapters are largely chronological, with chapters 2 and 3 constituting Medicare's prequel. Born in Scotland to a working-class family in 1904, Douglas was one of many immigrants who adapted to life on the prairies of Canada. As a Baptist preacher in Weyburn, a town in southeastern Saskatchewan with a population of 5,000, Douglas witnessed the full force of the Great Depression, an experience that would redirect him from a clergyman to a social activist and radical politician. Chapter 3 covers his time as a CCF member of Parliament, from 1935 until his ascension as leader of his party in Saskatchewan and its election victory in 1944, an outcome that would send shock waves through the Canadian establishment. During these years, he concluded that health care should be a service available to all rather than a commodity purchased only by those able to pay.

Chapters 4 to 11 cover T.C.'s time as premier of Saskatchewan. When the Saskatchewan CCF was elected in a landslide victory in 1944, T.C. made the introduction of fundamental health reforms his government's key priority and appointed himself as minister of health to make certain of their timely implementation. These reforms, the two ambitious tracks on which they are organized, and the brilliant individuals T.C. lured to Saskatchewan to spearhead change, are the focus of chapter 4. At the same time as these major changes were occurring, Douglas was preoccupied with the Dominion-Provincial Reconstruction Conference of 1945–6. As shown in chapter 5, the Douglas government did everything in its power to support the federal government's Green Book proposals, which included an offer of federal shared-cost funding for comprehensive health insurance. To T.C.'s great regret, the federal government withdrew its offer when it was unable to obtain the agreement of the governments of Ontario and Quebec to a more permanent tax-rental agreement.

Douglas ultimately decided, despite the fiscal risks involved, to proceed alone. As described in chapter 6, the decision to forge ahead with universal hospital and diagnostic services coverage required expert planning and management. To achieve these, Douglas recruited

Dr. Fred Mott, an experienced health program administrator in the Roosevelt New Deal, who then spearheaded a major effort to get the program ready in a few short months. Once implemented, Saskatchewan's hospital insurance plan quickly became recognized as a model program. At the same time, the Douglas government became a world-leading innovator in other areas such as mental health (chapter 7), while still struggling with its ambitions for a more integrated model of health care through organized health regions, polyclinics, primary care centres, and its plans for a school-based children's dental program (chapter 8).

How the Saskatchewan model of hospital insurance became the template for the rest of the country is covered in chapter 9. After almost a decade of inaction on national health insurance, the federal government was pressured by a coalition of provincial governments into making a proposal on federal cost sharing of provincial programs. Ottawa's offer ultimately set eligibility conditions for provincial participation, conditions that were drawn directly from the Saskatchewan model.

Chapters 10 and 11 describe the momentous struggle to introduce and implement universal medical care coverage in Saskatchewan. From the beginning, the Douglas government faced off against organized medicine, which was determined to stop the program. Douglas was equally determined to push ahead. However, his time, energy, and focus were soon diverted by the movement drafting him as the national leader of the NDP. Unable to mitigate the growing opposition to the provincial government's medical care plan, Douglas was forced on the defensive. Chapter 12 covers the year following his departure from the premier's office in November 1961, marked by a series of political defections and setbacks and his humiliating defeat in his Regina riding in the federal election of 1962. One of the causes of T.C.'s defeat was the growing opposition to his medical care insurance bill, which precipitated a twenty-three-day doctors' strike in the province. This strike and the impact of the compromise reached between the government and the medical profession is explored in chapter 13.

Chapter 14 changes focus to the national scene and the Royal Commission on Health Services, commonly known as the Hall Commission. Eventually, to the surprise of many, the Hall Commission recommended the extension of universal health coverage. T.C. adeptly used the commission's report to put pressure on a minority Liberal government in a political landscape that shifted to the left in the early 1960s. As shown in chapter 15, this led to a federal cost-sharing proposal and the adoption of universal medical care coverage by all provincial governments. Chapter 16 covers Douglas's final years as a politician, his retirement from Parliament in 1979, and his death in 1986. During these years, he was a notable public defender of Medicare, even if his direct political influence had diminished. It is only after his death that he emerged as potent symbol of Medicare, and his legacy remains inextricably tied to his role in making this the country's defining social policy.

# 1 Medicare: The Agony and the Ecstasy

*In this short life*
*That only lasts an hour*
*How much – how little – is*
*Within our power*

                                                    Emily Dickinson

**Friday, the 13th of October 1961, the Saskatchewan Legislative Assembly**

As T.C. Douglas sat bolt upright in his seat in the Saskatchewan legislature as the member representing Weyburn, he carefully observed the members of the opposition across from him, the speaker to the left, and the gallery high above him to his right. It was his seventeenth year in the Legislative Assembly and his seventeenth year as premier. That morning, his government's minister of health, Walter Erb, introduced a bill on universal medical coverage – popularly known as "medicare."[1] He, his government, and his party, the Co-operative Commonwealth Federation (CCF), had been yearning for this day for almost two decades, since his government was first elected in 1944.

    This was T.C.'s crowning moment in a political career that had begun in the depths of the Great Depression, first as a member of Parliament, then as provincial leader of the CCF, and finally as premier of Saskatchewan when the CCF was elected in a landslide victory. The election of the first "socialist" government in North America had stunned political watchers in Canada and the United States. Under his charismatic leadership, the CCF won another four successive elections, becoming the perennial governing party in Saskatchewan in this period.[2] In seventeen years, he achieved many of his original objectives, but one that had remained elusive was a comprehensive health program. Fourteen years earlier, in 1947, his government had implemented universal hospital insurance – a major step in this direction, but still only one step.

T.C.'s government had called for a special fall session to get two pieces of legislation through the assembly. The first was a bill on income tax, necessitated by the federal government's termination of its tax-rental arrangement and the province's resumption of control of personal and corporate income taxes. The second was the Saskatchewan Medical Care Insurance Act, the bill that would draw almost all of the attention during the short session. With his government holding a comfortable majority in the assembly, Douglas knew both bills would pass, but there had been a fiery conflict over medicare in recent months, and he knew the bill would inflame passions on both sides of the aisle.

Passing the medical care bill would be easy, but he knew that implementing it would be arduous, the most difficult challenge ever faced by the CCF government. The prospect of a government-administered program of medical care insurance deeply divided the population, and Douglas was in a life-and-death struggle with organized medicine, the business lobby, and the local newspapers for the hearts and minds of the population beyond his diehard supporters.

The constant criticism of the CCF government from the business and professional establishment and the Liberal-dominated daily newspapers in Saskatoon and Regina had been a fact of life since 1944.[3] However, the medicare bill threatened his government in a much more dangerous and existential way. For the past several months, Douglas himself was being demonized by almost all the doctors in the province and their allies across the country and beyond. And the doctors had talked to their patients about how the government's plan for medicare would result in the mass exodus of medical practitioners from the province. This prospect terrified Saskatchewan residents, including even some of those who had voted for Douglas and his party in previous elections. However much he disliked the tactics of the doctors, he still needed them – as the main providers in the proposed program – to cooperate, however grudgingly, if medicare were to become a reality.

He knew he could rely on his own troops. The CCF party faithful welcomed medicare, which they saw as a long-needed and long-overdue change. Despite the constant attacks on the government, Douglas felt that the cabinet and his backbenchers were holding firm, although some grumbled about Walter Erb, hoping he would be moved to a less important job, replaced by a more resolute cabinet minister who would be firmer with the College of Physicians and Surgeons of Saskatchewan

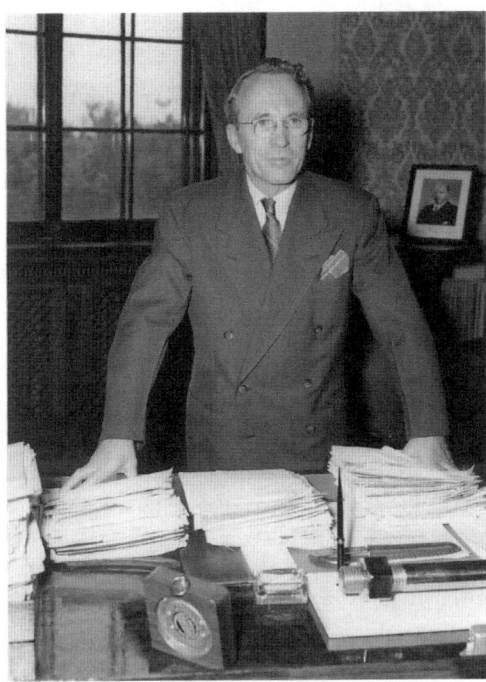

T.C. in the premier's office, 1961 (PAS R-A10679(3))

(CPS). However, Douglas put loyalty first and refused to demote or fire Erb, despite his own growing concerns about the health minister.

On the positive side, medicare had mobilized party supporters. Even his party's most left-wing activists had been encouraged by what they perceived as renewed feistiness in the government. They were now energized by the possibility of major change and almost giddy at the prospect of confronting a clear and present enemy. For his part, T.C. was buoyed by the left wing's new energy. He was also grateful for the temporary reprieve from their constant harping about how far his government had drifted from its earlier socialist ideals. He felt their aspirations had been ably reflected in the speech given by Marjorie Cooper two days earlier in reply to the short Speech from the Throne that had opened the special session.

Cooper was one of T.C.'s experienced backbenchers and the only woman on the government side of the house.[4] She took issue with the doctors on a host of issues, including their arguments in favour of subsidizing private health insurance based on a means test, user charges, and the need to have doctors involved in the administration of any medicare scheme.[5] She had also taken great pains to point out some of the deficiencies of the fee-for-service payment model, which she felt discouraged physicians from spending adequate time with patients. While the bill accepted the doctors' strong preference for fee-for-service, Cooper argued that it was important to at least allow for the possibility of salary and capitation payment down the road.[6]

Douglas did not mind Cooper's pointing out some shortcomings in the bill. He even agreed with the substance of her argument and her hope that eventually the practice of medicine would not only become more responsive to the needs of patients but would focus on keeping patients healthier, not just treating their illnesses and injuries. However, his government needed to compromise to avoid the threatened exodus of doctors from the province. In this case, perfection was the enemy of good, as forcing physicians to embrace a model of care they would not yet accept would make medicare impossible to implement. This was something the Labour government in Britain had understood when it implemented the National Health Service (NHS) in 1948. There, the government had to find a compromise with the British Medical Association, and, while the Saskatchewan plan was not perfect, it was the best that could be done at the time to "meet the needs of the people." It was only a start. The government needed to keep working at it, improving the plan year by year, so that "in ten or twenty years," it would have a better plan, one that came much closer to achieving the government's original objectives. In this, Douglas expected that "succeeding legislatures and succeeding governments will keep evolving that plan to meet the needs of our people."[7]

Marjorie Cooper had ably dispensed with the most common arguments against medicare as unnecessary, given the number of people in the province who already had private health insurance.[8] The doctors, through the CPS as well as the Canadian Medical Association, said that the only useful role for the government was to subsidize the purchase of private health insurance by those unable to afford the premiums. Douglas derided this alternative as "tin cup medicare" because it required what he viewed as a humiliating means test.

Those advocating a needs-based subsidy approach also favoured user fees – generally called deterrent fees – to keep people from overusing medical care. While T.C. admitted that some people might seek unnecessary care, these cases would, he believed, be few and far between. After all, little about going to a doctor was inherently pleasurable. As for the few potential cases of abuse, deterrent fees would prevent only those with limited means from seeking physician care, while the

Medicare: The Agony and the Ecstasy 15

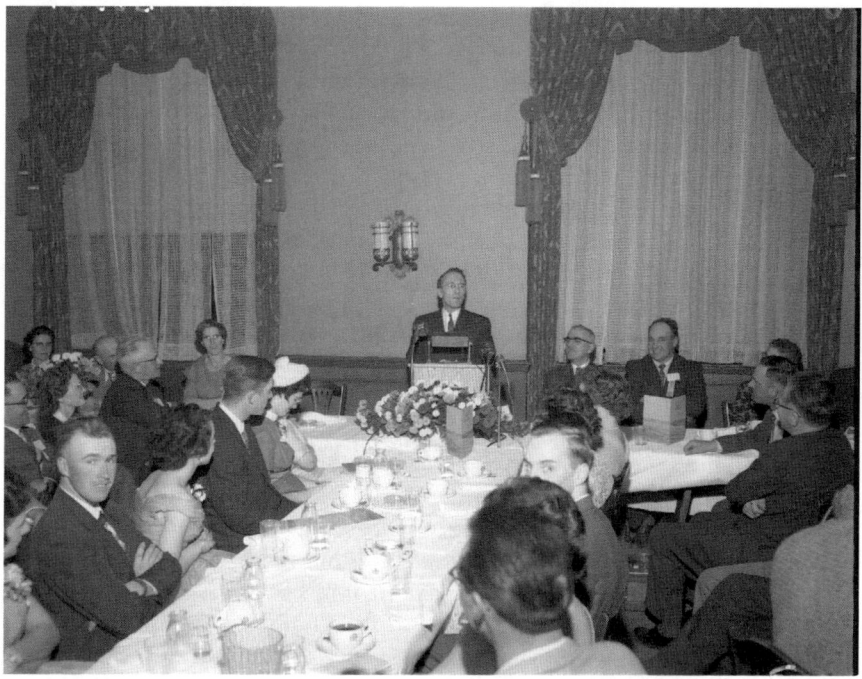

T.C. speaking at a Canadian Medical Association banquet in Saskatoon, October 1959 (SPL B-6561)

reasonably well-off could abuse the system with impunity. Still, the CPS was insisting on both private health insurance and deterrent fees.

A little less than a month earlier, the college's doctors had voted overwhelmingly – 444 to 1 – to oppose the medicare plan.[9] Despite this, T.C. remained hopeful the doctors would eventually accept the government's plan if their concerns were met halfway. He was willing to allow them to continue to practise as small businesses, receiving a fee for each of their services, as long as they agreed to having the government pay all their bills on behalf of patients and all residents having access to the same insurance coverage. He would not insist on any changes to the way in which they practised medicine, and he always made it clear that he would ensure that their clinical autonomy was respected. Based on his past willingness to engage with organized medicine, he remained confident the doctors would become more conciliatory once the bill was passed and they understood that the government could not be dissuaded from its implementation.[10]

But time was working against Douglas. Having announced his intention of establishing medicare in March 1959, he had hoped to have the bill in the Legislative Assembly well before autumn 1961. Early in 1960, he had established a public advisory committee – the Thompson Committee – to work with doctors and other stakeholders on the program design. Then, in the provincial election of June 1960, he promised that, if re-elected, his government would implement medicare based on the committee's report. Converted into a de facto referendum on the initiative, with significant and well-funded opposition from the CPS, it was the toughest of the CCF's five provincial elections. When his party won by a solid margin of seats, T.C. felt he had received the democratic mandate to proceed.

The other remaining difficulty was the Thompson Committee itself, which had been dragging its feet after the election, largely due to the stalling tactics of the doctors representing the CPS on the committee. Douglas originally thought the extra time would be enough for the doctors to come to their senses, realize the futility of their opposition, and work out a design they could live with, however grudgingly, through the committee. Instead, the doctors filibustered by pushing the committee to investigate issues well beyond its original mandate on medicare, purposely wasting valuable time in the process. Consequently, the most his government could get from the committee – and only after demanding it – was an interim report, in which the majority recommended universal medical care coverage. But unanimity proved impossible, and the three physicians representing the profession, joined by an ally representing the business community, released a dissenting minority report.

T.C. used the majority report to proceed, even though most doctors in the province, as represented by the CPS as their official bargaining agent, remained opposed. He felt he could not wait any longer. Fourteen weeks earlier, he had been elected leader of his national party, now rebranded as the New Democratic Party (NDP). Although hardly in love with the idea of languishing on an opposition backbench in Ottawa, Douglas felt obligated to lead the national party. However, he would not relinquish his post as premier until the Saskatchewan CCF convention at the beginning of November, where he would formally resign and his successor would be selected.[11] Passing the medicare bill was the only unfinished business he had left before the convention and his move to Ottawa.

In addition to resistance from the medical profession, T.C. faced a determined adversary in the assembly. After seventeen years of often desultory opposition, the provincial Liberals were getting their first taste of blood. The groups opposed to medicare were actively supporting the

Liberals in an informal anti-socialist coalition as the most viable option to defeat the CCF.[12] They rejoiced in Douglas's imminent departure as premier and provincial CCF leader. They would no longer have to contend with the man they portrayed as a malevolent magician slavishly worshipped by his followers. They intended to take full advantage of the opportunity presented by his removal to Ottawa. Liberal leader Ross Thatcher, a former CCF MP with a tough, calculating streak, was dedicated to kicking the "socialists" out of office so he could institute a more business-friendly government that would encourage more private investment in the provincial economy.[13]

The opposition was far from dispirited following its election loss in 1960: medicare combined with T.C.'s decision to give up the premiership for the federal NDP leadership produced the opposite result, and the Liberals under Thatcher seemed more alert and skilful than ever. They played a nuanced game, opposing the government's management of medicare and questioning its potential cost, but being careful to seem in favour of medical care insurance in principle. However, they refused to provide any details on the type of program they would support.[14] These tactics gave the doctors the impression that the Liberals were on their side, but, at least in the legislature, the party would not commit to any one model.

As for the doctors, T.C. had miscalculated. He thought their counterproductive involvement in the election of 1960 would have taught them a lesson. Instead, the experience politicized rank-and-file doctors who had paid little attention to politics in the past, turning a number of them into determined foes of his government. Still, he believed that many doctors were of good will, particularly the family doctors living outside the cities and away from what he saw as the more corrosive influence of the self-interested specialists in the cities, who were in charge of the provincial medical association. He still hoped these "more reasonable" doctors would put pressure on the leaders of the CPS to come to their senses.

Douglas had seen such opposition before. When working on his bill on universal hospital coverage fifteen years earlier, organized medicine had been far from keen on what they saw as a first step towards socialized medicine. Yet, by focusing the bill on paying hospitals rather than doctors, and by making it clear that he had no intention of forcing doctors into the salaried service of the provincial government, T.C. avoided a major confrontation that would have blocked the implementation of publicly administered hospital insurance. Now, once again, but with far more force, doctors claimed that he intended to turn them into bureaucrats.

The doctors in the province were not alone. The coalition supporting the College of Physicians and Surgeons was powerful and included many others in the business and professional community. In addition, organized medicine outside the province, including the Ontario Medical Association and even the American Medical Association, threw its support behind its Saskatchewan colleagues. The most powerful backer was the Canadian Medical Association. All wanted to prevent a beachhead for what they called "socialized medicine" in North America.

The doctors and their allies were being manipulated very adroitly by Ross Thatcher. Adept at drawing media attention to himself, Thatcher was proving to be the Saskatchewan Liberal Party's most effective politician since Jimmy Gardiner, who first became leader and premier in 1926. Thatcher had already drawn together a sizeable anti-CCF coalition, including individuals who would otherwise have supported Social Credit or the Progressive Conservatives. Thatcher was politically astute enough to avoid outright rejection of the bill – medicare was popular among many middle-of-the-road voters he was hoping to bring into his camp – even while turning the fear of a possible exodus of doctors and the establishment's anti-medicare sentiment into a general attack on Douglas's government.

T.C. knew Thatcher well. While he despised the Liberal leader as a political turncoat, he respected his formidable political skills. First elected to Parliament in 1945, Thatcher had been part of the Saskatchewan CCF caucus in Ottawa. Unlike other political parties, there was virtually no separation between the federal and provincial branches of the CCF, and, as premier, Douglas kept in close touch with all CCF MPs, including Thatcher. Ten years after he became an MP, Thatcher left the CFF, opposed to the party's views on corporate taxation. Coming from a business family, and a businessman in his own right, Thatcher had always been in the right wing of the CCF caucus, and he found himself increasingly uncomfortable in the party. After breaking with the CCF, he ran for the Liberal Party of Canada but was defeated by the CCF candidate in the federal elections of 1957 and 1958. In 1959, he shifted to provincial politics, taking over the leadership of the Saskatchewan Liberal Party.[15]

The day before the medicare bill was introduced in the legislature, Thatcher complimented T.C. on his long service to the province, recognizing "his ability, his integrity, or his sincerity." Still, claiming that Douglas's departure was bound to help the Liberals, Thatcher said he was not sorry to see him go. Moreover, he had no intention of wishing "him good luck in his new job" because he did not want him to "be too successful" in Ottawa.[16] Thatcher then went on to attack Douglas for not resigning the premiership the moment he had been elected federal leader. The remarks got under T.C.'s normally thick skin. When he finally stood to speak, he began with an attack on Thatcher in the withering yet humorous style that had been his trademark since his first appearance in the House of Commons in 1935:

> Here is a man who changed his political party. He was three times elected as a CCF member for Moose Jaw–Lake Centre. Then he walked across the floor of the House of Commons and sat as an independent. He made some advances, first to the Social Credit party and then to the Progressive Conservative party and when he found the welcome sign wasn't out, he joined the Liberal party. Many of the people in his constituency demanded that he should resign and come back and face his constituents, and this he refused to do. As a matter of fact when the 1957 elected rolled around he didn't even go back to that constituency which he had deserted, in order to give his constituents an opportunity to express their opinion about what he had done. Instead he went to another constituency where he was defeated in both 1957 and 1958.[17]

Douglas then pointed out that "in his address yesterday," after throwing "cold water" on the government's plan, Thatcher had recommended it wait for the federal government, which had just launched the Royal Commission on Health Services chaired by Justice Emmett Hall. The opposition's argument "that we should wait for a national plan," Douglas said, "is to ask the people of Saskatchewan to drag along and wait, as they have waited for thirty or forty years, for the federal government to act and knowing full well that they are not likely to act unless some province leads the way."[18] Why, he asked, wait for a royal commission report that the federal government was not obligated to implement?

T.C. took particular offence at Thatcher's charge, one made regularly both in the Legislative Assembly and in the media, that he was rushing the medicare bill through the house to give him, as national NDP leader, an advantage in the next federal election:

> He [Thatcher] said the government is just hurrying this plan through for the publicity effect in the federal election. Yet, I remember at the last regular session of the legislature, that at least two or three members opposite asked the government when we were going to get on with the medical care plan. They pointed out that the government had promised it in the election of 1960. They wanted to know what we were waiting for – how long was the medical advisory committee going to take to gate [get] a report

down – what was holding us up? Mr. Speaker, this is surely a disorganized army. The rank and file are saying forward, and the leader is saying retreat. They had better make up their minds. Does the Liberal party believe we should have a medical care plan? Do they believe we should have it now? Do they want to postpone it? They can't be "forwards-backwards" all the time. They've got to take a stand. I think the people of the province have a right to know where they stand on this question. When the House votes on this matter they'll have a chance to see, and their constituents will have a chance to see what they think about a medical care plan.[19]

Seizing on Thatcher's statement that there was "not a shred of evidence to show that any person in the province has been unable to get medical attention," T.C. retorted that Thatcher was "out of touch with the people."[20] His comment, Douglas argued, was "like Marie Antoinette at the time of the French Revolution when the people were crying for bread, saying, 'Why don't they eat cake.' To say that there is no evidence to show that any person in the province has been unable to get medical attention" is to defy the evidence:

The Canadian Sickness Report, 1951, conducted by the Government of Canada shows clearly that the lower income groups in the period under study had more illness and more days of disability than did the higher income groups. It shows, conversely, that the volume of medical care received by the low income groups is much less than that received by higher income groups. The low income groups because of poor diet, poor housing conditions and harder working conditions have more illness and have more disability. Yet the records show that they are the people who get the least medical care.[21]

Even if doctors provided charitable care to the poor, this depended on the goodwill of individual doctors and therefore the luck of the draw for patients. This T.C. knew well, having received surgery as a child because a surgeon decided it would make a good teaching case for medical students. He reminded Thatcher and all members that "patients are reluctant to go to the doctor if they know they can't pay." Moreover, they "fail to seek medical counsel and medical advice when they should get it and they leave it until the situation is serious and even dangerous."[22] Contrary to the argument that medicare was all about helping the poor, Douglas pointed out that the financial barriers to access affected many who could be described as middle class:

The ... fact is that many people who do go to doctors incur bills and debts which cripple them for years to come and this does not just apply to poor people. There are thousands of people in Saskatchewan and across Canada living on reasonably comfortable incomes who are able to make the payments on their houses and their cars and on their television set and who can get by providing two things, firstly – they don't lose their jobs and secondly, that the bread-winner doesn't get seriously ill. For such people, doctor bills amounting to large sums of money can put that family in a serious financial predicament for years to come.[23]

T.C. then defended the very concept of universality, answering the question of why his government was making a sizeable public investment in a universal plan as opposed to taking a targeted approach, where the government would pay private health insurance premiums for residents who passed a means test. He argued that the idea that access to basic health care was a right of citizenship – the essence of universality – was hardly a communist concept and, indeed, had become accepted in several "Western" capitalist countries:

> This is not a new principle. This has existed in nearly all the countries of western Europe – many of them for a quarter of a century. It has been in Great Britain since 1948; it has been in New Zealand since 1935; it has been in Australia. The little state of Israel that only came into existence in 1948 has today the most comprehensive health insurance plan in the world. It has more doctors, and nurses and dentists per thousand of its population than any other industrialized country or any country for which we can get statistics.[24]

Implemented in 1947, Saskatchewan's program of universal hospital coverage had proven that universal health insurance was affordable, even though Saskatchewan was one of the poorer provinces in the country. And it had been done within a balance budget. T.C. had always insisted on never running a deficit – part of his ongoing effort to prove that socialists could be better fiscal managers than the governments run by the business-friendly Liberals and Conservatives. But what was a stake was more fundamental than money, a point he had consistently repeated since his days as the resident Baptist minister in Weyburn, when the Great Depression was devastating vulnerable townspeople and farm families:

> To me it seems to be sheer nonsense to suggest that medical care is something which ought to be measured just in dollars. When we're talking about medical care we're talking about our sense of values. Do we think human life is important? Do we think that the best medical care which is

available is something to which people are entitled, by virtue of belonging to a civilized community?[25]

Douglas conveyed what he felt would be the impact of the medicare bill on the future evolution of Canada. If his government's program were successful, it would "be the forerunner of a national medical care insurance plan" and "the nucleus around which Canada will ultimately build a comprehensive health insurance program" covering "all health services," including "dental care, optometric care, drugs and all the other health services which people require." T.C. believed "such a plan operated by the federal and provincial governments jointly" would not come about unless Saskatchewan led the way. "I want to say that when the history of our time is written, it may well be recorded that in October, 1961, the Saskatchewan legislature and the Saskatchewan people" had the courage to take "a first step towards ultimately establishing a system of medical care insurance for all the people of Canada."[26]

He then provided a personal reflection on what he had learned as the premier of Saskatchewan:

> I would be foolish if I were to say that in all these seventeen years no mistakes have ever been made, or that my judgment or the judgment of my colleagues has always been right. Any human being who would make such a statement would either be foolish or dishonest. But I do believe that in these seventeen years, we have done some things to make this a better province for the ordinary man and woman to live in; that there are more of the amenities of life; that there is a greater measure of security and a greater measure of equality of treatment; that there is greater freedom from discrimination; and that our people have, working together, moved forward. No government, of course can take all the credit for this. A government may give leadership, but in a democracy, unless there are people – thousands of them – who are prepared to work together for the mutual good of their community …, no government can accomplish very much.

He closed with a personal thanks and tribute to the people of Saskatchewan and their past achievements, which permitted such a bill to exist in the first place:

> They were the first people to set up union hospitals on this continent; the first people to set up municipal doctor plans; and the first people to establish an Anti-Tuberculosis League. They are people who have learned that they must help each other. They learned it in the hard days when neighbors had to co-operate with one another, or face the possibility of

starvation, or freezing to death. Fortunately, the traditions of our forefathers had stayed with them. Ours is a great province of self-help and mutual co-operation.[27]

The introduction of the medicare bill in October 1961, and Douglas's impassioned defence of it in the legislature, is arguably the apotheosis of his political career. It was certainly a watershed: the debate on the bill continued for weeks, and by the time it was passed in mid-November, Douglas was no longer a sitting member of the Legislative Assembly. In the months that followed passage, the controversy over medicare grew in size and intensity, culminating in a twenty-three-day doctors' strike in July 1962. Meanwhile, in the rest of the country, Canadian citizens and their governments weighed the merits and demerits of national medicare. As leader of the national NDP, Douglas would be at the centre of this debate. Still, 13 October 1961 formed a dividing line between what T.C. had achieved in Saskatchewan as premier and what he could influence and shaped on the federal level, as the leader of a small national party unable to attain office.

# 2 The Making of a Preacher-Politician

Then let us pray that come it may
(As come it will for a' that,)
That Sense and Worth o'er a' the earth
Shall bear the gree, an a' that,
For a' that, and a' that
It's coming yet for a' that,
That Man to Man, the world o'ver
Shall brothers be for a' that

                Robert Burns, "A Man's a Man for A' That"

Let the river run,
let all the dreamers
wake the nation.
Come, the New Jerusalem
        Carly Simon, "Let the River Run" (inspired by Walt Whitman)

Born on 20 October 1904, in Falkirk, Scotland, between Glasgow and Edinburgh, Thomas Clement Douglas took his first and last name from his father and his middle name from his mother, Annie Clement. By family tradition T.C.'s father, his grandfather, and all first sons before them were named Thomas. His father and grandfather worked at the iron works first established in 1759 on the banks of the River Carron near Falkirk. Producing pig iron and cast-iron products, including canons, the Carron Company had been in the forefront of the Industrial Revolution in Britain and for almost 150 years was the largest iron works in Europe.[1] Douglas's father, Tom, and his grandfather, Thomas, were skilled iron moulders, making the moulds that were used to cast the iron products.

The family of T.C.'s mother were originally weavers living in the Highlands west of Perth. While in their early twenties, his mother's parents moved to Glasgow, where T.C.'s grandfather worked as a freight driver for the Scottish Co-operative Wholesale Society. Speaking only Gaelic when they arrived, they quickly learned English.[2] Both the Douglas and Clement clans were working class and Protestant, but there were differences between them. The Douglases were members of the Church of Scotland while the Clements were devout Baptists. Even after T.C.'s father stopped attending church services (although he continued to identify himself as a Presbyterian), T.C., his mother, and his two younger sisters remained devout members of the Baptist Church.

Tom Douglas's work as an iron moulder at the Carron Company was interrupted by war. Then still a single man, he volunteered with the 91st Argyle Highlanders to fight in the South African War. Since he had to remain in service for three years, he finished out his time in India before returning home to Scotland and resuming his job at the iron works. At the end of the summer of 1903, Tom Douglas married Annie Clement.[3] Almost fifteen months later, T.C. was born, followed by a daughter Annie (Nan), born in 1907, and a final child, Isobel (Billie), born in 1911. Tom's experiences in Africa and India made him uneasy of what he came to perceive as his family's limited future in Scotland. He yearned to live in a country with a less rigid class system and more opportunity for his children. He decided to emigrate to Canada with his younger brother Bill, who had already worked for some time in the iron foundries of the rapidly growing city of Winnipeg before returning briefly to Scotland.[4] T.C.'s father would go ahead with Bill to get job and house sorted in advance of his wife and children coming over.[5]

**From Scotland to Canada and Back Again**

In early April 1912, a seven-year-old T.C., his mother, his sisters, and an uncle climbed aboard a ship in Glasgow to make their passage to Saint John, New Brunswick, at about the same time that the ill-fated *Titanic* left Southampton for New York. T.C. remembered the heavy fog, which forced a major delay, as the ship was surrounded by icebergs – a precaution that allowed the vessel to avoid the *Titanic*'s fate. The family then boarded a train and made their way to Winnipeg in a third-class settlers' car with wooden seats and a wood stove at the end to cook meals.[6]

As a British citizen, T.C. was not officially an immigrant, but by virtue of his "old country" Scottish accent, the obvious traces of which he kept for a lifetime, he always had a degree of separation from native-born

Canadians. Indeed, he referred to himself as an immigrant. But this identity would share space with another identity in Winnipeg. There, he would be deeply marked by the working-class, immigrant, and politically radical culture of the North End in what was at the time the most "polyglot" but also most class divided city in Canada.[7]

The Douglas family lived in a series of rented houses all near the Vulcan Iron Works, where his father plied his trade as an iron moulder. He attended what he described "a little Norquay Street school."[8] His home and school were close to All Peoples' Mission, where Douglas and the immigrant children who lived around him would congregate to swim, play sports, and use the library. This Methodist mission gave North End youngsters a place to go outside of their overcrowded homes, and T.C. was impressed by the enormous difference the mission made in his life and the lives of the children of his neighbourhood. The mission also took in used clothing that could be redistributed to poor families in the North End. T.C.'s mother, Annie, an active churchgoer and occasional attendee at the mission's chapel, was a volunteer worker at the mission and highly influenced by its superintendent, J.S. Woodsworth.[9]

According to T.C., his mother had "great regard" for Woodsworth, and his near saintly reputation provided both with a model of a life dedicated to serving the poor and marginalized.[10] Like most social reformers of his time, however, Woodsworth perceived immigration from regions of the world with different languages and cultures – particularly those from Eastern Europe – as a potential threat, with Winnipeg as the "storm centre" of the problem. Indeed, he saw All Peoples' Mission as an instrument to assimilate and make "worthy citizens" of immigrant children by offering their mothers English classes as well as instruction in childcare and nutrition.[11] T.C., in contrast, never seemed to share Woodsworth's fear of immigration, in part because of his experience with the immigrant kids he grew up with in the North End.

Although T.C. had fond memories of All Peoples' Mission, he was often physically unable to participate in its sporting activities because of a painful medical condition caused by the extreme inflammation of his knee bone. He had cut his knee on a stone while playing as a child in Falkirk. When the resulting wound did not heal properly, an inflammation of the bone known as osteomyelitis set in, and a local doctor decided that surgery was required. Placed on the family's kitchen table, he was sedated with a chloroform gauze mask. The doctor then cut into his leg just above the knee to expose the bone and then scraped the femur with a knife. Shortly after the doctor left, the suture let go and the wound bled heavily and had to be staunched by his parents.[12]

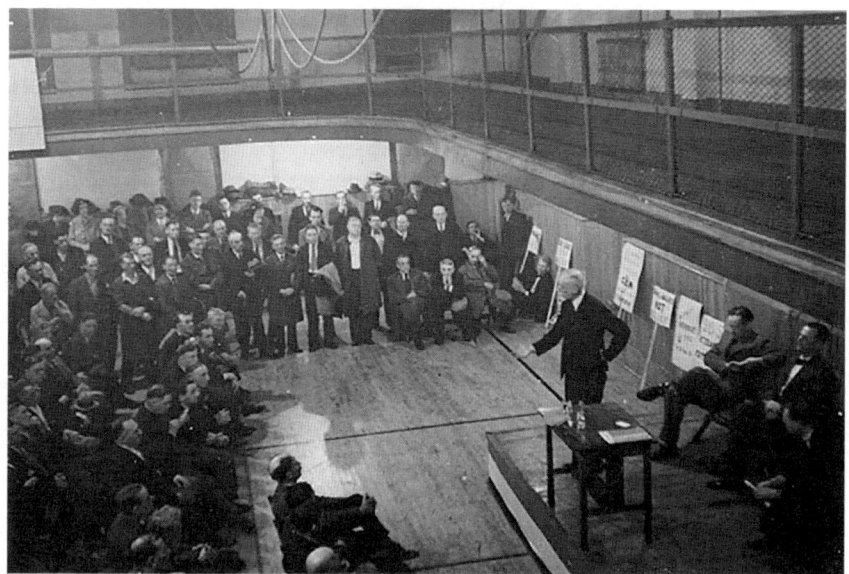
J.S. Woodsworth addressing a meeting of the unemployed, 1935 (LAC c55451)

The operation proved ineffective, and T.C.'s condition worsened shortly after the family arrived in Winnipeg.[13] With the infection flaring up, he had to walk on crutches. When winter came and the icy conditions prevented him from hobbling to school on his crutches, two neighbourhood boys from Poland and Ukraine talked to T.C.'s mother and offered to pull him back and forth to school on a sleigh. She readily agreed.[14] As he later recounted, this act of kindness reinforced his lifelong rejection of what were then commonly accepted ethnic hierarchies, particularly among settler families originating from the British Isles.[15]

T.C.'s condition deteriorated to the point that he was hospitalized continually and subject to more surgeries, all ineffective.[16] This, of course, was in the public ward of the hospital, which had limited resources and time to deal with his case. Finally, his family was notified that his leg had to be amputated.[17] Fortunately, he happened to be seen by Dr. Stanley Smith, a talented young orthopaedic surgeon at Winnipeg's Children's Hospital who offered to perform a complicated (and expensive) corrective procedure for free as part of a "teaching project" for his medical students.[18] The operation saved his limb, even if T.C. would be plagued, intermittently, by pain in his knee and leg for the rest of his days.[19]

T.C. would return to this episode over and over in his life. He used it in his speeches to explain why universal health coverage was essential. If he had not been lucky enough to obtain the charity of the surgeon, he would have had to go through life with only one leg. In his mind, his operation, or any other medically necessary procedure, should be automatically available to all, and not only to those able to pay or to those, like himself, who were saved based on the ultimately arbitrary decision of a generous individual. In an interview conducted in 1958, T.C. expressed his gratefulness to Dr. Smith but also spoke to the larger lesson he took from his experience.[20]

> I always felt a great debt of gratitude to him [Dr. Smith]; but it left me with this feeling that if I hadn't been so fortunate as to have this doctor offer me his services gratis, I would probably have lost my leg. My parents were having quite a difficult time ... Money was very scarce, and they couldn't possibly have hired a man of Dr. Smith's standing. I felt that no boy should have to depend either for his leg or his life upon the ability of his parents to raise enough money to bring a first-class surgeon to his bedside. And I think it was out of this experience, not at the moment consciously, but through the years, I came to believe that health services ought not to have a price tag on them, and that people should be able to get whatever health services they required irrespective of their individual capacity to pay.[21]

A few years later, when he was twelve, T.C. left Winnipeg with his mother and two young sisters to join Annie's family in Glasgow. T.C.'s father, Tom, despite his negative experiences in the war against the Boers, had enlisted with the Canadian Expeditionary Force in April 1916.[22] At thirty-six years of age, Tom was assigned to a field ambulance unit in France. Allowing for the possibility that Tom might be killed, leaving her on her own, Annie sought the support of her parents.[23] For over two years, T.C. would live with his grandparents in their flat in Glasgow's Clydeside.[24] It was a tough working-class neighbourhood, and T.C. had to join one of the local gangs to gain at least some protection on the street.

Initially, T.C. attended school and made extra money by helping his grandfather, Andrew Clement, in his deliveries for the Scottish Cooperative Wholesale Society. Clement was also a lay preacher, and T.C. regularly heard him preach sermons to Baptist congregations.[25] A year later, T.C. decided not to return to school in the fall of 1918. Not quite fourteen, he had begun working earlier that summer at a cork factory and decided to work on a more permanent basis to help his mother and grandparents with expenses.[26]

## Back to the North End

Just after the armistice of 11 November 1918, Tom Douglas joined his family on leave and began to make plans with Annie for the family's return to Winnipeg. He was upset that T.C. had quit school so young, and he remained insistent that the boy have a future beyond that of a simple wage worker like himself.[27]

Although the family intended to return as a unit, Tom was deemed unfit to be demobilized and instead was sent to a Canadian military hospital in Britain. He was treated for soldier's heart, a largely psychological condition that created physical symptoms such an irregular heart rate and uncontrollable shaking, which he had first exhibited in 1917. His illness was hardly surprising. As a stretcher bearer often on the front lines, Tom Douglas not only shared the physical dangers of over two years of trench warfare but had to provide first-line treatment to hundreds of horribly injured soldiers.[28]

Not knowing how long her husband would be kept, Annie and her children went ahead. Arriving back in Winnipeg in January 1919, T.C. went to work as a printer's apprentice. With his mother making very little in her job, T.C. made a pact with his sisters to work until they could buy a house for their parents, at which point they would be free to leave home.[29] As demobilized soldiers began to return to Canada in the following months, however, fewer jobs were available. When he finally made his way back to his family in early June 1919, Tom Douglas found that he faced a lack of steady work, despite being a skilled labourer.[30]

Winnipeg became a tinderbox of unemployment and discontent.[31] T.C. watched the Winnipeg General Strike unfold in mid-May 1919. The climax of the strike came five weeks later, on 21 June, or "Bloody Saturday," when returning soldiers paraded down Main Street to protest the arrest of strike leaders.[32] Douglas was walking home from work and climbed up the wall of a building in time to see the Royal Northwest Mounted Police attack the protesters. Years later, he described the police firing on the crowd and killing "a man who stood on the corner of Main Street and Williams Avenue" and "then reforming on Portage Avenue and coming back down again, riding the strikers down and break up ... their parade."[33] His sympathies lay with the workers, soldiers, and the unemployed, and he was highly upset when J.S. Woodsworth was jailed on the charge of seditious libel for his editorials in the pro-worker *Western Labor News*.[34]

While T.C. was not yet politically partisan in the sense of joining a party, his sentiments were already clear. In Scotland, his father was an outspoken supporter of the British Labour Party and discussed politics at almost every family meal.[35] His father's political stand caused strained relations with T.C.'s paternal grandfather, Thomas. A radical liberal, Thomas supported the Liberal Party for years, a party that, until the 1920s, held more parliamentary seats in Scotland than the Labour Party, although he ultimately switched his allegiance to Labour.[36]

From his father, T.C. would have heard much about fellow Scotsman Keir Hardie, trade unionist and founder of the Labour Party as well as its first parliamentary leader. Kenneth O. Morgan, one of Hardie's most prominent biographers, described Hardie as an idealist and pragmatist, in words that could just as easily be applied to T.C. Douglas's own life as a politician.[37] Hardie was willing "to work with radical Liberals whose ideology he largely shared, subtle in building up the Labour alliance with the trade unions and other socialist bodies, and supremely flexible in his political philosophy, a very generalised socialism based on a secularized Christianity rather than Marxism."[38]

As for Tom Douglas, it would take a few years before he was able to return to his work as an iron moulder. He had come back from war a sick man. His physical and mental injuries were such that for "the rest of his life he would suffer bouts of despair." Unable to sleep, he would walk through the city for hours at night. His army pension was a miniscule $12 a month, so he went back to the iron foundry whenever work was available. To survive, Annie, T.C., and his sisters had to pool their earnings.[39]

T.C. would work in a printer's shop for the next five years.[40] At the beginning, when he was only sixteen, he was already operating a Linotype machine – the hot lead typesetting system that remained the dominant technology for mass printing until the 1950s. He went to night school to improve his technique as a printer and passed the necessary tests to make his full $44 a week union wage.[41]

T.C. was an enthusiastic member of numerous church groups and a leader in their activities. He also took up boxing. Although short and rail thin, the "wee Scotsman" (as he was often called) developed into a very good fighter, and he was the lightweight championship of Manitoba for 1922 and 1923. The sport offered T.C. an outlet for his adversarial nature, which, in future years, only politics would replace.[42] All of this bustle squeezed out any time for rest and reflection. Perhaps it also limited the time he had to spend at home with his ailing father.

His interest in religion was largely a product of his mother's influence. Living with the Clement family in Glasgow had reinforced T.C.'s affiliation with the Baptist Church. A small minority in Scotland, different Baptist congregations forged the Baptist Union of Scotland in 1869, based on "common concerns for temperance, education, and youth work."[43] Annie was active in social outreach activities and inculcated the motto of the Baptist Women's Auxiliary, "By love serve one another," in her son.[44]

Near their home in Winnipeg's North End was the Beulah Baptist Church, where Annie, T.C., Nan, and Billie all were regular attendees. For T.C., Beulah offered more than church services and Sunday School. He attended "Beulah for Scouts on Tuesday nights, Prayer Meeting on Wednesdays, Young People's Meeting on Friday and the Christian Endeavour youth group outings on Saturdays."[45] He became a Scout leader and was given chances to lead youth groups as well as to help plan Sunday evening services. In 1922, he was given his first opportunity as a lay minister to preach at a church service.[46]

Acting and the art of elocution fascinated young T.C. He became a chaplain in the Order of DeMolay – an international fraternal society (associated with the Freemason) for young Protestants – in part so he could perform monologues at the order's public events.[47] It was at a DeMolay meeting that another member of the order noted his talent and convinced him to finish high school and continue his education. T.C. was helped in this decision by Mark Talnicoff, a member of the Beulah congregation and ministry student who had T.C. assist him with church-sponsored activities for boys. Stopping in at the Douglas home on a regular basis, Mark became romantically attached to T.C.'s sister Nan, whom he would later marry.[48]

T.C. and Talnicoff chatted regularly about religion, the betterment of society, and the ways in which they could achieve something more in life. Followed his friend's lead, T.C. enrolled as a ministry student at Brandon College, then affiliated with McMaster University, a Baptist institution, for the fall term of 1924.[49] For T.C., the real advantage of Brandon College was that it offered a pre-college curriculum, permitting him to complete the years of high school he had missed. He would pay his way by filling in as a relief preacher in rural Manitoba. This work, like his five years of experience with urban workers in a printer's shop, gave him considerable insight into the culture and psychology of the farmers and small-town merchants on the prairies.[50]

**Brandon College, Supply Preaching, and Marriage**

At Brandon College, T.C. was taught by a group of liberal-minded professors who eschewed the fundamentalist perspective held by many other Baptists, at a time when the church was being riven by an ongoing

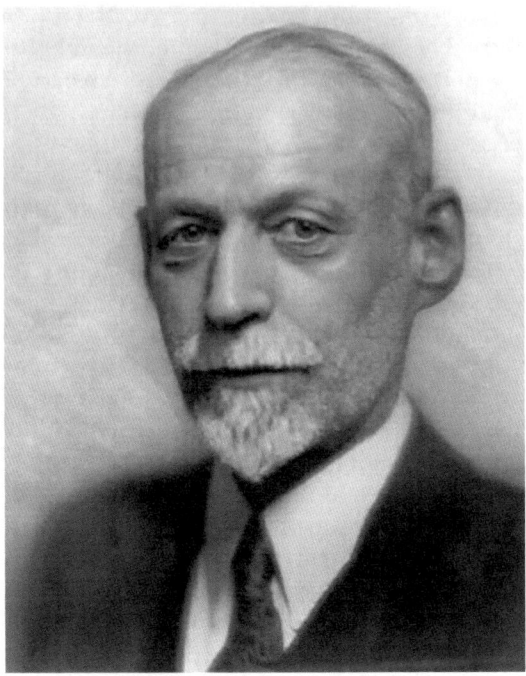

J.S. Woodsworth, c. 1930s (Wikimedia Commons)

debate between progressives and fundamentalists.[51] He was most influenced by one professor, Harris Lachlan MacNeil, who rejected a literalist approach and insisted on each text being treated as a poem to be "interpreted in the light of the purpose for which they were written."[52] Although T.C. had become quite familiar with J.S. Woodsworth's viewpoints on religion and politics while in Winnipeg, he had not had the education to fully understand the tenets of the social gospel. Professor MacNeil and the progressive clique at Brandon College would allow him to explore the social gospel and its implications, exposing him to ideas that would shape his political ideology for the rest of his life.[53]

Douglas made a long-long friend and political ally while studying at Brandon. In September 1927, Stanley Knowles arrived from Winnipeg to begin his studies. They entered the three-year BA program at the same time. Although Douglas had already been at the college for three years, he had only completed his required high school credits.[54] Beyond both having slight physiques, they had much in common, including dealing with the adversity of childhood illnesses, apprenticing in the printing trade, and having to work their ways through college.[55] In terms of personality, however, Douglas and Knowles were opposites. Knowles was quieter and less social, as well as more studious and cerebral, than T.C.[56] It was T.C., not Knowles, who ran for student association president in their final year at Brandon College, with Knowles as his "greatest cheerleader" in the campaign. Drawn to both the social gospel and socialist ideas, they teamed up to lead a student protest to get a course on socialism reinstated after it was cancelled.[57]

From later descriptions of his part-time preaching during these years, it was obvious Douglas was already infusing immediate social concerns into his sermons. He was, in fact, an adherent of what he would later call "practical Christianity," a belief system that emphasized the importance of positive action relative to spiritual reflection.[58] Interested in the "social and economic questions" of the day, T.C. was drawn to a Christianity that emphasized "building a society and building institutions that would uplift mankind, and particularly those who were the least fortunate."[59] His sermons as a relief preacher often connected current social problems with the moral message implicit in Jesus's life and teachings.

Among the Manitoba towns where T.C. regularly preached was Carberry, just east of Brandon on the way to Portage la Prairie. Here, he had also been recruited to preach at a Presbyterian church every Sunday for two years, an unusual arrangement for a Baptist minister but one that he would accept with increasing frequency in the years to come. In Carberry, he first met Irma Dempsey, who, although a Methodist, had begun to attend the Presbyterian church with her family. Like many in the community, she was curious to hear the "boy preacher."[60] Beyond preaching, T.C. was also responsible for community work in Carberry, directing various youth groups such as athletic clubs, Boy Scouts, and Girl Guides. It was through such youth groups that T.C. and Irma got to know each other.[61]

Already earning money as a music teacher, Irma subsequently attended Brandon College to study music, likely influenced by the fact that T.C. was there.[62] On at least one occasion, they opposed each other in a college debate competition. Irma's team may have won the debate that day, but this only fortified T.C.'s belief that she was the one for him. Reserved and of a quiet nature, Irma was drawn to the young man with an outgoing personality, a zest for life, and a quick wit. For his part, T.C. was drawn to the petite, brown-haired woman with "shining eyes."[63]

Within the year of meeting, T.C. proposed to Irma, just after he and Stanley Knowles graduated from Brandon College in the spring of 1930.

On 30 August 1930, T.C., then twenty-six, and Irma, eighteen, got married in a small ceremony at a boarding house owned by Irma's parents in Brandon. Stanley was T.C.'s best man. The ceremony was officiated by Mark Talnicoff, who by this time was married to Nan and was himself the Baptist minister in Portage la Prairie.[64] That summer, T.C. was doing relief preaching in Weyburn, Saskatchewan, while Stanley was doing the same at First Baptist Church in Winnipeg.[65] They swapped positions for two weeks after the wedding so that T.C. and Irma could spend two weeks in Winnipeg for their honeymoon, even while T.C. continued to work.[66]

Thinking back to his early career as a preacher and his marriage to Irma, T.C. recalled that the faculty and staff at Brandon would "warn the girls at college to stay away from the theologs or they'd end up in a drafty manse somewhere, getting their clothes out of a missionary box."[67] Although she would not suffer great deprivation herself, Irma would be greatly pained by the hardship she witnessed as a "steady stream of people" showed up at their church and home to get food and spare clothing. As she later recounted, she and T.C. "never turned anybody down. I – still almost weep. Some poor soul always turned up – oh gosh, they never stopped coming."[68]

While honeymooning in Winnipeg, T.C. and Irma stayed with T.C.'s family, after which they moved to Weyburn, where T.C. had been hired as a full-time preacher.[69] Both T.C. and Stanley Knowles had done some relief preaching at Calvary Baptist Church in Weyburn, and both were considered for the position when it became available. However, Knowles took himself out of the running by letting the congregation know he was, in fact, a United Church adherent and would be seeking a pastoral position in Winnipeg.[70] The Weyburn post was therefore offered to T.C., whom the church probably wanted more anyway. He had greatly impressed the congregation with his dramatic, yet down to earth, style of preaching, with a sense of humour perfectly suited to a rural prairie town. But Weyburn was a community in the first stages of what would become a decade-long crisis.

**Drought and Depression**

Two images come to mind when the Great Depression of the 1930s is mentioned: the desert-like conditions on the Great Plains and the long lines of unemployed in the cities. While drought and depression were hard on vulnerable Canadians wherever they lived, those residing in the three Prairie provinces were dealt a particularly heavy blow, with Saskatchewan the worst off. While provincial per capita income fell by

44 per cent in Ontario and Quebec between 1929 and 1932, it dropped by 49 per cent in Manitoba, 61 per cent in Alberta, and 71 per cent in Saskatchewan over the same period.[71]

One word explains Saskatchewan's greater weakness during the Depression – wheat. The province's economy had become almost exclusively tied to the international sale of wheat, and exports markets went into a tailspin as continental European countries imposed ever larger tariffs on wheat imports in the late 1920s, causing prices to drop by almost 70 per cent between 1928 and 1933.[72] Farmers who had invested heavily in machinery and land could not make their loan and mortgage payments. This was no small matter, as nearly seven out of every ten people in the province lived in rural areas, according to the census of 1931.[73]

Of course, the economic devastation was hardly limited to farms. Since the businesses in smaller urban centres like Weyburn, with its population of some 5,000 souls, were dependent on the health of the farm economy, they too suffered severely. Even the prosperity of the province's largest city and capital, Regina, with a population of 53,000, was dependent on King Wheat – the name used in Saskatchewan to describe the province's dominant monoculture – despite the government being the larger employer.[74] By 1931, one in four adult male workers in Regina was unemployed.[75]

These conditions were exacerbated by years of drought, which resulted in a major decline in crop yields.[76] A region in southwestern Saskatchewan and southeastern Alberta, known as the "Dry Belt" within the Palliser Triangle, had always been prone to drought, but prolonged and severe drought became a feature of almost all of southern Saskatchewan and Alberta and even the far western part of Manitoba, the northern reaches of what became known as the Dust Bowl in the United States and Canada.[77] Although receiving sufficient rainfall throughout much of the 1920s, the farms around Weyburn suffered severe drought for most of the following decade. Farmers were going bankrupt, and their families forced to go on relief to avoid starvation.[78] The businesses that served farmers in the area laid off employees to stave off bankruptcy, and the town doctors saw their incomes shrink, as farmers and others could no longer afford even the most basic medical care.

The difference between the parkland and forest of the more northerly areas of the province and the dried-out southern grasslands, including places such as Weyburn, was striking. John G. Diefenbaker, then a young criminal lawyer based in Prince Albert who had clients throughout the province, described it best: travelling south from Prince Albert, which was hundreds of kilometres north of Regina, to the Palliser Triangle "was like moving from the Garden of Eden to the Dead Sea."[79] Dust storms were a regular feature of life. In May and June 1931, the dust storms in Weyburn and the surrounding region were so bad that they warranted successive front-page stories in the weekly *Weyburn Review*.[80]

In the early 1930s, the safety net for farmers and the unemployed was almost non-existent. Municipalities were responsible for the indigent, and most provided relief payments. Relief, in these instances, was in fact a loan by the local government provided to those residents who could prove extreme need, and carried an expectation of repayment in the future. Programs were far removed from contemporary concepts of social assistance or unemployment insurance, and getting relief during the depression was a humiliating experience. Despite the meagre provisions, local governments, including the urban municipality of Weyburn and the rural municipalities surrounding it, were overwhelmed within the first two years of the depression, and provincial governments were forced to step in with their own relief efforts.[81] The largest of these in Canada was the Saskatchewan Relief Commission. Once they proved that their families were barefoot and virtually starving, farmers on relief received vouchers for essential seed, fuel, food, and clothing that could be redeemed at local businesses on a one-time basis.[82]

Children in parched regions of the province, including the Weyburn area, were hit particularly hard. While relief may have allowed families just enough food to survive – although there was one report of starvation – malnutrition was common. In a survey of 34,564 students early in 1931, the provincial Department of Public Health found that 5.2 per cent were suffering from nervous disorders, almost 13.75 per cent were underweight, 19.4 per cent had unhealthy throats (likely from inhaling dust), and 42 per cent required dental work.[83] This was a mere snapshot of the health of children taken early in the Great Depression. Their health could only worsen as the droughts continued and the years of depression lengthened.

The problems for children went far beyond their physical health, with young people suffering terribly from a lack of stimulation during these years. Before the Great Depression, teenagers in towns like Weyburn had small paying jobs that kept them occupied, but these jobs disappeared after 1929. Seeing the problem, Reverand Douglas, as he was known in the small prairie community, started a boys' group in conjunction with United and Presbyterian pastors and with congregations supporting the venture. One evening a week, T.C. ran a sports program that included boxing as well as baseball and basketball, and devoted another evening to discussion and study – his effort to not only keep the boys "off the street" but also to keep them focused on completing school so that they might have a better future.[84]

One of the boys most impressed with Douglas was a fourteen-year-old by the name of T.H. (Tommy) McLeod. His father was a printer in town, and his mother, originally from the North End of Winnipeg like T.C., had worked for J.S. Woodsworth. Part of Douglas's boys' group, McLeod was a frequent visitor to his office in the church and to the Douglas home. When T.C. made his first federal electoral bid a few years later, he entrusted McLeod to canvass throughout the surrounding rural areas and organize public meetings, even though he was only in Grade 11. Later, T.C. was instrumental in getting McLeod into Brandon College, which then led to graduate studies in sociology in the United States. McLeod would be one of the first officials hired by Douglas after his government's landslide election victory in 1944.[85]

Weyburn was ground zero for the Great Depression in Saskatchewan, suffering intensely from what T.C. called the "double whammy" of global economic collapse and the Dust Bowl.[86] In late November 1930, he preached a sermon entitled "Hard Times in Weyburn," in which he addressed the question of how the community might meet what was going to be a difficult winter.[87] Months later, he tried to provide a glimmer of hope with a message entitled "God's Promise for Hard Times."[88] However, as the depression deepened, T.C. felt he needed to do much more than appeal to the spiritual, but he also found that asking his parishioners to be more generous to those in need hardly helped.

T.C. and Irma took direct action, tapping individuals and organizations to donate food and clothing. From their stocked church basement, they redistributed all they could to the needy. They led multi-denominational charity drives. Soon, the young preacher was working with other ministers to get clothes and food shipped into Weyburn from other parts of Canada to support desperate families in the area. But the scale of the problem made T.C. question the system itself and realize the limitations in his education. To remedy this, he decided to pursue graduate work at the University of Chicago.

**Transition to Political Activist**

In the summer of 1931, Douglas obtained leave from Calvary Baptist Church to begin his studies in Chicago. As part of his course in Christian sociology, taught by well-known sociologist and theologian Arthur E. Holt, he did fieldwork in what was known as the hobo jungle of Chicago – a vast slum city built by 75,000 unemployed men.[89] The experience radicalized T.C. and, upon his returned to Weyburn later that summer, Irma noticed a major change in him.[90]

T.C. had concluded that the economic system itself was at fault for the Great Depression and needed to be changed. Before Chicago, he had never seriously "asked what's wrong with this economic system." Despite his leanings towards the social gospel and his previous reading on socialism and capitalism, he had still accepted the basic assumptions underpinning the economic order. The Great Depression, with its "poverty, misery, lack of medical care, and lack of opportunity for a whole generation of life," shattered his acceptance and fuelled a new belief in the need for thoroughgoing change.[91]

From this point forward, Douglas focused more on social actions aimed at improving the situation faced by the poor and destitute. In Weyburn, he set up a labour exchange so that men and women could exchange skills without the use of cash. T.C.'s activities inevitably spilled into the political arena. In September 1931, during the protracted Estevan coal strike in southeastern Saskatchewan, he and Irma toured the mining towns in the area. Both were "appalled by the poor housing and living standards of the miners." Douglas then "spoke at a mass rally of the miners in Bienfait," just east of Estevan. Although uncomfortable with the communist-led Worker's Unity League, he nonetheless "considered it a mistake to 'give up on a good cause because there are a few communists in it.'"[92]

In a confidential summary of his experience, which he shared with like-minded progressives, T.C. described the mine owners and their efforts to label the workers as Bolsheviks as "merely an excuse to cover a multitude of sins." In his view, after making a visit to the village of Bienfait, where six hundred of the miners lived, all the men were "asking for is a union which would provide a decent wage scale, rules and regulations for their employment, or dischargement, the option to buy provisions for their home wherever they wish [beyond the company stores], some provision for clean sanitary conditions, a fair weighting system [for piecework] and good government inspection." However, as far as he was concerned, the provincial government was "too messed up in party politics to be very interested in fair mine treatment," noting that whenever the provincial mine inspector "proposed to visit the mines he notifies the owners a day or two ahead."[93]

Immediately upon his return from Estevan, T.C. gave a Sunday sermon entitled "Jesus the Revolutionist." In the *Weyburn Review* notice advertising his Sunday service and a rally to support the miners followed by an evening service, T.C. asked how Jesus would "view the coal miners' strike in Estevan" and whether Jesus would "revolt against our present system of graft and exploitation."[94] Douglas then "organized a truckload of food for the strikers and their families," an action that upset some of the pro-business members of the church.[95] The growing perception of T.C. as a "Red" by some of the more conservative residents of Weyburn was not helped when he chaired a talk by George H. Williams, the province's leading leftist farm leader, who, based on a recent tour, gave a glowing report on the Soviet Union's progress.[96] Some of T.C.'s own congregants asked him to stick to preaching the gospel and not concern himself with politics.[97] However, the events about to unfold only strengthened his resolve.

On 29 September 1931, while miners and their families walked from Bienfait to Estevan to draw attention to their strike, they were met with lines of Royal Canadian Mounted Police (RCMP) officers. Upon entering the town square in Estevan, the police opened fire on the strikers, killing three and injuring twenty-seven others. A riot ensued. The next morning, the RCMP raided some miners' homes to arrest the leaders of the strike on charges of rioting.[98] For T.C., this was additional proof that the Canadian establishment, including the federal government and the national police force, was aligned against ordinary workers and their families.

Beyond the violence of the coal strike, day-to-day life in southern Saskatchewan was getting harder. It was heartbreaking for T.C. to witness the ways in which people would refuse to see a doctor or go into the hospital in Weyburn. They simply could not afford to do so. When he noticed a particularly serious case, Douglas would try to get some money from the relief office or tap some of Weyburn's wealthier residents to pay the doctor or hospital bill on the needy individual's behalf. However, he knew that such one-off measures could not be sustained and that he could not continually call upon the same individuals. Nor did he blame the doctors – they too had to make a living – or the hospital, for that matter, as it had to pay the staff and keep the lights and heat on.[99] He witnessed a case of a ruptured appendix where the individual had died due to "delayed surgery and care" and no antibiotics.[100] He was again reminded of the limits of charity and the need for a permanent program that would make medical care a public good rather than a market commodity.

**The Formation of the Co-operative Commonwealth Federation**

Early in 1932, Douglas established the Weyburn Independent Labour Association (WILA). As noted in the weekly *Weyburn Review*, the purpose of the association was "to influence public opinion by peaceful and legal methods in favour of organized labour and to secure legislation in the interests of the working class."[101] WILA soon brought him into direct contact with a new political movement that was beginning to emerge in Canada. In early February, WILA sponsored a talk by M.J. (Major James) Coldwell, the president of the Independent Labour Party (ILP) of Saskatchewan. Douglas had already hosted the province's most prominent farm leader just a few months earlier, making him a part of a grassroots movement that would soon see a coming together of these reform movements in a farmer-labour-thinker triangle.

The first point on that triangle comprised the farmers, who had already upset the status quo by establishing the Saskatchewan Wheat Pool and numerous other consumer and producer cooperatives in the province. And some, such as George Williams through the Saskatchewan Section of the United Farmers of Canada, were promoting more direct participation in electoral politics. Urban reformers who focused on organizing workers and lower-paid professionals (Coldwell himself was a teacher) were the second point of the triangle, while leftist intellectuals, largely based at Canadian universities, constituted the third point. As a well-educated preacher in rural Saskatchewan who had come from a labouring background, T.C. was in regular contact with representatives of all three groups.[102]

Although he had no direct background in farming, T.C. was beginning to extend his activities further into the countryside. In rural communities surrounding Weyburn, he would regularly speak to local farmers on the material and moral impacts of drought and depression and what could be done to alleviate them. He was selected as head of a couple of rural delegations to meet with J.T.M. Anderson, the Conservative premier of Saskatchewan, to lobby for remedial measures.[103] Years later, he reflected on the "physical suffering" he witnessed on the farms of southeastern Saskatchewan and the humiliation of getting a "pitiful little bit of relief" from local and provincial governments. The sheer "hopelessness of the situation" for so many pushed him to act.[104]

He wrote J.S. Woodsworth, by then the leader of a leftist group of MPs in Parliament, about his desire to do more for the unemployed. Woodsworth suggested that he contact Coldwell. A schoolteacher and elected city council member in Regina, Coldwell drove to Weyburn to talk to Douglas.[105] At their meeting, he suggested that Douglas have WILA become the Weyburn branch of the Independent Labour Party. T.C. readily agreed, and WILA morphed into the Weyburn Independent Labour Party.[106] T.C. then used his previous contact with George Williams to get the United Farmers of Canada to cooperate with his Weyburn branch of the ILP.

The first step in the formation of what became the Co-operative Commonwealth Federation (CCF) was a meeting of socialist, progressive,

The Making of a Preacher-Politician 41

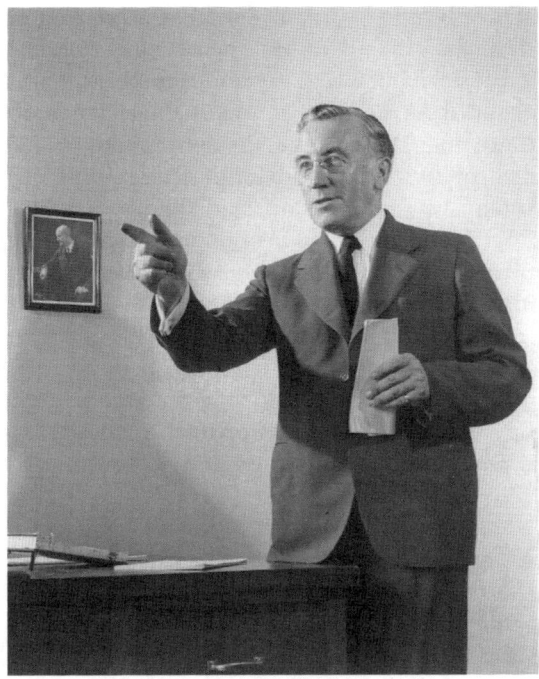

M.J. Coldwell speaking, c. 1930s (PAS R-B4315)

and reform-minded MPs in the parliamentary caucus room in Ottawa on 26 May 1932. The brief meeting resulted in the provisional establishment of the party, with Woodsworth as leader, and the intention to bring together farmer, labour, and reform-oriented socialist groups together in Calgary that summer.[107]

The second critical step was the agreement between Coldwell's ILP and the Saskatchewan Section of the United Farmers of Canada to form the Farmer-Labor Group and to send Coldwell as its representative to the meeting in Calgary. That one-day conference was intended to set the agenda and program for a meeting the following summer in Regina to form a new federal political party that would encourage the affiliation of social democratic parties, such as the Farmer-Labor Group in Saskatchewan, in the provinces.[108] To this end, it established a platform, the seventh point of which was "socialized health services," the meaning of which was left largely undefined by the delegates.[109] At the meeting in Calgary, Woodsworth was confirmed as leader and managed to secure agreement for his preferred name – the Co-operative

Commonwealth Federation – for the incipient party, a name that T.C. would later describe as "an awful mouthful."[110] The Farmer-Labor Group affiliated with the CCF to become the party's representative in Saskatchewan, and it formally appended CCF to its name.[111]

Douglas did not attend the Calgary meeting. However, he was implicated directly in the work plan developed there when he was named as one of the seven ILP members on the CCF council. He and the other labour representatives were joined on the twenty-one-member council by seven members of the United Farmers of Canada and an additional seven individuals picked by the delegates at the Calgary meeting. On Labour Day 1932, Douglas co-sponsored an ILP event in Weyburn, at which he and Coldwell were the main speakers.[112] T.C.'s ringing speech focused on "the tragedy of so much poverty in the midst of so much plenty" and the need for "thinking men and women to rally under one banner to end the poverty by drastic redistribution of the country's wealth."[113]

**Master's Thesis and Eugenics**

Although his political activity was absorbing more of his time, T.C. still had a church to run and a congregation to serve. He continued to devote significant time to directing the local organizations he had created to help those stricken by the depression. At the same time, he continued his graduate studies. Putting aside (temporarily, he thought) the program at the University of Chicago, he enrolled in a master's program in sociology at McMaster University through its affiliate, Brandon College.[114] He also took some courses in economics at the University of Manitoba to fill what he felt were significant gaps in his education. Even with summer leaves from preaching, he had to devote every extra hour to his various studies.

Fortunately, he was able to base his master's thesis on case studies drawn from Weyburn: twelve local women and their large families constituted the core of his study. These were among the poorest and most marginalized people in the small prairie city, many of whom had criminal records and were eventually confined in Weyburn's mental hospital, one of only two such institutions in the province. Perceived variously as thieves, lazy, violent, and drunks, these poorly educated and often jobless individuals were shunned by the "respectable" majority. Douglas knew some of these families from previous charity work and spiritual outreach, and had already built some rapport with his case subjects. To provide an assessment of the material, mental, psychological, and spiritual condition of his subjects, he had to conducts

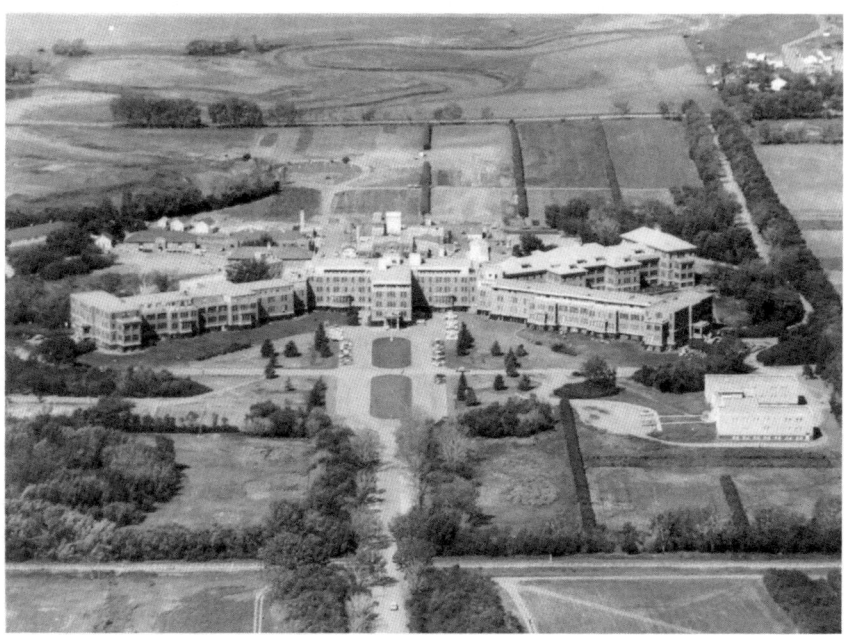

Aerial view of the psychiatric hospital in Weyburn (PAS R-LP194)

interviews at the mental hospital in Weyburn, the town's largest employer. T.C.'s growing familiarity with the institution during the Great Depression would be the wellspring for his government's leadership in reforming the treatment of mental health in the early postwar era.[115]

In March 1933, Douglas completed his thesis, entitled "The Problems of the Subnormal Family."[116] Extremely short – thirty-five pages, with an additional fifteen-page appendix – even by the standards of the day, his thesis was divided between a description of the enormous challenges faced by these families in their day-to-day lives and how best to address these challenges. The second half, devoted to remedial measures, was divided into three sections: changes in public policy through the government; changes in educational approaches and methods; and, finally, a discussion of how churches and their respective ministers might better address the problems faced by this underclass.

With respect to governmental action, he proposed that marriage laws require a medical certificate confirming the absence of sexually transmitted disease; the segregation of these underclass families in a separate community, where more structure and support might be given to them; and the sterilization of those described by Douglas as "mentally defective," an imprecise yet widely employed term meant to embrace those who were deemed to be afflicted with permanent mental illness or cognitive limitations and who likely required long-term institutionalization and other social supports. At the time, it was commonly believed, based on the science of the day, that genetics played a large role in causing mental illness and learning disabilities. Sterilization was a mainstream, even popular, idea in the first half of the twentieth century and was promoted by progressive Canadian reformers such as J.S. Woodsworth and Nellie McClung.[117]

Connections between progressive politics and eugenic ideas were later severed, spurred by post-war outrage at Nazi mass sterilization and extermination policies. Forced sterilization of the "mentally defective" would afterward become a discredited policy in most of Canada, with some notable exceptions such as Social Credit Alberta, which continued the policy until the late 1970s.[118] Douglas himself soon changed his mind on the issue of sterilization and, by the time he came to office in 1944, had already abandoned the policy of forced sterilization, even before its use by the Nazis had been fully revealed. As premier and minister of health, he rejected the recommendations of two experts – one liberal and the other radical left-wing – who promoted eugenic-style programs to reform the mental health system in Saskatchewan.[119]

As for what schools could do, Douglas suggested in his thesis that children with serious behavioural difficulties due to a difficult home life be placed together "under the care of a teacher specially trained to manage such problems" and that a special curriculum be designed with those children in mind.[120] He also recommended other educational initiatives, including recreational programs. Here, Douglas invoked his own experience with the church-based outreach programs he had established and managed since arriving in Weyburn in late summer of 1930. A group of eight boys had been released on probation into T.C.'s care. To build a sense of collective trust and loyalty, he got the boys accustomed to group games that required team work.[121] Such programs, rather than jail or other punishments, could, T.C. believed, begin to heal their broken lives.

At the same time, Douglas felt that changes in public policy and education were not enough. At the base of the problem was a lack of social belonging and sufficient self-respect to care about the future. In his mind, organized religion, what he called "the Church," was in the perfect position to offer both. In his view, the key challenge was that the "sense of worth" of the poor and marginalized "has been impaired." The only thing that can change this is their own "re-evaluation" of their worth, both in terms of having a sense of belonging and some belief in a greater purpose in life. This spiritual dimension was critical, according to T.C., as the penultimate paragraph of his thesis attests:

> When education and legislation have failed, there is still One who can take the broken earthenware from life's garbage heaps and make them vessels of honor in His temple of love. If the Church would play its part in the salvaging of these social outcasts, it must bring to the problem its belief in the regenerating power of the Christ, the "explosive force of a new affection" and the assurance that "He maketh all things new."[122]

## The Regina Manifesto and Socialized Health Services

T.C. was so occupied with his studies that he missed most of the CCF's founding convention in Regina in July 1933. Although not a delegate, he attended for a short time as an observer on the conference's third day, describing it at the time as "the finest thing I have ever seen."[123]

The convention produced the Regina Manifesto, which contained a ringing statement of principles in its introduction and conclusion, with a set of reforms constituting the rest of the document. At the request of J.S. Woodsworth on behalf of the delegates at the CCF's inaugurating Calgary convention the year before, a draft of the manifesto was prepared in advance by the members of the League for Social Reconstruction (LSR). With Woodsworth as honorary president, this group of intellectuals concentrated at the University of Toronto and McGill University provided a rough draft, written by Frank Underhill and edited by Frank Scott of McGill University and other LSR members. The LSR draft was then reshaped by the delegates at the Regina meeting.[124]

Just before the founding convention, T.C., as part of a CCF party committee, reviewed the draft manifesto. He was pleased with the content but concerned that the language would not be readily understood by average farmer or unemployed worker.[125] There is no record of his reaction to the Regina Manifesto other than his discomfort, registered in later years, with the incendiary statement added by the delegates at the end of the manifesto that was soon weaponized by the CCF's opponents: "No C.C.F. Government will rest content until it has eradicated capitalism and put into operation the full programme of socialized planning which will lead to the establishment in Canada of the Co-operative Commonwealth."[126]

The CCF's opponents' preoccupation with this rhetoric ignored the considerable content at the heart of the document. As part of the Regina Manifesto, the CCF delegates put forward a sweeping fourteen-point program, including the need for economic planning, a central bank and public investment board, public ownership of utilities, security of tenure for farmers, encouragement of cooperatives, a national labour code, constitutional and legal reform, and unemployment relief.[127] Article 8 of the manifesto was entitled "socialized health services," the same phrase used at the Calgary meeting. In this case, the original LSR text was ratified with minimal discussion or change.[128]

The Regina Manifesto's health program would become Douglas's own platform in his subsequent political campaigns, from 1934 until his campaign as the Saskatchewan CCF's party leader in 1944. Article 8 emphasized the importance not only of removing cost as a barrier to medical care but of maintaining a healthy population through emphasizing the prevention of illness. After the assertion in the first sentence that "the maintenance of a healthy population" is a collective responsibility, the next two sentences focus on the role of the state in removing cost as a barrier to health services, although the means to be used to achieve this are not specified. Finally, the article asserts that a "properly organized system of public health services including medical and dental care, which would stress the prevention rather than the cure of illness should be extended to all our people in both rural and urban areas."[129]

While illustrating the general philosophy of the CCF, which focused on population health as much as treating illness and injury, Article 8 hardly provided programmatic detail. This vacuum is what T.C. would have to fill over a decade later when his government was first elected in Saskatchewan. At the same time, he would strive to do more than remove cost as a barrier to access, as he tried to improve the health of the provincial population through public health and illness-prevention measures.

With the energy released by the 1933 CCF convention, Douglas and his fellow party members in Saskatchewan, such as Coldwell and Williams, though still a small group, had great confidence in the new party's ability to change the political landscape of the province and the country.[130] As a first step in attracting voters in his region, T.C. convinced Woodsworth to travel down to Weyburn after the conference and speak to potential CCF members and voters.

**The Unsuccessful Provincial Candidate**

By the fall of 1933, T.C. was being encouraged to stand as the Farmer-Labor Group (CCF) candidate for Weyburn.[131] As the founder of the Weyburn chapter of the ILP, Douglas had worked hard to forge close ties with left-leaning local farm organizations, in particular the United

Farmers of Canada (Saskatchewan Section). In the eyes of the leaders of Saskatchewan's growing CCF movement, he seemed the obvious candidate.[132]

The nominating convention began in Weyburn in the afternoon of 4 November 1933. In addition to Douglas and other nominees giving speeches, there were guest speakers, the most notable being Clarence Fines.[133] Although only twenty-eight years of age – ten months younger than T.C. – Fines was already a seasoned political organizer. From his base as a teacher and city councillor in Regina, he had worked closely with Coldwell in establishing the ILP and had been instrumental in organizing the CCF's founding conventions in Calgary and Regina.[134] Douglas was drawn to Fines – a sentiment fully reciprocated by Fines, who reported back to the CCF's provincial executive on how impressed he was with the thirty-year-old preacher from Weyburn.[135]

While three candidates had put their names forward, one withdrew at the nomination meeting, leaving the seventy-seven delegates with two choices. T.C. won easily on the first ballot and, according to the *Weyburn Review*, received a "tremendous ovation" when the results were announced. Taking the stage, Douglas admitted that it was "not customary for ministers to" enter politics, but then said he "would not be worthy" of his redeemer if he "did not take up the sword on behalf of the underpaid and underprivileged." He made it clear where he stood in terms of his "obligation to the great working class from which I have come and to which I belong."[136] Fines was amazed by Douglas's "electrifying" speech that afternoon: "I knew then, as I listened to him, that we [the CCF] had made a great discovery. In the game of politics some candidates are capable of making a one-base hit, sometimes even a double. Occasionally you find one you can count on for a home run practically every time he comes up to bat. That was T.C. Douglas."[137]

To prepare for the 1934 provincial election, Douglas began speaking to farmers and townspeople in southeastern Saskatchewan as well as to CCF clubs and associations recently established in the province's capital.[138] However, in March that year, he tangled himself up trying to defend and explain his party's platform on land reform – a complicated policy called "use-lease" to protect farmers against bankruptcy, through which the government purchased farm property in distress and then leased it back to farmers.[139]

Douglas and his fellow Farmer-Labor candidates were targeted by provincial Liberal leader Jimmy Gardiner and the Liberal-friendly newspapers as anti-democratic, anti-religious, and anti–private property revolutionary socialists. Of these three charges, the Farmer-Labor Group (CCF) was most vulnerable on the issue of private property, given the Regina Manifesto's stated purpose of "eradicating capitalism." Such rhetoric allowed Gardiner to mastermind a Red Scare campaign: it was in Gardiner's political interests to associate the CCF with the Communist Party of Canada (CPC) and equate the CCF's policy on use-lease with the elimination of private farm land policies by the Communist Party in the Soviet Union.

The Farmer-Labor Group (CCF) always placed the party name in parentheses to ensure that everyone knew the Farmer-Labor candidates were constituent members of the CCF and therefore different from labour or farmer candidates associated with the CPC or other left-wing groups.[140] Although the CCF was expansive in terms of which groups were allowed to affiliate with the party, it rejected the Communists because of their insistence on violent revolution rather than gradual reformism through parliamentary democracy. The CCF would face a stiff ideological and organizational challenge from the CPC throughout the Great Depression, especially after the CPC endorsed the Popular Front strategy of cooperating with (and co-opting, where possible) socialists and social democrats.[141] As noted by political historian Nelson Wiseman, this competition had an ethnic component. Both parties "championed the interests of poor working class immigrants ... [but] the CCF received most of it support from 'British-born Protestant immigrants'" – people like Douglas and his parents – and to a lesser extent from native born "Anglo-Protestants, Scandinavians, some Jews, and a few others," while the CPC's "support came overwhelmingly from Eastern European immigrants."[142] In response to this division, the CCF did everything it could to make headway into the Ukrainian and other Slavic communities.

Despite the CCF's efforts to separate itself, organizationally and ideologically, from the CPC, the Liberals and Conservatives regularly framed CCF socialists as adjacent to Soviet-style communists. Douglas easily swatted away the anti-democratic arguments. Incredibly, despite his status as an ordained Baptist minister, he was charged with being a godless atheist in at least one open debate.[143] He was amused by a Conservative newspaper's description of the Farmer-Labor Group as subversively socialist, led by a brain trust of "school teachers and Hebrew lawyers," coming, as it did, from a party that had the support of the Ku Klux Klan when it defeated the Liberals in the 1929 provincial election.[144] But the use-lease issue became toxic months before the election, with confusion reigning as to what the policy did or did not mean in terms of farmland ownership. It precipitated an acrimonious exchange in print, through letters to the *Regina Leader-Post* editor that only served to underline the political maxim that when you're explaining, you're losing.[145]

Due to the Great Depression's punishing impact on Saskatchewan residents, the deliberations and campaign of both Douglas and the Farmer-Labor Group focused on economic problems and their proposed solutions. Health care was given limited attention in the CCF's electoral platform. The Farmer-Labor position as set by the party's members early in 1933 referred to the "socialization of all health services." In its handbook for speakers, the Farmer-Labor Group, far from expounding on the Regina Manifesto's health program, was even more rudimentary on the question, defining the socialization of medicine as "medical treatment" that is "available to people, not in proportion to the amount they can pay for it, but in proportion to their need." Douglas and his fellow candidates called for "a medical service" made up of "doctors, nurses and hospitals" that would be "available for the treatment of all cases" based on need rather than ability to pay.[146]

Douglas understood that he was in an uphill battle against the Liberal machine in Saskatchewan. In addition, the local Liberal candidate, Dr. Hugh Eaglesham, was a long-established and respected family doctor who knew almost everyone.[147] Even the local Conservative incumbent, a well-liked lay preacher, could be counted on to get considerable support, despite the plummeting popularity of his party, which bore the brunt of the population's discontent at the ongoing malaise wrought by the depression. Still, Douglas was convinced he had a chance, based on the enthusiastic crowds that he spoke to in over a hundred campaign events in Weyburn and the surrounding villages.[148]

Since 1929, Conservative premier James T.M. Anderson had been leading a coalition government comprising Conservatives, progressives, and independents. By 1934, though, the coalition was becoming unglued by the relentless misery caused by drought and depression.[149] By that year, most farmers and townspeople in the Weyburn area had gone on relief just to get sufficient seed grain for spring sowing and the basics to feed their families.[150] In the end, however, such discontent and dislocation were not enough to seriously upset the political status quo, and when the votes were counted on 19 June, T.C.'s hopes for a political change were dashed.

In the optimism of the campaign, T.C. thought the CCF had a chance to get "at least twenty to twenty-five seats."[151] Voters, many of whom seemed to be attracted to the Farmer-Labor platform, nonetheless migrated to the Liberals to get rid of the Conservative-led coalition government. Under Gardiner, the Liberals swept fifty of the fifty-five seats in the province. The Conservatives were wiped out, and would be shut out of power in the province for another half-century.[152] This left a measly five seats for the Farmer-Labor Group (CCF), all drawn from rural

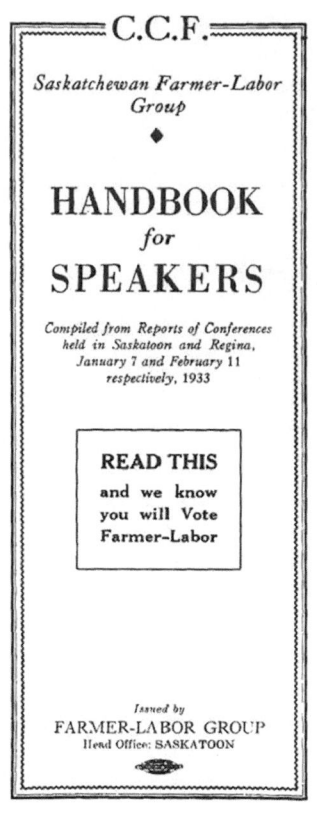

Cover page of a Farmer-Labor Group handbook for speakers, 1933 (USAS, CCF fonds)

Saskatchewan. Farmer-Labor candidates from urban centres, whether they were large urban seats such as Coldwell's riding in Regina or small like Douglas's riding of Weyburn, were defeated. In fact, like Coldwell, Douglas came in third behind the Liberal and Conservative candidates. He scored a mere 1,343 votes or 25.8 per cent of the total, 201 votes shy of the Conservative candidate and 983 votes behind Dr. Eaglesham.

Of the five successful Farmer-Labor candidates, only George Williams managed to get a bare majority (50.5 per cent) of the vote. The others squeaked in thanks to vote splitting between the Liberals and Conservatives. The election result would soon cause internal dissention in the CCF, when Coldwell suggested that he take the place of one of the five elected members so that he could remain the Farmer-Labor Group's leader. Rejecting Coldwell's idea out of hand, Williams assumed the leadership of the caucus, creating a schism in the party that was only

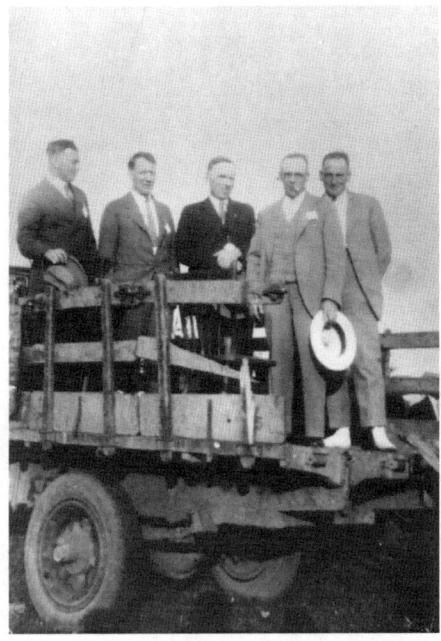

George Williams (second from right) at a wheat pool picnic, c. 1925 (PAS R-A15273)

papered over through a temporary agreement in which Williams was forced to share leadership with Coldwell, who would remain the nominal president of the provincial party, although real power lay with Williams as caucus leader.[153] The strained relationship between the two men would drive an enduring wedge between their respective supporters, which, as will be seen, Douglas could not avoid.

Reflecting on the reasons for his defeat many years later, Douglas pointed to two key factors. The first was a lack of resources, in terms of both campaign funding and the people willing to take time off to conduct door-to-door and farm-to-farm canvassing right up to election day, an assessment backed up by the party's provincial constituency organizer, who contrasted the "well-attended" and "enthusiastic" meetings with the very limited canvassing.[154]

The second problem was the platform, especially the complicated use-lease plank. Although this was an effort by the Farmer-Labor Group (CCF) to save farmers from losing their land, it was easily used by opponents to scare many farmers away from Farmer-Labor candidates and

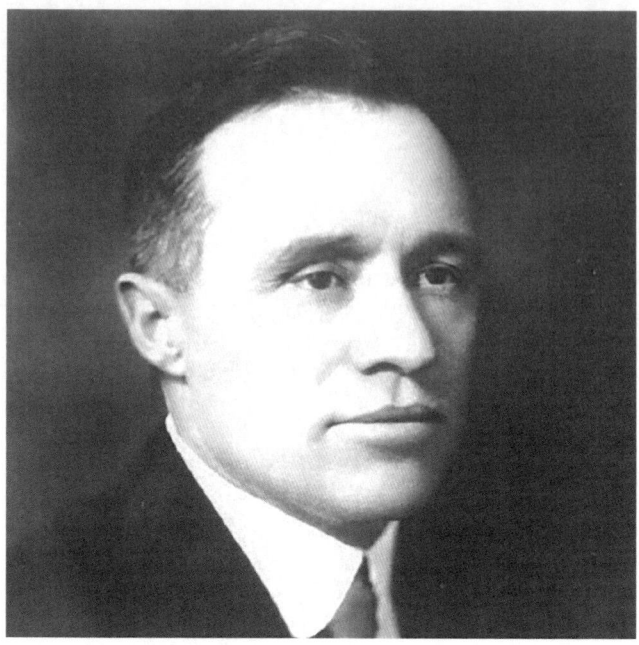

Jimmy Gardiner (Wikimedia Commons)

to support a narrative that the CCF would be little different than Soviet communists in collectivizing and expropriating private property.[155] As Jimmy Gardiner explained to his supporters leading up to the election, the key factor to be repeated, over and over, was that the objective of the CCF, as reflected in its own platform, was "the social ownership of all resources," including farmland. As Gardiner routinely communicated to potential voters, the Farmer-Labor Group (CCF) would implement "state socialism" if elected, "and not the Christian socialism that Mr. Coldwell speaks of."[156] Despite the best efforts of Coldwell, Douglas, and other Farmer-Labor candidates, this Liberal campaign tactic worked – the first but not the last time that the spectre of communism would be used against the CCF.

Despite the defeat, Douglas was undeterred. Disappointed though he may have been, he was determined to become even more politically active. Less than six weeks after the provincial election, he travelled to Winnipeg to attend the second convention of the national CCF in mid-July 1934. This convention turned out to be disorganized, with delegates not nearly as cohesive and productive as they had been the year before in Regina. Part of the reason was the roughly one hundred delegates representing a new affiliate of the CCF – the Co-operative Commonwealth Youth Movement (CCYM). Some of these young delegates adopted Marxist revolutionary positions at odds with the CCF's reformist majority and its focus on electing CCF members as the first step towards being able to form governments at the provincial and federal levels.[157]

When radical CCYM positions were rebutted by Woodsworth and others at the Winnipeg convention, these delegates threatened to secede from the CCF. Woodsworth, Coldwell, and Fines took Douglas aside and convinced him to challenge the leadership of the youth group. On the third day of the convention, after listening to numerous CCYM speeches in which he carefully inserted his own observations, Douglas put his name forward, and he was elected president by the majority of more moderate CCYM delegates. He too was convinced that the radical secessionists he had defeated in the CCYM were in fact being manipulated and controlled by the Communist Party of Canada.[158] As he put it in an interview just before he died, these young individuals had attended "Communist schools ... week-long seminars ... where they were really drilled in what I would call sabotaging social democratic movements, and moving them to the left or breaking them up."[159] These summer schools were a key instrument used by communist organizations to recruit and ideologically mould young people in the United States and Canada, and were soon emulated by the CCYM.[160]

At the same time, Douglas did his best to represent the CCYM, and this meant supporting to a limit its willingness to collaborate with numerous other political organizations, including the CPC, in response to the dire crisis of the Great Depression and the threat posed by the fascist dictatorships in Germany and Italy. The Canadian League Against War and Fascism was one of the more prominent Popular Front organizations of the time and was heavily supported by T.C. and the Saskatchewan-based CCYM. But this organization and other Popular Front creations were eyed suspiciously by Woodsworth and other more senior leaders within the CCF.[161] When the league held a major gathering in Toronto in early August 1934, Douglas spoke to its 275 delegates on behalf of the CCYM, a decision for which he was taken to task by the CCF's national council under the watchful of Woodsworth as national president and Coldwell as national secretary.[162]

Still, T.C. continued his participation in the Canadian League Against War and Fascism for years, rising to the position of vice-chair of its national council under a chair, A.A. MacLeod, who was a prominent member of the Communist Party of Canada.[163] Douglas was far less concerned than Woodsworth and Coldwell about the ability of the CPC to harm the CCF. This did not mean he was naive about the methods used by the CPC to infiltrate the CCF and then draw off members.[164] However, T.C. seemed more confident than most of the party establishment that the public would easily distinguish the CCF from the CPC and would, in most cases, support a party that promised a democratic path to socialism through the ballot box and would readily work within the traditions of a parliamentary Westminster system of government.

This confidence only grew with time as T.C. parlayed his growing political experience into a bid for nomination and then election as a federal member of Parliament for the CCF. As will be seen in the next chapter, he would abandon the notion of doing doctoral studies at the University of Chicago and pursuing an academic career alongside theology. Deep down, he knew he was not suited to a quiet, contemplative life. He yearned to be in the thick of the action rather than observing from the sidelines. Leaving his life as a small-town preacher behind him, he would seize the opportunities and the challenges that awaited him, and for the next four and a half decades he would be a full-time politician.

# 3 Federal Member of Parliament, 1935–1944

> It was the best of times, it was the worst of times, it was the age of wisdom, it was the age of foolishness, it was the epoch of belief, it was the epoch of incredulity, it was the season of light, it was the season of darkness, it was the spring of hope, it was the winter of despair.
>
> Charles Dickens, *A Tale of Two Cities*

As 1935 approached, Tommy Douglas was beginning to make choices that would soon transform him into a life-long politician. At this early stage, however, his career could still have gone in another direction. While a Baptist ministry in isolation had never been enough for him, he could easily have combined his life as a pastor with a scholarly career. While enrolled at the University of Chicago, he discovered he could finance his doctoral studies by teaching part-time and moving to a church ministry located near a major university.[1] But when offered the ministry at Strathcona Baptist Church, located a short distance from the University of Alberta – T.C. referred to it as Edmonton's "university church" – he turned down the position.[2] He had decided to become a politician in Saskatchewan.

In numerous interviews over the course of his life, T.C. never disclosed why he chose a political life over a religious and academic vocation, but the explanation for his choice can be adduced from his own character.[3] Douglas was hardly the kind of person who could have lived with the isolation necessary to become a top-notch scholar. He was simply too gregarious and too action oriented for such a contemplative life. Scholastically, he did very well at Brandon College, but not as well as his closest friend, the more introspective and scholarly Stanley Knowles. T.C. preferred action to study, particularly the kind of collective action to which he was drawn like a moth to a flame. In this, he generally played a leadership role, as evidenced by the many youth clubs and labour organizations he established early in his ministry career. As he explained later, a political leader was like the conductor of an orchestra, providing direction and a sense of cohesion to all members so that they could create a result otherwise impossible to achieve, despite each member's individual virtuosity.[4] As a clergyman and politician, he consistently gravitated to being a conductor – of youth groups and benevolent associations in his early years, and subsequently of a political party and government.

In all of this, Douglas was far more interested in improving conditions in this world than in preparing himself and others for an unfathomable life after death, however much he believed in what he called the Kingdom of God. In fact, he could be impatient with adherents to dogmatic theologies and ideologies, whether Christian or Marxist. What mattered most to him was what could be accomplished in the here and now – what he described as building the New Jerusalem in this lifetime – not a revolution that promised to change everything in the future and not an eventual heaven. This sense of immediacy was particularly apposite in the depths of the Great Depression, when a once-prosperous society on the Canadian prairies was being torn apart by poverty and hopelessness. One of his sermons revealed the social gospel basis of his political philosophy: "When one sees the church spending its energies on the assertion of antiquated dogmas, but dumb as an oyster to the poverty and misery all around," it was apparent that "a new interpretation of Christianity" was needed. Far better, he urged, "to build a heaven on earth rather than live in misery in the hope of gaining some uncertain reward in the distant future."[5]

The standard account, repeated in most biographies of Douglas, is of someone who only reluctantly entered the political fray. This was not the case when he became a candidate in the provincial election of 1934. It was even less so when he decided to run for the CCF in the federal election of 1935. While Douglas's own version, in which he was convinced to run in order to defy a threat from a senior Baptist official that he would never again be given a ministry if he became a candidate, may make for a good story – one that he often repeated – it was far from the deciding factor.[6]

**Politician by Nature**

T.C. had been preparing for his direct entry into politics since at least 1932, as is obvious by his early organizing efforts for the Independent

Labour Party that year.[7] To this must be added a flurry of keynote speaking engagements at clubs and organizations scattered far beyond his Weyburn constituency in the years leading up to his provincial election campaign. These activities reflect the effort and focus of someone investing considerable time in a movement and its associated political parties, with the intention of becoming one of their leading figures. Despite the romantic story about a reluctant hero pulled into the fray, Douglas was in fact drawn to the cut and thrust of politics more than to a more passive and cerebral life of a church minister or an academic. He preferred the concreteness of political action as opposed to more amorphous and arguably ephemeral modes of influencing people, whether through a sermon, lecture, or book.

For the rest of his life, he believed that, while intellectuals had a role to play in bettering society and reminding his party of its values and long-term goals, they would be far finer human beings if they occasionally rolled up their sleeves and worked with actual people, to really see if their "great ideas" on how to improve society could be accepted and then implemented in a workable fashion. He had little time for standoffish, rigid intellectuals who criticized people of action like himself for doing things that deviated from some ideal political ideology or axiom.[8] To his mind, the worst offenders were intellectuals so convinced of the rightness of their beliefs that they could accept no compromise on some idealized notion in their heads.

T.C. was convinced that what drove this commitment to theoretical rigidity was a distinct lack of modesty about the limits of human understanding and knowledge. Moreover, some of the intellectuals in his own party could not seem to accept that, in a democracy, politicians like himself had to appeal to those citizens who did not share their values and views. In his opinion, "none of us is always right" and "every one of us has been wrong on some occasion." To understand that no one has a monopoly on the correct course a society should take is the essential foundation of democracy. The right course, he argued, is produced through a "clash of ideas" and "different points of view," after which we may "finally emerge with a sort of consensus which is usually closer to the truth than any of the extreme views that are expressed."[9]

T.C. was restless by nature. Barely able to sit in one place for longer than an hour or two, he preferred a hectic schedule that brought him into regular contact with new people. Crowds energized him; when he spoke to a full room, he would always feel the mood and play on it. At the same time, he drew on his considerable skills as an actor and speaker, as well as knowledge gained from years of study, to galvanize people to join the forces for change. He felt that his greatest skill was reaching out to those who might not share his perspective, or even his values, and convincing them to support change on the most practical of grounds – that their own lives, and those of their families and neighbours, would improve.

**The Regina Riot**

At the same time as his 1935 nomination, a movement known as the On-to-Ottawa Trek was picking up steam. It had all started in April, when 1,500 unemployed men in a federal relief camp in British Columbia went on strike. The federal Conservative government, led by Prime Minister Richard Bedford (R.B.) Bennett, had, under the aegis of the Department of National Defence, begun setting up these relief camps in 1932 to concentrate single unemployed men some distance from urban centres to guard against violent insurrections. In this case, the men left the camp and travelled to Vancouver to protest their living conditions, their confinement under the supervision by the Department of National Defence, and their miserly payment of fifty cents per day.[10]

On 3 June, more than a thousand strikers left Vancouver and began riding boxcars eastward to personally present their demands to the Bennett government in Ottawa. By Wednesday, 12 June, the trekkers had made it to Moose Jaw, by which time the Bennett government had decided to use the Royal Canadian Mounted Police (RCMP) to pen in the protestors when they arrived in Regina and prevent them from carrying on to the national capital. This prompted the Regina branch of the CCF to forward a resolution for J.S. Woodsworth to present in Parliament supporting the trekkers and condemning the "highly provocative" attitude of the federal government in building up a police presence and attempting to stop the marchers.[11]

By the time they reached Regina, the trekkers ranks had swelled well beyond the original thousand, as hundreds of other unemployed men joined them. Bennett feared the possibility of a revolutionary mob descending on Ottawa.[12] In Regina, residents were polarized, with some recognizing in the trekkers their own frustrations as well as desire for a more hopeful future, with others convinced that the trekkers were a dangerous mob led by communists fomenting violent revolution.

Consistent with his position during the Estevan Strike four years earlier, T.C. was on the side of the trekkers. As he would explain subsequently in the House of Commons, the problem was not the strikers but an economic system that could not offer jobs to young men and a government that preferred to spend money on policing the unemployed rather than creating public works to employ them. The solution,

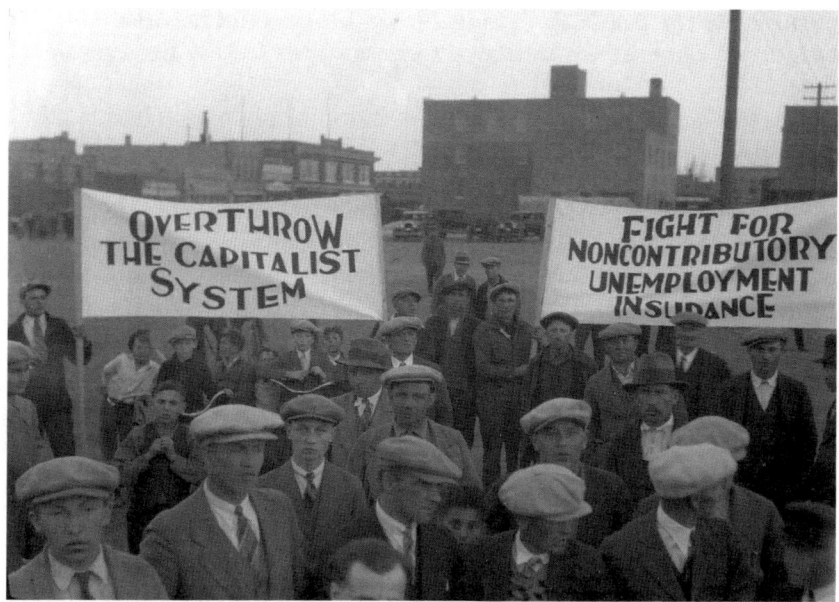

On-to-Ottawa trekkers in downtown Regina just before the Regina Riot of 1935 (PAS R-A27560(1))

he argued, was not to lock up the unemployed in relief camps but to give "these young men opportunities to live" instead of refusing "to realize the urgency and dangerous nature of the situation until it is upon us."[13] He bristled at the perception of the trekkers as bums who did not "want to work."[14]

The CCF and the Co-operative Commonwealth Youth Movement (CCYM) supported the trekkers during their stay in Regina through an organization known as the Citizens' Emergency Committee (CEC), which sought to provide food and other necessaries for the young men.[15] Although the CEC included a broad coalition of leftist organizations, from church groups and trade unions to the Young Communist League, it was the CCF and CCYM that drove the committee from the beginning. Local CCF-Labour politicians in the city such as Clarence Fines and CCF house leader George Williams regularly organized and spoke on behalf of the CEC and the trekkers.[16] At the first CEC meeting, on 13 June, M.J. Coldwell spoke on behalf of the CEC at radio stations to publicize events and to solicit donations of food and money. Jack King, the Saskatchewan secretary of the CCYM, was appointed chair of publicity for the CEC.[17] Months later, King would become the chief organizer of the CEC's initiative to raise funds for the trekkers' legal defence.[18]

The trekkers first rally in Regina was organized largely by the CEC. A local CCFer, Peter Mikkelson (who was about to be elected on the Labour ticket to Regina City Council), gave the first speech at the rally. When Mikkelson pointed out that the Liberals and Conservatives were not represented at the rally, the crown booed to express their derision for the two establishment parties. Coldwell came on stage to speak, promising the trekkers the "unqualified support" of the provincial CCF and demanding the withdrawal of the RCMP, which was assembling in large numbers nearby, and the lifting of the ban preventing the strikers from travelling to Ottawa.[19] To great cheers, Coldwell vowed that "no power will be able to stop your onward march."[20]

In the ensuing days, the trekkers case was vigorously advocated in Parliament by Woodsworth and his tiny caucus. In response, the Bennett government relented slightly, allowing a direct meeting in Ottawa between officials and eight representatives of the trekkers. However, this meeting proved fruitless. Bennett had no intention of negotiating with the strike leaders, so the On-to-Ottawa Trek delegates returned to Regina, frustrated and angry, on 26 June. Further efforts by strikers to leave the city and continue to Ottawa were blocked by the RCMP. According to the *Regina Leader-Post*, 1,075 trekkers from relief camps in the four western provinces plus another 335 trekkers who had rode the rails with them to Regina had been bottled up in Regina by this time.[21] By 1 July – Dominion Day – a public rally of roughly 1,500–2,000 strikers as well as city residents in Regina's downtown market square turned into a bloody riot when RCMP and baton-wielding city police charged the crowd from all sides in an attempt to arrest the strike leaders. While the attack was unprovoked, this initial assault and arrests caused a "stampede as people sought to escape," and some demonstrators returned the violence with "stones, fence posts or anything that could be hurled" at the RCMP and city police.[22]

By the time the Regina Riot ended, a trekker and a policeman were dead, and hundreds of trekkers, police officers, and residents were injured. During the riot, T.C. was at a political meeting in Kronau, a town a little less than thirty kilometres from Regina, at the northern edge of the federal constituency of Weyburn. When he drove into the city later that evening, he saw the debris and damage left by the riot. He joined Dr. Hugh MacLean, who had won the Regina City nomination for the CCF the week before, at the Regina General Hospital, where MacLean was treating those injured in the riot.[23] He told T.C. how he

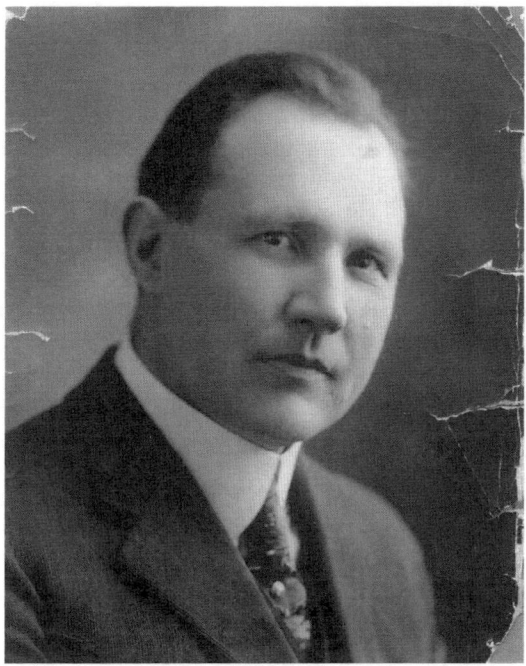

Dr. Hugh MacLean, c. 1920s (PAS R-A3399)

believed the riot was caused by the government and the RCMP and city police commanders who were under orders to attack and arrest the trek leaders that day. In Ottawa, Woodsworth took the Bennett government to task for its handling of the On-to-Ottawa Trek and for creating the conditions for the Regina Riot. Months later, he would be joined in Parliament by Douglas, who would lead the debate for a full enquiry.[24]

In the weeks before and after the strike, T.C. came to know and respect Hugh MacLean. A generation older than Douglas, MacLean had emigrated from Glasgow to Canada while still a boy. He went on to the University of Toronto, where he was conferred an MD degree in 1906. In 1921, he ran, unsuccessfully, as a Progressive Party candidate in Regina in the federal election.[25] He migrated to the CCF when it was formed in 1932 and soon became the CCF's resident expert on all things medical. T.C. was impressed by the way in which MacLean put his Hippocratic Oath first by regularly treating poorer patients for free and by offering "his services as medical attendant to the strikers' army" even before they had arrived in Regina.[26] True to his oath, MacLean spent weeks after the riot treating a seriously injured city police inspector, despite the doctor's support for the trekkers.[27] MacLean regularly spoke on the need for socialized medicine, what he sometimes called "state health services." In this, he predated by a few years the State Hospital and Medical League, a civil society pressure group dedicated to convincing the provincial government to reorganize health services and make them universally available.[28] Like T.C., MacLean had felt from an early age that health care should be a public service rather than a private commodity.[29]

Perhaps identifying with the relative youth of the trekkers – many of whom were in their late teens and early twenties – the CCYM was even more supportive of the strikers than was the CCF itself, if that were possible. As the CCYM's president, T.C. found himself embroiled in the aftermath of the Regina Riot.[30] Jack King, the CCYM's secretary, took the Citizen's Defence Committee national, rebranding it as the Citizen's Defence Movement and spinning off the Citizen's Legal Defence Committee. These organizations featured prominent CCF members, including Coldwell, Fines, George Williams, and Frank Scott.[31] As for T.C., he became the parliamentary point man for these organizations once he was a member of Parliament.[32]

**Candidate in the Federal Election of 1935**

Douglas's position as CCYM president exposed him to CCF clubs and organizations throughout the country.[33] This position also "made him the most prominent CCFer" in Weyburn and area, and "a natural choice to run" for the party in the federal election of 1935.[34] Before he put his name down as a potential nominee, however, he sought advice from his Weyburn congregation.

Pitching his candidature as a cause that would likely fail, T.C. said he still felt a duty to use the election to publicize the plight of farmers and the unemployed. Many in his congregation agreed, as long it was clear that he would make being a clergyman his full-time vocation afterwards. However, the treasurer of his church, a local lawyer, felt that politics and the ministry were completely incompatible, and resigned his position in protest against T.C.'s proposal. In addition, when the executive members of the Western Canadian Baptist Union got wind of T.C.'s intention to run for Parliament, they dispatched one of their senior members to Weyburn, who informed T.C. that if he insisted on running, the Baptist Union would block him from being posted to any other church in western Canada. Rather than dissuade Douglas, the threat only served to strengthen his resolve to run.[35]

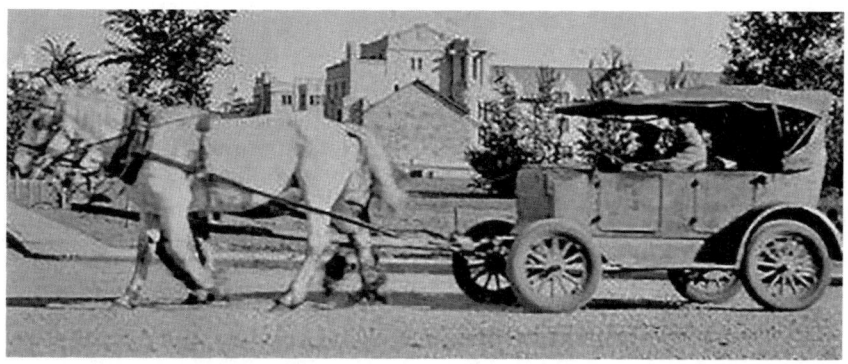

A Bennett buggy near the University of Saskatchewan campus, 1935 (Wikimedia Commons)

On a Saturday in mid-June 1935, standing before four hundred CCF members, T.C. and each of the other candidates explained why they deserved the nomination.[36] In the end, Douglas won the vote by a sizeable margin. As was required at that time by local CCF constituency associations, he also had to sign recall papers, which gave his local constituency members the right to force his resignation if they felt that he did not represent their wishes in Parliament.[37] Douglas had great hopes for himself and the party. After five years in office during the Great Depression, the Conservatives were highly unpopular, and the Regina Riot delivered the final nail in the coffin of Bennett's government.[38]

A serious man, Prime Minister Bennett did not take kindly to criticism, much less ridicule but, by 1935, he had to endure much of both. A good example was the sarcastic term that Canadians used for converted cars or trucks pulled by livestock. Without money for gas or engine repairs, some Canadians – especially prairie farmers – stripped their vehicles down to a weight more easily pulled by one of their farm animals. Blaming the prime minister for their plight, the owners called such contraptions Bennett buggies. Similarly, in the United States, such makeshift vehicles were known as Hoover mobiles or Hoover wagons, named after the president in office during the first four years of the Great Depression.[39]

Like most world leaders at the time, Bennett assumed the depression would be of short duration, but, as it dragged on, he faced increasing criticism for not doing enough for the unemployed or for prairie farmers facing prolonged drought and disastrously low wheat prices. Canadian critics contrasted the limited actions of the Bennett government with Roosevelt's New Deal south of the border and demanded more government assistance. As the clock ticked down towards the end of his electoral term, Bennett finally reversed course and introduced his own version of a New Deal. However, it was too little and too late to salvage his government's political fortunes.[40]

Due to the deep divisions within his own party, Bennett had been reluctant to call an election in 1935. But his government was at its five-year mark – one year beyond the conventional term – and he finally had to face the music from voters fed up with the suffering, turmoil, and chaos wrought by the depression. The Liberals and the CCF were both keen to take advantage of the Conservative Party's weaknesses and Bennett's image as an unfeeling plutocrat who cared little for the suffering of so many in the country. Both parties derided and dismissed his last-minute unveiling of a Canadian New Deal in January 1935 as political chicanery, a cheap effort to buy votes.[41] For his part, Bennett saw the CCFers as little different than communists, whom he had already promised to crush under "the iron heel of ruthlessness."[42] Meanwhile, Liberal leader Mackenzie King focused on Bennett's shortcomings but offered little to address unemployment and the farm crisis. When it came to the CCF, King resorted to name calling, dismissing it as a fringe group of "pseudo-intellectuals, monetary cranks, advocates of 'Socialism in our time,' and faddists."[43]

Like the Liberals, the CCF understood that the Conservatives had already been defeated by the unhappy state of the country, and both parties had been preparing for an election since 1934. The issue had been obvious to many for years: what could the government of Canada do to alleviate the suffering and unemployment so acute in the drought-ravaged Prairies reeling from the international collapse of wheat prices?[44] When it became clear that the Liberals would rely on a mild reform package (much milder than even Bennett's New Deal), the CCF felt that it had been given a golden opportunity for its ambitious program of fundamental economic and social reform. CCF activists believed that both establishment parties had demonstrated their inability to deal with the exigencies of the Great Depression – the Conservatives by their proven ineffectiveness after five years in office, and the Liberals by their policy timidity in the face of the greatest economic and social crisis the country had faced since Confederation. With so many Canadians desperate for change, the time seemed right for a new protest party with an ambitious agenda for social and economic change.

As for Douglas, he completely altered his own style of campaigning. In the 1934 provincial election, he described himself as lecturing audiences "like a university professor giving a course in sociology." In 1935, in contrast, he would start with a few jokes and once he got their attention, move into the serious part of his speech.[45] However, instead of reciting the details of dry policy solutions, he would use dramatic licence and his preaching skills to paint a vision of a New Jerusalem, with the role of the CCF in pushing the government in power to take bold action.[46] There was no point in talking about forming a government at this point, since the party was not running enough candidates in central and eastern Canada to be a viable contender.

While changing the health system was central to Hugh MacLean's personal campaign in Regina, there is little evidence that this was the most important issue in Douglas's Weyburn campaign. No doubt he was aware of the ambitious program then being put forward by the League for Social Reconstruction (LSR). Although not an official affiliate of the CCF, the LSR acted as the CCF's brain trust. Moreover, several of its members were also party activists, and a few had even become CCF candidates in the 1935 federal election.[47]

In September that year, just weeks before the election, the LSR published *Social Planning for Canada*, a comprehensive policy tome that exceeded five hundred pages. The authors, collaborating under the name the Research Committee of the LSR, included luminaries such as Frank Scott, Frank Underhill, Leonard Marsh, King Gordon, Eugene Forsey, and Graham Spry; J.S. Woodsworth contributed the preface. Despite its intimidating size, the book instantly became the go-to policy resource for serious CCF candidates. According to T.C., it was "a classic," a book he consulted for many years.[48] In the chapter on health and welfare services, eleven detailed pages critiqued what it called "private enterprise in medical practice" and included numerous recommendations on the public system that needed to replace it. From the LSR's perspective, the Great Depression had delivered the final blows to a private system that had "failed so lamentably that the State has already been forced to appropriate the public health field almost entirely and to render a great deal of service also in the field of curative medicine."[49]

The LSR argued for the need for comprehensive health insurance. Contrary to social health insurance as already implemented in a few countries in Europe, such as Germany, Britain, and Sweden, this insurance should not be limited to a sub-population of unionized male workers. The right to coverage would be based on the simple fact of citizenship rather than being a contributing member of a health plan. In contrast to existing social health insurance, which workers paid for through payroll deductions from their employers or contributions to their trade unions and similar organizations, the plan would be financed out of general taxation or a special premium tax.

For the LSR, "comprehensiveness" referred to both the population and to the services embraced in the package of coverage. *Social Planning for Canada* advocated for the inclusion of curative, diagnostic, and preventative services, including all necessary hospital, physician, nursing, and dental services, as well as laboratory services and all pharmaceuticals and surgical supplies. General practitioners would be central to the system, regulating patient access to more specialized services and prescription drugs, with doctors migrating from solo practices to group practices over time. Indeed, provincial health ministries "should explore thoroughly the possibilities of group practice and ... organize clinics, medical centres, collaboration between specialists, the pooling of equipment and other methods of group practice by doctors and dentists so far as this proves feasible and desirable."[50] The LSR was open to various remunerations systems for doctors and other health professions but pointed to the capitation scheme then being used in Britain's social health insurance schemes, a method of payment based on the number of patients being served in a doctor's practice. At the same time, the league was clear that it supported doctors' clinical autonomy and patients' right to choose their own doctors:[51] this is the policy detail upon which Douglas and MacLean relied in the 1935 federal election.

Unlike the 1934 election campaign, during which Douglas had been eager to discuss the details of CCF policy, this time around he kept things simple. He proclaimed that health care "should be made at least as freely available as are educational services today," almost a direct quotation from the Regina Manifesto of 1933.[52] The only additional detail he offered was to repeat from the federal CCF campaign platform that health should be part of a comprehensive national system of social security.[53] Earlier in 1935, a CCF MP from Alberta named Henry Spencer had made a motion in Parliament for a national health policy in which the federal government would work with the provinces in establishing state medicine. His arguments were supported in a CCF pamphlet entitled *Canada through C.C.F. Glasses* disseminated the year before.[54] From time to time, T.C. raised the issue of socialized medicine, especially when he shared campaign events with MacLean.[55] However, health policy was secondary to the main economic issues of the day and did not figure prominently in Douglas's campaign.

On 25 September, at a debate with his chief rival, the Liberal incumbent E.J. Young, in front of 5,000 people at the Weyburn rink, Douglas opened with a plea aimed at supporters of both the CCF and Social

Credit (the new party of protest that had just been elected in Alberta), saying that the main priority of the federal government should be to put purchasing power in the hands of the people: "Right here in Weyburn constituency, the purchasing power of the people is so low that people are, in some instances, forced to wear gunny sacks for clothing and go about in worn out shoes." He point out that, in Sweden, the central bank provided social allowances, and he purposely used the Social Credit term "national dividend" in his argument. Then he took a page out of the Roosevelt New Deal and advocated for a program of public works to put people back to work and for support for farmers in the form of raising farm prices. He then urged the introduction of public pensions at age sixty and of a national health plan. Ending his speech on a humorous note, he referred to Young's political philosophy as the "survival of the slickest," sparking an explosion of laughter.[56]

A poor and humourless speaker in comparison, Young began by arguing that the country would be bankrupted by the cost of the CCF platform. When he referred to a CCF pamphlet and its proposed national planning commission that would, in Young's words, "tell the famers what to do on their own farms," Douglas pounced. Knowing that Young's campaign manager, a local high school principal, had actually stolen the pamphlet from the print shop, he told the crowd that "any man who would stoop to such methods is unfit to be a teacher of the youth of this country! And any man who would make use of stolen property on a political platform is unfit to represent the people of this constituency in Parliament!"[57] The statement enraged Young's campaign manager, who rushed the stage, intending to punch Douglas, only to be stopped by some CCF supporters who swarmed to protect their candidate. For the pugilist preacher, it was a "great wind-up" to the debate.[58]

**Election Victory and Controversy**

Although unable to organize much beyond western Canada, the CCF nonetheless hoped it could have a sizeable caucus from this region and perhaps even displace the Conservatives as the official opposition to the Liberals. However, on 22 August 1935, a political earthquake shook the CCF when Social Credit, a rival western protest party, swept to victory in Alberta. Led by fundamentalist preacher William "Bible Bill" Aberhart, Social Credit won a stunning fifty-six out of sixty-three seats. The two establishment parties combined managed to eke out a paltry seven seats. The results were even worse for the CCF, which had not run as a separate party, as the Farmer-Labor Group in Saskatchewan had done the year before. Instead, it lost out completely through its affiliation with the discredited United Farmers of Alberta and the unpopular Alberta branch of the Canadian Labour Party.[59]

This Social Credit victory led to the fielding of federal candidates by the new Social Credit Party of Canada.[60] Like the provincial movement in Alberta that spawned it, the Socreds combined conservative Christian social values with the social credit monetary theory and policy of Major C.H. Douglas (no relation to T.C.'s family), a British engineer. Aberhart was a convert to Major Douglas's social credit doctrine of ending the Great Depression by increasing purchasing power through issuing credit directly to the public, an idea that had also appealed to many within the CCF, including T.C., well before the advent of Canada's social credit movement.[61] He knew that many cash-strapped farmers within his constituency were also attracted to the notion of social credit. Much larger than the provincial constituency, his federal constituency included more farmers than townspeople, the former being the base of support for the idea of social credit, which reached into Saskatchewan through a new national party.

Until Aberhart's victory, T.C. thought he would automatically reap all the votes of those discontented with both the Liberals and Conservatives, and that this might be just enough to get him elected. As the election the year before had taught him, active CCF partisans were a minority, so he needed to reach beyond them to voters with limited or no party affiliations. In the 1934 election, those same voters had gone back to what they knew – the provincial Liberals – and at least some of them would likely migrate to the federal Liberals. And now these voters were being attracted to a brand-new party of protest whose messages overlapped to some extent with those of the CCF. Moreover, with Aberhart's landslide victory in Alberta, Social Credit (unlike the CCF) had demonstrated that it could win an election.[62]

When T.C. became aware that the Liberals were trying to find a dummy candidate who, in return for sizeable sum of money, would run under the Social Credit banner to bleed votes away from the CCF, he made his move. His campaign team put together twenty or thirty Douglas supporters, who then held their own "Social Credit" convention, which then announced that, since they had no candidate of their own, they would endorse Douglas. His team also got Aberhart to denounce the Liberal-sponsored "Social Credit" candidate, leaving Douglas as the sole candidate to be endorsed by the Social Credit Party of Canada's organizer in Saskatchewan.

In return for this endorsement, T.C. pledged in writing that he would "initiate and support legislation in the House of Commons which would make possible the Social Credit system being operated in any province caring to do so."[63] Although Douglas argued that being endorsed by Social Credit was different than accepting a Social Credit nomination, Liberal newspapers such as the *Regina Leader-Post* and the *Saskatoon Star-Phoenix* portrayed Douglas as being nominated by both parties.[64] Worse still, his CCF colleague George Williams took great offence at Douglas's actions and called for an immediate review by the CCF executive. When they met, after a withering cross-examination of Douglas by Williams, the majority urged the repudiation of T.C.'s candidature. Coldwell, however, threatened to resign if the executive pulled Douglas's nomination. Williams decided to put the matter on ice until after the election.[65]

Under fire in the press just days before the election, T.C. responded vehemently to what he viewed as the Liberal influence exerted through what was known as the Sifton press – the main city newspapers in Regina (*Leader-Post*), Saskatoon (*Star Phoenix*), and Winnipeg (*Free Press*), all owned by the family of Sir Clifford Sifton.[66] The Sifton press, Douglas charged, was misleading "the people into believing that" he was "a joint candidate," when he was in fact only a CCF candidate who had received another party's endorsement. While he admitted that his constituency association had, on 25 September, passed a resolution stating that he would support legislation in Parliament that would allow "the social credit system being tried in any province caring to adopt it," he argued that this did not mean he had adopted Social Credit's entire platform, although that distinction was far from obvious.[67] Yet, he was not the only CCF candidate to make such a promise: six others in Saskatchewan had also "pledged themselves to support social credit legislation if elected."[68]

In the end, the benefits of locking up the Social Credit vote far outweighed the controversy it had triggered. The election results on 14 October 1935 gave Douglas his first political victory. Considered the biggest upset across Saskatchewan constituencies, his triumph was headlined in the *Regina Leader-Post*.[69] And to T.C.'s great delight, Coldwell won the Rosetown-Biggar seat.[70] Significantly, "these two constituencies polled the lowest Social Credit tallies of all constituencies" in the province. Coldwell himself had turned down the Social Credit nomination, but potential Socred supporters "gravitated to the CCF" after the Socred's chief organizer in that riding resigned, accusing his own organization of being nothing more "than a bogus front devised by the Liberals and Conservatives for the purpose of splitting the 'progressive' vote." And there was little to distinguish Coldwell from Aberhart, when the former "lashed out at the 'Fifty Big Shots'" who controlled Canada's financial system as being the major cause of the Great Depression.[71]

Despite their personal victories, T.C. and Coldwell were disappointed with their party's overall performance. They were the only two CCF candidates elected in the province, with only five more – three in British Columbia and two in Manitoba – elected elsewhere. In contrast, Social Credit was able to elect seventeen MPs, two of them in Saskatchewan and the rest in Alberta. From the CCF's perspective, there was better news in the fact that it had obtained 8.8 per cent of the popular vote compared to Social Credit's 4.1 per cent.[72] Clearly, the fight was on between the two new protest parties of the West. The results confirmed Douglas's intuition that he needed to secure a considerable part of the vote that would otherwise have gone to Social Credit. He had won 44 per cent of the vote, beating Young by only some three hundred votes, an amount that would easily have been exceeded by any official Social Credit candidate endorsed by William Aberhart.[73]

Regardless of its success, his strategic arrangement with Social Credit continued to upset his party's political purists as well as Social Credit party members who felt that Douglas should have taken his seat in Parliament as part of the Social Credit caucus.[74] Jacob "Jake" Benson, the defeated CCF candidate in the Yorkton riding, had been similarly accused of running as a joint candidate. The controversy continued to bubble within the party until mid-December, when the Political Directive Board of the provincial CCF met in Regina to hear evidence from T.C. and Benson. In reviewing all the relevant correspondence, it emerged that Coldwell had encouraged both candidates to seek endorsement from Social Credit that stopped short of an alliance. The CCF executive then focused on whether Douglas's and Benson's actions crossed the line into a formal alliance with Social Credit. After an "exhaustive" discussion, the CCF executive found that both had crossed the line.[75]

The party then passed a "motion of censure on Jacob Benson and T.C. Douglas and their respective constituency committees for actions" that caused "the general public to come to the conclusion that an alliance with Social Credit Party was formed in their constituencies." The motion then referred to "the ill-advised distribution of handbills and posters during the heat of the campaign describing" them as joint CCF-Socred candidates," which "had the unfortunate effect of embarrassing ... [CCF] candidates throughout Saskatchewan." However, the executive added that its motion of censure did "not in any way cast any reflection on the personal integrity of either Mr. Jacob Benson or Mr. T.C. Douglas, who have assured the board that they owe no allegiance to, or are [not] associated with, any other political party."[76] Clearly, the party was trying to get beyond the controversy and simply hoped that such "alliances" would be avoided in the future. As for Douglas, he hoped the controversy was finally behind him and that he could finally take his seat in Parliament as a CCF member.

**Federal Member of Parliament**

T.C., Irma, and their nineteen-month-old daughter, Shirley, travelled to Winnipeg to join the Douglas family that holiday season.[77] The plan was then to take the train on to Ottawa, where Irma would help her husband settle in before she and the baby returned to Weyburn. The plan was interrupted by a shock. Shortly after New Year's, on 5 January 1936, Douglas's father died.[78] He was only fifty-seven years old.[79]

Reflecting on his father's death later in life, T.C. said that it was, up to that time, "probably the greatest personal loss" he had "ever sustained," and certainly more significant than any of his political disappointments and regrets.[80] The episode was made more poignant due to the fact that Tom Douglas had never recovered from the injuries he sustained in the First World War and had lived out his last years profoundly sad and largely uncommunicative.[81] At least he had the satisfaction of seeing his son elected to Parliament, which gave the aging Scottish Labourite one last opportunity to give his son some laconic advice, in words that Douglas remembered decades later: "Now remember, laddie, the working people have put a lot of trust in you, you must never let them down."[82]

Although the life of an MP today seems exciting, if not glamorous, it was less so in the 1930s. In the days before air travel, MPs, particularly from far-flung parts of the country, had to put up with days of train travel between their jobs in Ottawa and their constituencies at home. They were required to have two residences, both paid for with what were then quite modest stipends. They received $25 for each day Parliament was in session, up to a maximum of $4,000. Unlike today, the only perk they received was an unlimited rail pass. Sometimes the railway would give a free pass to the MP's immediately family as well, but not for the sleeper carriage. MPs had to pay personally for other modes of travel within their own constituencies.

For T.C., whose rural constituency was vast (roughly 4,000 square kilometres), from the American border to near the city limits of Regina, this meant three months of travel by car for political meetings in hamlets, villages, and towns, all of which he paid for out of pocket. T.C.'s salary of $4,000 exceeded his minister's salary by $1,000, but he and Irma were actually worse off because of constituency work and the need to pay for two residences. Irma never complained, even when T.C. found that he was flat broke and had to get a personal bank loan for $1,500 in 1940 just for him and his family to travel to, and live in, Ottawa that year.[83]

In the latter half of the 1930s, Ottawa was still a small, sleepy city of fewer than 100,000. While the excitement of politics and being on the national stage of Parliament greatly appealed to T.C., life would have been more difficult for Irma and Shirley in their small apartment. Work life permeated personal life, as Douglas's closest political colleagues also made up his family's social network. Of the seven MPs who made up the tiny CCF caucus when Parliament opened in 1936, T.C.'s closest friend was Coldwell, with whom he shared an office in the Centre Block and whom he sat alongside in Parliament. Douglas idealized Coldwell, seeing him as an exemplary parliamentarian and a great intellect. Irma also became very close to Coldwell, driving him on local errands and taking him out to the Gatineau Hills when he needed a break. As T.C. recounted later, he loved Coldwell like an "older brother or father."[84]

T.C.'s first impression of Parliament was one of shock. He could not believe that there seemed to be so little understanding of, much less concern about, the devastating drought and depression in the Palliser Triangle among MPs from outside the region. When Parliament opened, Mackenzie King spoke on behalf of the Liberal government for hours about the benefits of a low-tariff regime. Speaking for the Conservative opposition, Bennett's speech in reply focused on the need for higher tariffs to both protect Canadian industry and retaliate against countries such as the United States, which were imposing higher tariffs on goods. In Douglas's mind, King, Bennett, and most of the MPs in the two major parties had "no appreciation of the fact that there were a million people living in the direst poverty, unemployment, and that there were thousands of people on the farms who were slowly starving."[85]

As the two CCF MPs from Saskatchewan, Coldwell and Douglas took the few precious opportunities they had in Parliament to call for major change. They put forward motions for major public works, like those created by the Roosevelt New Deal, to "put the unemployed to work" and offer part-time jobs to farmers in areas hard hit by drought. King's finance minister, Charles Dunning, had been premier of Saskatchewan from 1922 until 1926 and was good friends with Coldwell, despite their partisan differences. Dunning treated T.C. with great kindness, even patting the young MP "on the shoulder" in the corridor. However, in the House of Commons, Dunning would look across at Coldwell and Douglas and remind them that money for such projects did not "grow on gooseberry bushes." T.C.'s rebuttal was that, while he did not "know what kind of bush money" grows on, he did know that, if Canada "went to war," the minister of finance "would find the bush."[86]

This response highlighted the other issue T.C. faced in Parliament – the growing threat of war. In his maiden speech in the House, Douglas went beyond the need to address the suffering and human upheaval of the Great Depression and called for economic sanctions against Fascist Italy for its invasion of Ethiopia the previous October.[87] At the same time that Mussolini's Italian forces were conquering Ethiopia, Adolf Hitler was sending military aid to support another fascist, General Francisco Franco, in the bloody Spanish Civil War. Although T.C. sought ways to be not far out of step with the pacifism of the CCF's federal leader, J.S. Woodworth, he personally felt that force was required to stop fascism. Moreover, disagreeing with the isolationist position taken by many other members of his party, such as Frank Scott, he became a fervent believer in the need for collective action through the League of Nations.[88]

While MP, T.C. continued to serve as vice-chair of the Canadian League Against War and Fascism, despite Woodsworth's and Coldwell's ongoing concern about communist influence in that organization.[89] Whatever his differences with communists in the league, Douglas nonetheless concluded that they were his allies in the fight against fascism.[90] T.C. remained vice-chair even after the Molotov-Ribbentrop non-aggression pact between Nazi Germany and the Soviet Union in August 1939, but he split with the communists in the league when he publicly decried the Soviet invasion of Finland in November of that year.[91]

**The Winds of War**

T.C. had a first-hand opportunity to see the situation in Europe when he was selected by his party to be part of a three-person parliamentary delegation to attend the World Youth Congress in Geneva. Involving seven hundred delegates from thirty-six country, the congress, sponsored by the League of Nations, was held from the end of August until mid-September 1936.[92]

T.C. was the CCF's natural choice. Not only was he national president of the CCYM, but he was also closely connected to the local chapter of the Canadian Youth Congress and had been a keynote speaker at its Toronto gathering in 1934.[93] Douglas was joined by two other young MPs selected by their respective parties, Denton Massey from the Conservatives and Paul Martin Sr. from the Liberals.[94] Coming from the governing party, Martin was appointed head of the delegation. The three were expected to chaperone thirty-five delegates from Canada who were members of various youth organizations, some of whom were aligned with the Communist Party.[95] The three MPs got along well, and both Martin and Massey were impressed with Douglas, even if the two central Canadians had some difficulty understanding his evangelizing brand of prairie socialism.[96]

At the time, the World Youth Congress and its country chapters were perceived by critics as a Popular Front organization ultimately controlled by the Communist Party in the USSR. And, in fact, two Canadian Youth Congress delegates were associated with the Communist Party of Canada. However, the World Youth Congress movement was more than a Popular Front organization dominated by Moscow, and the delegates in Geneva faithfully reflected the common anti-fascist and pro-peace agenda shared at the time among liberal internationalists such as Martin and Massey, democratic socialists such as Douglas, and young communists.[97] In his memoirs, Martin admitted having some concerns about this communist influence in the Canadian delegation, but he felt that the outcome of the conference was well worth the price.[98]

The trip would have a profound impact on T.C.'s perspective on developments in Europe, in particular his realization that, irrespective of how much he desired peace, a world war was fast becoming inevitable.[99] Douglas took advantage of the World Youth Congress to spend a further three months in Europe, travelling to numerous countries. Prime Minister King arranged for Douglas, Martin, and Massey to join a separate Canadian delegation at the League of Nations, where he saw Anthony Eden, the head of the league's British delegation. Sympathetic to the Republican cause, Douglas went to Spain, where he met with socialists, communists, and liberals supporting the Republic in the war against Franco's Nationalists.[100] In Paris, he met with France's socialist prime minister Léon Blum; in London, he met with a few Labour Party leaders: in both cases, he was appalled at the lack of official support for the Spanish Republic expressed by these fellow socialists.[101]

T.C.'s first port of call after leaving Geneva had been Germany. He went to Nuremberg, where he witnessed a major Nazi rally, with German bombers flying over tanks and goose-stepping troops, and with Hitler at the podium speaking and giving the Nazi salute.[102] Douglas had letters of introduction to some Baptist ministers but found that these individuals, along with Jews and other members of religious minorities, had been arrested. When he returned to Canada in late October, he gave a series of lectures on what he had witnessed in Germany and the rest of Europe.[103] Many of these talks were given in Saskatchewan, where he was threatened by some recent German immigrants belonging to the pro-Nazi Deutscher Bund Canada.[104]

One of the longer-term consequences of the trip was the bond that formed between T.C. and Paul Martin Sr. Both saw the Nazi state as a major global threat, and, despite disagreeing about the Spanish Civil War (Martin backed the pro-Catholic Franco forces), they nonetheless became friends, in that limited way that marks most relationships that cross partisan lines.[105] As will be seen later, their relationship between 1946 and 1957, when Martin was the minister of national health and welfare, would benefit both men and their social policy ambitions.

In the period immediately preceding the outbreak of the Second World War, Douglas had to walk a difficult tightrope between his party's official position on the prospects of war and his personal view that war was both inevitable and necessary. On this question, the CCF was deeply split into three identifiable factions.[106] The pacifists, such as J.S. Woodsworth, were, as Douglas put it, "opposed to war in any shape or form."[107] The isolationists believed that Canada need not, and should not, involve itself in European problems: they saw the war as a fight among imperial powers defending their capitalist interests. And then there were hawks, like Douglas, who believed that fascism at that point could be stopped only through war and who watched with horror as Italy invaded Ethiopia, Japan brutally occupied Manchuria in northeastern China, and Nazi Germany annexed Austria and Czechoslovakia.[108] In each of these cases, Douglas gave speeches in Parliament, calling for the King government to not allow Canadian metals and other resources to be shipped and sold to the aggressors.

Although Douglas and other like-minded MPs could never have convinced Woodsworth of the need for war, they did manage to get him to at least allow Douglas to put forward a parliamentary motion on the need for collective security through an international police force under the League of Nations.[109] Following the German invasion of Poland on 1 September 1939, and the declaration of war by Britain and France two days later, Mackenzie King announced in a nationally broadcast radio speech that he would be calling for a special session of Parliament in which he would recommend a declaration of war.[110]

In response, the CCF quickly called a national council meeting involving the caucus and all CCF provincial leaders to work out a consensus position for the special session of Parliament.[111] What emerged was a tortured compromise, the CCF agreeing with the country's re-arming and recruiting to defend its shores but not with sending troops to Europe.[112] When the extraordinary war session of Parliament opened on 7 September, M.J. Coldwell spoke on behalf of the CCF caucus.[113] As for Woodsworth, although the national leader, he had to speak for himself on his objection to Canada's declaration of war.[114] "I am opposed to all war," he said, first because he was a socialist who believed that war is the inevitable outcome of capitalism, and second because he was a Christian, and war "is against my ideals."[115]

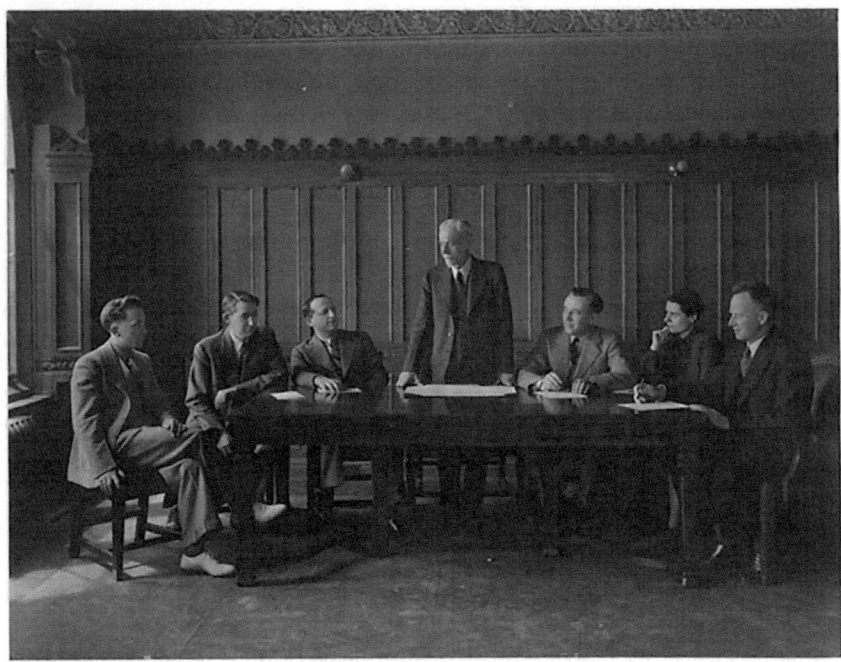

CCF parliamentary caucus meeting in June 1938 led by J.S. Woodsworth (standing in middle), with M.J. Coldwell sitting to his right and a snappily dressed T.C. at far left with white shoes (LAC, Yousef Karsh, e010751833)

Despite disagreeing with this position, Douglas greatly admired Woodsworth's courage in the face of a handful of Conservative MPs shouting "shame." Although few knew at the time, Woodsworth had recently suffered a major stroke that had partly paralyzed one part of his face and made him almost blind.[116] When he rose to speak, Douglas "moved down to sit beside him" in a chair normally occupied by H.H. Stevens, the renegade leader of the recently formed, and even more recently disbanded, Reconstruction Party, who had opted to rejoin the Conservative caucus. Douglas described the profound impression Woodsworth made on him that day, perhaps sensing that there would come a time when he too would stand against the majority before both Parliament and the country. Because of Woodsworth's stroke-impaired vision, "his wife had written out his notes with a crayon in great big letters, an inch or two inches high" and "he had several sheets of these notes, each with just a few words to remind him of what he was going to say." T.C. "passed these notes up to him one by one" so that Woodsworth could make "his great declaration of faith" that war under any circumstances was wrong.[117] Coldwell then stood up to present the compromise position hammered out by the CCF's national council.

Outside of Parliament, T.C. was increasingly perceived as pro-war. When accused by Saskatchewan CCF pacifist Carlyle King of being "practically an imperialist,"[118] Douglas felt compelled to explain his reasoning to the party faithful:

> There is a distinction in Jesus' teachings between individual ethics: turning one's cheek, giving one's coat, going the extra mile – and social ethics ... When someone attacks a small child whom I have pledged to defend with my life, then the lion becomes me best. I can give my coat, but I have no power to give away an old man's coat at the command of a well-clad bully. I can give up some of my rights, but when a group of lawless men endeavour to destroy the fabric of law and order by which alone human society is possible, then I have a responsibility to discharge.[119]

On 10 September, with Parliament's approval, Canada declared war against Germany, one week after Great Britain. So convinced was he of the justice of the war, Douglas tried to enlist with the First Battalion of the South Saskatchewan Regiment. A thirty-five-year-old suffering from chronic osteomyelitis, Douglas was rejected in favour of younger, healthier men. However, he was able to join the training group (Second Battalion) for the South Saskatchewan Regiment, first as a corporal and then (after officer training) as a lieutenant, eventually reaching the rank of captain. He took time from his duties as an MP to be a training officer at a winter training camp in Weyburn. Although he volunteered to be an officer accompanying the Winnipeg Grenadiers to Hong Kong, he was held back after the Winnipeg miliary doctor turned him down because of his bad leg.[120]

The men he would have joined were being sent to defend Hong Kong, and many of them died, either in 1941, when the city was seized by Japan, or later as a result of the appalling conditions of Japanese captivity. In Parliament, Douglas's criticism of the King government's decision to send young men with almost no training or adequate equipment was, thus, personal. He described putting these men up "against seasoned, trained Japanese troops" as "just a little short of murder."[121] When his comments were condemned as aiding and abetting the enemy, Douglas deftly responded that if there was "inefficiency and incompetence at Hong Kong," there seemed "little point in keeping it from the Japanese" as they already "know all about it."[122]

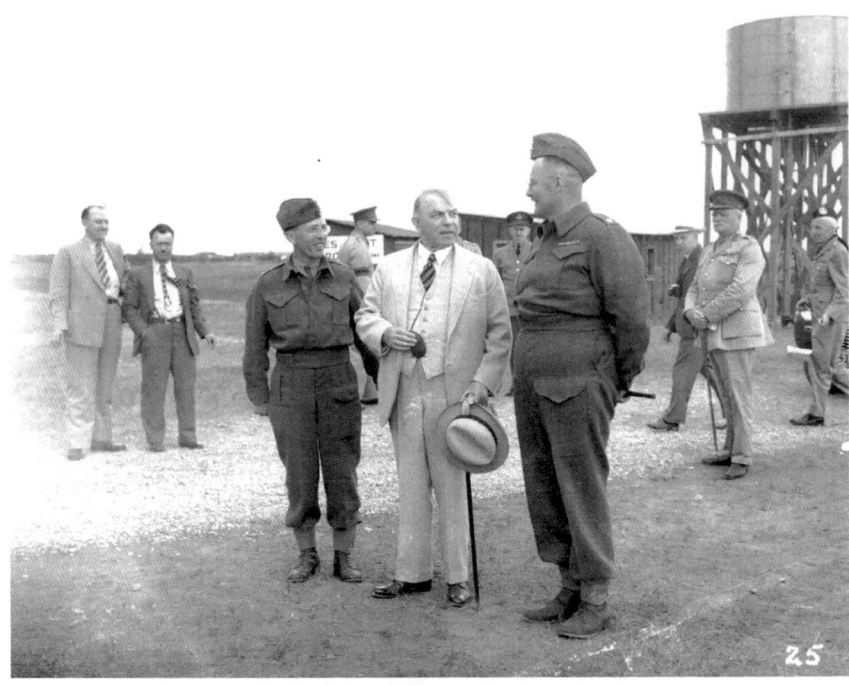

Lieutenant T.C. Douglas (South Saskatchewan Regiment), MP, with Prime Minister Mackenzie King on 5 July 1943. Walter Tucker, Liberal MP and, from 1946 to 1953, leader of the Liberal Party in Saskatchewan, is on the right (SPL B-2973)

## Cradle-to-Grave Welfare State: The Beveridge, Marsh, and Heagerty Reports

By 1942, with the Soviet Union and the United States both in the war against the Axis powers, the tide was finally beginning to turn in the Allies' favour. By the end of that year, the landmark Beveridge Report had been released in the United Kingdom, sparking discussion about the role of the state in providing social and economic security in a post-war world. Similar activity in Ottawa would soon become the subject of parliamentary committees, which received the rapt attention of Douglas and his CCF colleagues. Mackenzie King encouraged this work, in part because he saw political advantage in taking the initiative. Witnessing how government expenditures during the war created full employment, Canadians were changing their views on what governments could do in the future to avoid a catastrophe like the Great Depression. The CCF was gaining electoral ground because it was the one party speaking to this desire for a reconstructed welfare state, and King wanted to convince Canadians that his party and government was just as capable of delivering reform, but without what he saw as the dangerous socialist claptrap of the CCF.

When the subject of the Beveridge Report came up in King's cabinet in January 1943, the prime minister said that the proposed work of Leonard Marsh on social security and the Advisory Committee on Health Insurance's work, led by J.J. Heagerty, would be presented to Parliament in March 1943.[123] A former member of the League for Social Reconstruction (he had been its president from 1937 to 1939) and one of the authors of the league's 1935 policy opus *Social Planning for Canada*, Marsh had also been Beveridge's student at the London School of Economics.[124]

Douglas was captivate with Heagerty's work on health insurance, which had been central to the advisory committee's voluminous report.[125] A federal public servant, Heagerty was the director of public health in the Department of Pensions and National Health.[126] Douglas was so impressed with Heagerty's report that, when he was about to leave Ottawa to take up his role in provincial politics in 1944, he asked for Heagerty's advice on which international experts he might tap to help him implement health insurance and a new health system in Saskatchewan.[127]

Heagerty's report recommended that the federal government provide the provinces with conditional transfers equal in value to up to 60 per cent of the estimated costs of comprehensive health insurance. The items to be covered included hospital, medical, nursing, dental, pharmaceutical, and diagnostic services.[128] Unlike the Marsh Report, which recommended that the federal government rather than the provinces be responsible for the administration and financing of health insurance as part of a larger social security program made possible through a constitutional amendment, Heagerty preferred a provincially administered program that would not require any constitutional amendment, a formulation that Douglas much preferred.[129]

While the Marsh and Heagerty reports were being digested by the King government, which had established a cabinet committee on reconstruction, Sir William Beveridge paid a visit to Ottawa. After he arrived in the last week of May 1943, he gave a radio address that not only summarized his report but argued that winning the war was not enough for the Allies: it was the duty of all governments, including the government of Canada, to make plans for peace that included the establishment of a welfare state.[130] Beveridge then spoke to a House of Commons and Senate joint committee on his report and post-war planning.[131] He put his remarks in the context of the Marsh and Heagerty Reports. When asked by the press whether he had read the Marsh Report (no one asked if he had read the much longer Heagerty report), Beveridge stated that he had read it and could hardly believe that such "a remarkable document" could have been produced so quickly after his own report was tabled.[132] After the session, Beveridge made sure to have a private meeting with Marsh.[133] Then he was off to Montreal to receive an honorary doctorate from McGill and speak to the Canadian Club, and to Quebec City, where he met with Liberal premier Joseph-Adélard Godbout and his cabinet.[134]

The trip to Canada was a small detour from Beveridge's two-month tour in the United States sponsored by the Rockefeller Foundation so that he could discuss his report and the concept of a welfare state providing security for an individual from the cradle to the grave and thereby help support the extension of social security in that country. Beveridge's first stop after his few days in Canada was New York City, where he and Mackenzie King received honorary doctorates from Columbia University. After the ceremony, Beveridge and King had dinner with the president of Columbia University.[135] Beveridge's trip to Canada and the time he spent with the prime minister in New York no doubt reinforced the Canadian government in its view that it was on the right track. However, unlike Britain's unitary state, the structure of Canada's federation required Ottawa to work closely with provincial governments of varying ideological stripes, including those who saw the Liberals as their chief rivals, to construct a welfare state. In this context, T.C. was well on his way to changing the political landscape in Canada, not from his position as an MP in Ottawa, but from his position as premier of the first so-called socialist government in North America.

**CCF Leader in Saskatchewan**

Ever since George Williams took over the presidency of the Saskatchewan CCF from M.J. Coldwell at the end of 1935, tensions had been growing between the national CCF and its provincial section. When Coldwell became the de facto national leader after Woodsworth's illness forced him to step back, he felt the time had come to replace Williams with someone who would work more effectively with the federal party.

Other disaffected party members also began to turn on Williams, including Carlyle King, who had run against his leadership at the 1940 provincial convention. Although King failed, it was becoming evident that Williams was losing the confidence of many in the party. In 1940, Coldwell wrote, "I am sorry to say I have no confidence in George. His actions over the past six months have disgusted me completely. With another leader we could carry the province next time."[136] The person he wanted as that leader was T.C. Douglas.

When Williams, who had enlisted almost immediately after the declaration of war, was stationed in Europe, the time seemed ripe for the change. Although a federal MP, Douglas had successfully challenged Williams for the presidency of the provincial party in July 1941. Clarence Fines, a Regina alderman and Douglas supporter, was elected vice-president. However, holding the office of president did not automatically make Douglas the provincial party leader. That position still belonged to Williams until he finally relinquished it in 1942. Even then, Douglas had to run against John Brockelbank, one of Williams's most stalwart partisans, in an election for provincial leader that year.[137]

Douglas won by a sizeable majority, partly in recognition of the work both he and Fines had done in rejuvenating the provincial party even while a federal MP. Dividing his time between Ottawa and Saskatchewan, Douglas then spent the next three years coordinating his team on the ground, which was headed by Fines. The first task was to increase party membership, which had dropped during Williams's tenure. By April 1944, Douglas and his team had increased provincial party membership to 26,000 from the 5,000 members it had when Williams was in charge in 1941.[138]

The second job was to work up a policy program that would not only be attractive to voters but would be substantive enough to demonstrate the CCF's readiness to become the government in Saskatchewan. By establishing subcommittees that focused for many months on six defined policy subjects – education, social services, housing, natural resources, agriculture, and health – the provincial CCF was able to develop a very detailed program. The subcommittees reported to two main committees, on planning and budgeting. Douglas headed up the Planning Committee, and Fines led the Budgeting Committee. Individuals on both committees would become the key members of Douglas's first cabinet. This structure produced a real shadow cabinet, one that would be ready to govern after the 1944 election.[139]

Early in 1943, Douglas used the health proposals that were being worked through by the health subcommittee in a provincial radio address:

> We believe that by extending our present socialized health services ... to cover more and more kinds of illness, we can ultimately give our people a completely socialized system of health services. This would have to be done in a series of stages. The first might be to make the hospitals available to all who require hospitalization. The second might be to set up cancer clinics and gradually to extend them to cover other ailments and diseases. Other stages will include the steps by which the doctors, dentists

and nurses, through some form of health insurance, would make their services available ... irrespective of ... individual ability to pay ... When we [consider] that a properly planned health system would place the emphasis on preventive medicine rather than curative medicine, we can see why the cost should be less than what we are now paying.[140]

Built on the work of numerous party committees, the CCF's electoral platform "Humanity First" was published in late 1943 as a twenty-page booklet. Roughly a page and a half, under the heading "Health for All," was devoted to what was called "socialized health services." The CCF proposed "to set up a complete system of socialized health services with special emphasis on preventive medicine, so that everybody in the province" would "receive adequate medical, surgical, dental, nursing, and hospital care without charge." The booklet commended the planning work already done by the province's State Hospital and Medical League (SHML) but would not commit itself to some of the details of the SHML's proposed plan, including putting physicians on salary. Although creating "a complete network of health services covering all parts of the province" would take "considerable time," the CCF promised to begin right after it was elected to "provide minimum services at once, perhaps by means of travelling health clinics." However, beyond promising more educational opportunities for new doctors, nurses, and dentists, and pledging that it would hire its health managers and advisors based on ability and competence (a direct swing at the partisan appointment system that underpinned the provincial Liberal machine), the booklet left unanswered the question of what exactly would be done if the CCF were elected.[141]

CCF canvassers were provided with pocket-sized cards that summarized their platform, which they could refer to when knocking on doors. This simplified version of the commitment on health simply said that a CCF government would provide nine things, including, as number four, "medical, dental and hospital services irrespective of the ability of the individual to pay." Some voters took this to mean the immediate implementation of comprehensive universal health coverage, even though Douglas repeatedly explained in his speeches that public coverage would be extended in stages. The platform did not provide details on financing and avoided the issue of how doctors would be paid. As will be seen, these ambiguities, especially on the question of physician payment, would later cause problems with some of the CCF's left-wing supporters.[142]

The Liberals too had a health plank for the election. Just before the final session of the legislature ahead of the election, the government had put forward a health insurance bill that simply said that the province was prepared to enact a program when the federal government

Federal Member of Parliament, 1935–1944   83

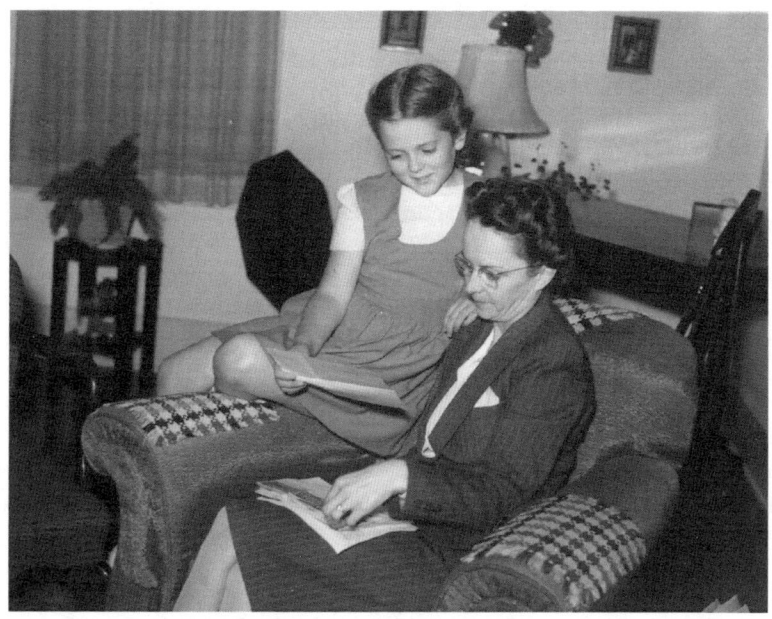

Shirley and Irma Douglas at home in Weyburn, 1944 (PAS R-B2908(2))

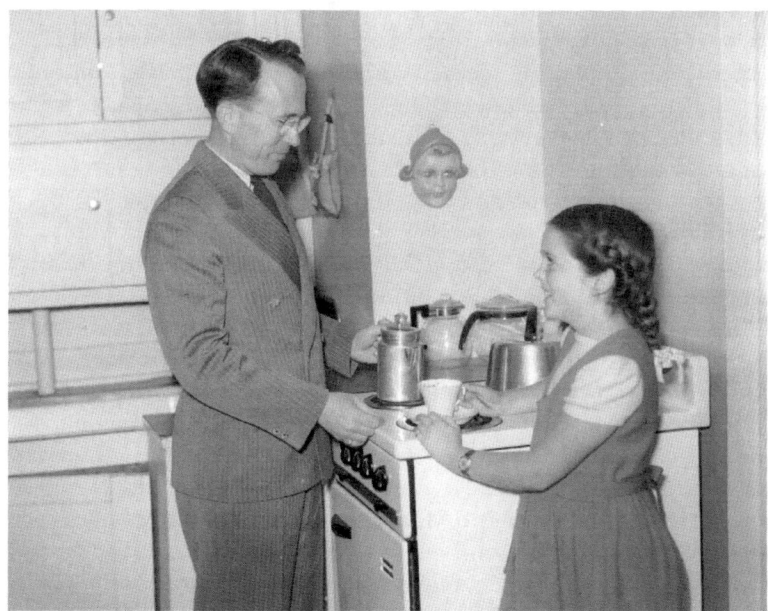

T.C. and daughter Shirley at the family home, 1944 (PAS R-B2908(3))

negotiated a federal-provincial deal to cost share such a plan. This federal program was, of course, based on the Heagerty proposal, which had already been much discussed in Parliament. The Heagerty Report and the possibility of it becoming national policy allowed Jimmy Gardiner's Liberal successor, Premier William J. Patterson, to say that, when Ottawa was ready, the province could bring in a complete package of coverage "including medical, surgical, obstetrical, dental, pharmaceutical, hospital and nursing benefits" for all Saskatchewan residents.[143]

Although the CCF questioned the sincerity of this bill, given its lack of detail – and the government's unwillingness to make any move without Ottawa taking the first step – the CCF members of the legislature voted in its favour. To distinguish the bill from the proposals of his party, Douglas emphasized the fact that his government would "commence at once to move in the direction of socialized health services with a view to making them available to all citizens irrespective of their ability to pay." He also was more specific than the campaign literature in outlining that this would "necessitate a series of stages beginning with assistance to the municipalities in financing municipal doctors and municipal hospitals, making municipal doctor service available to the two-thirds of our rural areas which are still without it. Health clinics will also be set up as a beginning in the C.C.F. program."[144]

On 15 June 1944, election day in Saskatchewan, Douglas was confident of victory. A Gallup poll had predicted a CCF victory, even though the *Regina Leader-Post*, a long-time supporter of the provincial Liberals, had predicted a Liberal win based on another, suspiciously unidentified, poll.[145] In the event, the scale of the CCF's victory was a surprise to all. Douglas was at his Weyburn CCF office listening to the radio when it was announced that all but five seats had gone to the CCF. The CCF won 53 per cent of the popular vote, compared to the Liberals' 35 per cent and the Progressive Conservatives' 11 per cent. Douglas easily won his seat in Weyburn, and the Liberal Party leader and premier, William Patterson, came within a hair of being defeated in his riding by CCF candidate Gladys Strum.[146] According to long-time CCF activist and candidate Clarence Fines, the Saskatchewan public was so desirous of change that the CCF could have won a bare majority even without Douglas, but "the enthusiasm generated by his leadership" ensured the landslide.[147]

The Saskatchewan election results sent shock waves through the country. Under Douglas, the avowedly socialist CCF had won its first victory, creating the impression that the CCF was on the cusp of gaining power in other provinces and even threatening Mackenzie King's Liberal hegemony in Ottawa. Douglas's victory appeared to signal a left turn in the country, causing a surge in support for the CCF nationally and provincially.[148]

# 4 Sigerist, Sheps, and Socialism

*The C.C.F. is determined to make a demonstration of what a socialist government can do for the people. They find that the health field is best suited because the people are aware of the problem and ready for a plan.*
　　　　　　　　　　　　　　Henry E. Sigerist, diary entry, 8 September 1944[1]

*It is most pleasant to deal with this government. They are simple and honest people, idealists with a realistic approach. Everything is very informal and that makes it so pleasant.*
　　　　　　　　　　　　　　Henry E. Sigerist, diary entry, 13 September 1944[2]

It was a far from forgone conclusion that health reform would become the CCF government's most important policy in its first term of office (1944–8) in Saskatchewan. In fact, based on the campaign literature and especially the CCF program released before the election, health seemed secondary to some other programs and policies. Unlike education, for example, which had been worked up by the CCF into a full-fledged program of larger school units to improve and extend primary and secondary education in the province, CCF strategists had given health far less policy attention in the year leading up to the election.[3]

Nevertheless, the rhetoric of the CCF electoral platform, promising to "immediately begin" to establish "a complete program of socialized health services," created high expectations for the fledgling government.[4] While the CCF tried to set some limits by admitting that the setting up of "a complete network of health services covering all parts of the province" would "undoubtedly take considerable time," CCF activists and voters expected the government to deliver, even if "the details of such a system" would, as stated in the campaign literature, "have to be worked on in consultation with, and upon the advice of, specialists in public health administration."[5]

Given his promises during the election campaign, T.C. felt that his government had to have an implementable health program within the shortest time possible and that he, relative to any other elected member of the party, was in the best position to coordinate and push it forward in the initial stages. He drew on what he saw as the emergence of a trend, as nascent as it was, towards universal health coverage in a few countries led by social democratic administrations, such as the Labour government in New Zealand and the Labour contingent in the wartime coalition in the United Kingdom.[6] Despite some positive signs, nothing tangible had yet been achieved in the United States or in Canada, and Douglas was excited about the possibility of Saskatchewan becoming a pilot project for North America.[7]

As premier and minister of health, T.C. could force health reform to the very top of his government's agenda. However, he would be unable to keep it there for long without soon suffering significant dissension within cabinet, his sizeable backbench, and the party grassroots. After fifteen years of depression and war, government attention and spending was needed in numerous other areas, including education, economic development, local government reform, agricultural safety nets, transportation infrastructure, and social welfare. These needs were subsumed under cabinet portfolios led by ministers equally committed to making real change. T.C. had to convince them to accept the urgency and strategic importance of health reform when so many other matters were crying out for attention as well.

Part of T.C.'s argument was that health care should be available to all as a basic human right, simply by virtue of citizenship or, in the case of Saskatchewan, of residency. This idea fit well into the CCF government's rights-based agenda, including labour rights and individual freedoms. The introduction of the Trade Union Act (1944), which extended the right of collective bargaining to civil servants for the first time in Canada, was one of the first major legislative steps of the Douglas government.[8] This was followed three years later by the protection of individual freedoms through the country's first Bill of Rights, put into law one year before the United Nations General Assembly adopted the Universal Declaration of Human Rights.[9]

**Picking a Cabinet**

The first and most important decision in the running of any government in a Westminster parliamentary system is the selection of a cabinet. To have any hope of translating his party's ambitious objectives and the sentiments of his supporters into effective programs with

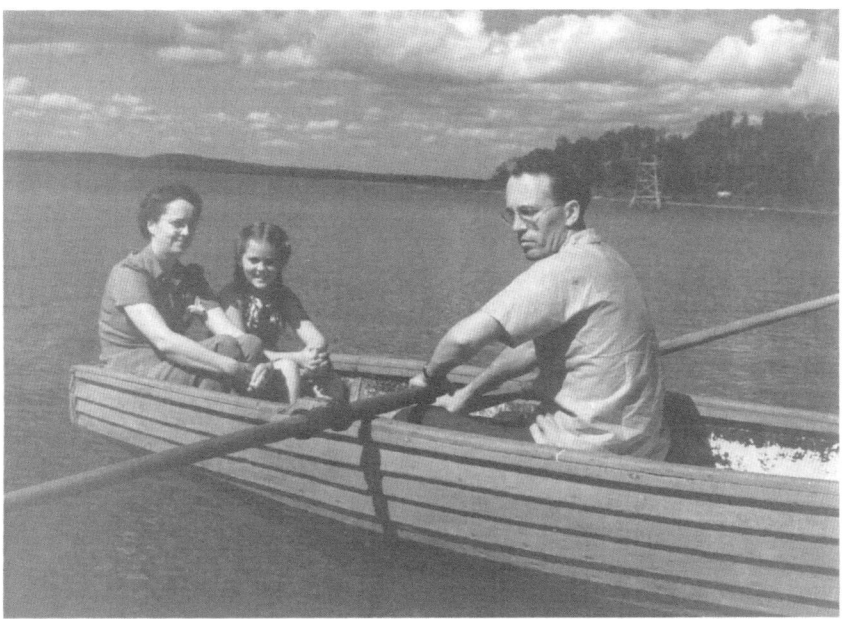

The Douglas family at Carlyle Lake, 1944 (PAS R-B2907)

accompanying legislation, organization, and personnel, T.C. needed ministers who were not only effective at directing their respective departments but able to work together to make the best decisions possible for the government. Due to the government's extremely limited fiscal resources, these collective decisions involved difficult and delicate trade-offs, and could be heartbreaking for individual ministers committed to major changes in their area of responsibility.

During the four weeks when the Liberals were moving out of office, Douglas took the time he needed, including a couple of days at the family cottage at Carlyle Lake, to select from among the forty-seven elected CCF members the individuals who would have the right to make decisions at the cabinet table. As part of assessing existing knowledge and potential leadership skills, he had already seen how some had performed in terms of their respective contributions to the CCF's comprehensive electoral platform.[10]

Clarence Fines, the president of the provincial CCF, organized the work on the platform and masterminded the preparations for the election. It was only natural that T.C. relied heavily on his advice for the selection of members for the first cabinet.[11] Fines had amply demonstrated his great abilities as a fiscal manager, fundraiser, and organizational manager since the CCF's inception. From Douglas's perspective, Fines was the perfect choice as the government's chief operating officer. T.C. wanted to focus on setting his government's broad direction while being its principal cheerleader inside and outside the province. To accomplish this, he needed Fines, an individual who paid close attention to details, to manage the day-to-day operations of the government, both as the provincial treasurer and de facto deputy premier.[12]

There were other obvious choices, including Woodrow Lloyd as education minister. Although only thirty-one years old, Lloyd had already accumulated fifteen years of teaching experience. He had led the policy proposal on educational reform, including a bold proposal for larger school units, the goal of which was to deliver a consistently higher standard of primary and secondary education in the province through better-educated and -paid teachers. Another clear choice was Attorney General John Corman, the only lawyer in the CCF caucus, who had a habit of quipping at the end of his regular radio broadcasts, "You are born into the old parties. You have to think your way into the CCF. Good night."[13] Douglas respected Corman's ability to read the public mood and would use him as a barometer on the popularity of his government.[14] Joe Phelps, a farmer, was Douglas's pick for minister of natural resources, as he had been one of the most effective MLAs in the CCF opposition since 1938. Phelps championed direct government ownership, including some questionable small manufacturing enterprises that fared poorly and would cause the government some embarrassment in its first term of office.[15]

The other cabinet choices were less obvious and more difficult, as they involved factors beyond existing knowledge and potential leadership skills. One of these factors involved healing a long-standing rift within the Saskatchewan CCF that dated back to the conflict between M.J. Coldwell and George Williams following the Saskatchewan election of 1934. Putting aside his own past grievances with and concerns about his former rival, T.C. calculated that if he put Williams in cabinet, he could bury the persistent factionalism that had inflicted so much damage within the CCF. Douglas visited Williams at home and asked him to choose his own cabinet post. Also eager to end the feud, Williams requested agriculture, to which Douglas immediately agreed. The meeting was, according to Williams's biographer, "a significant first step in the reconciliation of the two men."[16] To further mend the rift, Douglas followed up with John Brockelbank, appointing him minister of municipal affairs, a key portfolio in an agrarian province given the sheer

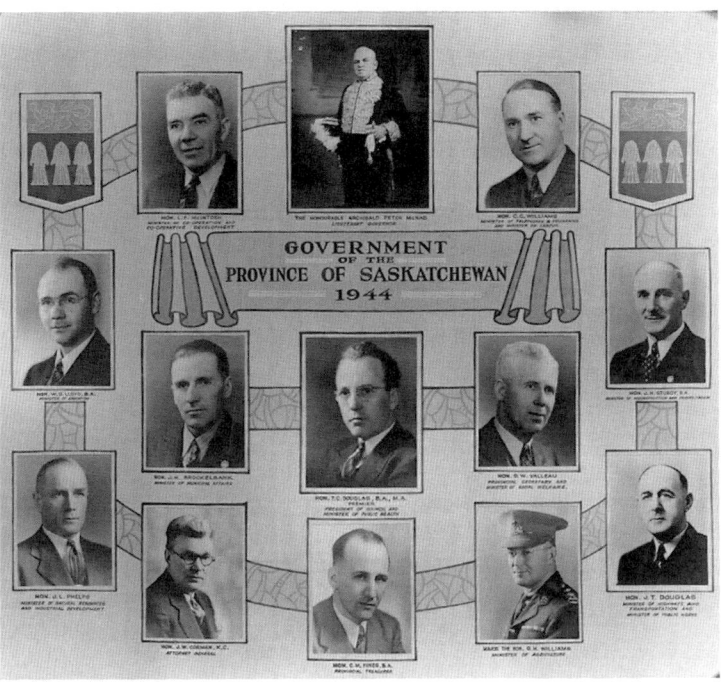

The Douglas cabinet of 1944 (PAS S-B1203)

number and (at that time) political clout of local governments. (Several provincial CCF caucus members, including Fines, had entered politics through local governments and continued to be linked to municipal politicians and issues.) Brockelbank had been one of George Williams's main supporters in the past, and Douglas felt he had to include him in the cabinet no matter how much the anti-Williams faction hated the idea.

T.C. also had to address the question of ensuring adequate geographical and religious representation in cabinet. Given the CCF's very limited appeal to Roman Catholics – in part due to the church's official statements against socialism – he needed a member of that faith in his cabinet to build bridges to Catholic voters.[17] On these and other issues concerning cabinet, Douglas sought the advice of CCF party officials and representatives.

In considering issues of representation, though, there was one area that was either ignored or actively dismissed: T.C. appointed no women to cabinet, despite the election of Beatrice Trew, a long-time

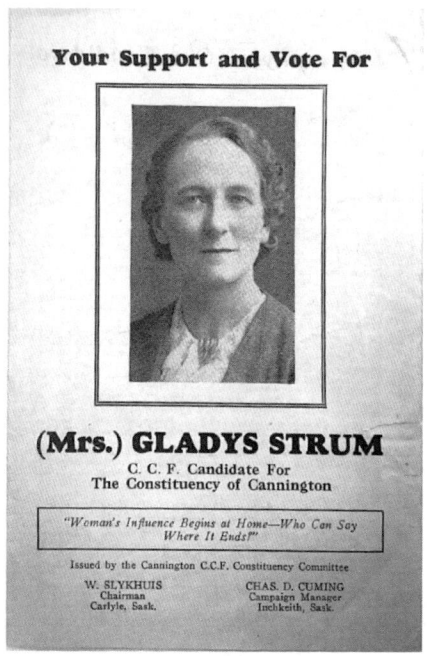

Gladys Strum campaign poster from the 1944 Saskatchewan election campaign (USAS, Sophie Dixon fonds, box 6, file CCF election materials)

CCF activist from southwestern Saskatchewan.[18] In this decision, unlike so many others he would take over the next few years that would stake out new ground, Douglas was very much a product of his times. While women played a major role in the CCF, in part because of the promise of greater equality within leftist parties, few were encouraged by their male counterparts to participate directly in electoral politics.[19] In not selecting Trew as a member of his first cabinet (or other women in any of his subsequent cabinets), Douglas reflected the social conservatism of his rural province and a distinct lack of progressivism that clashed with his forward-looking position in other areas. The civil service too would reflect this conservatism.[20]

Outside of his caucus, T.C. relied on Thomas H. McLeod, the local Weyburn boy he had mentored and who had since gotten a university education and become a lecturer in economics at Brandon College. Tommy McLeod was the first official hired by T.C. He was expected to provide a broad range of policy and administrative advice as well as

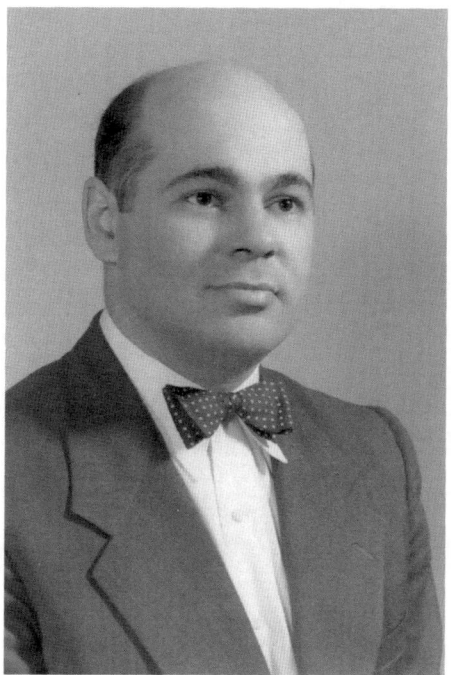

T.H. (Tommy) McLeod, T.C.'s Weyburn boy and first hire in 1944 (PAS R-A5335)

to find and hire other officials to implement his boss's extremely ambitious agenda.[21] McLeod prepared a memo suggesting some changes to the departmental structure in order to create three new portfolios in the areas of labour, cooperatives, and social welfare that reflected the priorities of the new government.[22] He also began to redesign the machinery of government to better serve the cabinet, including creating new central agencies and cabinet committee processes. This new machinery would establish the benchmark for the modernization of public bureaucracy throughout Canada in the post-war era.[23]

T.C. personally took over the health portfolio, an unprecedented decision. While some provincial premiers in the past had appointed themselves attorney general or treasury minister, depending on their own skill set and desire to personally control a central agency within the government, public health, as it was then known, was a narrow portfolio requiring technical skills and was almost always offered to a physician. Beyond this convention, public health was generally seen as

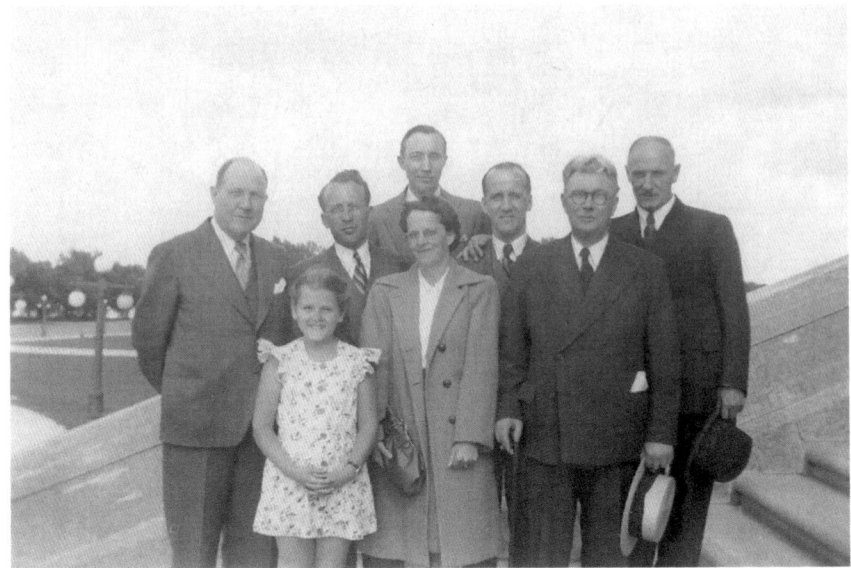

T.C. on the steps of Legislative Assembly with (from left) Dr. Hugh MacLean, Shirley and Irma Douglas, Frank Scott, Clarence Fines, Jack Corman, and Joe Phelps, 10 July 1944 (PAS S-B8178)

a portfolio that had little impact on the overall direction and management of the government and thus was of little interest to most premiers. The fact that Douglas assumed the job of health minister himself signalled that he felt compelled to implement key aspects of the CCF's election promises on health reform in the first years of his government. If he had had a determined expert like Dr. Hugh MacLean in his cabinet, he no doubt would have considered giving him the job. However, since MacLean had moved permanently to Los Angeles years before, and there were no doctors in a cabinet composed largely of farmers, teachers, and preachers, Douglas took on the job himself.[24]

To allow as many supporters as possible to witness the inauguration of Canada's first socialist cabinet, Douglas wanted the swearing-in ceremony to immediately proceed the provincial CCF's convention in Regina. On 10 July 1944, eight hundred CCF supporters, members of the media, and curious observers crammed into the legislative chamber to see thirteen MLAs, including T.C. himself, be sworn in by William Martin, chief justice of the Saskatchewan Court of Appeal (Martin had also been the province's Liberal premier from 1916 until 1922), in front of the lieutenant governor (and former Liberal cabinet minister), Archibald McNab.[25] The cabinet members walked up the staircase, which had been carpeted in red for the occasion, and then through the oversized wooden doors into the chamber. T.C. took a seat beside Irma, their daughter, Shirley, and his mother, Annie, who was "resplendent in a formal gown and big hat" and beaming with pride.[26] In the order decided by Douglas, each minister gave his oath of office, and, after everyone was done, the oaths of office were signed by Douglas and countersigned by the lieutenant governor. All the CCF party members attending that day then decamped for the CCF convention at the Hotel Saskatchewan.

## Dr. Hugh MacLean's Convention Speech

To emphasize the centrality of changes in health care and public health in the new administration, T.C. recruited his old friend and ally, Dr. Hugh MacLean, to deliver the keynote address on health reform at the CCF convention at the Hotel Saskatchewan immediately following the swearing-in ceremony.[27] The purpose was to prepare his supporters, especially his backbenchers and cabinet members, to understand why health reform would be so central in the new government. Douglas had already asked MacLean's advice on how best to "tackle" the health portfolio and had a very good idea of what the doctor would likely tell his jubilant troops.[28] MacLean readily agreed and gave a speech that combined his own ideas with those being advocated locally by the Saskatchewan State Hospital and Medical League (SHML), a non-governmental pressure group whose membership included CCF activists, and by Henry E. Sigerist, a world-renowned academic, based at Johns Hopkins University in Baltimore, whose ideas on "socialized medicine," expressed in publications, lectures, and speeches, were internationally influential.[29]

MacLean's speech achieved exactly what Douglas had hoped it would. It put health reform under a spotlight for the party faithful. He began by recounting past achievements in the province, such as tuberculosis control, cancer treatment, the municipal doctor plan that allowed municipalities to hire doctors on salary to work in underserviced rural areas, and the union hospital scheme that enabled multiple municipalities to pool their resources to construct a single, centrally located hospital to serve their residents. MacLean argued that these advances provided Saskatchewan with the necessary foundation on which to build a socialized health system. He then pointed to a future with approximately fifteen health regions, each with a referring hospital along with a more specialized outpatient clinic providing a range of medical services not available in the basic clinic, including laboratory, diagnostic, and pharmaceutical dispensing services to support primary health centres throughout rural Saskatchewan. This pattern of organized care owed much to Henry E. Sigerist and his key elements of "socialized medicine."[30] Rooted in the needs, concerns, and language of the 1930s, Sigerist's vision of a highly organized health system overlapped in some very important respects with that of the SHML, which had as it objective the "socialization of medicine and hospitals in the province," even if it had not yet laid out a vision as detailed as the one already put forward by Sigerist. In a groundbreaking speech at Yale University in 1938 on what socialized medicine might look like in a North American context, Sigerist highlighted the importance of organized health regions and accompanying hospitals and primary clinics.[31]

MacLean's speech also introduced a few of his own ideas, some of which differed from those of the party's left wing, particularly those who were prominent members of the SHML. Perhaps the most significant difference was his flexible attitude towards the remuneration of physicians. Both the SHML and Sigerist insisted on the need for doctors to move from fee-for-service remuneration to a salary base, in part because the former was associated with a private business model of physician practice that emphasized volume rather than quality, and treatment rather than prevention. For MacLean, however, the form of payment was less important than the fact that, for any plan to be successfully implemented, it would have to have the voluntary agreement and cooperation of doctors, especially the College of Physicians and Surgeons of Saskatchewan (CPS), the self-regulatory body that had been doing double duty as the doctors' political advocate – that is, the Saskatchewan Division of the Canadian Medical Association (CMA) – as a cost-saving measure since 1936.[32] In taking this position, MacLean presaged T.C.'s flexibility on the issue of payment of doctors and his desire to get the medical profession onside with his reform objectives.[33]

Since the province was so poorly resourced with clinicians and facilities, especially in rural areas, the government would need to move in a stepwise fashion to achieve socialized health care. One key element was to create the first medical school in the province in order to increase the supply of doctors. To finance the scheme, MacLean preferred to see the government rely almost exclusively on general revenues rather than targeted taxes or premiums, since income taxation (both personal and corporate) was more progressive than the alternatives. He also urged the government to get the appropriate experts to conduct surveys on the management of hospitals in the province as well as similar surveys for dentistry and nursing.[34] T.C. had the same idea, except he wanted a much broader survey than that suggested by MacLean, and he wanted Henry Sigerist to head it up.

## Henry Sigerist and Socialized Medicine

Like most on the left in Canada, T.C. was a keen student of the Beveridge Report. He saw how the British report had encouraged even the Liberal government of Canada to formulate its own version of the future welfare state through the Marsh and Heagerty Reports.[35] While these new ideas were percolating in Ottawa, Henry Sigerist came to Canada to extol the merits of socialized medicine to parliamentarians as well as the Canadian media and public.[36]

The tiny CCF parliamentary caucus had been particularly excited about Sigerist's visit in February 1944. A CCF MP, Sandy Nicholson from Saskatchewan, commended Ian Mackenzie, the minister of pensions and national health, for having the foresight to call upon Sigerist for advice.[37] Referring to the professor's address to the parliamentary Social Security Committee that was then reviewing the Marsh and Heagerty Reports, Nicholson "exhorted all elected representatives to attend" Sigerist's public speeches.[38] Interest in Professor Sigerist was so great that his first public address in Canada, "Medical Care for All," was published in the Canadian Public Health Association's journal.[39] His luncheon parliamentary address – sponsored by Ian Mackenzie – was on developments in Soviet medicine, the same topic of his public lecture that evening at Glebe Collegiate in Ottawa.[40]

T.C. was so impressed with Sigerist that he convinced his CCF colleagues to ask him to undertake a Canadian lecture tour, under CCF auspices, on the organization and delivery of medicine in the Soviet Union.[41] Despite receiving advice from his academic colleagues that he should not accept an invitation offered by any political party, Sigerist quickly accepted, stating in his formal reply that the CCF "stands for the ideals that I have always been defending." He noted that he would "welcome an opportunity to see the present organisation of medical services" in Canada and that he might "be able to make a few constructive suggestions for their future development."[42]

Sigerist was an international celebrity long before his 1944 Canadian tour. In January 1939, his portrait appeared on the cover of *Time* magazine, accompanied by a breathless profile that described "him as the world's greatest medical historian" and, at least according to earnest health reformers, the nation's most widely respected authority on

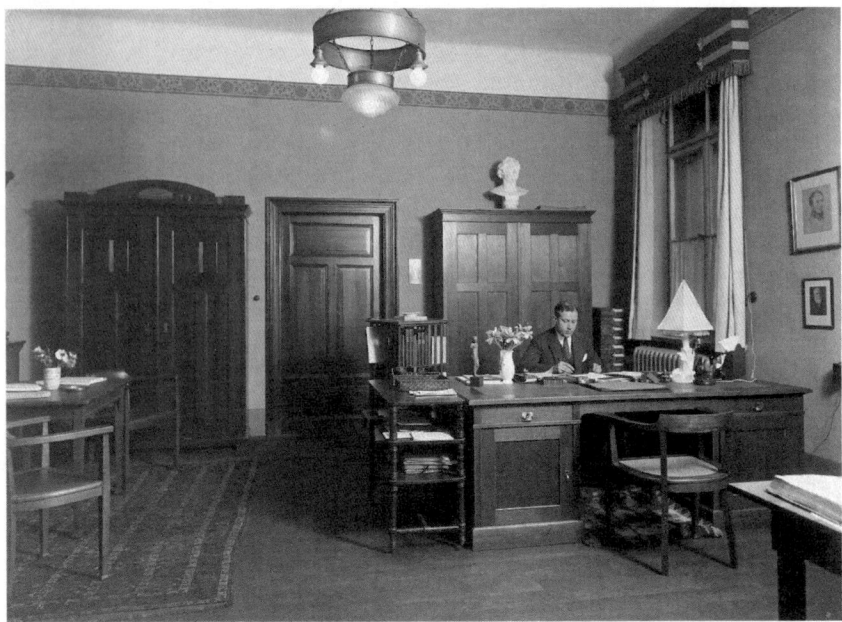

Professor Henry Sigerist before his move from Europe to Johns Hopkins University (Wikimedia Commons)

health insurance and health policy.[43] A cosmopolitan with sweeping interests and research knowledge, Sigerist lived for years in France, Germany, and Switzerland before moving to the United States to become a professor and the director at Johns Hopkins University's Institute of the History of Medicine, a position he kept until the Cold War made him unwelcome in the United States, forcing his return to Switzerland in 1947.

Although the history of medicine was a recurring subject for Sigerist, he was constantly preoccupied by questions of contemporary health organization and policy and spent much of his time advising and writing on issues of health policy. Watching the Great Depression's impact on workers and farmers in the United States and following his visits to the USSR in the mid-1930s, he became a tireless advocate of socialized medicine in North America. In particular, he was "struck by the discrepancy between" the "highly developed technical capacities" of American medicine and the "very limited access to health care" by the urban and rural poor.[44] At the same time, Sigerist was a realist. He understood that only a tiny minority of Americans had the political appetite for a comprehensive, government-run health service. So, instead, he advocated in favour of government-mandated and -financed health insurance as a modest first step towards a more organized system of socialized medicine.

Sigerist was lionized by health reformers within the Roosevelt administration. Very early on, in 1933, he attended a roundtable on national health planning and medical care sponsored by the Milbank Memorial Fund, a private foundation headquartered in New York City that funded research and public discussions on health reform. In his speech entitled "Trends towards Socialized Medicine," Sigerist told his audience that compulsory health insurance was simply a recognition of the duty owed by all citizens to each other, and he lauded Roosevelt's new Federal Emergency Relief Administration (FERA) as an acceptance of the role of government, on behalf of all its citizens, in maintaining the public health of the population.[45] The first federal aid program of the New Deal, FERA funnelled $500 million to state and local agencies to pay for emergency nursing, dental, and outpatient acute care for relief recipients.[46] Also at the Milbank roundtable was FDR's main advisor, Harry Hopkins, who had been asked to give a speech reflecting the views of the Roosevelt administration. In it, Hopkins conveyed his optimism "that with one bold stroke we could carry the American people with us, not only for unemployment insurance but for sickness and health insurance, and that it could be done in the next eighteen months if we only have the courage to go after it and do it."[47]

Sigerist believed that the Roosevelt administration was on the cusp of introducing compulsory health insurance through its social security legislation.[48] However, the next year, the administration quietly dropped any reference to national health insurance from the social security legislation it presented to Congress. By this time, Sigerist was becoming more radicalized by the Great Depression and what he began to see as a shining example of fundamental health system change in the Soviet Union. In 1935, he went on a study tour of the USSR and, like many other Western leftist intellectuals of his time, returned home highly impressed with the country's achievements. He was particularly struck by the organized way in which the government provided basic medical and hospital care through its health centres and tiered hospital system. Like so many other sympathetic visitors to the Soviet Union during the 1930s, he was carefully shielded by his handlers, and Sigerist showed little sign that he had glimpsed the ugly reality of Stalinism.[49]

Sigerist's book *Socialized Medicine in the Soviet Union* appeared in 1937 to great acclaim and became as well-known among the Canadian left as it was among progressives in Europe and the United States.[50] Not surprisingly, those opposed to socialism of any kind had the opposite reaction. Due to its "consistently laudatory tone" towards the Soviet Union, no book that Sigerist wrote before or after "brought him more notoriety" among establishment figures in the West.[51] Although never a communist himself, Sigerist was deeply impressed by what he saw as the Soviet Union's achievement in providing basic medical and hospital care for all its citizens. Most of all, he was struck by the way in which the Soviet health system was organized and how health services were provided as a public service, free of charge, as a right of citizenship.[52] How different this was than even the most advanced Western European countries, where access to health was determined by social health insurance, with benefits limited largely to premium-contributing workers and their families.[53]

A year after the publication of his book on health care in the Soviet Union, Sigerist gave his famous lecture on socialized medicine at Yale University. He began by arguing that, while Americans had been divided on whether health was a right or "a commodity to be sold on the market to whoever can afford to purchase it," the exigencies of the Great Depression combined with New Deal programs providing medical care to the indigent, had gradually moved public sentiment towards the idea that medical care should be a universal right.[54] In response to outspoken members of the American Medical Association who had pilloried the idea of universal health coverage, Sigerist ridiculed a prominent physician and medical school professor for stating that he did not "believe that a patient" was "entitled to free medical service any more than" an individual was "entitled to free housing, free clothing, and free feeding." Given that the United States was incapable of providing full employment, Sigerist argued, did this mean it is "perfectly normal for the unemployed to be evicted" from their homes, "to run around naked, sick, and starving?" In Sigerist's view, it was both "barbaric" and "foolish" not to accept the need for universal health coverage.[55]

Identifying the health services already being provided through the public sector, including New Deal programs, Sigerist posited that extending these services to the entire population was not only possible but highly desirable, from both an economic and ethical standpoint. He attacked the notion that "socialized medicine" had deteriorated into "a term that smelled of socialism or even Bolshevism" and therefore come to mean "something utterly un-American."[56] As he would argue in Saskatchewan, "socialized medicine" was just another term for organized medicine and could be implemented as easily in a liberal democracy as in a totalitarian system, whether communist or fascist.[57]

Making sure that everyone had access to medical care was the essence of socialized medicine, but it was more than simply figuring out a way for patients to pay for hospital and medical care. According to Sigerist, the chief objective of socialized medicine was a health system that allowed society to give everyone, wherever they lived and whoever they were, access to "the best possible medical service," combined with illness prevention, health promotion, and public health services. He laid out what he felt was the ideal way to achieve this in the United States, describing a system of health regions (what he called districts) with tertiary care hospitals and health centres. The latter would be polyclinics that combined curative, diagnostic, and preventive services. The health workforce would consist of general practitioners (GPs) and specialists working on salary, nurses, nutritionists, public health doctors and nurses, social workers, and others, while the infrastructure would include a polyclinic facility in which the providers would work as a team, a pharmaceutical dispensary, a tuberculosis station, an anti–venereal disease station, and educational equipment and space for health promotion and physical exercise.

This infrastructure and associated health providers would support outlying clinics serving people in more rural and remote areas. These "outposts," as he called them (and which would be renamed rural health centres in his 1944 report to the Saskatchewan government), would be staffed by a minimum of two physicians plus nurses and technicians. The outposts would work in "close cooperation" with the more urban polyclinics. Each region would itself be led and directed by a chief medical officer, who would be responsible and accountable for the health of everyone within the region.[58]

To his audience at Yale, Sigerist admitted that he leaned heavily on the Soviet model for some of the organizational elements of his idealized system of socialized medicine, but he also made it clear that the Soviet system was very much a work in progress, still lacking the quality and quantity of infrastructure and human resources to implement the ideal socialized medicine system.[59] In 1941, Sigerist launched the *American Review of Soviet Medicine*, a journal that showcased scientific and organization developments in the Soviet Union, which he continued to admire even after his view on Stalinism soured.[60] The new journal was particularly attractive to physicians who had joined organizations that were sending medical and other aid to the USSR following Nazi Germany's invasion of that country in 1941, and who, like Sigerist, had earlier supported anti-fascist groups, including those aiding Spain's leftist Popular Front government against Franco's fascist Nationalists in the Spanish Civil War.[61] Indeed, he travelled to Canada in 1941 to support similar Canadian organizations providing medical aid to the Soviet Union at the very time the Nazis were laying siege to Moscow.[62]

Sigerist became a celebrated icon of the medical left in the United States, Canada, Europe, and Australasia, in part because of his sympathetic view of the Soviet Union.[63] Yet this sympathy meant that he was distrusted, even hated, by those fearful of socialized medicine, especially the influential physicians who ran the American Medical Association. Their criticism was temporarily muted by the fact that the Soviet Union's war effort was critical in slowing Nazi Germany's victorious drive through Europe.

Sigerist had immediately agreed to the CCF request to tour Canada on its behalf, but, following the CCF's provincial election victory, T.C. and his colleagues in Ottawa decided that Sigerist was particularly needed in Saskatchewan.[64] Writing Douglas from California, Dr. Hugh MacLean also felt that Sigerist was the best person to review conditions in Saskatchewan and recommend the practical steps the government would need to take in order to implement a socialized health system.[65] On 20 July 1944, just one week after MacLean's speech to the CCF convention and the swearing in of Douglas and his cabinet, Douglas cabled Sigerist and asked him to review the situation in Saskatchewan and recommend the next steps the government should take in creating an organized health system capable of providing access to needed services for all residents, especially those who lived in the vast rural areas of the province.[66]

Sigerist was excited about the possibility of working in Saskatchewan. He had had links with Canada since his first visit in 1933 and had subsequent tours involving both government work and lectures in 1941 and 1943.[67] His interest in the country was further piqued when the CCF was elected, noting in his diary that this was the "first time that a socialist party has full control of a Canadian province," which presented the possibility, for the first time in North America, "of organizing medical services in a sensible way."[68] Douglas's telegram was the antidote that Sigerist needed to snap out of a depression caused by "a lack of sleep" and "too much work." But most of all, he was delighted with being put in charge "of a fact-finding committee" that involved a "good opportunity to do some field work and a really constructive job." Still, like all highly productive authors, Sigerist always saw such assignments through the prism of his own writing, and he confided in his journal how the experience was likely to give him "good material for the book" he was then working on.[69]

For his part, T.C. knew intuitively how best to use Sigerist's celebrity to advance his government's ambitious health reforms. In recounting this episode years later, Douglas pointed to the two things he expected to achieve by bringing Sigerist to the province to head a commission to survey health services. First, it would underline the fact that he intended to focus his government's attention on health in its first years of office. Despite being premier as well as minister of health, he still needed to justify, both to his party and his cabinet members, why his proposed new health spending deserved a privileged claim on the province's very constrained revenues.[70] Second, Sigerist would draw talent to the province. In Douglas's words, "it gave the people in the health field who were interested in the type of program we had in mind a terrific amount of encouragement; because suddenly here is a world authority coming to this little province of Saskatchewan to make recommendations about a health program."[71]

As Esyllt Jones concludes in her history of the CCF government's health system ambitions and innovations in its first term of office, T.C.'s use of Sigerist "was a stroke of public relations genius" that "ensured that the eyes of the world – at least the North American media – would be focused on events in the province."[72] Sigerist was paid a flat fee of $1,000 plus expenses, a reasonable charge given the four weeks expended by Sigerist on the project (the typical deputy minister in Saskatchewan was paid an annual salary of $4,000 in the mid-1940s), but a bargain given the international spotlight placed on Douglas's ambitions for health reform.[73]

Douglas made it clear to Sigerist that while he would be solely responsible for the report, he was to be assisted in his survey by a few "technical experts."[74] In Sigerist's mind, this did not dilute his own role. In his diary, he wrote that Douglas had conferred on him "the status of Beveridge, that is, I, alone will be responsible for the report and the other members [will] act as technical advisors."[75] Without input from Sigerist, T.C. appointed four technical advisors to assist in the survey, drawing on four different areas of health services. Dr. J. Lloyd Brown, a pediatrician from Regina, was vice-chair of the College of Physicians and Surgeons of Saskatchewan's Health Insurance Commission. Ann Heffel, a public health nurse who had worked in the province for years, represented the nursing profession and provided some public health expertise. The dental perspective was supplied by dentist Dr. J.L. Connell, while advice on hospitals and acute care was furnished by Clarence Gibson, the former superintendent of the Regina General Hospital (the largest in the province) and former president of the Saskatchewan Hospital Association.[76] Although these advisors were less than enthusiastic about socialized health care, they complemented Sigerist's deep knowledge of health systems around the world with detailed local

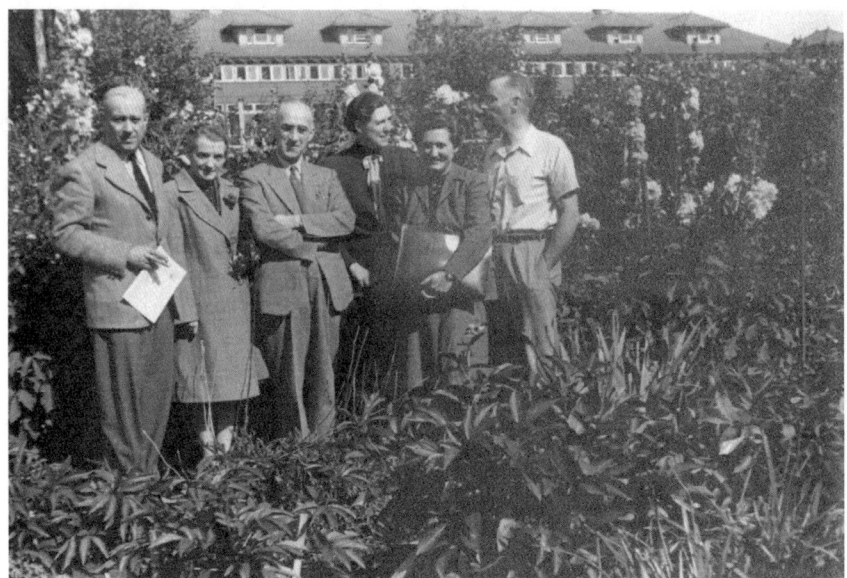

Henry E. Sigerist (far left) and Mindel C. Sheps (second from right) with members of Sigerist Commission, Saskatchewan, September 1944 (JHCA)

knowledge, a factor important to T.C., who was sensitive to the charge that he was reliant on "outsiders" who knew little of the province and its people.

T.C. had already hired Dr. Mindel Cherniack Sheps, a recently graduated doctor and CCF activist from Winnipeg, as secretary of the commission. She was both impressed and highly influenced by Sigerist and his articles and books extolling the virtues of socialized medicine. Sheps's appointment raised some eyebrows among the province's doctors. She was, in their view, too young – she was just entering her thirties – and too political. Worse, she was a female Jewish doctor in a place that had never seen anyone like her before. But, as a dedicated socialist who heartily agreed with Sigerist's views on the advantages of an organized health system, she had Douglas's confidence.

Before he had commissioned Sigerist and Sheps, T.C.'s two main advisors on the health file were MacLean, who had returned home to California shortly after the CCF convention, and Tommy McLeod, who was quickly overwhelmed with the job of getting the machinery and people in all the central agencies, boards, and departments of government in place for Douglas and the rest of cabinet. The Department of Public Health was itself of limited help. The public servants were a holdover from the previous government, and, while some were adequate administrators, they possessed little policy breadth or vision. Under the Liberals, they had had the same minister, Dr. John Uhrich, from 1923 and 1944, interrupted for a few years by the Conservative coalition government.[77] As a result, the senior people in the department were of a conservative nature, used to decades of managing the status quo. Unlike Dr. Sheps, they were unable to facilitate the fundamental changes that Douglas was seeking.[78]

**Mindel C. Sheps and the Sigerist Commission**

Mindel Cherniack Sheps was born in Winnipeg in 1913 to Jewish immigrants from southern Russia. In the old country, her father, Joseph Alter Cherniack, had been a Labour Zionist, and her mother, Fania (née Goldwin), a socialist who had been jailed for her political activities. In Canada, they both remained involved in numerous progressive Jewish organizations, which eventually attracted both Mindel and her younger brother, Saul, who would, in the late 1960s, become a cabinet minister in Manitoba's first New Democratic government.[79]

Dr. Sheps was responsible for providing Sigerist with the necessary financial and health data as well as other essential details on the current organization of the province's health and dental services and human resources. She was fully committed to the CCF's goals for health reform, which she saw as consistent with Sigerist's brand of socialized medicine. In her letter of introduction to Sigerist, she noted that she and her husband, Cecil Sheps, also a leftist Jewish physician from Winnipeg, had "been very great admirers of yourself ever since we first read your book on Soviet Medicine in 1937 – an impression which has been fortified by everything of yours we've read since then."[80]

Upon arrival in Regina, Sigerist visited Douglas and then was introduced to the cabinet for a discussion. As table 4.1 illustrates, what followed was a whirlwind of public hearings throughout the province, punctuated by hospital and other facility tours, as well as luncheons and dinners often accompanied by one of Sigerist's lectures. The commission was met everywhere with considerable interest and was reported assiduously in the province's media. At the very centre was the rotund Dr. Henry Sigerist, his intense eyes taking in all around him. Showing great interest in the oral presentations of hospital managers, local government officials, and community activists, Sigerist was careful to relate these local experiences in his summaries of the conditions

Table 4.1. Henry Sigerist's daily itinerary in Saskatchewan, September 1944

| Location | Description | Date |
| --- | --- | --- |
| Regina | Meets members of cabinet and some officials | 7 Sept. |
| Regina | Meets members of his commission; gives luncheon speech to Regina Board of Trade entitled "Medicine Today and Tomorrow" | 8 Sept. |
| Regina | Visits two Regina hospitals (Regina General and the Grey Nuns hospitals) and the Regina Cancer Clinic | 9 Sept. |
| Regina | Chairs hearings in the Saskatchewan Legislative Assembly building | 11–12 Sept. |
| Strasbourg | After chairing meeting in the town hall, visits a doctor's office and nursing home | 13 Sept. |
| Wadena | Visits the Wadena Union Hospital in the morning; chairs open meeting at the town's Legion Hall in the afternoon | 14 Sept. |
| Tisdale | Visits Catholic hospital (Ste. Therese); chairs open meeting in the town hall arranged by the State Hospital and Medical League; speaks at dinner hosted by the local board of trade | 15 Sept. |
| Prince Albert and North Battleford | Visits tuberculosis sanitorium in Prince Albert and the North Battleford Mental Hospital | 16 Sept. |
| Saskatoon | Chairs open hearing at city hall; visits St. Paul's Hospital and City Hospital; gives speech entitled "Medicine for Today and Tomorrow" at annual meeting of the CPS of Saskatchewan | 18 Sept. |
| Saskatoon | Chairs open hearings at city hall; present for T.C. Douglas's speech at CPS annual meeting | 19 Sept. |
| Saskatoon | Chairs open hearings at city hall; guest at City Hospital luncheon; speech to Canadian Club in the evening | 20 Sept. |
| Eston | Visits Eston Union Hospital; chairs open meeting at Eston Theatre; gives evening speech entitled "Medicine in the Soviet Union" at Eston Board of Trade banquet | 21 Sept. |
| Shaunavon | Visits Shaunavon Union Hospital; holds open hearings at the town's courthouse | 22 Sept. |
| Regina | Gives Saturday evening CBC radio broadcast, "Saskatchewan Plans for Health" | 24 Sept. |
| Regina | Chairs open hearings at the Saskatchewan Legislative Assembly building; gives address at the local Kiwanis Club | 25 Sept. |
| Regina | Chairs open hearings; gives evening speech entitled "Planning for Post-War Health" to Women's Canadian Club | 26 Sept. |
| Moose Jaw | Addresses public meeting arranged by the State Hospital and Medical League; gives evening speech entitled "Planning for Post-war Health" at public library | 27 Sept. |
| Regina | Addresses meeting arranged by the Junior Board of Trade | 28 Sept. |
| Regina | Appears on CBC Saturday evening radio broadcast, "Planning for Post-War Health" | 30 Sept. |

Sources: Provincial Archives of Saskatchewan, Health Services Survey Planning Commission (Sigerist Commission), R-251, file 28, daily diary of the Health Services Survey Commission 1944. The subject titles and sponsors of Sigerist's speeches were found in the *Regina Leader-Post*: "Committee Plans Public Hearings," 23 Aug. 1944, 3; "Board to Hear Dr. Sigerist," 6 Sept. 1944, 3; "Dr. Sigerist Club Speaker," 22 Sept. 1944, 6; 4; "Post-War Health," 27 Sept. 1944, 5; "Report Due Next Month," 28 Sept. 1944, 3; "Eston Board of Trade Banquets Member of Health Commission," 28 Sept. 1944, 6; advertisement for Sigerist broadcast, 30 Sept. 1944, 4.

in other countries. In between the public hearings, Sigerist and other commission members visited hospitals, doctors' offices, and a nursing home, and then spent an extra day of travel to visit a tuberculosis sanitorium and a mental hospital.[81]

The Sigerist Commission achieved exactly what Douglas had hoped in terms of public attention. Here was a world-renown figure talking to business owners, farmers, labourers, housewives, doctors, and lawyers in their hometowns about the many potential benefits of a socialized health system and paving the way for radical action by the government. Not everyone agreed with everything Sigerist said, especially about the Soviet Union, but it was hard not to be persuaded by the logic of his vision of a more organized and effective health system. His guest appearance on the Canadian Broadcast Corporation's national radio broadcast on a Saturday evening immediately after he completed the public hearings only added to his allure. By this time, Sigerist was hard at work on his report for the Douglas government.

## The Sigerist Report

Sigerist's time in Saskatchewan was limited, and so, working closely with Mindel Sheps, and with very limited input from other members of his commission, pieces of the report were cobbled together while the commissioners travelled from town to town and in the few spare minutes between public hearings and speeches. The public hearings were largely completed by 25 September, the day that Sigerist rolled up his sleeves and began the work of revising the rough draft of various sections into a coherent report. He completed his draft by 4 October and immediately handed it over to Douglas.

Once published, the final report proved to be a short read, the main body merely twelve pages in length. The report avoided a conclusion in favour of eight recommendations for "immediate action." It repeated the Douglas government's election platform promise "to set up a complete system of socialized health services with special emphasis on preventive medicine, so that everybody in the province will receive adequate medical, surgical, dental, nursing and hospital care without charge."[82] However, since this long-term goal might "have to wait until the Province" received "subsidies from the Dominion" or could obtain other "sources of revenue," the report focused on what could be done immediately, especially in terms of improving health services in the rural areas, where two-thirds of the population was living.[83]

Sigerist's recommendations returned to the design he had originally laid out in his Yale lecture on socialized medicine in 1938. A health system could be rationally integrated only if it was planned and coordinated by the visible hand of government rather than the invisible hand of the market. This approach involved at least four components: the regional integration of facilities and providers; the integration of public and population health with personal health care services, including the integration of illness prevention into the delivery of treatment services; the direct linkage of education and research into the organization, management, and clinical delivery of health services; and the scientific treatment of mental illness in a manner parallel to the treatment of physical illness and injury.

Sigerist saw regionalized integration as the way forward for improving access and the quality of care in the province's vast rural areas. He recommended the coordination of inpatient and outpatient care through a connected infrastructure of hospitals, primary care clinics, and polyclinic-type health centres. Although a term more common in the United Kingdom than in North America, "polyclinics" went well beyond providing GP services, offering more specialist examinations and treatments for a wide variety of diseases as well as diagnostics and drug dispensing.[84] Influenced by what he had observed in the Soviet Union as well as by the health centre (polyclinic) movement in the United Kingdom and the New Deal's rural health initiatives in the United States, Sigerist recommended a highly organized system with a large regional hospital as the base from which the polyclinic and the primary health centres radiated.[85]

Although Sigerist had been advocating this structure for years, the idea was becoming more popular in health reform circles. On the same day that Sigerist presented his report to Douglas, the American Public Health Association formally recommended that American states and local governments adopt a regionalized health system, including the "construction of needed hospitals, health centers, and related facilities," as part of a national health insurance plan.[86] Moreover, this hub-and-spoke system was identical to one that was about to be recommended for rural areas by the US Public Health Service.[87] Advocating this model for Saskatchewan, the commission recommended that each region have a tertiary care hospital hub that would also have offices for specialist outpatient medical and dental care. These "district hospitals" would support smaller polyclinics – what Sigerist called rural health centres – a combination of small rural hospitals with up to ten maternity and general beds, a diagnostic services centre, an operating theatre for deliveries and minor surgeries, and a small clinical laboratory. Doctors would be paid a salary based on years of service as well as a sum for travelling to see patients in outlying villages and farms.[88]

The first task for the government was to figure out the number of health regions and their geographic boundaries. To accomplish this, Sigerist recommended the establishment of a Health Services Planning Commission (HSPC), which not only would work out the boundaries of health districts but would also determine the health needs and resources of local governments and set up two pilot project health regions.[89] A more rudimentary version of this hub-and-spoke regionalized system had previously been promoted by the province's State Hospital and Medical League in an eight-point plan that it had release three years earlier.[90]

As for integrating personal health care services with public and population health, Sigerist started from the principle that socialized medicine should do away, as he felt it already had in the Soviet Union, with the "traditional distinction between preventive and curative medicine."[91] As for how such an approach could be implemented in Saskatchewan, he recommended that his proposed health regions could lead in this endeavour. Responsible for coordinating the delivery of public health services, each would be assigned a full-time medical officer of health by the Department of Public Health. He also recommended the establishment of two new divisions in the Department of Public Health, one for venereal disease control and the other for health education and promotion. The treatment of sexually transmitted diseases should be provided free to all residents to better protect the population, he argued. Sigerist also recommended the inclusion of health education in the curriculum of provincial schools and suggested that teachers could play a more direct role in prevention and early diagnosis by notifying "local health authorities" when observing students who might require medical attention. He also suggested that health regions collaborate with civil society groups to shape and deliver physical activity programs.[92]

A major proponent of what we would today call evidence-based medicine, Sigerist was a fervent believer in the progressive role of education and research in transforming health systems. While capitalism restricted the benefits of medical science and technology, socialized medicine would produce new attitudes towards medical teaching, research, and knowledge.[93] The new health professionals and scientists would be integrated into the health system in a strategic manner. In the municipal doctors scheme in Saskatchewan, he saw a nucleus of a salaried profession whose priority would be practising medicine rather than running a business. He recommended that the province's future medical school (ultimately established in 1952) at the University of Saskatchewan be upgraded into a "grade A Medical School" that could set "a new pattern" for medical education" in Canada by being open to all irrespective of "race, sex or economic status" at a time when ethnic, gender, and class discrimination were common attributes of medical schools throughout the country. Taught about the social as well as the technical dimensions of medicine, graduates would bring more progressive attitudes to their clinical practices. Numbers would be increased through scholarships for qualified students with limited means who would agree "to spend a certain number of years in rural practice" staffing the province's new rural health regions. A major teaching hospital needed to accompany the medical school to facilitate "scientific teaching, clinical instruction and research."[94]

These medical graduates would be joined by a new cadre of dentists, nurses, and social workers attracted to well-remunerated positions in the health regions. Referring to the extremely poor oral health of Saskatchewan residents – the worst in the country at the time – Sigerist recommended dental scholarships and the establishment of a school of dentistry at the University of Saskatchewan. As for nurses, including public health nurses, recommendations included a new regime of better pay, improved working conditions, and pensions. In addition, there should be scholarships and arrangements for student nurses to gain experience in the small rural hospitals that would become polyclinics in the regionalized system that Sigerist envisioned. He also wanted to see social workers attached to the district hospitals within his proposed health regions, with a course for the training of more specialized "medical social workers" set up at the University of Saskatchewan.[95]

**Implementing the Sigerist Report through Local Governments**

Shortly after the Sigerist Report was issued, Mindel Sheps was joined by her husband, Cecil, in Regina. They had married in 1937, shortly after the two had graduated from medical school at the University of Manitoba. They then travelled to England on postgraduate fellowships. When they returned, Mindel went into general practice in Winnipeg and became active in community organizations, the Winnipeg school board, and the provincial CCF.[96] When she accepted Douglas's offer to work for his government, she was in Calgary, where Cecil was a captain in the Royal Canadian Military Corps and stationed as director of venereal disease control for the troops in Alberta. Immediately after the Sigerist Report was tabled, T.C. announced that he was creating a new division for venereal disease within the Department of Public Health. He put Cecil in charge, after negotiating his secondment to the province from the federal government.[97] With the return of Canadian soldiers

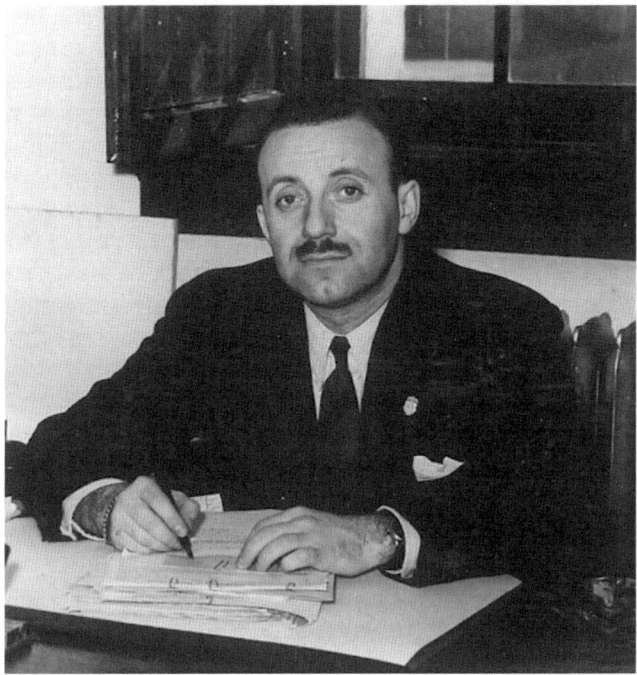

Cecil Sheps, c. 1946 (PAS R-A3008)

from Europe, syphilis was becoming a national epidemic, and the "situation in Saskatchewan" was, in Douglas's view, "alarming." Under Cecil Sheps, Douglas posited, the efforts of the Canadian army and the provincial government could be combined to "wipe the disease out of this province inside of five years."[98] Unofficially, T.C. also wanted Cecil to assist Mindel and Tommy McLeod in implementing other aspects of the Sigerist Report.

Although deferring to the Shepses on what he saw as the bureaucratic and technical details of creating a socialized health system, T.C. took direct charge of what he considered to be the system's political dimensions. As premier and health minister, he felt it was his responsibility to manage the stakeholders, from the demands of leftist farm and labour groups for a complete socialized health system, to the fears the doctors had about even the most incremental changes. However, the line dividing the political from the technical dimensions was hardly distinct. Often, when he met with various provincial stakeholders, Douglas found himself negotiating not just the boundaries of the new system but also its very substance, something about which his advisors were supposed to be providing expert advice.

On the basics, Douglas was in complete agreement with Sigerist (and Mindel Sheps), especially with respect to the two-track strategy the government needed to adopt to make progress on its ambitious health agenda. The first track was to change the delivery of services to create a system that shifted the emphasis from the treatment of illness to improving health and preventing illness in the first place, as had been advocated by Sigerist and the State Hospital and Medical League. The foundation of this would be to work with local governments in setting up public health regions, each of which would have full-time public health staff, including a medical officer of health, public health nurses, and sanitarians (public health and safety inspectors).[99] The provincial government was responsible for the hiring of this staff and paying the lion's share of their salaries.[100]

The second track was to improve access to treatment services. Most of all, this meant figuring out how to get more doctors, nurses, and dentists into rural areas, and providing more accessible hospital care and diagnostic services in the larger towns. While the ultimate goal was to provide coverage of all necessary health services for all Saskatchewan residents, doing so would be pointless unless there were enough clinicians and facilities to service the province's mainly rural population. Of Saskatchewan's almost 833,000 residents in the census of 1946, 62 per cent lived rurally. The four largest cities – Regina (60,246), Saskatoon (46,028), Moose Jaw (23,069), and Prince Albert (14,532) – together constituted only 17 per cent of the total population.[101] The other so-called urban centres were little more than market towns dependent on the surrounding farms and were themselves some distance from the tertiary hospitals in the four major centres. By providing grants to both rural and urban municipal governments, the HSPC would encourage new hospital and health centre construction in these agricultural towns and get more doctors to join municipal doctor plans to serve the province's extensive rural population.[102]

As for the election promise that the CCF would "provide every resident of Saskatchewan with all necessary medical and hospital care, regardless of his or her ability to pay for it," Douglas needed to make some immediate progress on improving access.[103] He decided to focus on providing full coverage for hospital and medical care for three groups by 1 January 1945. The first group consisted of the roughly 25,000 residents who were already considered dependants, the recipients of "mother's allowances" or old age or disability pensions. They were to be covered under what would soon be called the Public Assistance

Medical Plan. Second, the provincial government would underwrite all diagnostic and treatment costs for cancer patients. Finally, the families of all mental health patients in the province's two psychiatric hospitals and the psychiatric wing of the Regina General Hospital would no longer have to contribute towards accommodation or treatment costs.

Mindel Sheps and Tommy McLeod worked day and night with the municipalities to expand the number of medical facilities and personnel in rural Saskatchewan, even while they were writing and amending legislation to extend hospital and medical care coverage to these three groups.[104] At the end of October, just weeks after he had been presented with the Sigerist Report and negotiated with the College of Physicians and Surgeons on how doctors would be reimbursed, Douglas presented to the legislature Bill No. 58 – the Health Services Act – for first reading, a bill written largely by McLeod under Mindel Sheps's watchful eye.[105] A week later, the bill went through second reading and debate before being passed on 10 November 1944.[106] Even more remarkable than the speed of this particular legislation was the fact that Douglas's government put forward more than seventy other bills covering social welfare, education, labour rights, and farm income protection in the special fall sitting between 10 October and 10 November 1944.[107] It was an explosive start, announcing the most ambitious provincial government in Canadian history.

In addition to setting up the legislative framework for the provincial government to work with local governments in establishing health regions and to provide grants for municipalities to ramp up hospital construction and hire new doctors, the Health Services Act officially created the Health Services Planning Commission, with Mindel Sheps immediately put in charge as secretary. She hired a tiny staff, which was supplemented by Tommy McLeod, who divided his time between the HSPC and his work on structure and personnel for the entire government. All the work obligations shouldered by the two Shepses and McLeod required the three to get together in the evenings. McLeod would meet the couple at their house, and they would work while cooking dinner and continue after eating until well after midnight. McLeod found that both Mindel and Cecil were "brilliant people" who exerted an "influence" that was "hard for anyone to resist." Anyone, that is, except the doctors representing the College of Physicians and Surgeons, whose world view "was so at odds" with that of the HSPC and the Shepses that conflict was inevitable.[108]

Although T.C.'s relationship with the CPS was somewhat better, it was "a fragile one" from the beginning. In McLeod's view, Douglas was never "as successful as he thought he was in winning" the college leadership "over to any extent to the ideas of a universal scheme." The "gap" between the CPS and Douglas "was just too great," as would be demonstrated when the relationship between the two shattered fifteen years later over the issue of medical care insurance.[109]

In December, the Shepses and McLeod gave T.C. a first and very lengthy draft of their blueprint.[110] They then prepared an abridged version of their report for the HSPC's Advisory Committee, a document that was completed in mid-February 1945, a little over two weeks in advance of the committee's meeting.[111] The "abridged" forty-four-page plan focused on how best to organize health services for the population living outside the major urban centres. The HSPC argued that the key to making health care accessible to all and to optimizing health outcomes was for the provincial and local governments to build a predominantly public health system. At its core would be fourteen geographic health regions, which would provide fulsome public health infrastructure and personnel. These regions would receive provincial grants to build more hospitals and add more doctors.

The report began by describing the great deficiencies in current health services – both public and private – available to rural residents. To determine the gap in primary care, the HSPC used what was then thought by physician and public health organizations in the United States and Canada as the minimum standard of one GP for every 2,000 individuals. Overall, the province had one GP for every 2,882 people, but, outside the major centres, the ratio was one for every 3,471 residents. As for the specialists, the vast majority were concentrated in Regina and Saskatoon, close to the main tertiary hospitals. There was also a shortage of nurses to service the province's existing hospitals as well as its two psychiatric hospitals, and there were far too few public health nurses to serve the entire province. Patients had to come to them, as they rarely, if ever, ventured into rural Saskatchewan. As for hospital beds, the minimum standard advocated by hospital associations in Canada was 5 beds per 1,000 people, while Saskatchewan only had 3.4 beds per 1,000 residents, and these were concentrated in the cities.[112]

Before the election of the CCF, municipal governments had done what they could to improve health services for their residents. Local governments were responsible for establishing union hospital districts, which required the cooperation of contiguous municipalities for the funding and construction of hospitals that could draw on a population large enough to make the operation feasible. Local governments also hired doctors on contract to provide basic medical services to their residents, especially in areas with dispersed populations unable to support a sustainable fee-for-service practice.[113]

Since their establishment shortly after the province was created in 1905, the almost three hundred rural municipalities (RMs) constituted the core of Saskatchewan's local government system in the twentieth century. Each RM was made up of nine townships, and a township encompassed thirty sections (a section was 640 acres). RMs were like "perforated squares," organized completely independently of hamlets, towns, and villages, which had separate government structures. But considerable political power rested with the RMs and their primary organization, the Saskatchewan Association of Rural Municipalities (SARM), much more than was held by the urban municipalities, despite their greater number, and their provincial organization, the Saskatchewan Urban Municipalities Association (SUMA).

Individual RMs had initiated municipal doctor plans in 1919, providing salaries to doctors who were prepared to work in sparsely populated rural areas if they received a guaranteed income, which they then supplemented with fee-for-service arrangements for patients living in the villages and towns located within the RM as well as with private patients from adjoining municipalities without municipal doctor contracts. Through SARM, the RM governments lobbied the provincial and local governments to pool their financing to create rural hospitals, beginning in 1916. By 1929, SARM had facilitated a program for the free treatment of all tuberculosis patients, which was funded partly by local governments.[114] These rural municipal governments had shown great creativity in the face of the adversity of the Great Depression, and some continued to be proactive in establishing union hospital districts and municipal doctor plans with the return of prosperity in the early 1940s.

Douglas's election victory was a product of the organizing capacity of the CCF, which in turn rested in the hands of an able corps of individuals with considerable experience working in local governments and cooperative enterprises. The political culture forged by municipal politicians – equal measures of agrarian activism, pragmatism, and fiscal conservatism – was fully shared by Douglas and many members of his cabinet who had spent years working in elected local government positions.[115] Indeed, the CCF in Saskatchewan was "firmly rooted at the time in a tradition of agrarian, democratic populism" that predated the party.[116]

A modest majority of the elected members of local governments had voted for the CCF in 1944, and T.C. wanted to work with them to establish the health regions, health centres, and rural hospitals that would underpin what would eventually become a "complete system of socialized health services."[117] The challenge was that, with increasing agricultural mechanization came an ever-shrinking rural population, diminishing the fiscal and administrative capacity of RMs to deliver services, which in turn created pressures on the province to centralize the financing and management of services.[118] Indeed, the Douglas government had just bypassed local governments in enacting the Larger School Units Act to equalize the quality of education, standardize teacher income, and improve school infrastructure in the province. Although the reform raised the standard of education while improving working conditions and remuneration for teachers, larger school units were implemented over the heads of local governments, and they let Douglas know how dissatisfied they were with the process.[119]

To avoid upsetting these municipal leaders any further, T.C. ensured that they retained the responsibility to establish new health regions through referendums. He tried to make the option to create a health region as attractive as possible by providing most of the funding for the public health personnel and infrastructure required, but he had to leave the decision of whether to form a region up to local governments. Through radio broadcasts, he encouraged municipal residents to vote in favour of regionalization, explaining the benefits that would flow from organizing health services within their respective health regions.[120] Despite his efforts, there was limited enthusiasm at the local level for regions, and it would take more than a decade before even half the province's population were in organized health regions.[121]

At the two-day meeting in March 1945, twenty-one of the thirty-two members of the HSPC Advisory Committee assembled in the legislature in Regina. The doctors were easily outnumbered by representatives of farm, labour, and women's organizations as well as SARM, SUMA, and SHML delegates. In welcoming the Advisory Committee members, T.C. emphasized the importance of "being able to consult with the people most concerned in health services" in order to get the HSPC's "plans off to a good start." During the discussions over the next two days, the lay (non-physician) members of the committee enthusiastically endorsed the HSPC's blueprint and pushed for the government to establish "at least one region in the very near future."[122] In contrast, the CPS's representatives, Dr. Clarence Houston and Dr. J.F.C. (Jack) Anderson, hated the plan. To block any potential vote on the plan by the Advisory Committee, Anderson said that he and Houston had no authority to decide anything on behalf of the College of Physicians and Surgeons and would instead take the blueprint back to the college for further discussion.[123]

Just days after the meeting, the CPS passed a resolution rejecting the HSPC plan. It was, the doctors argued, nothing less than a blueprint for a government-run health system, rather than what the doctors had expected, a proposal for government-subsidized health insurance. Thus, the blueprint was contrary to the Canadian Medical Association's position. Moreover, it went far beyond the ambit of the federal government's Heagerty health insurance plan. Two items particularly galled the CPS. The first was the HSPC's strong endorsement of a salaried medical service, and the second was its insistence that only a government could (and should) administer such a health system. The CPS was worried about the provincial government's potential control over the system but also argued that municipal governments would have too much potential control over doctors and that this "local interference" was "not good" for doctors and the care they needed to provide to patients.[124]

The CPS enumerated other clear limits to any scheme to which the doctors would agree. The first was that "state-aided Health Insurance" had to be based "on a reasonable fee-for-service basis"; the second that "the administration of such arrangement is put into the hands of a non-political independent commission on which the Medical Profession is adequately represented."[125] Although the final paragraph of the CPS resolution dismissed the HSPC plan as not meeting "the needs of the people of the province," or of "those rendering the services," the college nonetheless left the door open by restating its desire "to assist the Government in preparing suitable plans to meet the medical needs of the people."[126]

**Meeting with the Medical Profession, 21 March 1945**

In a meeting that started on the afternoon and ended in the evening on 21 March, the CPS resolution was personally handed to Douglas by a delegation led by Anderson and Houston.[127] It was significant that Douglas managed the meeting with only one official present, Dr. Clarence Hames, the new deputy minister of public health hired by Douglas.[128] Neither of the Shepses nor McLeod were invited, likely at the college's request, due to CPS antagonism towards the three, especially Mindel. Years later, McLeod recounted the two main reasons why Mindel in particular was disliked by the doctors. First, she was a woman in a profession where the female sex was not accepted, a fact fortified by prevailing attitudes in Saskatchewan, which were shared by many in the CCF.[129] Second, she was Jewish at a time where "there was ... a fairly strong strain of anti-Semitism" not only in the medical profession but in Canadian society more generally.[130]

To create a little distance between himself and the HSPC blueprint, Douglas began the meeting by saying that he and Hames had not had time to carefully study the document. However, he openly questioned why the CPS was so critical of the plan when, for their part, the doctors had never presented any concrete alternative. He also took issue with the charge that his government had not properly consulted the CPS, arguing that, "since his government had taken office, the medical profession had been consulted on all matters concerning the practice of medicine."[131] Douglas then shifted gears, trying to allay the fears of the profession. According to the account published in the college's journal, the *Saskatchewan Medical Quarterly*, T.C. said his main concern was "to provide medical services for everyone as rapidly as possible," while the method used to achieve that goal "did not matter." In addition, his government's "policy [was] to provide stated-aided health insurance for the cities and municipal doctor plan in rural areas." While salaried municipal doctors might be needed to serve the poorer and more rural areas, this left "a very large place for private practice" in the province.[132]

When pressed on the issue of remuneration, Douglas showed some openness to the government providing funding not only to municipalities paying doctors on salary but those who might be willing to offer fee-for-service contracts to physicians. However, he shut down the idea of a commission independent of the provincial and local governments managing the municipal doctor plan and any future health insurance scheme, pointing out that he intended that the HSPC would administer any future plan to ensure democratic accountability through him as minister reporting on the spending of public funds in the provincial legislature. At this point, the CPS representatives launched a personal attack, stating that it "had little confidence in the Health Services Planning Commission and particularly in the Commission's medical member" – that is, Dr. Mindel Sheps. In response, Douglas quickly shifted to the fact that the position of HSPC chair remained vacant because he was still searching for someone "sympathetic to both the government and the medical profession."[133] These words served to undercut Sheps's authority with the doctors and would cost Douglas dearly because each time the college disagreed with the HSPC, it would bypass Sheps and insist on meeting with Douglas directly to sort things out.[134] And, as T.C. soon realized, he did not have enough time in a day for endless discussions and debates with the college.

As a final grand gesture, the CPS threatened to oppose provincial grants to municipalities for additional doctors if "used as a means of coercion to force a salaried system of medicine in rural areas." Rather than continue to rebut and assuage, Douglas suggested that Anderson, Houston, and a third doctor at the meeting form a subcommittee of the Advisory Committee to work out the issue of future remuneration for municipal doctors. The CPS enthusiastically agreed.[135] While this suggestion may have closed the meeting on a more positive note, it was only because the college had won a major concession. T.C. understood the disadvantages of fee-for-service payment but concluded that he could not even convince salaried municipal doctors, many of whom were zealous about protecting their outside fee-for-service income, much less the college's leadership, of the advantages of a purely salaried service.[136]

**Initiating Health Regions and a Pilot Project**

T.C. needed the cooperation of organized medicine, not just farm organizations, labour unions, and local governments, if he wanted to see a few health regions set up before the end of 1945. As he told the HSPC Advisory Committee members in early March, the HSPC was ready to meet with local government officials within the boundaries of the geographic regions already sketched out. If most of their electors were agreeable, they could set up a health region board and apportion costs for all the local governments within the region.[137] Initially, the local governments most responsive to the HSPC's calls to establish health regions were in the more southern areas of the province, Health Regions No. 1 (Swift Current), No. 3 (Weyburn-Estevan), and No. 6 (Moose Jaw).

In the HSPC blueprint of 15 February 1945, each health region was designed to be a complete health services unit, including public health infrastructure and services, regional, district, and local hospitals, and health centres all connected by the region's medical officer of health and regional health boards drawn from local governments. Physicians working in outlying areas, supported by public health nurses and specialists at the regional and district levels, would be responsible for school health, immunization, as well as maternal and child welfare.[138]

This kind of primary health care, which combined population-based preventive services with individual patient consultation and treatment, required salary rather than fee-for-service remuneration to work effectively. However, given T.C.'s compromise with the CPS, the best that Mindel Sheps and her tiny staff could do was continue to encourage municipalities to hire doctors on salary. To this end, she prepared a model physician salary contract for use by the RMs.[139] To countervail Sheps, Clarence Houston rapidly prepared a competing "model" fee-for-service municipal doctor contract, but the HSPC provincial grants continued to go to municipalities hiring doctors on salary.[140]

Despite hiring new staff into the HSPC by the summer of 1945, Mindel Sheps simply did not have enough personnel to carry out the commission's bold plan for rural Saskatchewan. As she explained in a letter to Henry Sigerist in August 1945, such limitations meant that the HSPC could not arrange, much less attend, enough meetings in the many

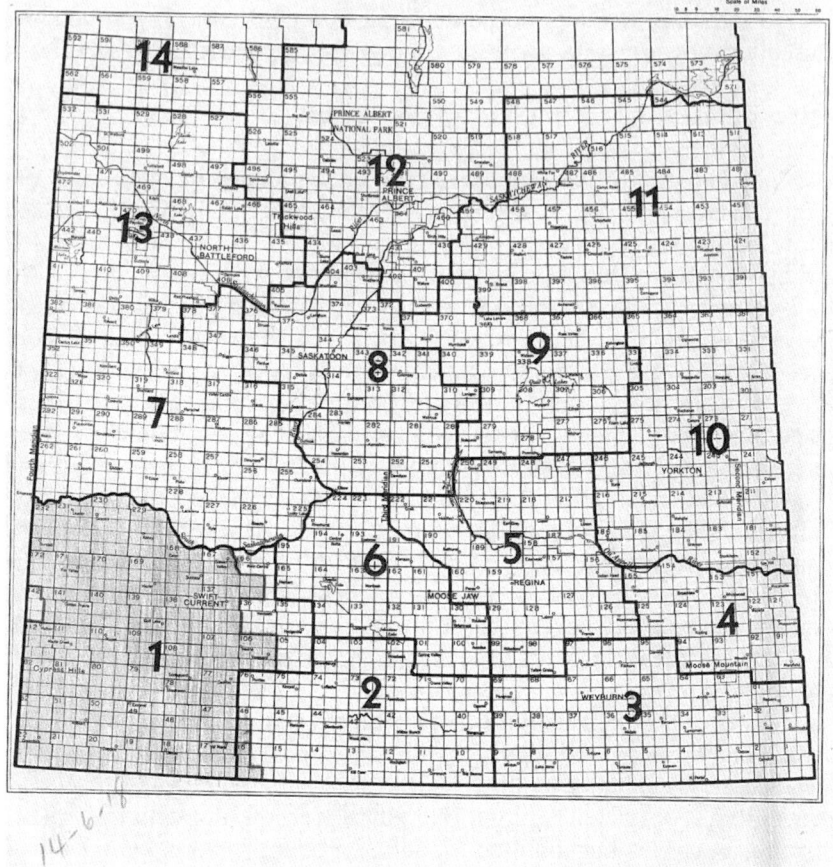

The Health Services and Planning Commission's tentative map of fourteen health regions, 24 November 1945 (PAS, T.C. Douglas fonds, R-33.5, III.122a)

communities interested in the idea of setting up a health region. "We have been forced" she explained to Sigerist, "to deal with Municipal councils largely by letter" – in her view, "not a very satisfactory way of doing things."[141] She decided it was time to try a different approach.

Working in partnership with the provincial government's newly formed Adult Education Division, Sheps hoped to set up citizen conferences in the areas where local governments were interested in becoming part of a health region. She designed a template agenda for each of these conferences addressing: 1) the organization of health services in other countries; 2) the social aspects of medicine – what she and Sigerist understood as socialized medicine; 3) federal-provincial plans for health services; and 4) panel discussions on the particular health service problems most prominent in the area where the conference was being held. She hoped that "from these conferences there will grow communities" who will be more prepared "to see that their local services are surveyed and that a health region is organized."[142]

That summer, the Adult Education Division and the HSPC held citizen conferences in the towns of Kamsack, Saltcoats, Canora, and Sturgis to drum up local support for the establishment of a health region.[143] Little did Mindel Sheps know that Watson Thomson, director of the Adult Education Division, would soon be fired by the government and the division shuttered. By the time she had developed her conference arrangements, the Adult Education Division was already in the bad books of cabinet.[144] At least some members of cabinet believed that Thomson had close ties to the Labour-Progressive Party – the legal front for the Communist Party of Canada after the latter was banned during the Second World War. But Douglas had hired Thomson despite complaints from a few of his colleagues in the national CCF about the latter's ideology and loyalties. Within months, however, Woodrow Lloyd, Douglas's minister of education, who had originally encouraged the establishment of the Adult Education Division, was beginning to have his doubts. Douglas was also contacted by M.J. Coldwell, who raised further concerns. Coldwell wrote Douglas that, while Thomson might "not be a communist – or even a fellow traveller – the Communist Party is out to wreck the CCF" and was manipulating sympathetic activists such as Thomson to do its bidding. Coldwell and the national executive had clear evidence that Thomson had been speaking at events he knew full well were co-sponsored by the Labour-Progressive Party. By supporting the communists in this way, Thomson "ought not to be in a position of trust anywhere in our movement," warned Coldwell.[145]

Not aware of the extent to which Thomson and the Adult Education Division had come under a cloud, Mindel Sheps continued work on the citizen conferences to help get regionalization back on track. She begged Sigerist to consider either coming to Saskatchewan to present in person, or at least record, a twenty-to-thirty-minute speech on health systems throughout the world that could be accompanied by film visuals.[146] Although Sigerist liked the idea of the citizens' conferences, he very courteously declined due to his many publication commitments and deadlines, the pressures of which were, as always, causing him perpetual insomnia and periodic bouts of illness.[147] In the end, his absence didn't matter, because the whole effort collapsed when Thomson was fired and the Adult Education Division permanently shuttered.

The episode seemed emblematic of Mindel Sheps's growing frustration at the time. She simply had too few staff to meet the premier's ambitious timelines for forming health regions. Moreover, Douglas's insistence on working through, and compromising with, the existing structures and interest groups, from the hundreds of local governments to the professional associations, especially the physicians, presented enormous daily challenges for the HSPC. Adding to Sheps's workload, he also wanted one of the new health regions to act as a pilot project for what he soon hoped would be a provincial health insurance plan.

In response to Mindel Sheps's attempt to focus the HSPC's limited resources more effectively, Paul Dodd, a consulting economist from the University of California, Los Angeles, was hired to do an analysis of the health region most likely able to set up and manage a program of health coverage.[148] By the time Dodd delivered his report, however, local governments were pushing the pace and making decisions that would determine the pilot project. Local governments in proposed Health Region No. 1 (Swift Current) and No. 3 (Weyburn-Estevan) were both prepared to go beyond the public health and health centre mandate of health regions to introduce health coverage for their populations. In local referendums, each promised to establish universal hospital coverage programs, but local governments in Swift Current had gone even further, with a pledge to also cover all physician care.[149]

Given its limited local resources and infrastructure, Swift Current was far from the ideal model, but this mattered little to the very energetic local politicians in the region and the farmers, ranchers, and small-town business owners they served.[150] Weyburn-Estevan was a little better, but still hardly ideal. According to the detailed analysis by Dodd, proposed Health Region No. 6 (Moose Jaw) was preferable for a health insurance pilot, as it had better hospitals, more doctors, better-off farmers, a deeper tax base, and a less dispersed population than other potential health regions.

The southwest corner of Saskatchewan bordering Montana and Alberta, which encompassed the Swift Current health region, had suffered more than any other part of the province from the drought and depression of the 1930s.[151] Residents there responded by using their local governments to provide essential health services. By the time the Douglas government had been elected, four RMs in the region (and some participating village governments within their respective boundaries) were running municipal doctor plans. There were three existing union hospitals, while the hospitals in Maple Creek and Swift Current were in the process of being converted into union hospitals to serve the surrounding population.[152]

For William J. Burak, an entrepreneurial official in an RM located just northwest of Swift Current, such local efforts, while laudable, were not enough. Burak immediately saw the potential benefit of working with the Douglas government and, in January 1945, he wrote to every local government in the region proposing they work together to establish a health region offering a comprehensive suite of health services. They agreed but had to wait, impatiently, for six months before the regulations under the Health Services Act on the process of setting up a health region were finalized. Once the process was set out – a petition with a required number of signatures followed by a local referendum – Burak and other local politicians went right to work.

In August 1945, when Mindel Sheps was in Swift Current to discuss the establishment of a union hospital district, she was shocked by how much groundwork had already been laid by the municipalities to establish the health region.[153] She informed her boss, and both readily accepted the inevitable: the provincial government would fully support Swift Current in its bid to become the province's experiment in health insurance.[154] After Mindel Sheps returned to Regina, the organization of Health Region No. 1 moved at breakneck speed. Five days after his meeting with Sheps, Burak sent a long letter to the thirty-one RMs and forty-three city, town, and village governments in the region.

In mid-September in Swift Current, Burak hosted a meeting involving forty-one of the eighty-eight local governments in the region. He was assisted by two key HSPC officials – Tommy McLeod and a new employee, Dr. Orville Hjertaas, a recent medical graduate. At the meeting, Burak stressed the merits of comprehensive health insurance, while McLeod and Hjertaas tried to get Burak and the local government representatives to focus more on the need for more doctors, hospitals, and public health personnel and facilities before jumping to health insurance. Yet, even the HSPC officials realized as they travelled throughout the region in the weeks following that the principal reason for support from the new region was the provision of health insurance.[155]

The municipal vote was scheduled for 26 November, a day on which electors in the Swift Current and the Weyburn-Estevan regions would decide the fate of the government's regionalization plan. While Douglas, Sheps, and McLeod prepared radio broadcasts to promote the merits of regionalization, Hjertaas made the same arguments in person at farms and in villages and towns.[156] In his radio broadcast, T.C. emphasized the desperate need in rural communities for public health and preventive services. He downplayed the utility of regions providing health insurance at that point because he thought the provincial and federal governments were on the cusp of concluding an agreement for the provision of comprehensive health coverage for all Canadians. In this, and will be seen in the next chapter, he would soon be proven wrong.[157]

To the relief of T.C. and his HSPC team, electors in both areas voted in favour of establishing health regions, with 71 per cent of voters in the Swift Current region approving the initiative. This percentage would have been higher except for the lukewarm support of residents in the urban municipalities of Swift Current and Shaunavon, who perhaps were not keen about sharing their municipal hospitals with those who resided outside their towns. A few rural municipalities in the northeastern part of the region had also voted against the proposal and were excluded from the scheme. In early December, the Douglas government passed an order in council to authorize the establishment of the two health regions.[158] Now, the only thing left was to form a regional health board. In the Swift Current Health Region, each local government council appointed representatives to the four district councils in the region, with the members of the district councils forming the regional health board. For the HSPC team, "this democratic structure" provided "a very useful two-way channel from the local municipal council" to the health region board.[159]

**Showdown with the Doctors, December 1945**

The way seemed clear for progress on more health regions, except for the continuing opposition by the College of Physicians and Surgeons. After demanding (yet another) private meeting with Douglas without the presence of the HSPC team, a six-person delegation from the college trooped in the premier's office at 8:00 p.m. on 30 December 1945. Beside T.C. was his deputy minister of public health, Clarence Hames. Once again, the CPS threatened to withdraw its support for the government's efforts to set up health regions and health centres unless Douglas disbanded the HSPC.

Douglas was blunt in reply. In the absence of any concrete evidence demonstrating the incompetence and inflexibility of Sheps and McLeod, T.C. refused to get "rid of any personnel," even if the college placed "a pistol" to "his head." The doctors changed the subject by repeating some gossip that Mindel Sheps would soon be leaving the HSPC for "family reasons." T.C. confirmed that Mindel had decided to step back in order to care for a recently adopted child and that he would appoint her husband, Cecil, as the temporary chair of the HSPC. The suggestion was poorly received, as Douglas must have known it would be, although the CPS was somewhat assuaged by the information that Cecil would soon be leaving Saskatchewan to pursue graduate education in the United States.[160]

Hames then intervened with a surprising statement – that the government was hoping to hire Dr. Fred Mott, the deputy surgeon general in the United States, because of his experience in organizing six agricultural regions as a senior New Deal official. Douglas jumped in, making it clear that there was no guarantee that Dr. Mott would "be available" for the position. At this point, other names for the chair were suggested by the CPS. Unwisely, though, the college members then attacked Tommy McLeod, and T.C. lost his temper, insisting that McLeod had always acted properly, and testily remarking that he himself was not an idiot and knew very well what was going on in his own government. If the college no longer had "confidence in his judgement" or "integrity," then "he would be glad to consider any other member" of his cabinet for the "position of Minister of Health." Adjourning the meeting to the next day on this sour note, he informed the CPS that his HSPC officials would be joining him for all future meetings.[161]

The following day, Douglas led the discussion with the doctors but deferred to HSPC staff on technical matters, even allowing himself to be corrected on details by Mindel Sheps. He "opened the discussions by pointing out that votes taken in the Swift Current area and the Weyburn-Estevan area had favoured the organization of Health Regions." While the doctors supported the new public health functions of health regions, they were against health regions organizing and administering curative care through health centres, reorganized hospitals, and health coverage programs.[162]

Despite his difficulties with organized medicine, Douglas was optimistic. Federal-provincial negotiations for a pan-Canadian program of comprehensive health insurance were going well, and soon, he thought, his government would have a substantial influx of federal cash to fund the comprehensive health services he had promised in 1944. It was all going so fast that his original need to get Swift Current operating as an experiment in health insurance might not even have been necessary. He would soon see how wrong he was.

# 5 Rise and Fall of the Green Book Proposals

Between August 1945 and May 1946, Tommy Douglas was absorbed by successive meetings of the Dominion-Provincial Reconstruction Conference convened by Prime Minister Mackenzie King. The ultimate failure of this conference would force him to revise his own ambitions to provide all Saskatchewan residents with full and free access to a comprehensive range of health services. The choice was stark: either he abandon his promise and wait patiently for a future federal proposal or go it alone with a more modest program of coverage. He would choose the latter, designing, financing, and delivering North America's first universal hospital insurance program.

Before that story is told in the next chapter, it is important to understand the nature of the Green Book proposals – a set of federal proposals covering public infrastructure investments and new social welfare measures – in the federal-provincial context of the day. This chapter examines how T.C. thought he could use Green Book proposals to achieve comprehensive health coverage during the CCF's first term of office in Saskatchewan and put in place other aspects of a modern welfare state, including a public pension plan and more extensive unemployment insurance. Notwithstanding the failure of the Dominion-Provincial Reconstruction Conference, Douglas would use the Green Book proposals for the rest of his political career as the gold standard for what he felt should have been the country's post-war aspirations.

## Saskatchewan and the Origins of the Dominion-Provincial Reconstruction Conference

While the Dominion-Provincial Reconstruction Conference of 1945–6 provided a national venue for Douglas to expound his vision of a post-war Canada, the context for the conference long predated the election

Table 5.1. Ratio of relief costs to revenues: Severity of fiscal burden in provinces, 1930–7

| Province | Total relief spending in province relative to total provincial revenues (%) | Relative severity of burden index (national average = 100) |
|---|---|---|
| **Saskatchewan** | **13.3** | **367** |
| Manitoba | 4.2 | 115 |
| Alberta | 3.6 | 100 |
| British Columbia | 3.6 | 100 |
| Quebec | 3.2 | 90 |
| Prince Edward Island | 2.8 | 76 |
| Ontario | 2.7 | 76 |
| Nova Scotia | 2.5 | 70 |
| New Brunswick | 2.4 | 67 |
| **All provinces – average** | **3.6** | **100** |

Source: *Report of the Royal Commission on Dominion-Provincial Relations: Book I – Canada 1867–1939* (Ottawa: King's Printer, 1940), 164 (table 58).

of the CCF. In brief, the near bankruptcy of the three Prairie provinces during the Great Depression produced a federal review.[1] When William J. Patterson's Liberal government presented the Saskatchewan case in 1937 to the Royal Commission on Dominion-Provincial Relations, commonly known as the Rowell-Sirois Commission, the case was made that provincial revenue sources were incapable of dealing with the crisis, including the cost of providing relief to destitute farmers and the businesses that supplied them with seed, fuel, clothing, and food. Moreover, as explained by the Saskatchewan government, provincial and local governments were increasingly being asked to subsidize hospitals and even physicians whose patients were unable to pay their bills. Even the opposition CCF under George Williams was pleased with the provincial government's arguments to the royal commission.[2]

These arguments were not exaggerated. Based on the evidence amassed by the Rowell-Sirois Commission, it was clear that the burden of relief facing provincial and local governments was inversely related to those governments' abilities to pay. Based on the ratio of provincial relief spending to provincial revenues, Saskatchewan was in a league of its own, with over 13 per cent of all provincial revenues spent on relief from 1930 to 1937. As illustrated in table 5.1, even among the other beleaguered provincial governments in western Canada, the fraction of revenues spent on relief was miniscule compared to that of Saskatchewan. In its presentation to the commission, the Saskatchewan government urged Ottawa to "assume exclusive rights to income and corporate taxes and succession duties" and, in return, give the provinces "unconditional grants" adjusted for "fiscal need."[3]

In the end, the Rowell-Sirois Commission would use the imbalance between provincial revenue capacity and growing social program responsibilities to recommend a permanent system of national adjustment grants to enable provinces like Saskatchewan to provide "adequate" public services "without excessive taxation," based on the "average Canadian standard."[4] These adjustment grants would be large enough for provincial governments to finance growing social expenditures, especially given, as the royal commission put it, "the economic and social changes of the past seventy years," which "have made necessary state activities and state expenditures on health matters to an extent undreamed of by the Fathers [of Confederation]."[5] In return for these adjustment grants from Ottawa, "the provinces should withdraw entirely" from the fields of income tax (personal and corporate) and inheritance tax.[6]

The 1940 Rowell-Sirois Report was well-received in Saskatchewan by the governing Liberals. It was also welcomed by Douglas, who was spending almost as much time in the province as he was in Ottawa. Book II of the report began with a statement that accorded with Douglas's view of the world: the "maximum welfare" of all citizens was the goal of government, which should not only facilitate economic growth but also distribute the fruits of that growth more effectively and provide greater social and economic security. The Canadian constitution should serve these purposes; if it did not, it needed to be changed. The commission's view of a modern Canadian society in which government – not the market – would largely be responsible for the provision of health services reflected the position staked out by Douglas and the CCF since the 1933 Regina Manifesto.[7]

In January 1941, Prime Minister King convened a meeting with the provincial premiers to consider the Rowell-Sirois recommendations. While both Premier John Bracken of Manitoba and Premier Patterson of Saskatchewan made a concerted pitch for Ottawa to adopt the commission's main recommendations, the fiscal recommendations were strongly opposed by the premiers of Ontario, Alberta, and British Columbia, who, while allowing for a temporary "renting" of tax fields, given the wartime emergency, would not countenance a permanent change.[8] In the end, the governments of Saskatchewan and Manitoba were denied the fiscal changes they were seeking, and it would take almost two decades more before the adoption of a system of adjustment grants – what became known as equalization. As an MP in Ottawa and then as premier of Saskatchewan, Douglas continually advocated in favour of implementing the recommendations of the Rowell-Sirois Commission.[9]

In the years following the Dominion-Provincial Conference of 1941, the King government would, for some time, tack to the left in its social policy thinking. In part, this was a response to a rethinking of the role of the state that was part of a larger transnational movement, of which the 1942 Beveridge Report in the United Kingdom was the most impactful.[10] The Liberals under King were also responding to political trends, especially the growing popularity of the CCF in Ontario and the West.

**The Federal Government's Health Insurance Proposals**

After spending close to a decade in the House of Commons, from 1935 until 1944, Douglas was familiar with various members of the federal cabinet through their speeches and actions. In the small, clubby atmosphere of Parliament in the 1930s and early 1940s, he had gotten to know some well. While he respected and even liked some of the more progressive Liberal MPs, he disliked others for their constant defence of the status quo.

Among those parliamentarians T.C. disliked, the MP who stood in a league of his own was Jimmy Gardiner. As the former Saskatchewan premier and Mackenzie King's long-time minister of agriculture, Gardiner ran a patronage system in Saskatchewan that was a continuing annoyance to Douglas. T.C.'s disdain was fully reciprocated by Gardiner, who felt that the Weburn MP had fooled the electorate into believing that the CCF's brand of socialism was benign. In T.C.'s mind, Gardiner exemplified the attitude among some Liberals that they were entitled to power. The debates between the two men in the House of Commons were legendary for their sarcasm and low blows.[11] In one stormy encounter in the House, after being constantly interrupted, Douglas finally stopped the diminutive Gardiner by saying: "I don't want any more interruptions. If the Minister of Agriculture will sit up in his chair and dangle his feet, I'll go on with what I have to say." According to Douglas, Gardiner never forgave him for the slight, despite the fact that T.C. himself was no taller.[12]

T.C.'s attitude towards Mackenzie King was more complicated. During his years as an MP, he had got to know King better than did most opposition MPs. He came to see him as a do-nothing PM who avoided any decision or action unless forced into a corner. As Frank Scott would later remark, under the heavy "smoke-screen of his politics," King was also ingenious in his "ambiguity, inactivity, and political longevity."[13] At the same time, T.C. respected King's political savvy and his graciousness in the corridors and the chamber of Parliament. For his part, King thought Douglas was a remarkable politician with great skills as a debater. He liked Douglas and occasionally even confided in him to an extent, perhaps in part because T.C. appeared to resemble King's only brother, who had died years before.[14] In his diary, King described him as "a man of high ideals" and a far "better leader" than William Patterson, Gardiner's Liberal successor in Saskatchewan, whom King described as "heavy, lethargic and less idealistic."[15] Under King, the federal government had done extensive work on social security and, as discussed in chapter 3, had seen considerable promise in the Marsh and Heagerty Reports of 1943.[16]

In 1943, King made Brooke Claxton his parliamentary secretary. He soon assigned Claxton the task of being a liaison between his cabinet committees on reconstruction and an interdepartmental committee of senior officials who were working almost full-time on a set of proposals for a new welfare state inspired by the Beveridge Report but highly adapted to Canada's federal context. The Marsh and Heagerty Reports were used as the starting point for the drafting by these officials of what would become known as the Green Book (the colour of the cover). The Green Book's social welfare measures were made up of two new programs, one for comprehensive health coverage and the other for public pensions, as well as an expansion of the existing unemployment insurance program.[17]

Having rubbed shoulders with members of the League for Social Reconstruction in the early 1930s, Claxton was one of the more progressive MPs in the Liberal caucus. He struck the prime minister as an effective administrator and, in October 1944, King appointed him minister of the brand-new Department of National Health and Welfare. Claxton was largely responsible for iterative drafts of the Green Book proposals as they moved from the bureaucrats to the cabinet committees, each word scrutinized, changed, or approved.[18] The resulting fifty-two-page document would be tabled with the premiers and their delegations at the opening of the Dominion-Provincial Reconstruction Conference in August 1945.[19]

In advance of King's formal letter of invitation to the conference, all the provincial premiers received a memorandum of suggestions for the agenda, which featured the topic "Public Welfare and Social Security," under which was placed "health insurance and disability benefits." Douglas's copy of the memorandum features his scribbled marginalia referring to two items most on his mind at the time, the Heagerty Report and Saskatchewan's continuing need for additional health personnel and facilities.[20] Coverage alone, without adequate hospital facilities, diagnostic equipment, and a sufficient number of doctors, nurses, X-ray technicians, and many other specialized health workers, would be a chimera.

The precise timing of the proposed conference was another sore spot. King initially delayed having the meeting in 1944 after the Normandy landings had shifted the tide in favour of the Allies. This date would have coincided with the CCF's election in Saskatchewan. Yet when George Drew, the Progressive Conservative (PC) premier of Ontario, proclaimed that his main purpose was to bring down the federal Liberal government, King delayed the conference until after the 1945 Ontario and federal elections, in the hope that Drew would be defeated and King himself would be re-elected.[21] In an effort to throw the PCs off their game, King set the federal election for 11 June, the day that Drew had already selected for the Ontario election, prompting the furious premier to reschedule the provincial election a week earlier. The grudge match between the two would continue after the elections, which returned both of their governments.

**Breakthrough Denied: The CCF and the Federal Election of 1945**

CCFers throughout the country believed the 1945 federal election would be the party's great breakthrough. Beyond the momentous victory in Saskatchewan the year before, the party had gained enough ground in the 1943 Ontario election to become the official opposition, a status it had also enjoyed in British Columbia since 1941.[22] A *Toronto Star* editorial captured the prevailing sentiment: "Whatever else the electors may have known or felt about CCF policies, many did feel that this party was facing forward, and that its older rivals, though moving somewhat, were still looking back wistfully over their shoulders to a social order which is no longer acceptable."[23]

In the preface to their 1943 book *Make This Your Canada*, David Lewis, the CCF's national secretary, and Frank Scott, its national chair, emphasized not only the gains in Ontario but the fact that the CCF had won two federal by-elections only five days after the 4 August provincial election in Ontario.[24] The party's momentum was growing. In the months following the Ontario election, Gallup public opinion polls showed the CCF growing rapidly in popularity among voters, with one poll even showing the CCF slightly ahead of both the Liberals and the Progressive Conservatives.[25]

In anticipation of the 1945 federal election, M.J. Coldwell's *Left Turn, Canada* was rapidly published. In it, the federal leader of the CCF pointed to Saskatchewan as a key example of the progressive

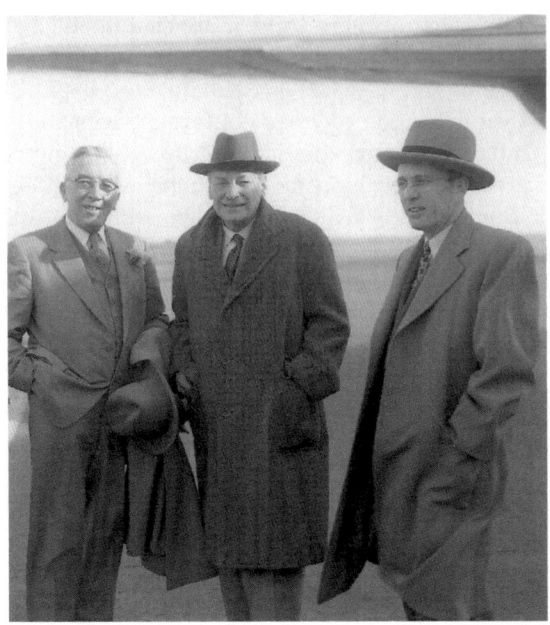

From left to right, M.J. Coldwell, British prime minister Clement Attlee, and T.C., during Attlee's visit to Canada in November 1945 (PAS R-LP1705)

governance Canadians could expect if the CCF gained national office or held the balance of power in a minority government.[26] *Left Turn, Canada* presented the party's lengthy election manifesto, which included a "socialized health service aimed at providing a national standard of health care in every part of Canada." Contributing to the party's momentum was the media's reporting on the growing popularity of the Labour Party in the United Kingdom under the leadership of Clement Attlee and the general feeling that social democracy was on the rise with the end of the war.

The federal CCF's platform on comprehensive health insurance included "full medical and dental care" and full hospital coverage in regular hospitals, psychiatric hospitals, tuberculosis sanitariums, and rehabilitation facilities. The CCF promise also included the establishment of "health centres in rural as well as urban communities, to bring medical care within the reach of all" – in order words, the regionalized health centre system that Douglas was trying to implement in Saskatchewan. Encompassing preventive and public health services, the CCF's commitment included regular medical "check-ups for all citizens, particularly school and pre-school children," a "national food policy, based on modern nutritional standards," and the funding of programs for "research in health and medicine" and public "education in health and nutrition." Public funding would be made available for the education and training of "doctors, dentists, and nurses," and the supply of health professionals in Canada would be increased.[27]

The CCF's platform on socialized health service, endorsed by the Canadian Labour Congress as well as the country's largest farm lobby, the Canadian Federation of Agriculture, pushed the Liberals into action. Mackenzie King and his Liberal candidates promised to work out a deal for national health insurance with the provinces at the Dominion-Provincial Reconstruction Conference scheduled for after the election.[28]

Similarly campaigning on a promise to establish socialized health services, the Ontario CCF were also facing an election slated for early June 1945. To support the Ontario candidates, M.J. Coldwell as national leader and Douglas as the only CCF provincial premier went on a speaking tour in Ontario while simultaneously seeking support for the imminent federal election. At the same time, the Labor-Progressive Party (the renamed Communist Party of Canada) contested thirty-seven seats, twenty-seven of which were held by CCF members of the Provincial Parliament, in a bid to destroy its closest rival in that province. Scheduled one week before the federal election, the Ontario election outcome would set the stage for the national contest.[29] Despite its best efforts, the results were disastrous for the CCF. It lost twenty-six of the thirty-four seats it had won in the previous election, while its share of the popular vote dropped ten points, from 33 to 23 per cent. Within weeks, the Ontario CCF had gone from looking like it would form the second provincial social democratic government in Canada, to a minor third party.[30]

Even though the provincial Liberals had also lost to Drew's Conservatives, Mackenzie King understood immediately that the CCF no longer posed a threat to the federal Liberals and that his party's victory was assured. Coldwell too realized that momentum had shifted from the CCF to the Liberals. Both were correct. In the national election, the CCF won twenty-eight seats, an increase of twenty and better than Social Credit's thirteen, but far less than the advance polling had suggested and certainly far beneath the party's hopes and expectations.

Like his counterparts in Parliament and the CCF's National Office, T.C. was deeply disappointed in the election results. After years of public opinion surveys showing national CCF gains at the expense of the establishment parties as well as provincial gains west of Quebec, especially the victory in Saskatchewan, the CCF was unable to gain the seats required to form the government in another province. Worse, just when it seemed that the CCF had a real shot at becoming the official opposition in Ottawa, it had to accept third-party status in a Parliament controlled by a Liberal majority.[31]

The election over, the King government felt confident going into the Dominion-Provincial Reconstruction Conference. Before this election outcome, King had felt pressure to initiate CCF-style reforms to channel to itself some of the momentum of the socialist juggernaut.[32] However, after the election, his enthusiasm for national health insurance faded with the removal of the CCF as a major political threat.[33]

**The Dominion-Provincial Reconstruction Conference Begins**

The initial session of the conference in August 1945 was T.C.'s introduction to the federal-provincial relations stage. Desiring federal financial support for a comprehensive program of health insurance, old age pensions, and income supports, he mobilized his advisors in advance to prepare Saskatchewan's position and draft his opening speech. He saw the conference as an opportunity to build a new welfare state that reflected the values and policy elements of the CCF. Among these elements was federal responsibility for the economy, including the willingness to keep unemployment to a minimum through two means: first, a system of social security that would help fund provincial health programs; and second, Keynesian counter-cyclical fiscal spending to prevent the repeat of another Great Depression.

From the beginning, the federal government's quid pro quo was clear. It would cover 60 per cent of provincial costs of comprehensive health insurance. In return, the provinces would have to agree to a more permanent version of the temporary wartime tax agreements that had bolstered the government of Canada's share of tax revenues relative to that of the provinces.[34] T.C. felt that this was a reasonable demand. Now it was time to work out the details.

The first session lasted five days. Douglas already had Frank Scott call upon his friends and contacts in Ottawa to get some advance intelligence on the federal negotiating position.[35] Joined by five ministers, two senior public servants, and two advisors, Douglas's provincial delegation was comparable in size to the other Western provincial delegations but considerably smaller than Ontario's thirty-member contingent. But most striking of all was the size of the federal delegation, which numbered fifty-nine advisors and civil servants as well as twenty ministers, including Prime Minister King.[36] The federal government,

## Rise and Fall of the Green Book Proposals   133

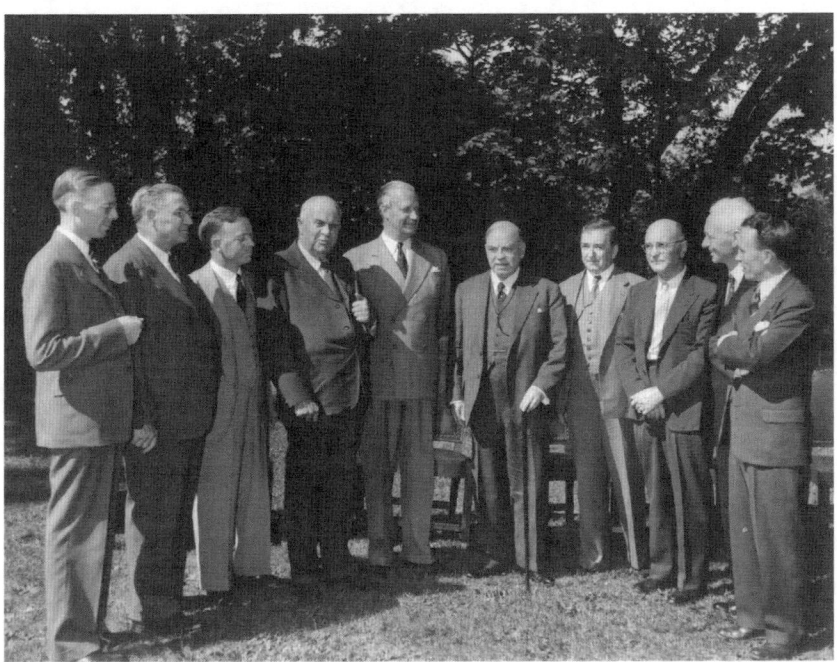

Prime Minister Mackenzie King and premiers at the Dominion-Provincial Conference on Reconstruction (Ernest Manning at far left and T.C. at far right), August 1945 (PAS R-B28897)

having grown by leaps and bounds during the war, was at the peak of its influence over the provinces and was supported by a corps of public service mandarins with a scope and expertise unmatched in the provinces, although Douglas was quickly assembling a group that would, in quality if not quantity, be regarded as equal to the Ottawa bureaucracy.[37]

From the beginning, Douglas understood that he would have few allies among the provincial premiers. Based on the intelligence he had received in advance of the conference, he knew that George Drew of Ontario and Maurice Duplessis of Quebec would oppose the federal proposals. Both premiers were hostile to any major expansion of the welfare state and to federal authority over what they viewed as provincial jurisdiction.[38] Knowing he could never convince them otherwise, Douglas set out to find common ground among the other premiers. It was a tall order.

While the three Maritime premiers, all Liberals, were more flexible in their views, they were not especially enamored of embarking on any bold welfare state experiments, especially Alexander MacMillan of Nova Scotia, who was the oldest first minister and about to retire. MacMillan and his successor, Angus Macdonald, were closer to Drew and Duplessis's views on the federation than were the Liberal premiers of New Brunswick, Prince Edward Island, and Manitoba.[39] John Hart of British Columbia, the head of a Liberal-Conservative coalition directed against the CCF, could hardly be expected to support a CCF premier.[40] And then there was Ernest Manning, the Social Credit premier of Alberta. A conservative evangelical Christian, Manning was fundamentally opposed to both Douglas's brand of Christian socialism and the idea of the welfare state. However, Manning, who grew up in rural Saskatchewan during the Great Depression, recognized the inadequacies of the status quo and agreed that the poor needed better access to health insurance.[41]

Like all the other premiers and their delegations, Douglas had been presented with a copy of the federal government's Green Book proposals at the beginning of the conference. The "National Health Programme" was the first of three major items in the book under the broad heading of social security.[42]

On 6 August, with the delegations convened in the House of Commons chamber, King called on the provinces to work in "partnership" with the federal government for "the maintenance of a high level of employment and income" along with "the promotion of the welfare of the Canadian people." These measures included the establishment of "a comprehensive system of social insurance, partially federal and partially provincial, through which the community will share with the individual in meeting the variations of income and expense to which the rise and fall of business activity, natural disasters, accident, ill health and old age render us all liable."[43]

King's words matched T.C.'s hopes for the conference, but he also knew that the support of other provinces would be necessary to push the prime minister into action. These were costly measures, and King could simply blame the premiers if the proposals were never enacted, while taking credit for the initiative. If some of the premiers argued against the permanent tax transfer and others were against the health insurance proposal and other Green Book social measures, they, not him, would be responsible for the failed discussions.[44]

After his opening remarks, King had hoped to have his key ministers present the details of the federal proposals. Instead, George Drew sprang to his feet, citing objection after objection concerning the agenda and the procedures King wanted followed at the conference. Although annoyed, King's personal frustration with Drew was temporarily assuaged when two pieces of news were delivered to him while the Ontario premier was speaking. The first was that King had won his by-election in the Ontario riding of Glengarry (after having been defeated in the Saskatchewan constituency of Prince Albert in the 1945 election), and the second was that the Americans had dropped an atomic bomb on the Japanese city of Hiroshima, an event he felt was bound to hasten the end of the war in the Pacific.[45]

According to Tommy McLeod, who was in the room with Douglas, King "arose from his place at the end of the conference table and said he was about to make one of the most important announcements of his career." Some of the premiers "snickered, thinking that King might be jokingly preparing to pass on a trivial message" but, instead, he "read a statement" informing the stunned group about the dropping of the first atomic bomb. During the break that followed King's announcement, McLeod found one of Saskatchewan's part-time advisors, Frederick Cronkite, the dean of the law school at the University of Saskatchewan and a holdover from the previous Liberal administration, speaking to "the white tile wall in front of him" that the atomic bomb was "the end of God."[46]

After King's astonishing news, the premiers rose to speak in order of their province's entry into Confederation – a long-standing convention in federal-provincial relations in Canada. As Drew had already spoken, Duplessis was next. Uncompromising in his demand for the return of fiscal powers and tax authority to Quebec and for Ottawa to respect the constitutional division of powers, Duplessis argued that the "Federal government is the child of Provincial governments" and expressed his "hope that the child will never undertake the absorption of the mother."[47]

By the time the premiers of Nova Scotia, New Brunswick, Manitoba, British Columbia, and Prince Edward Island had spoken, it was close to 3:30 p.m., and Douglas's turn at long last. He jumped straight to the point that his province was "not only desirous of co-operating with the Dominion government and the other provincial governments" but that he was "prepared to do everything" in his government's "power to ensure the success of the Conference."[48] With his carefully prepare remarks in front of him, Douglas then suggested that any written provincial proposals also be made public, given the fact that the federal government had just released its Green Book proposals. The idea did not go down well with Duplessis, who formally opposed Douglas's recommendation on the basis that the provinces "were not called upon to produce memoranda" and that this procedure would prejudice those provinces, like Quebec, that had not prepared a formal written proposal.[49]

Of course, the real reason for Duplessis's objections was that he was vehemently opposed to Ottawa trying to horn in on programs and policies that, for him, were clearly within the constitutional jurisdiction of the provinces. Moreover, he was ideologically and instinctively against the kind of welfare state envisaged in the Green Book proposals and did not want to see provincial proposals expanding upon, or refining, the Green Book proposals to make them even more acceptable to the premiers around the table.[50] Douglas, as the country's sole CCF government leader, represented a trend towards socialism, which the premier of Quebec abhorred. For his part, Douglas regarded Duplessis as a fascist, a perception reinforced by Frank Scott, who had been outraged by Duplessis's infringement of civil liberties, including through the infamous Padlock Act of 1937, which had empowered the Quebec attorney general to close, for one year, any building used for propagating "communism or bolshevism," terms that the act did not define.[51]

In the evening session after the premiers' speeches, Douglas's attention was focused on the federal government's proposals on social security, including health insurance, as presented by Brooke Claxton. The time had come, Claxton stated, for Canada to adopt a system of health insurance. Given the federal nature of the country and its constitution, this meant that the provincial governments should administer the program but under some basic national standards and principles, in return for which the federal government was prepared to make a major grant contribution.

Comprehensiveness would be achieved in two distinct stages. In the immediate term, health insurance would include hospital care, primary care as provided by general practitioners, and nurse-based home care. In the next phase, coverage would be extended to all specialized medical services, other nursing (mainly institution-based long-term care), prescription drugs, dental care, medical appliances, and diagnostics, including X-rays and the laboratory results for blood tests. He laid out a detailed estimate of the per capita cost of all these services along with the federal contribution as well the federal transfers to each province in the first and second stages of the plan.[52]

Even if he disagreed with some of the details, T.C. was impressed with the degree of precision and planning in the Green Book proposals. In fact, the careful preparation went far beyond anything that had ever before been presented at a federal-provincial conference and reflected the deep expertise that had been developed within the federal

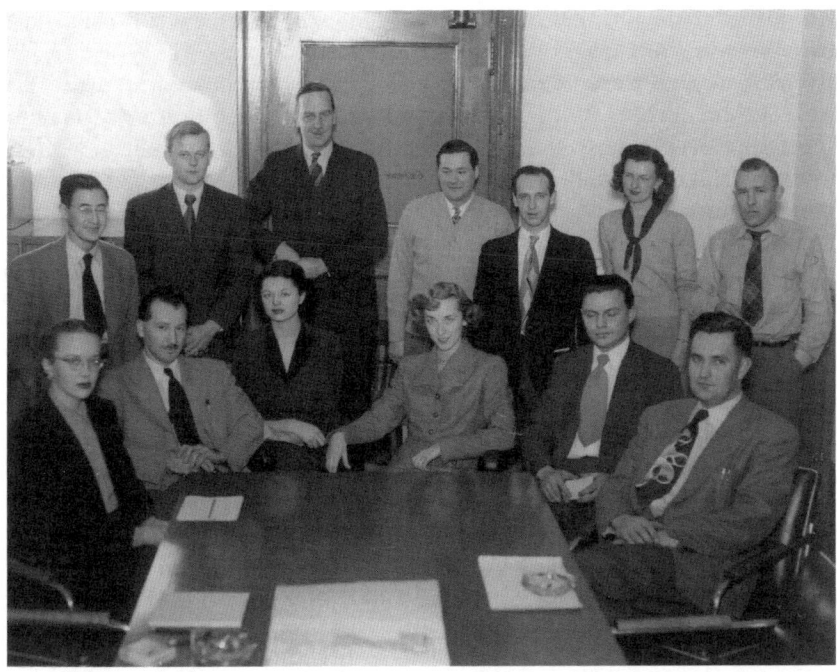

George Cadbury (standing third from left) and the staff of the Economic Advisory and Planning Board, the most powerful central agency in the Douglas government, c. 1948 (PAS R-A8840)

bureaucracy during the depression and Second World War.[53] For his part, Douglas was building the finest provincial public service in the country so that his government would be capable of planning and implementing an even more ambitious agenda of policy change. Just before the conference, he had written Frank Scott at McGill University in Montreal to tell him his plans, including that, until Scott and others could make themselves available, he would continue to retain the services of two noted academics from the University of Saskatchewan, Frederick Cronkite, who was dean of law, and economist George Britnell. Although these two men had helped his government prepare for the conference, neither could connect their sharp analyses of problems to a solution pertinent to the design, implementation, and management of the Douglas government's programs. Douglas needed scholar-practitioners who had these skills. He revealed to Scott that he was about to hire George Cadbury, a British socialist who had originally trained as an economist under John Maynard Keynes and who also had extensive business experience. At this point, Cadbury was working for the British government in the United States. Douglas wanted him to work with Tommy McLeod to assemble a team of economic experts who would be on par with the Ottawa mandarins and their highly skilled personnel, some of whom were providing constant advice to King and his ministers at the Dominion-Provincial Reconstruction Conference.[54]

The conference's second day was focused on fiscal relations, in particular the desire of the federal government to continue the wartime tax-rental agreement and the proposal for a system of regional fiscal redistribution. The latter would allow provinces, such as Saskatchewan, with lower taxation capacity to be able to offer public services such as health insurance at rates of taxation comparable to those of wealthier provinces with deeper tax capacity, such as Ontario and British Columbia. But none of this could ever happen if other first ministers followed the lead of the oppositional premiers of Ontario and Quebec. Douglas tried to convey what he felt was at stake, reminding everyone around the table that they were "meeting at what may well be a turning point in Canadian history." After "ten years of economic depression and five years of war," he went on, Canadians were "looking to this conference for leadership." Failure to reach agreement would have "disastrous results" for all Canadians, while success would "see the Canadian people launched upon an era of economic expansion and social well-being."[55]

It was a cry in the wilderness. T.C. was largely isolated. Even the four Liberal premiers seemed reluctant to support the federal government, prompting Douglas, during a break, to say privately to the prime minister that he and King were "the only Liberals" at the conference.[56] Indeed, the Liberal premiers seemed lukewarm at best on the need for a new and ambitious welfare state as envisioned in the federal Liberals' Green Book proposals.[57] Despite this, Douglas still hoped that the federal money associated with the Green Book proposals – a 60 per cent cost-sharing formula in the case of health insurance – would work its magic, not only among the Liberal premiers but also among the others. In this, he agreed with Alex Skelton, the conference's federal secretary, who originally assumed that the federal offer was "so favourable to the provinces that none could refuse it."[58]

After five days of debate, the conference adjourned, on the understanding that discussions between provincial and federal officials would continue on the details of the federal proposal. At this point, T.C. remained optimistic that an agreement would be reached in the weeks and months ahead. Before the adjournment, it was agreed that an executive committee, the Continuing Coordinating Committee – made up of the prime minister; his finance minister, J.L. Ilsley; his justice minister, Louis St-Laurent; and the nine provincial premiers – would meet when necessary.

## Hopes Rise and Fall

Two weeks after the adjournment, Brooke Claxton asked for T.C.'s advice on the social security portion of the Green Book proposals, while Alex Skelton asked for Tommy McLeod's input on the financing of health insurance and old age pensions.[59] As Ottawa's staunchest ally on the Green Book proposals, the Saskatchewan government began to help the Liberal government tweak the federal proposals in an effort to make them more palatable to the other provinces.

By the time of further in-person meetings in Ottawa in September, Douglas realized that Ontario and Quebec would never agree to a permanent fiscal transfer to Ottawa. Working on the assumption that he might be able to at least salvage the health proposal, T.C. asked Mindel Sheps to prepare a full analysis of the health insurance portion of the Green Book before the meeting.[60] In November, when the Continuing Coordinating Committee met in Ottawa, T.C. made his pitch for a "full consideration" of the health insurance proposal, "irrespective of whether or not agreement" could be reached on the full federal proposal.[61] By this time, the other premiers were picking apart the details of the social security proposals, even as Nova Scotia joined Ontario and Quebec in opposing any continuation of the Wartime Tax Rental Agreement, the legislative vehicle that had transferred tax authority from the provincial governments to the federal government.

For Ottawa, the proposals stood or fell as a package deal. The federal government produced an amended version of its original proposal on the understanding that a further meeting would be held in January to iron out any continuing differences.[62] T.C. and his officials spent weeks carefully preparing a written submission, by far the lengthiest and most detailed provincial response.[63] Going beyond the Green Book proposals with which it agreed, the Saskatchewan brief recommended an additional change drawn from the report of the Royal Commission on Dominion-Provincial Relations in 1940. Douglas wanted a system of equalization, what he called "adjustment grants to assist those Provinces which are exposed by nature to wide fluctuations in income."[64] He was wasting his breath. The January meeting would be derailed by Ontario, which released its own counter-proposal, which was nothing less than a major attack on the Green Book proposals and a resolute rejection of any extension of the Wartime Tax Rental Agreement.

Premier Drew surprised even King and Claxton because, before the meeting, Skelton had led them to believe that Ontario's position had been softening.[65]

Things went from bad to worse by the end of January at the next meeting of the Continuing Coordinating Committee. With Duplessis's full support, Drew doubled down on his criticism of the amended federal proposals, and the meeting ended in acrimony. While the first ministers agreed to reconvene that April, it was all over except for the crying. When the Continuing Coordinating Committee met again on 25 April, some premiers outside central Canada seemed a little more willing to compromise, but when the public portion of the conference began on 29 April, any notion of flexibility disappeared, and the conference was adjourned five days later, never to be reconvened.[66]

In the ensuring months and years, Douglas did everything possible to pressure the King government into reconvening the conference or at least kick-starting a national health insurance program.[67] As he put it to King in November 1946, while there was no value to discussing a possible federal-provincial tax agreement, he nonetheless felt that there could still be "agreement in matters of social security, unemployment, health insurance and old age pensions."[68] Not prepared to take on the extra spending responsibility without a revenue quid pro quo, King rejected the idea. Moreover, he had no intention of calling the premiers back together again unless he knew in advance that the outcome would be successful. One failed conference was enough.

T.C. would never give up trying to get King to reconvene the conference, and, when King was succeeded by Louis St-Laurent, Douglas tried to convince the new prime minister to call a conference on the health insurance portion of the Green Book proposals. By this time, Saskatchewan's hospital plan had been in operation for a year and a half, and British Columbia had just implemented its own plan. These plans, Douglas argued, "are placing a very heavy financial burden upon the individual taxpayer and upon the provincial treasury." But the "widespread acceptance of these hospitalization plans are [sic] ample proof, if proof were needed, of the keen desire on the part of the Canadian people to have some system of prepaid health services established." He believed that "most of the provinces would welcome an opportunity to discuss a health insurance program and the immediate steps that might be taken toward its implementation."[69] From Douglas's perspective, the federal Liberals only wanted the illusion of change – enough to get them re-elected in 1949 – and were never keen on the substance of the economic and social changes in the Green Book proposals.[70]

## Opportunity Lost, Opportunity Gained

In the words of one Canadian historian, the Dominion-Provincial Conference on Reconstruction "was one of the most important in Canadian history – not for what it accomplished, but for what it did not."[71] In the eyes of reformers, its failure marked one of those great lost opportunities in Canada's history, one that would force a piecemeal and glacially slow approach to the emergence of the welfare state in Canada.

Among historians, there has been a polarized debate about who was responsible for the failure of the conference. Was the cause a risk-averse federal government and a prime minister no longer desirous of a welfare state, or was it the intransigence of the governments of Ontario and Quebec?[72] In T.C.'s view, the fault lay mainly with the Liberal government, especially Mackenzie King, whom he felt always had the option of concluding a successful agreement with all the provinces outside of central Canada, leaving open the possibilty for the governments of Ontario and Quebec to enter the agreement later. For Douglas, the failure of the King government to implement the Green Book proposals with a willing coalition of provinces like Saskatchewan "was a tragedy."[73]

The conference's failure triggered more immediate concerns about the future of the Douglas government's agenda. Without federal cost sharing for comprehensive health insurance, T.C. was forced to trim his sails considerably. This had two immediate consequences. The first was that he would have to lengthen the timelines for the establishment of health regions and the associated infrastructure, health personnel, and grants to local governments that were integral to improving the quality and orientation of Saskatchewan's health services, particularly in rural parts of the province. More importantly, the failure of the Green Book proposals forced his government to fund a more modest plan of hospital insurance out of the province's limited revenues.

The reconstruction conference and its accompanying Green Book proposals present a major "what if" in Canadian history. What if the federal government's social policy proposals had been accepted and implemented by both orders of government? Would the country have saved two decades, implementing in the immediate post-war years measures that would take until the late 1960s to finalize? Would Canada have gone even further in evolving the welfare state, to become, along with the Nordic countries, among the most equitable and prosperous societies in the world? Would the country have created a universal health coverage system incorporating a much broader range of services than those ultimately included? Might it even have been able to go beyond health insurance to establish a pan-Canadian health service, thereby anticipating the National Health Service in the United Kingdom? Or would the health insurance program as then enacted have been so defective in terms of value for public money or in meeting its original objectives that it would have been rejected by the 1960s or 1970s, pushing the country in a more pro-market, neoliberal direction?

These questions could produce many alternative histories, but one thing is sure: If the Dominion-Provincial Reconstruction Conference had succeeded and comprehensive health insurance had been introduced immediately after the war in all provinces, Tommy Douglas would have been a far less significant figure in the history of Canada. Universal health coverage, however it evolved over time, would have been initiated by Ottawa rather than Regina, and Douglas might have been just one premier among many implementing a federal design. Our historical attention would have focused far more on Mackenzie King and his ministers of health and welfare (Brooke Claxton and his successor, Paul Martin Sr.), and one key civil servant, J.J. Heagerty, the original author of the federal health insurance proposals, rather than on Douglas. But it was precisely the shelving of the Green Book proposals that created the vacuum that would be filled, largely, by one provincial government led by a rookie premier in his first term of office.

# 6 Universal Hospital Insurance in Saskatchewan

*Unless the electorate is given the opportunity to change the experts as well as the politicians, elections will lose much of their significance.*
    Tommy Douglas, 1940s[1]

*Planning offices are generally not effective as such. They are effective only, if at all, if they are an arm of the boss.*
    Werhner Von Braun, Apollo space program chief[2]

With comprehensive health insurance no longer an immediate possibility, due to the failure of the Dominion-Provincial Conference on Reconstruction, it was time for the Douglas government to shift to Plan B. As premier and minister of health and as head of a party that had made ambitious promises in the 1944 election campaign, T.C. felt he had to deliver something concrete before the next election. His plan for building up services through the health regions was dependent on local government cooperation, making it too uncertain and slow a process to be considered a promise kept. Further, providing full hospital, drug, and medical care coverage for public assistance recipients and cancer patients affected only a minority of Saskatchewan residents. To make concrete progress on his policy ambitions and to keep his political promises, something much bigger, something that applied to everyone, was needed, and that was universal insurance for hospital care, which Douglas saw as a first essential step towards comprehensive health coverage.

From the beginning, T.C. intended to use his hospital plan as leverage to convince the federal government to reopen negotiations with the provinces.[3] The gambit of going it alone was risky. He knew that a hospital plan would stretch his government's financial capacity to the breaking point, so he needed the federal government to help underwrite the program within a couple of years. If Ottawa did not come through, he would be forced to impose an enormous increase in sales tax, as provincial income taxes had been turned over to the federal government as part of a wartime agreement that had been extended after the war. The other options were even more distasteful. His government could run a large deficit, but this was something he had vowed never to do, as it would be tantamount to making the province hostage to Eastern financial interests, as it had been during the Great Depression. A third option, of beginning a hospital insurance plan only to abandon it a few years later if Ottawa refused to assume some of the financial burden, would be unacceptable to the people of Saskatchewan, who would be just as likely to blame the provincial government as Ottawa for the withdrawal.

Initially, despite these risks, taking on hospital insurance alone seemed a very reasonable gamble when the federal government's Green Book proposals in early August 1945 included cost-shared health insurance with the provinces. However, after the collapse of the Dominion-Provincial Reconstruction Conference in early May 1946, it seemed an extremely poor bet. In the best-case scenario, it could take many years to reach a federal-provincial agreement that would permit federal money to flow to Saskatchewan. In the meantime, if Douglas proceeded before cost sharing was available, spending on this one program would prevent countless other social spending and infrastructure investments. This would be hard on his ministers, who had their own policy ambitions associated with their respective portfolios. It would also test the credibility of his government, given the ambitious policy agenda his party had developed and then unveiled in the 1944 election campaign. At the same time, he knew he could count on his provincial treasurer, Clarence Fines, to find some way to raise the money needed in the immediate future as well as to constrain ministers and their spending plans. This fiscal discipline would allow the hospital program sufficient funding not only to proceed but to succeed.[4] Still, in the long term, the province could not fiscally sustain such an expensive program without federal cost sharing.

**Why Start with Hospital Coverage?**

Why did the Douglas government select hospital insurance as the first step towards comprehensive health coverage? Of all health services, the two most costly items were hospital stays and doctors' fees, and the purpose of coverage was to remove cost as a barrier to access. However, without federal cost sharing, the provincial government could afford coverage for only one of these two services.

T.C. and Fines were committed to two operating principles. The first was not to raise taxes beyond a level acceptable to the average taxpayer: otherwise, they would create a popular backlash that would decimate the CCF in the next election. The tax issue was made worse by the fact that, due to the tax-rental agreement, the provincial government was largely limited to increasing sales tax or earmarked per capita taxes, like a separate earmarked tax on individuals and families, to fund social programs.[5] The second principle was their commitment to never allow ongoing programs to be financed through government debt, a commitment based not in political necessity but in the experience of the Great Depression and a deep-seated fear of being indebted to the central Canadian banks.

On a conceptual level, it might have made sense to first cover doctors' fees, particularly those for general practitioners (GPs), who provided almost all the primary care in the province. In the case of Saskatchewan in the mid-1940s, however, the rural areas were still so poorly served by doctors that insurance for "medical care" – the term commonly used for all physician services – would have been a major benefit only to residents in urban areas. Given the few doctors serving the vast rural areas of the province, coverage for physician fees would be of limited use to most of the population.

In other words, the province was not ready for physician care insurance. Instead, the Department of Public Health provided medical grants and encouraged local governments to recruit salaried municipal doctors and procure the needed medical equipment and facilities. Introducing hospital insurance first would buy the time needed to add more doctors and facilities to prepare for the eventual introduction of medical care coverage. In the meantime, beginning in January 1945, the government paid for the medical care of residents on public assistance as well as everyone needing cancer treatment or psychiatric care.[6]

Beyond these considerations, the key factor that propelled the Douglas government in the direction of hospital rather than medical care insurance was the potential opposition of the College of Physicians and Surgeons of Saskatchewan (CPS). T.C. knew from the beginning "that the doctors were going to create problems" when it came to any government involvement in paying for their services. In contrast, they were willing to go along with the government providing hospital and diagnostic services coverage. Not only did this not require them to change anything about their practices, but universal hospital insurance put more money into their pockets.[7] When they no longer had to pay

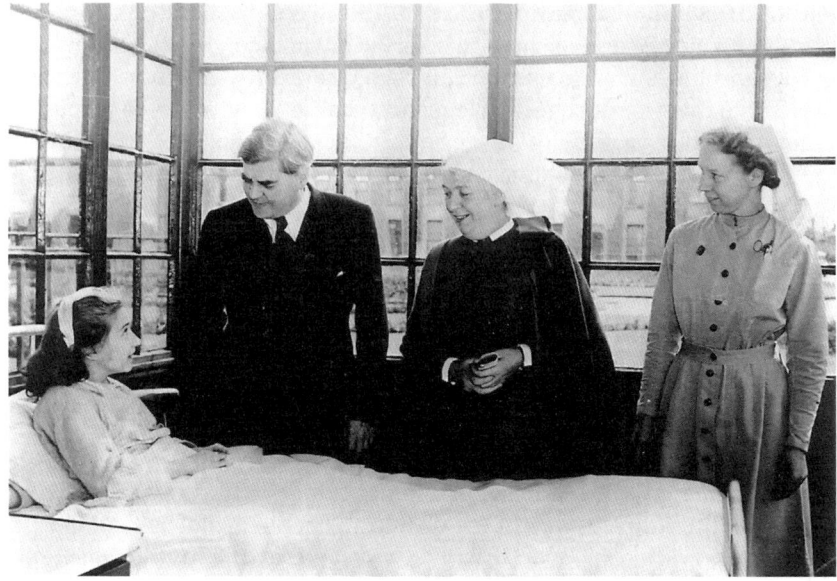

Aneurin Bevan, the British minister of health, on the first day of the National Health Service, 5 July 1948 (Wikimedia Commons)

for their time in hospitals, patients would be more able to pay for the physician care they needed. This logic also propelled the CPS to accept government payment for public assistance beneficiaries, covering individuals who would otherwise forego medical services or be treated for a discounted fee or even for free by an attending doctor.[8] All things considered, then, publicly financed hospital insurance was the path of least resistance.

The Saskatchewan hospital plan was one of the first universal plans of its type in the world. The social health insurance systems in continental Europe originated by Chancellor Bismarck of Germany in the late nineteenth century were largely limited to industrial workers and their families.[9] The National Health Service (NHS) in the United Kingdom, the rudiments of which had appeared in the Beveridge Report, would begin operating on 5 July 1948, eighteen months after Douglas had scheduled the implementation of his more limited hospital plan.[10]

The plan that was closest to what Saskatchewan was attempting was in New Zealand, a tax-based universal program closely studied by Douglas and his Health Services Planning Commission (HSPC) staff.[11]

Implemented during the Second World War by a Labour government similar in ideology and objectives to the CCF, the New Zealand social security scheme provided free hospital care, diagnostics, and prescription drugs for all citizens in public hospitals and subsidized coverage in private hospitals, in addition to providing non-contributory pension, disability, and unemployment assistance. These social and health benefits were paid for from general taxation and were non-contributory in design. The Labour government's objective was to make these health benefits a right of citizenship.[12]

In practice, the New Zealand scheme had serious problems.[13] Although the government's original intention had been to also offer free medical care, organized medicine in New Zealand fought the scheme for years, highly resistant to the subsidized scheme that covered only half of the fees charged by GPs and even less for specialists.[14] Other problems with the plan included a design that incentivized the excessive use of diagnostic tests and insufficient public payment to fully cover hospital administrative costs. These issues were communicated to T.C. by his old friend Hugh MacLean, who, along with a colleague at UCLA, had obtained the research funding necessary to conduct a fact-finding mission to New Zealand and publish their findings.[15] As a result, the Saskatchewan planners did not use New Zealand as a model and instead figured out a unique design calculated to give hospitals adequate revenues with effective costs controls, and to put in measures to prevent unnecessary and potentially harmful diagnostic testing.

**Preparing a Hospital Plan**

To design and implement a universal hospital insurance plan, Douglas knew he could not rely on his Department of Public Health. As a department still largely dominated by holdovers from the previous Liberal administration, officials were used to administering existing programs, not creating new ones, and certainly nothing as bold as the first universal hospital program. Instead, Douglas relied on the creative thinkers in the HSPC. Although it had originally been established in November 1944 as a strictly planning and policy body, Douglas made the HSPC responsible not only for designing the hospital coverage program but also for implementing and managing what would be the signature policy of his government.

Yet, in 1945, the HSPC secretariat was tiny in comparison to the Department of Public Health. It was stretched thin just trying to get the health regions established and the infrastructure and human resources in place so that an organized system of hospitals, clinics, and diagnostic services would better serve the province's rural population, a major task, given that 80 per cent of the population lived outside of the province's four cities that had a population of 10,000 or more. After the HSPC had presented Douglas with its planning on the establishment of rural health regions and all the personnel and facilities that were needed to support the plan, Douglas asked Mindel Sheps to shift the commission's focus to sketching out a hospital insurance plan. In June 1945, Douglas received Sheps's carefully thought-out memorandum on the subject.

Sheps argued that universal hospital coverage, while not in itself transformative, should be considered an essential part of any fundamental reworking of health care into a coordinated and accessible system – what she referred to as "socialized health services." She argued, first, that hospitals were "an essential component of good health services" and central to both the diagnosis and treatment of more serious illnesses and injuries, but that, without prepaid coverage, most residents could not afford the high cost of hospital treatment for serious illnesses that were, by their nature, almost impossible to predict and prepare for. If these costs were fully paid by the provincial government, a more predictable and higher revenue stream for hospitals would be created, allowing them to be "able to improve and expand their facilities and accommodation," thereby raising the standard of care. Sheps was also convinced that the considerable unmet demand for hospital service in the province would result in the cost of the hospital plan growing rapidly in the first few years. Still, in her view, the benefits from universal hospital coverage would become so obvious that Saskatchewan's residents "would be ready to bear any necessary" increases in taxation to keep the program.[16]

But there was also bad news in Sheps's memorandum for Douglas, who wanted to see the hospital plan translated into a program as soon as possible. The HSPC forecast that the expansion of hospital beds by local governments – supported by provincial grants – wouldn't allow the province to proceed with universal hospitalization for two years, warning that it would be a serious mistake to proceed any earlier. As it was, most hospitals in the province were "over-crowded" due to the increased demand placed on the system by old age pensioners and other public assistance recipients receiving free hospital and medical care since the beginning of the year. Sheps feared that the rapid introduction of universal hospital coverage might flood the already overburdened hospitals in the province with patients who had previously been unable to pay for hospital care. Instead, time was needed to increase the number of hospital beds as well as to fund additional nursing homes so that long-term-care patients would put less pressure on hospital beds, which should be reserved for acute care patients.[17]

Since both hospital beds and nursing homes were in the hands of local authorities, the provincial government needed to continue providing hospital, nursing home, and other health care grants to local governments both before and for years after it introduced universal hospital coverage. The HSPC estimated that the cost of such a program would be between $3.5 and $4 million, estimates that would turn out to be much lower than the actual costs.[18] On top of this, the government had to help fund hospital expansion so that it could actually deliver on the promise of universal hospital coverage. Between 1945 and 1949, the government rapidly increased its hospital construction grants and loans to municipalities, and the number of union hospitals shared among municipalities tripled from twenty-six in 1944 to seventy-eight by 1948.[19]

After he digested Sheps's memo, Douglas asked the HSPC to begin consulting key groups affected by the change, a huge task, given the number of actors and their capacity to veto the government's efforts. First, the HSPC had to work with local governments for the registration of their respective populations to facilitate the collection of annual premiums (the compulsory flat-rate taxes paid by individuals or families), a task that would take months to complete. Second, the HSPC had to consult the Saskatchewan Hospital Association, whose member hospitals would be receiving payments from the government rather than patients once the plan was implemented. Third, and most disagreeably for Sheps, the HSPC would have to continue to talk to the College of Physicians and Surgeons, even though its members were not directly affected by the plan. Although many specialists worked in hospitals, they would continue to bill their patients directly or, for the few with private health coverage, their insurance carriers. There were exceptions. Some radiologists, for example, were salaried by hospitals, and, under the plan, hospitals would be reimbursed for their services by the provincial government. Despite the lack of direct impact on most doctors, they continued to raise concerns, and Douglas wanted the tacit approval of the CPS in order to minimize opposition to the plan.

Originally, the plan, in its legislative form in 1946, had been designed to be eligible for a federal contribution under the Green Book proposals. Adopting a social insurance approach, the federal hospital insurance proposal required "that every person 16 years and over be registered and that there be some kind of contribution." Compared to relying strictly on general taxation, this "poll tax" – as Douglas publicly called it – was administratively "clumsy" and regressive but was a condition for eligibility for federal cost sharing if the Green Book proposals were ever resurrected following their failure in 1946.[20]

The tasks of registration and tax collection were one and the same. To register, a tax would have to be paid, either by an adult individual or the head of a family on behalf of all dependants. In return, the resident would receive a hospitalization card, which would have to be shown and recorded each time the resident (or a member of the resident's family) accessed any hospital or diagnostic service.[21]

To make the plan universal – that is, covering all eligible residents – registration needed to be compulsory. The provincial government readily accepted the offer of the rural and urban municipalities that their governments "serve as registration and collection agencies." The roughly nine hundred municipal secretaries who were already responsible for collecting municipal taxes constituted "a ready-made administrative structure," even if the HSPC would have to provide considerable training in new procedures to minimize administrative errors.[22] The HSPC agreed to provide local governments with a standard form setting out the information that had to be collected from each family or single individual. Each city and town needed to make an enumeration of all persons within their respective boundaries at the same time as they made the enumeration for their municipal voters' lists. Each village and rural municipality needed to do the same.[23] The HSPC agreed that it would provide all local governments the standard form with the information that needed to be collected from residents in order to register for the plan.

Next came the discussions with the hospital association and its member hospitals on how they were to be paid. This negotiation was conducted largely in the first half of 1946 after Mindel had stepped down and her husband, Cecil, was appointed acting chair of the HSPC on the understanding that T.C. would have the next six months to find a permanent chair. The Shepses had decided to move to the United States so that Cecil could pursue graduate studies in at Yale University. But the couple also had other reasons for leaving Saskatchewan.

**The Shepses Depart**

In September 1945, Mindel and Cecil had adopted a five-month-old baby boy.[24] From that time on, Mindel began to limit her time in the office to afternoons.[25] She then resigned as HSPC secretary in January 1946.[26] While the baby was certainly a factor in her decision, it may also have been triggered by some personal frustrations in dealing with the College of Physicians and Surgeons and perhaps with Douglas as well.[27] Dr. Orville Hjertaas, a relatively new member of the HSPC who had demonstrated his effectiveness in a few short months, replaced Mindel as secretary.[28] By this time, Mindel and Cecil were thinking of leaving the province.

Cecil had met with John B. Grant of the Rockefeller Foundation, who had been in Saskatchewan as part of an international survey of trends in medical care. Impressed by Cecil, Grant said that his foundation would be interested in providing him with financial assistance so that he could support his family while doing a graduate degree in public health at Yale.[29] In January 1946, Cecil travelled to New Haven and New York to make the final arrangements for his studies. He then travelled to Baltimore, where he had been invited by Henry Sigerist to give a seminar on Saskatchewan's reforms to Sigerist's students at Johns Hopkins University. When he returned to Regina, Cecil informed T.C. that he and Mindel would be leaving the province by the summer but that both would be willing to return to serve in his government after Cecil had completed his degree.[30]

While Cecil Sheps was away, Tommy McLeod worked on iterative drafts of enabling legislation for the hospital plan. As a broad framework for what the government was intending to do, the wording was purposely open on key issues. The legislation could not, for example, spell out how the hospital insurance tax – the individual family premiums – would be collected, since negotiations were ongoing with local governments through their peak organizations, the Saskatchewan Association of Rural Municipalities (SARM) and the Saskatchewan Urban Municipalities Association (SUMA). The eventual bill simply provided for the appointment of "one or more" premium tax collectors, Douglas admitting that, if his government could not get the local governments to take on the task of tax collection, the HSPC would have to set up "some machinery" to do so, an enormous job that would have resulted in delaying implementation of the plan.[31]

At the time the legislation was being drafted, T.C. was still optimistic about the outcome of the Dominion-Provincial Reconstruction Conference and the possibility of federal cost sharing. Therefore McLeod had to formulate the law so that it could work with any federal offer of cost sharing for health insurance more broadly defined, even while preparing for the possibility that the conference might end in failure, forcing the province to go it alone on hospital insurance.[32] Moreover, even after the conference permanently adjourned in early May 1946, T.C. continued to be hopeful that Ottawa might accept a separate federal cost-sharing deal on health insurance at some future date.

On 14 February, the Throne Speech opening the Legislative Assembly session of 1946 unveiled the government's intention to introduce a bill on universal hospital coverage, "an important step towards socialized health services for the Province."[33] One month later, Douglas introduced Bill 45, An Act to Provide Payment for Services Rendered to Certain Patients by Certain Hospitals and other Institutions – in its short form, the Saskatchewan Hospitalization Act – in the legislature.[34]

During the second reading, Douglas triumphantly declared that Saskatchewan was "blazing the trail," and he was "pleased and proud that Saskatchewan should be the first province to launch a complete province-wide scheme of hospitalization." Of course, hospital insurance was considered just the "first milestone" on the road to "complete socialized health services."[35] To some, this term meant universal coverage for all needed health services, including medical and dental care, but to others, particularly in the CCF's left wing, it also meant a completely regionalized health system with salaried GPs and other specialists working in an organized system of hospitals, polyclinics, and primary care clinics. At the time, there is little question that Douglas meant both, even if he thought the latter was on a slower track than health insurance.[36]

The Saskatchewan Hospitalization Act passed third reading on 2 April 1946 and received royal assent by the lieutenant governor two days later.[37] Although this meant it was the law of the province, the plan would not legally begin operating until 1 January 1947. Given its significance at the time, it may seem strange that it elicited relatively little discussion in the media and almost no criticism from the opposition parties. The only explanation is that everyone thought the government was astute in preparing the ground for a program that would have 60 per cent of its costs underwritten by Ottawa. Even more interesting is the fact that, based on the record of questions posed by Saskatchewan MLAs in the 1946 legislative session, there seemed to have been no criticism of the law and its objectives. Indeed, while opposition MLAs asked multiple questions about Mindel (even after she resigned) and Cecil Sheps as well as the management of the North Battleford Mental Hospital, they did not raise a single question or concern about the objectives of hospital insurance and the form it was to take.[38]

Yet, not everyone was pleased with the legislation. The College of Physicians and Surgeons was unhappy with two aspects of the law. The first was the use of the government as the sole payer of all hospital bills. The doctors preferred a multi-payer plan, one that allowed for private insurance carriers. However, they were willing to let this go if the government did not invade the field of insurance for physician services and the operations of its two newly established medical care insurance companies providing insurance for physician services: Medical Services Incorporated (MSI), which had been set up by Saskatoon doctors, and Group Medical Services (GMS), the company sponsored by Regina doctors.

The second and much bigger issue for the college was the fact that hospital coverage would be administered by the HSPC rather than by a non-governmental commission with key members whose appointment would be determined by the CPS. The college and the government had collided on this issue from the beginning, but, on this point, Douglas refused to yield. Since the scheme would be entirely funded by the taxpayer, in his view this required direct accountability between the health minister (and cabinet) and the people through the Legislative Assembly. The minister of health had to be answerable for the public money being spent, not an independent body over which he, as minister, had no control. A government body, therefore, whether it was the Department of Public Health or the HSPC, had to be accountable to the minister of health.

Initially, Douglas thought the college would prefer the HSPC to the health department, since doctors were represented on the HSPC's Advisory Committee. However, the doctors entirely rejected Douglas's logic. From their perspective, the HSPC, which reported directly to the minister of public health, was an integral part of the government and therefore not at arm's length, much less the independent commission they were seeking. Moreover, the influence of the college on the Advisory Committee was dulled by the presence of so many other stakeholders. As a result, the CPS actively tried to prevent the committee from providing guidance to the government and preferred to use its direct access to Douglas to bypass the committee altogether. And the college remained strongly opposed to Mindel Sheps.

Putting aside this last issue, Douglas knew the law was nothing more than a framework, and that the devil lay in the details. His government faced enormous implementation challenges. One was whether providing universal access would simply overwhelm the province's existing hospital capacity. Another serious challenge related to the administrative capacity and innovative planning required to pull off hospital insurance in a few months.

The tiny HSPC team was extremely creative and hard working, but, for the most part, team members had limited experience in the actual running of hospitals and clinics.[39] Moreover, as the temporary head of the HSPC, Cecil Sheps proved to be no more successful in dealing with the college than his wife had been. The burden of soothing relations with the doctors always seemed to fall on Douglas. However, this challenge paled in comparison to the failure of the Dominion-Provincial Reconstruction Conference. Without federal cost sharing, his "government faced extraordinary pressures on a seriously limited budget," even with 50 per cent of the hospital program financed through hospital taxes (premiums) levied on families and individuals.[40]

Some of the fiscal constraints were self-imposed. Neither Douglas nor Clarence Fines would countenance deficit financing, committed as they were to running a slight surplus every year so that the province could pay down the debt it had accumulated during the Great Depression.[41] And both men were keen to reduce the leverage of bankers on the province. At the same time, to limit the tax increase, the boundaries of hospital insurance had to be clearly delimited, and the program would have to be managed as tightly as possible to restrain cost escalation, two concerns that were embedded in the design of the program.[42]

Even assuming sufficient money and hospital beds as well as talented personnel were available, there was still the problem of time. A compulsory program of this type had never been implemented, and Douglas needed a viable, practical plan. Moreover, he needed it be to operational – with all the bugs worked out – well before the next provincial election, which he had planned for June 1948. For his government to have any chance of being re-elected, Saskatchewan voters would have to experience some of the benefits from this major investment of public money. From his perspective, he had to have the program begin no later than 1 January 1947. This meant his team only had months to work out the plan, including the form of patient registration, payment methods for hospitals, and numerous other details. Then, assuming there would be problems once it was implemented, they needed to determine how best to identify and fix the problems as quickly as possible. So much to do, so little time – and so few people he could really rely on not only to get it done, but to get it done right. The Sifton daily newspapers – "the voice of western Liberalism" in Regina, Saskatoon, and Winnipeg – were just waiting for the chance to seize on any implementation problems.[43]

For its part, the CPS had rapidly assented to government payment for providing health services for patients on public assistance, though it remained concerned about the precedent this set for future state intrusion into physicians' private affairs. In a letter sent to its entire membership in 1945, the college stated that it could "only hazard vague guesses as to where and how far similar further 'steps' may lead in the future."[44]

In August 1946, just months after his hospital bill had passed, T.C. summarized the rationale for comprehensive health coverage, starting with hospital care, to the province in a radio broadcast. He made it clear that only such a policy could ensure that the benefits of medical science would be available to all. Only a government plan could remove the near impossibility "for the average family to pay" when the service is required. Risk pooling across the entire population through publicly financed insurance was essential so that every resident could use such services regardless of "individual ability to pay." "The right to health," he declared, was "the very essence of a dynamic democracy."[45]

In the same address, Douglas looked beyond hospital insurance and argued that physician care should not "be allowed to remain the privilege and personal business of the individual doctor." He suggested the replacement of solo physician practice by group practices in a clinic environment. What remained unsaid was whether these clinics would be owned and operated by the provincial government in the newly forming health regions and whether doctors would become salaried employees within these health centres and clinics. The exact form that these developments would take depended on the new permanent chair of the HSPC.

## Fred Mott and His New Dealers

Many months earlier, Douglas had reached out to Henry Sigerist for advice on a suitable candidate for the HSPC chair. Without hesitation, Sigerist told him that "the ablest man on the continent" to lead the HSPC as well as implement a prepaid health insurance plan was Dr. Frederick D. Mott.[46] When Douglas reviewed Mott's background, he agreed with Sigerist. Mott seemed the ideal person to build up health services in rural areas through expanding the number of health regions, constructing new hospitals, recruiting more doctors, and establishing polyclinics and primary care clinics. He also seemed very experienced in planning and had already implemented and managed health insurance plans.

While Ohio-born Mott had obtained his undergraduate honours degree in history at Princeton University, he received his medical degree from McGill University in 1932, where he was awarded the Thomas Smith Wood Gold Medal for academic achievement. Already by this time, Mott was expressing positive views on the merits "socialized medicine," which, at the time, he defined as a "system for promotion of health and the cure of disease for all the people, organized by the medical profession, administered by the medical profession, and supported by the people through taxation."[47] After graduation from McGill, Mott was registered by the Medical Council of Canada as a practising physician but moved to New York, where he did a two-year internship in internal medicine at the Presbyterian-Columbia Medical Center, at the end of which he was licensed in New York State. After practising medicine for another three years, he entered government service in the Farm Security Administration (FSA), the most recent New Deal agency, first as an associate medical officer (1937–42) and eventually as chief medical officer and assistant chief of the FSA's Health Services Branch (1942–6).[48]

These titles underplayed Mott's role in the FSA. From the beginning, he was pivotal in creating the structures and organizations that would provide hospital, medical, dental, and public health services to hundreds of thousands of poor farmers and migrant farm workers throughout the United States.[49] Working with farm and community-based organizations to forge prepayment plans, Mott gained valuable experience in the implementation and management of publicly financed and administered health insurance programs, experience that Douglas intuitively knew he needed for the effective design and implementation of hospitalization in Saskatchewan.[50]

With the entry of the United States into the war, following the attack on Pearl Harbor in December 1941, many migrant farm workers joined the military, creating a labour shortage that forced the United States to rely on farmworkers from Mexico and the Caribbean. Mott was seconded by the FSA to the War Food Administration as chief medical officer, responsible for adapting the facilities and methods used in the FSA for foreign farm workers in 250 health centres.[51] The system Mott was central to setting up was described by New Deal historian Michael Grey as a "highly creative" health policy experiment in the United States.[52]

In addition to all his relevant experience, Douglas was attracted to Mott for two other reasons. First, Fred Mott, who was the same age as Douglas, was the son of John R. Mott, a world-famous Christian evangelist and long-serving leader of the Young Men's Christian Association (YMCA) who would win a Nobel Peace Prize for his work in 1946. Thus, the Mott name was already well-known to T.C., and this lineage could only have contributed to the premier's growing fascination with Fred Mott.[53] Second, exhausted from having continual meetings with the doctors, due to their refusal to accept either of the Shepses as his representative, Douglas yearned to have an HSPC chair with sufficient standing and respect to take over such meetings. And here was a distinguished American doctor and experienced health administrator. Moreover, Douglas likely thought, based on Mott's track record in dealing with organized medicine for many years in the United States, that Mott would be more diplomatic than the Shepses in his dealings with the college. Finally, given the prevailing anti-Semitism within the Canadian medical profession, Mott's prominent Christian pedigree, in contrast to the Jewish background of the Shepses, was no doubt more palatable to the CPS leadership.

In January 1946, Douglas flew to Washington, DC, to try to convince Mott to join his government. After giving him a pitch on the exciting challenges that would await him in Saskatchewan, Douglas encouraged him to get a second opinion from Henry Sigerist, knowing the professor's stature among progressive doctors in the United States.[54] Like Sigerist and many other New Deal supporters, Mott had lived in hope for over a decade that the Roosevelt administration would introduce national health insurance. He was inspired by Sigerist's speeches, books, newspaper commentary, and public lectures supporting such a policy shift. Although Roosevelt stopped short of pushing for broad health insurance, Mott, as a senior official in a New Deal agency, was able to implement at least some targeted coverage programs, which Sigerist applauded as important steps on the road to national health insurance, forging a close bond between Sigerist and New Deal health administrators such as Mott.[55]

The meeting in Washington went well, and Mott, suitably encouraged by Sigerist, wrote Douglas in mid-March 1946 to confirm the understanding that he would report directly to the premier rather than the provincial deputy minister of health. He also expected to have a free hand in bringing in whoever he felt he needed, including Dr. Len Rosenfeld, whom he had worked with in the past and felt was ideally suited to the challenges ahead.[56] Although Mott could not move to Saskatchewan until the last week in August, he wanted to hire Rosenfeld at the beginning in July to conduct a survey of "recent development in the United States having any bearing on all of the various aspects of organized health services which are contemplated in Saskatchewan."[57] In the meantime, Mott asked to be released from his role as a commissioned officer at the rank of senior surgeon in the US Public Health Service to take on the HSPC chairmanship.[58]

Once this was done, the Saskatchewan government issued a glowing press release to announce Mott's hiring. In the release, Douglas stated that "the government and the people of Saskatchewan are extremely fortunate in securing the services of one of the top public health figures on the continent and one who has specialized in instituting medical care programs in rural areas."[59] No doubt resonating with the many farm families in Saskatchewan who had suffered greatly during the Great Depression, the release emphasized Mott's leadership in the Farm Security Administration and its "extensive health and medical care activities among low-income farmers as part of its rural rehabilitation and farm ownership program." These activities included the "development of medical, hospital and dental service plans on a prepayment basis." The release pointed out that, under Mott, the FSA was managing "995 prepayment plans" for over 600,000 people by 1942.[60]

Even the Sifton press responded positively to Mott's appointment, repeating large chunks of the government's press release.[61] In an editorial, the *Regina Leader-Post* commended Douglas for his choice of Mott to "take over the reins of the government's largest social project," remarking that "such a prominent and highly qualified public health authority" should be of the "utmost value" to the province.[62] Such words stood in sharp contrast to the usual carping about outsiders that Douglas had brought into the province since the election. Douglas was even more delighted when he received word that the CPS itself had reacted favourably to the news of Mott's appointment, a welcome reprieve from the college's disapproval of Mindel and Cecil Sheps.[63]

The decision to move to Saskatchewan had not been an easy one for Mott. He had been toying with two other offers, including becoming the executive director of the National Health Council, a leading non-governmental patient advocacy organization based in Washington, DC, and a full professorship at New York University's School of Medicine. Douglas told Mott that he knew it "must have been a difficult decision for you to make and that it involves considerable personal sacrifice." He agreed to Mott's request to hire Rosenfeld, although he suggested that Mott should perhaps come to Saskatchewan first before making such a decision. Through such a visit, he might find among the current personnel "sufficient material out of which to build the kind of organization you want without bringing anyone else in from outside."[64]

Fortunately for Douglas, Mott did not follow his advice, and Rosenfeld accompanied him to Saskatchewan. The two New Dealers arrived in Regina the last week of August 1946 so they would have one week of overlap with Cecil Sheps before he and Mindel departed for Yale.[65] Mott and his wife moved in with the Shepses for the first few days, while Rosenfeld and his spouse stayed at the Hotel Saskatchewan until they could find a place to live in Regina.[66] Appointed as vice-chair of the HSPC, Rosenfeld was Mott's second-in-command, the person he most relied on to hammer out the key details for the working machinery of what would become the Saskatchewan Hospital Services Plan (SHSP). Although remaining in the province for only two years, Rosenfeld was key to Mott successfully implementing the plan. In the words of Tommy McLeod, who remained a core member of the HSPC, Mott and Rosenfeld worked like fanatics on the design and implementation

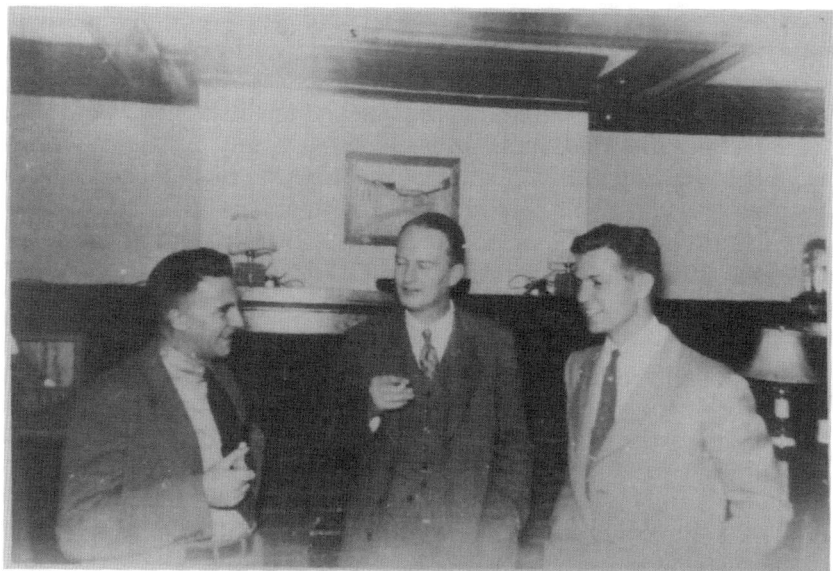

From left to right, Milton Roemer, Fred Mott, and Len Rosenfeld during Roemer's visit to Saskatchewan in 1947 (YUA)

of hospitalization.[67] They had little choice, given the circumstances. Although Mott had been given a free hand by Douglas to hire his own team, including outsiders like Rosenfeld, the reality was that recruitment took time, and he had only four months to get the plan ready to go before the start date of 1 January 1947.

Mott used the expertise of other New Dealers, including Milton Roemer, a public health physician and sociologist who had worked under Mott in the Farm Security Administration. Drawing on their FSA experience, Mott and Roemer had been working on a major book addressing rural health in the United States since 1945, which would eventually be published in 1948 as *Rural Health and Medical Care* in 1948.[68] The book was largely done by the time Mott landed in Regina but was subject to publishing delays caused by a backlash against left-leaning public health advocates such as Mott and Roemer, a story well-told by medical historian Jim Connor.[69] Their concern for poverty-stricken farmers during the Great Depression and commitment to universal health coverage mirrored T.C.'s own experiences and preoccupations.[70]

Roemer did not move to Regina, at least immediately. Instead, in 1947, at Mott's request, he obtained a short-term leave from the Public Health

Service in Washington, DC, so that he could work for a brief stint in Regina to review the province's public assistance coverage program.[71] A devoted disciple of Henry Sigerist and a member of the American Soviet Medical Society, Roemer faced persecution in the early Cold War years for his leftist views until, in 1953, he finally fled to Saskatchewan, where he was appointed director of medical and hospital services in the health department.[72] Roemer would eventually go on to enjoy a stellar academic career, a pioneer in the field of comparative health systems and a vocal advocate for universal health coverage in the United States.[73] The development of what became known as Roemer's Law – that, with hospital insurance, every new hospital bed would soon be filled – was first based on Roemer's observations of the Saskatchewan hospital plan.[74]

### Implementing the Saskatchewan Hospital Services Plan

Although Cecil Sheps had established a committee for the Douglas government to work with SARM and SUMA on registration and the collection of premiums, an agreement had not yet been finalized. The more politically powerful of the two peak organizations, SARM had long indicated its willingness, in principle, to "assume some measure of responsibility" for collecting the personal taxes needed to provide farmers and their families with health insurance.[75] These premiums were set at $5 per individual (adult or child), up to a maximum of $30 per family, and were intended to cover over half the cost of the plan.[76] A rapid agreement between the government and the municipalities was essential if there was to be any hope of meeting the January implementation deadline.

The roughly nine hundred municipal clerks in Saskatchewan constituted a "ready-made administrative structure," while the alternative – the setting up of provincial government offices to register residents and collect premiums – would have required many months.[77] To ensure that registration could be completed before the end of the year, Mott quickly concluded an agreement with SARM and SUMA on 3 September 1946. The city and town clerks said they would complete registration by the end of that month, while the rural and village municipal clerks would complete registration by mid-November.[78] The final agreement allowed the local governments to keep 5 per cent of the total sum they collect as compensation for the combined tasks of registration and tax collection.[79]

By the third week of September, Mott, Rosenfeld, and McLeod had finalized the regulations under the Saskatchewan Hospitalization Act, 1946. These detailed regulations identified exempt classes of beneficiaries (e.g., individuals already covered under the provincial assistance health plan and members of the Canadian Armed Forces covered under a federal plan), the minimum waiting period for new residents (six months), registration, form of payment, collection of premiums, and penalties in the event of non-payment, a necessary provision given that registration was compulsory for all residents in the process.[80]

Items as seemingly simple as creating a province-wide hospital admission-discharge form took weeks of preparation. Hospitals each had their own forms based on their own perceived financial and clinical requirements. Given that the provincial government would be the sole payer, this form not only had to be standardized so that it could be used to reimburse hospitals, but additional information needed to be gathered to facilitate the coordination of care between admission, diagnosis (including the ordering and clinical assessment of X-rays and blood results), and discharge back to a GP.

Douglas's ambition was to set up a coordinated system of health care to be managed by the government as a public service. Consequently, Mott and Rosenfeld struggled with how to extract information on individual hospital occupancy so that the admission-discharge forms would give the HSPC "a clear picture of the availability of hospital beds throughout the province."[81] While this required more detailed patient information than had been collected before, it was essential that the form still be short enough to be easily administered by the hospitals. To find the right balance, Mott, Rosenfeld, and their internal HSPC working group held several meetings, including on weekends, to meet a printing deadline of mid-October.[82]

By early October, both Mott and Rosenfeld were concerned about what they might have missed in terms of implementation details, so they flew in Edgar Clapp, a US-based management consultant with the depth of expertise they needed, to review their work and identify any gaps. In his first report, Clapp stated that the HSPC's "preliminary plans have been well made especially considering the time element involved in getting the plan under way by January 1st, 1947." In particular, the HSPC had already arranged for local governments to begin registration so that it could be completed by mid-November, and the hospital insurance premiums collected by the end of the year. However, this decentralized form of enumeration, registration, and collection of premiums suffered from "the lack of uniformity and understanding" that was the inevitable result of "so many people" – an "estimated 1,000–1,100 people throughout the province" – "handling the work of enumeration and collection."[83]

Clapp recommended that the HSPC immediately set up a unit "for the purpose of giving service to the districts on such matters that are not clear, answer correspondence, straighten out questions and incorrect or incomplete information on registration blanks, etc." In addition, based on a sample study Clapp had done of the registration conducted by one rural government and one small city government, he concluded that the HSPC needed to set up a centralized tax-payment record system to keep close tabs on registration and payment by local governments throughout the province. Although premiums were often paid by families on behalf of dependants (at that point, an average of 2.4 persons per registration based on the sample study), Clapp recommended separate registration and that a hospital insurance card be issued for each resident above the age of fifteen, irrespective of how the premium was paid.[84]

Despite the HSPC's best efforts, Mott realized by early November that many details still needed to be worked out. Tired and discouraged, he sat down with the premier and explained why they thought they could not have the plan implemented by 1 January 1947. Douglas said he could not change the implementation date. His election promises, combined with his recurring statements to the newspapers on the start date, meant that his own reputation and political future depended on the program's beginning on time. He understood that not everything would be in place in two months, and he knew there would be some problems; indeed, he had already prepared the public for some implementation mistakes, which he said would be understood as part of "blazing a new trail."[85]

Douglas was more concerned about potential opposition from the doctors and the hospitals than about potential administrative problems. The CPS was not just bothered by the fact that the government would administer the plan, but it also "felt this was the beginning" of a full-fledged plan of "socialized medicine," in which doctors would eventually become salaried employees. But the more serious threat came from the Saskatchewan Hospital Association (SHA). While the hospitals had been cooperating with the HSPC, they too were concerned about whether this was the first major step towards their absorption by the government. To assuage the SHA's concerns, Douglas and Mott both spoke at made the SHA's annual convention in early November 1946. Douglas began by rejecting the idea, common among the members of the SHA, "that it would have been better to postpone the scheme for another year." While he admitted that there might be some difficulties with implementation, "you could never accomplish anything ... if you always waited until the perfect conditions arrive" because "they never would." As for concerns about a point system the HSPC had devised to reimburse hospitals, Douglas tried to calm his audience: "While we are the guardians of the public treasury we are equally concerned that hospitals not be penalized by the plan. We are prepared to make adjustments as we go along. There is nothing rigid about the scheme, no fixed principles, techniques will have to be worked out" over time.[86]

In his own address to the SHA, Mott made a rare stumble. After thanking the association for its cooperation in determining a method of payment for hospitals, Mott added something that fed the anxiety of the SHA about the province's hospital plan. Future provincial funding for hospital and health centre construction, he stated, would be based on the priorities set by the HSPC.[87] The result was a confrontation early in December, when "the entire executive of the Saskatchewan Hospital Association marched into" T.C.'s office. No longer prepared to cooperate, the members claimed that the government was taking too much control. T.C. rebutted the claim, saying the government would simply "collect the money and then pay the hospitals for the care" they provided, but "the running of the hospital would continue to be in the hands of hospital administrators." The premier had no desire whatsoever to have the headache of managing all the hospitals in the province. However, Douglas went on, "if they couldn't run the hospitals under this plan then on 1 January," his government would be forced to "take over the hospitals."[88] The SHA instantly backed off its threat to not cooperate and from that point forward worked with Mott and his team to make the implementation work as well as possible for the hospitals.

In the end, the question of ownership would turn out to be the critical difference between Saskatchewan and the National Health Service that would be implemented in the United Kingdom in July 1948. In Saskatchewan (and as eventually adopted in the rest of Canada), the government paid for all hospital bills, but the delivery of services remained in the hands of others, while, in the United Kingdom, the government took over all the hospitals within its purview and operated them as part of a single national health service. Today, the former are classified as national health insurance systems and the latter as national health service systems.[89] It is interesting to speculate on what could have happened if Douglas had been forced, however reluctantly, to assume the ownership of all the hospitals in the province. If this additional step had been taken, then Saskatchewan would have been the first jurisdiction in the world to implement a national health service system (albeit with more limited coverage than the NHS), many months before the British NHS began operating.

Given the unique challenges involved in creating the new program, Douglas agreed to allow Mott to second the personnel he needed from other government departments and agencies in order to get the new plan into operation even while he continued to recruit permanent staff into a new HSPC operating division – the Saskatchewan Hospital Services Plan. One of the temporary secondments was a remarkably talented young civil servant, Al Johnson, who was then working under George Cadbury in the Economic Advisory and Planning Board but who would soon be transferred to the newly formed Budget Bureau under Tommy McLeod.[90] Johnson would come to play a central role in the federal-provincial negotiation for national medicare in the mid-1960s. In his account of the evolution on health insurance in Canada, Malcolm Taylor described the "feverish activity, reminiscent of mobilization in 1939," on the eve of implementation: "The only office space available was in an ancient, vacated store building: clerical desks were long rows of plywood-on-trestles, with clerks sitting elbow-to-elbow, processing the registration and tax collection payments according to a system that, although using mechanical tabulating equipment, was quite primitive."[91]

## The Launching of North America's First Universal Hospital Coverage Plan

On 20 December 1945, a short public ceremony was held at Regina City Hall. There, Hospitalization Card No. 1 was given to Premier Douglas as a prelude to the launch of the province-wide plan. As he handed over the card to the premier, City Assessor Arthur Robbins said that he considered this event "to be one of the most memorable occasions in the history of the province" because it represented "the official inauguration of a social hospitalization scheme never before attempted in any part of the Dominion." As the mayor of Regina noted in his remarks, the city assessor had earned the honour of presenting the card because he was responsible for collecting hospital insurance fees from the city's residents, which had included Douglas, for the scheme. Robbins beamed with pride when he noted he had already collected $161,000 out of the estimated $225,000 of individual and family premiums in the city, almost two weeks in advance of the plan going into operation.[92]

When he wished the premier many more years of health, hoping he would never be required to use the card, Douglas quipped that he hoped for the same. He then smiled back at the crowd, saying, "I see some of our hospital people present and they too, no doubt, will be hoping that not too many people require hospitalization." But, turning

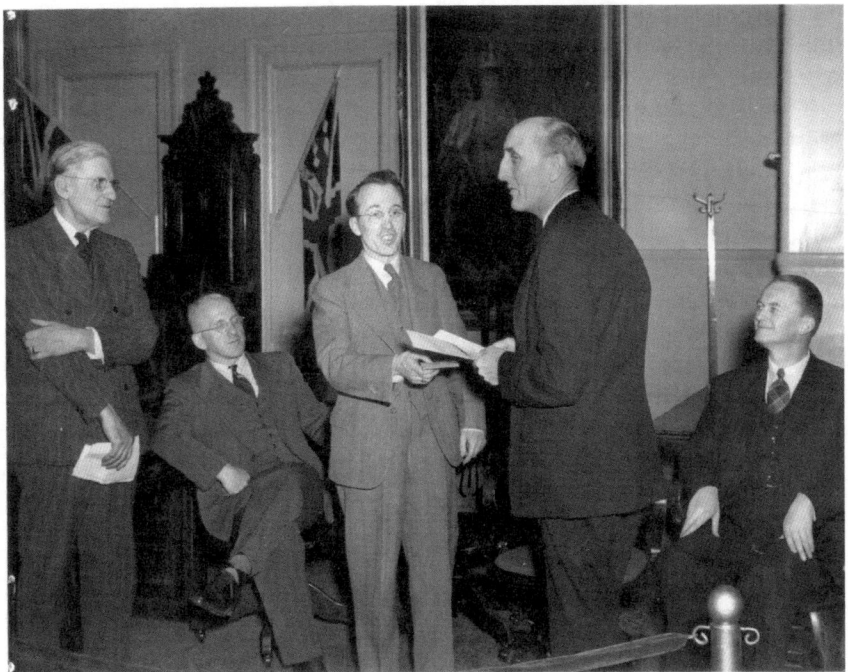

T.C. receiving Hospitalization Card No. 1 from City of Regina tax assessor Arthur Robbins, with Fred Mott looking on at far left, 20 Dec. 1946 (PAS R-A3256)

more serious, he told those assembled that, now, "services will be available to all those who need it [sic]." Given the unique nature of the plan, T.C. tried his best to reduce expectations by also warning that the scheme would inevitably have some implementation problems, and these could be successfully overcome only by patience and the cooperation of local governments and hospitals. At the same time, he emphasized that the world – in particular, interested observers in both Canada and the United States – was watching the province to see the results of this bold experiment.[93]

Ten days later, on New Year's Eve, Mott and his small team stopped to pick up T.C. at his home. They then went together to Regina General Hospital to see the first patient billing the Saskatchewan Hospital Services Plan, which happened to be the family of a baby boy born fifteen seconds after midnight.[94] The plan was off to a good start despite reaching only about 70 per cent of registrations and premium collections, a deficit that had to be closed as quickly as possible in the first weeks of the its operation.[95]

Although Douglas had been prepared that not everything would work perfectly, things went better than he expected. This was due in large part to the team Mott put together as the permanent staff of the SHSP. In a few weeks, the SHSP cobbled together the staff, equipment, policies, and procedures for overseeing registration and tax collection and paying hospitals, including the field staff to support municipal clerks and hospital managers throughout the province. For the first three months of operation, Rosenfeld, as head of the SHSP, guided the new staff in addressing implementation problems, which generally involved hospitals and local governments. Once the system became routinized, SHSP employees refined and simplified internal administrative procedures and worked with municipal officials to improve registration and tax-collection processes.[96]

Hospital utilization spiked the moment the plan was introduced, in part because of individuals and their doctors who, in the last months of 1946, purposely delayed surgeries until 1947 so that their patients would not have to pay for hospital care. This was a very short-term blip. The bigger challenge was posed by new patients who, in the past, had avoided hospital care because of its cost and would now be prepared to go into hospital whenever necessary. As shown in table 6.1, this pent-up demand drove the growth in the number of patients per capita and may have influenced the average length of stay in the plan's first two years.

This increase was bound to put pressure on existing hospital capacity, and the HSPC had to work double time to encourage the building and expansion of hospitals, especially in the rural and remote areas of the province. In 1947, supported by provincial grants distributed by the HSPC, fifteen new hospitals opened their doors to patients. In addition, the HSPC encouraged another ten existing hospitals, including those in urban centres, to add new buildings and extensions, which increased capacity by 736 beds. A further 507 beds were added in 1948. In 1946, the province had 4.8 beds per 1,000 people; by the end of 1947, this had increased to 5.1 beds per 1,000, and by 1948, to 5.6 beds per 1,000, a remarkable increase in only two years.[97] Since the hospital insurance plan included inpatient diagnostic services, the HSPC had also provided grants to numerous hospitals towards the purchase of new chest X-ray units.[98]

Throughout this initial period, the HSPC was encouraging municipal governments to continue working together to establish union hospital districts (UHDs), allowing for the creation of larger hospitals with more

Table 6.1. Hospital utilization in first two years of public hospital insurance in Saskatchewan, 1947–8

| Year | Patients admitted and discharged — Number excluding newborns (per 1,000) | Patient days — Number (per 1,000) | Average length of stay |
|---|---|---|---|
| 1947 | 121,951 (156) | 1,221,453 (1,565) | 10.0 |
| 1948 | 138,030 (178) | 1,455,744 (1,875) | 10.5 |
| | Newborns number | Newborn patient days | |
| 1947 | 20,415 | 187,092 | 9.2 |
| 1948 | 19,164 | 173,743 | 9.4 |

Source: Malcolm G. Taylor, "The Saskatchewan Hospital Services Plan: A Study in Compulsory Health Insurance" (PhD diss., University of California at Berkeley, 1949), 304–5.

doctors, nurses, and equipment that could better serve the residents of numerous rural and urban municipalities. In 1947, 8 new UHDs were established, including the Swift Current Union Hospital District, bringing the total number of UHDs to 67 by year's end. By the end of 1948, a further 11 new UHDs had been added, bringing the total to 78. This compared to only 26 UHDs in 1944, at the outset of CCF government, to 37 in 1945 and 59 in 1946. In other words, the number of UHDs had tripled in 4.5 years of CCF administration. The HSPC also helped local governments enlarge existing UHDs, and, in 1947–8, several municipalities without hospitals were added to ten existing UHDs. Their hospitals became a magnet drawing the farmers and townspeople within the enlarged UHD boundaries.[99]

This rapid growth in hospital infrastructure was essential to the success of the hospital plan. If the Douglas government had not begun its hospital construction and improvement efforts in tandem with the hospital owners, whether local governments, the Catholic Church, or the Red Cross, in 1945–6, and if it had not ramped up the program in 1947–8, the increased use of hospitals by patients with the advent of universal coverage would have swamped hospitals, created burdensome wait times for procedures and diagnostics, and undermined the entire program. Instead, the opposite happened. Hospital care was now available to all residents based on need. Patients could access any hospital in the province by simply showing their hospital services card.[100] The fact that this expansion occurred before the introduction of the National Health Grants Program, discussed below, meant that

Saskatchewan, unlike other provinces, relied on its own revenue base to increase hospital capacity.

From the day the Saskatchewan plan was introduced until the country's final universal hospital insurance plan was implemented in Quebec in 1961, "no provincial government failed to send its officials to Regina to learn at first-hand how the program operated" and how it "could be adapted to their home provinces."[101] Even at the design stage early in 1946, senior officials in the government of British Columbia exhibited considerable interest in the Douglas government's unfolding plans.[102] So impressed was British Columbia's Liberal-Conservative coalition that that government enacted a universal hospital insurance plan modelled on the Saskatchewan program in 1948. In politics, as in life, imitation is the sincerest form of flattery, and the fact that a provincial coalition government established to keep the CCF out of power adopted Saskatchewan's "socialist" plan spoke volumes about the popularity of hospital coverage.

In Ottawa, the new federal health minister, Paul Martin Sr., who had replaced Brooke Claxton, was also impressed. He was carefully observing the Saskatchewan experiment, as he had taken over the portfolio with the hope that, sooner or later, the federal government would underwrite a national hospital insurance plan.[103] As he saw it, Douglas and Mott had proven such a plan was viable, even in a rather poor province.[104] Martin's parliamentary secretary stated in the House of Commons that "the authorities and the people of Saskatchewan" deserved "a great deal of credit for what has been accomplished in the matter of hospitalization."[105]

**The 1948 Election and the Hospital Insurance Plan**

As he had planned from the time he insisted on the earliest possible implementation date, Douglas pointed to universal hospital coverage as a significant down payment on his 1944 election promise of access to a comprehensive suite of health services. Under the slogan "Progress with Security," in which the CCF also promised farm, labour, education, social, and democratic security, health security was itemized not only as hospital coverage but also an increase in hospital beds and the establishment of six health regions, air ambulance services, and free treatment of cancer, polio, venereal disease, and mental illness for all residents.[106] During the election campaign, CCF candidates made frequent references to hospital insurance, emphasizing the low premium cost for individuals and families, as illustrated in its one-page advertisement in the *Regina Leader-Post* on behalf of the two local candidates, Clarence Fines and Charles Williams.

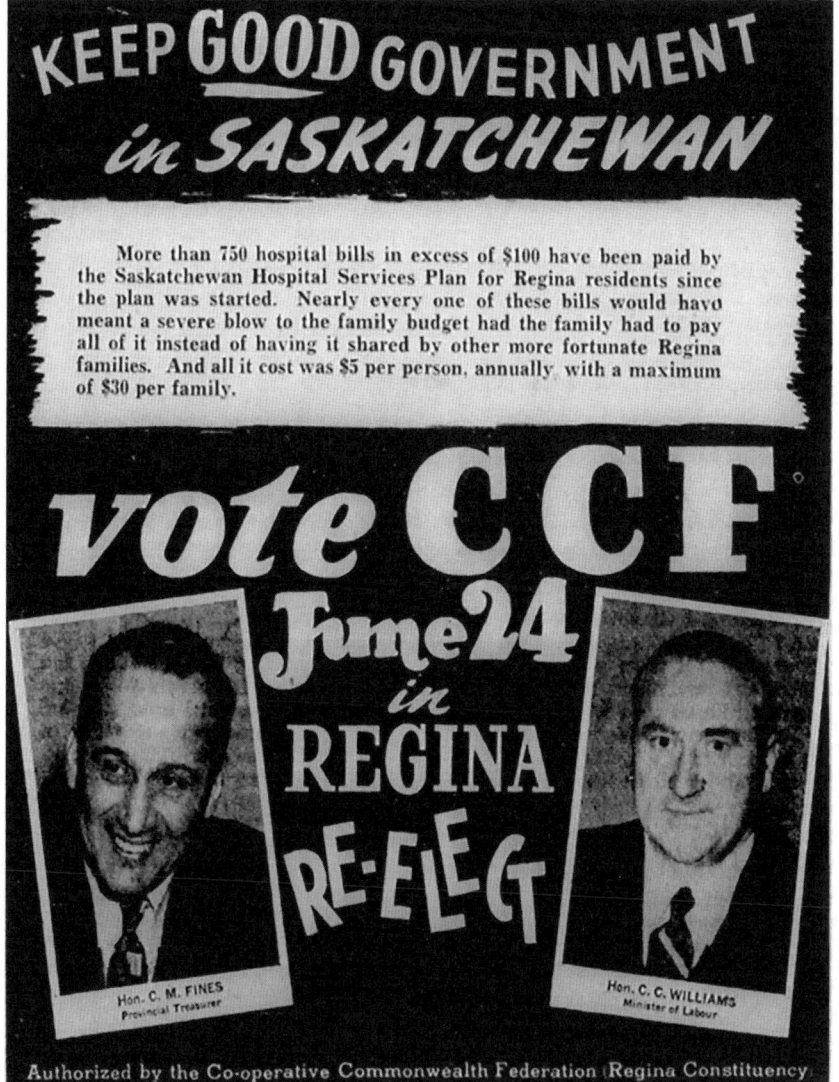

Full-page CCF election campaign ad, 1948 (*Regina Leader-Post*, 8 June 1948, 10)

The fact that the hospital plan was the CCF's best argument for a second term was reflected in the Liberal campaign. Walter Tucker, the Liberal's blustery leader, promised that his party, if elected, would not dismantle the program. Instead, he pledged to expand it while making it more cost effective and to decentralize to local governments what he described as the top-heavy administration set up by Mott and Rosenfeld in Regina.[107] Tucker and the Liberals relied on a crude Cold War hysteria, linking the CCF with communists everywhere, combined with a promise to end the tax-and-spend approach of the Douglas government.[108] One major Liberal newspaper ad placed in the major dailies proclaimed "Up Go Taxes! Down Comes the Iron Curtain."[109] This red baiting eventually prompted Douglas to issue a scathing response that was printed by the *Leader-Post* as part of an election series in which all political parties were invited to present their cases:

> Our opponents say that we are dropping an Iron Curtain around Saskatchewan; that we smack of Russia; that we plan to expropriate all industry, services and utilities; that we are working toward the kind of tyranny and despotism found in Russia; that our plans are laid to take over and regiment the farmer's life and to throw him on a communal farm; that our past four years' accomplishments are an absolute guarantee that Soviet collectivism is around the corner; that we will probably hold no more elections because we can brook no opposition, and if they are held the people will be able to vote only for official candidates; that first, will come the bridgehead then crash comes the iron curtain of dictatorship, terror and tyranny, and we are that bridgehead ...
>
> Actually, there is an iron curtain around Saskatchewan, but it is not [of] our making. It is similar to the iron curtain that exists today around Britain and its Labor government. It is an iron curtain that distorts and misrepresents the facts about an active, progressive government which is trying to give its people a better way of life but which, in doing so, runs directly counter to capitalistic and reactionary concepts and systems which have proved to be helpless in meeting today's problems.[110]

Even while attacking the Douglas government as socialists in bed with communists, the Liberals seemed to be imitating the detail of CCF programs as well as its progressive approach to government. In response to the CCF slogan "Progress with Security," the Liberals countered with "Progress and Security with Freedom," arguing that the choice for voters as either "Four More Years of Socialism in Saskatchewan, or a Return to Sound Democratic Government."[111]

When Tucker suggested that the CCF intended to socialize the province's farms, a throwback to the Liberal characterization of the

Farmer-Labor Group's land-lease platform in the 1934 provincial election, Douglas was quick to deny that his party ever had any intention of doing so.[112] "Only a stupid person would call any Social Democratic party Communistic," Douglas stated at his Weyburn nominating convention in early June. On the contrary, "Social Democrats are the only governments holding the Communists at bay" in Canada and Europe.[113]

In fact, Douglas argued, the lack of any new policy ideas on the part of the Liberals reflected the "do-nothing Liberalism" of their federal counterparts, who continued to refuse to establish a national, shared-cost comprehensive health insurance program based on the Green Book proposals. He told audience after audience that, while the federal and provincial Liberals had regularly used the Heagerty Plan and the subsequent Green Book proposals as political propaganda in elections, they never had the intention of carrying them out: "The Haggerty [sic] bill and Haggerty plan," he proclaimed, "are as dead as the hopes of the Liberal party in Saskatchewan."[114] As stated in a CCF advertisement, the issue was whether voters wanted to go "Backward to Do-Nothing Liberalism or Forward to CCF Accomplishment."[115] Moreover, the CCF reinforced that the federal Liberals' failure to implement the Green Book proposals was responsible for putting an unnecessary fiscal burden on the province and its financing of hospital insurance and was preventing the province from also covering physician services.[116]

Understandably proud of what had been accomplished in four years, Douglas fought the 1948 campaign based on the record of his government. The jewel in the crown – universal hospital coverage – had improved the life of most in the province. Confident of the outcome, he assumed his CCF administration would be rewarded on voting day, even if they would lose some votes for other policies that were not as popular, such as the larger school unit initiative, which had upset so many rural municipal officials because of its top-down imposition.

When the votes were counted, Douglas found his government had won not much more than a workable majority, a disappointing but, for Douglas, not unexpected result, given the lopsided nature of the CCF's landslide victory in 1944.[117] The party lost sixteen seats, dropping from forty-seven to thirty-one, with most of the losses in rural areas. The CCF's share of the popular vote, although still a respectable 47.6 per cent, had declined by 5.6 points. Why did this happen? According to many of the more right-wing members of the party, it was because the government had gone too far too fast in its first term and upset too many people who were comfortable with the status quo. According to the far left within and outside the CCF, it was because the government had not done enough or had compromised too much with certain interest groups, and they wasted no time turning their guns on the CCF. For

172   Tommy Douglas and the Quest for Medicare in Canada

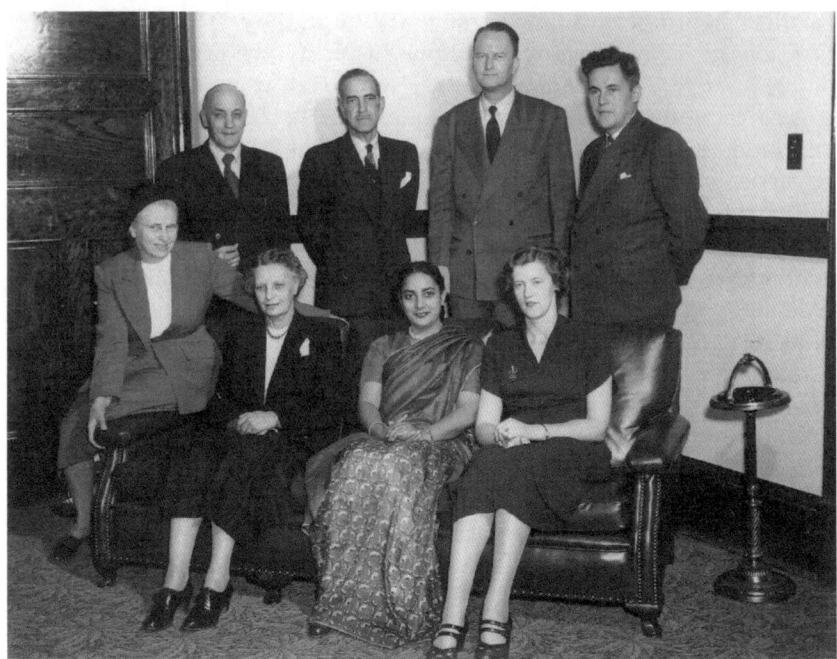

Fred Mott (standing, second from right) with foreign delegation examining the Saskatchewan Hospital Services Plan, 1950 (PAS R-A2935)

his part, Douglas refrained from attacking organized medicine directly during the election campaign, but he did state that while the wealthier doctors, mainly specialists in the cities, opposed the government's plans for the health care system, especially its plan for organized health regions, he nonetheless continued to have confidence that a majority of doctors would support his government's health reforms.[118]

Some in the party's left wing perceived the hospital plan as a retreat from a socialized health system of polyclinic health centres and primary care clinics staffed by salaried doctors. On this, Douglas's answer was that the government would continue encouraging the establishment of more health regions until the province was covered, but that the pace would be set by the municipal governments who were prepared to buy into the concept. Douglas was also unwilling to force salaried remuneration either on local governments or rural doctors.[119]

Douglas nonetheless felt that hospital coverage was a major factor in his government's re-election and would reverberate positively for successive elections afterwards. In the 1952 provincial election, which delivered a larger majority for the CCF, for example, Douglas was convinced that hospital insurance had been the single most important factor in keeping the CCF in government. Although Mott had left the province to return to the United States just months before the election in June 1952, he received a letter from Douglas just after that election in which the premier told him that the program he "left behind," in such excellent working condition was "more responsible for the [electoral] results than any other single factor."[120]

Following the election of 1948, the immediate challenge was not only to figure out how to finance the government's expensive social programs, the costliest of which was its hospitalization plan, but how to expand it to cover medical care, as T.C. had promised in the election campaign.[121] Douglas always understood that the downside of going it alone was the cost to the provincial treasury; indeed, his health department absorbed 22 per cent of the entire provincial budget. As George Cadbury, the government's most senior economic advisor and chair of the Economic Advisory and Planning Board, identified in a revealing letter to a close friend soon after the hospital plan had begun, this burden was beginning to cause serious problems both for Douglas and the government.[122] The financing of hospital insurance and other expensive department responsibilities increasingly seemed to be at the expense of other departments and the mandates of his other ministers. Moreover, given the fact that the provincial economy was almost wholly dependent on agriculture and the export of grain, both subject to uncontrollable factors such as rainfall and international markets, revenues could plummet if a drought occurred or if the global price of wheat suddenly dropped. This would cut public revenues and restrict public borrowing while health expenditures would continue to grow or, if the crisis was deep enough, begin to soar, given the inverse relationship between income and illness. Confiding to his UK friend, Cadbury said these considerations had forced the Douglas government to increase hospital premiums just months after the 1948 provincial election. The problem, according to Cadbury, was reconciling the Douglas government's rapidly growing health and education budgets with its limited financial means. Given the fact that the province was renting its individual and corporate income taxes to the federal government, the only way to finance this growth was through increases in regressive hospital and education taxes and by cutting costs or services in other programs.[123]

Despite his 1948 promise to extend universal coverage to medical care, Douglas knew this was impossible without the federal government sharing costs, and he devoted considerable time and political capital to trying to pressure the St-Laurent government into calling a federal-provincial conference and implementing a version of the original Heagerty Plan. Although he persisted in believing that federal assistance was just around the corner, he was to be disappointed again and again in the years to come.

It would take another decade before Saskatchewan received direct assistance, and this would be limited to hospital insurance, forcing him to proceed with medicare in the face of very constrained provincial finances. He was willing to take the risk of proceeding without federal cost sharing on both hospital and medical care insurance because he was convinced that the federal government would never consider cost sharing until a provincial government could demonstrate both the feasibility of a program and its political attractiveness. He had to make Saskatchewan the laboratory in which universal health coverage would be tested and proved so that it would become the model for the rest of the country and feed popular pressure on the federal government to act.

# 7 National Health Grants and New Frontiers

*To stay in office for twenty years and to win five consecutive elections is not the record of a mere protest movement. The CCF government, elected in 1944 under the leadership of T.C. Douglas, proved itself something much more than that. There was content in its program and method in its execution.*

George Cadbury, 1971[1]

Despite T.C.'s persistent lobbying for Ottawa to share the cost of the Saskatchewan hospital insurance program, the federal government under Prime Ministers Mackenzie King and Louis St-Laurent steadfastly refused. Instead, the Liberals inaugurated the National Health Grants Program in 1948. Although initially not keen on the program, Douglas had to admit its usefulness in funding new provincial initiatives in health as well as needed health human resources and infrastructure.

The federal health grants allowed the province to continue existing programs in public health, tuberculosis control, monitoring and control of infectious diseases, and health research in numerous areas. The provincial hospitalization program was buttressed by grants to construct new hospitals as well as to refit and expand existing hospitals. Despite the assistance they provided, T.C. always felt that the national health grants were a poor substitute for federal cost sharing of comprehensive health insurance. Yet, his government could not have financed such an ambitious program of health reform without the substantial financial support that came from these grants. While every province benefited substantially from the program – which was in place for over twenty years – the CCF government in Saskatchewan took greatest advantage of Ottawa's money to learn about, experiment with, and ultimately extend the frontiers of the organization and delivery of health services and the research base supporting these new developments.

More importantly, the health grants program would help pay for new health initiatives, including a detailed health survey and analysis of the province, which provided a baseline for health system planning and targeted interventions throughout the 1950s, as well as support for new mental health programs, policies, and research, among the most innovative in the world at the time. However, success created its own problems, including the rising expectations of mental health advocates and prominent psychiatrists working for the CCF government. Although T.C. resigned the health portfolio in 1949, health initiatives continued under the ministers he appointed. Moreover, as premier and the savviest health policy member of his own cabinet, he followed all developments in his old department with a sharp eye until he became leader of the federal New Democratic Party in 1961.

**Origins of the National Health Grants Program**

In the two years preceding the introduction of the National Health Grants Program, T.C. was so focused on resurrecting the Green Book proposals that he did not see such a program coming. He never for a moment considered the possibility that federal health grants would be offered in isolation from the health insurance proposal.

T.C. had begun his campaign in 1946, just after the Dominion-Provincial Reconstruction Conference was postponed indefinitely. He asked Mackenzie King to meet again with those premiers who were willing to accept the federal proposals. King said he would be willing to reopen the Green Book proposals, but only after all the provinces accepted the federal tax proposals – a non-starter, given the positions of Ontario and Quebec.[2] Douglas could not understand why the prime minister allowed the central Canadian provinces to prevent any progress. He felt that the federal government should simply enter into tax-rental agreements with willing provinces and move on to comprehensive health insurance and the other social security elements in the Green Book. King remained adamant, however, that the Green Book proposals were dead until the federal government received the fiscal security of a permanent tax transfer, something that would mean little if the country's two most populous and industrial provinces refused to endorse such an agreement.[3]

By 1947, T.C. was in full attack mode, telling Chris Higginbotham, a journalist close to him and his government, for public release, that the failure of the federal Liberals to implement the Green Book proposals was "a breach of faith," and would "almost certainly be the main issue on which the C.C.F. government" would fight its next election in

1948.⁴ Douglas seized upon Mackenzie King's statement that he would be prepared to call another first ministers' conference "as soon as there was sufficient acceptance" of a permanent provincial tax transfer to Ottawa. Based on his view that the six provinces that had accepted this transfer constituted "sufficient acceptance," Douglas threatened to ask Saskatchewan voters to show "that they disapprove of Ontario and Quebec running the Federal government."⁵

Then, in mid-May 1948, roughly a month before the provincial election, Fred Mott described to Douglas a Round Table on Social Security sponsored by the government of Canada he had just attended at the University of Toronto. The key figure attending was Paul Martin Sr., the minister of national health and welfare since his elevation in December 1946 from his previous position as a parliamentary secretary.⁶ An ambitious politician with his eyes firmly fixed on becoming leader of the Liberal Party of Canada and prime minister, Martin was determined to carve out a dynamic policy legacy. A social reformer, he was very much in the minority in the conservative cabinet under Mackenzie King, who was soon to be succeeded (to Martin's great chagrin) by King's preferred heir, Louis St-Laurent. As one journalist put it, Martin was isolated as "a Liberal in a sometimes high-Tory cabinet."⁷ According to Mott, Martin "aroused a storm of protest" from the provincial attendees when he "suggested that perhaps the thing to do was to make health grants [to the provinces] at the present time and then about five years later subsidize health insurance." Mott was taken aback and, in his words, "was among those who stated in no uncertain terms that there should be no delay in instituting financial assistance for provincial health insurance plans."⁸

Little did Douglas or Mott know that Martin's announcement of the health grants was based on a less than popular cabinet decision engineered over many months.⁹ Few outside the federal cabinet room could have fully appreciated Martin's struggle to realize the National Health Grants Program. When he first became minister of national health and welfare, Martin realized that the failure of the Dominion-Provincial Reconstruction Conference had scuttled the idea of national health insurance. Although he had one of the most smoothly running departments in the government when he took over from Brooke Claxton in 1946, he and his officials were nonetheless demoralized that the health insurance proposals first put forward by J.J. Heagerty had gone nowhere.

In the summer of 1947, Martin hired Harry Cassidy, a leading academic from the University of Toronto and expert on issues of social welfare and health, to "conduct a thorough rethink" of the original Green Book proposals and adapt them to the new political environment.¹⁰

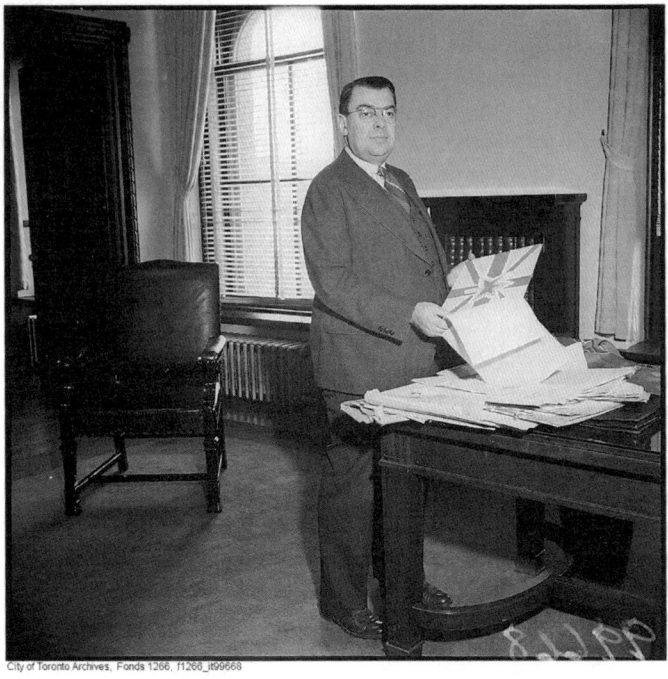

Paul Martin Sr. in his parliamentary office, 1945 (Wikimedia Commons)

During the 1930s, Cassidy had been a CCF activist and had worked as a director of social welfare for the government of British Columbia. Under the federal Liberals, he worked with the Department of National Health and Welfare's formidable research division to generate a series of studies that were presented in weekend workshops to senior officials, while the mandarins in the rest of official Ottawa "looked on from afar and wondered at the 'strange things happening in the health department.'"[11]

In December 1947, Cassidy presented his work to Martin. Although national health insurance was no longer a viable option, he recommended that the department act immediately and unilaterally with federal health grants to the provinces. These grants, originally presented as a supporting measure to the main health insurance plan in the Green Book proposals, would become the main vehicle to prepare for a comprehensive health insurance program in the future. The grants would be accompanied by other social welfare measures, including a contributory pension plan. Martin agreed and took the plan to King, who had just announced his intention to retire before the end of 1948.

Martin "wooed" the prime minister "with flattery," arguing that the retiring politician needed to pursue the measures so he could step down knowing that he had achieved the "humanitarian" goals he had set for himself when he entered the political arena as an idealistic young man.[12] Although King rejected the contributory pension part of the plan, he agreed with the health grants idea as long as it was trimmed down. Martin reduced the $40 million proposal to $30 million, but when he brought the matter before cabinet in April, and again in early May, his colleagues refused to make a final decision. Instead, the plan was sent to a committee of senior officials, who would agree only if the grants were renamed "to remove any implication" that they were "a precursor to national health insurance."[13] But once Martin had done this to the satisfaction of the committee, he found his cabinet colleagues implacably opposed.

Concerned about Martin's inability to convince his colleagues – and about his lack of political judgment generally – King decided he needed to step in and handle the matter himself. Martin had convinced him of the desirability of the federal health grants as a legacy policy in light of the failed dominion-provincial conference, but he despaired at Martin's inability to manage cabinet members who perceived him as overly ambitious and a media hound who had a tendency to leak matters under confidential discussion. To fix things, King met with Martin as well as his chief opponents for the party helm, Finance Minister Doug Abbott and Martin's chief rival for the post of prime minister, Louis St-Laurent. King then told each what their respective roles would be in the ensuing cabinet discussion. King would open the debate, framing the health grants program in terms of past Liberal promises, after which he would ask Martin to review the program in detail. King would then call upon the minister of finance. This would set up Abbott, who would then put up a *pro forma* defence of the treasury view, only to have St-Laurent (at King's prior request) swooping in at the end to support the health grants program, a finale that would be surprising to the rest of the cabinet, given St-Laurent's long-standing opposition to the idea.[14]

On 12 May 1948, this precise pantomime played out in the cabinet room in the East Block of the Parliament Buildings. To make sure no unexpected opposition arose that day, King adjourned the meeting after the various actors had played their parts, delaying the decision till the following day and making sure his message had sunk in. Cabinet then unanimously approved the plan and, the day after that, King personally made the announcement in Parliament concerning the National Health Grants Program.[15] It was a masterful orchestration by King but one that did little to improve Martin's relationship with the rest of cabinet, particularly Abbott and St-Laurent, who, if not for their boss, would have done everything in their power to block the program.[16]

T.C.'s initial reaction to the National Health Grants Program was also negative. In a letter to Martin, he stated his belief that health grants would be used to indefinitely postpone the introduction of national health insurance. Martin strongly refuted this interpretation. In a line Martin would repeat over and over for the next ten years, the grants merely represented "the first step in the development of a comprehensive Health Insurance Plan for all Canada."[17] There is no evidence on whether T.C. believed Martin but, without any doubt, he did not believe Martin's bosses – first Mackenzie King and then Louis St-Laurent.[18] And the program undoubtedly undermined to some extent the arguments T.C. had been using for reconvening the Dominion-Provincial Reconstruction Conference.[19] After all, the federal government, without any negotiation with the provinces, had introduced a portion of the Green Book proposals, with a promise to implement comprehensive health coverage in the future.

Douglas was also upset that all the money the province had already spent on hospital construction – over $1 million – between 1945 and 1948 was not retroactively eligible for the federal grants. Although he described this as the price his government paid "for being too progressive," he was nonetheless glad he had gone ahead. Without the grants for new hospitals as well as the medical assistance grants for municipalities to hire more doctors, the province could never have proceeded with universal hospital insurance in 1947.[20] This did not mean that Douglas was above trying to attack the Liberals for "replacing" the more ambitious Green Book proposals with the limited National Health Grants Program.

Although known as the National Health Grants Program by everyone outside Ottawa, Martin and his deputy minister, G.D.W. (Donald) Cameron, insisted on calling it the National Health Program for Canada.[21] False advertising for a more comprehensive program, the term "National Health Program for Canada" never really caught on, and I use the far more accepted label, "National Health Grants Program," here.

## National Health Grants in Action

Despite T.C.'s criticisms, his government would take full advantage of the National Health Grants Program.[22] In its first year of operation, in 1948, the federal government made available just over $30 million in health grants to the provinces, worth a bit more than $400 million in 2023 Canadian dollars.[23] By the summer of 1949, less than a year after the grants had begun to flow, Paul Martin gleefully told the press that his department was spending $5,000 per hour on national health grants.[24]

The federal government added considerably more money to the program in each successive year until it expired in the late 1960s. All the grants except one – a one-time grant to conduct a comprehensive survey of health services and population health in each jurisdiction – would continue until the late 1960s. Roughly 43 per cent of the total that first year were earmarked for hospital construction, although such expenditures were intended to decline rapidly relative to increases in the other health grants.

Beyond hospital grants and the one-time health survey, the money was distributed in the following eight categories, as described in the original phraseology and in descending order based on the size of allotted expenditures: 1) public health; 2) mental health; 3) cancer control; 4) tuberculosis control; 5) venereal disease control; 6) crippled children; 7) professional training; and 8) public health research.[25] Except for research, the potential amount each province could be allocated was based on a per capita calculation, although the actual amount received depended on the province providing a satisfactory proposal.

Thanks to the depth of expertise gathered by Fred Mott in the Health Services Planning Commission (HSPC), Saskatchewan proved extremely adept at putting together coherent proposals that the Department of National Health and Welfare could accept, confident the money was being well spent. Indeed, in the first few months of the National Health Grants Program's operation, Saskatchewan was able to secure 73 per cent of its per capita allotment, the largest proportion in the country.[26] Even though no province could exceed its per capita allotment, it was still up to individual governments to produce satisfactory proposals if they wanted to claim their share. These proposals had to indicate the objectives sought by the spending, how it built upon (and did not replace) existing provincial spending plans, and what the province was willing to bring to the table in terms of fiscal resources, both in cash and in kind.

Mott assigned Malcolm G. Taylor the task of spearheading the health grant proposals.[27] An Albertan by birth, Taylor had largely completed (though not yet defended) his PhD thesis at the University of California at Berkeley. In contention for an academic position at the University of Toronto, Taylor was drawn instead to Saskatchewan by Mott.[28] Mott had first met Taylor when he stopped in Regina while travelling from California to Toronto eighteen months earlier.[29] The stop was no

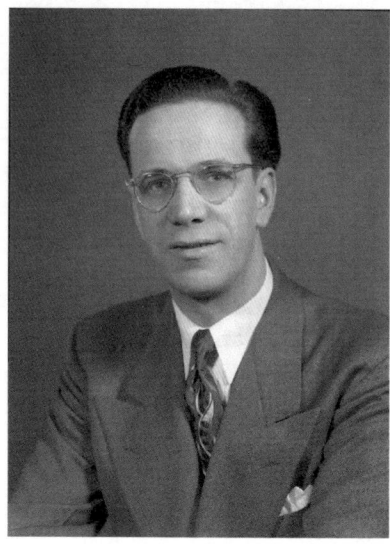

Malcolm G. Taylor, director of research for the Health Services Planning Commission (1948–51), in 1950 (PAS R-WS-A11567)

accident. Taylor's dissertation was on the origins and implementation of Saskatchewan's hospitalization program, and he was keen to do some on-the-ground research and interviews.[30] When Len Rosenfeld left the HSPC in August 1948 to take up a position in the United States, Taylor was appointed HSPC secretary.

As the research director for both the HSPC and the Department of Public Health (Mott assumed the role in deputy minister in addition to HSPC chair in 1949), Taylor was in the best position to understand ongoing developments in Saskatchewan across a host of health sectors and his department's planning and priorities in terms of the organization and delivery of health services. Both Mott and Taylor had a dedicated team of specialists, many of whom they had hired personally. When Taylor left the province in 1951 to join the University of Toronto, another accomplished planner, Dr. Murray S. Acker, Mott's personal assistant in 1947–8, would take on his role until 1956, when he left Regina for Singapore to work for the World Health Organization.[31] Without doubt, the high calibre of departmental leadership gave the province a major advantage in maximizing the take-up and effective use of federal health grants.

In the case of hospital construction grants, the federal government required a 50 per cent fiscal commitment from the provinces. While upset that the rules prohibited cost sharing of the enormous investment

Table 7.1. Provincial and federal contributions to hospital construction in Saskatchewan, fiscal year 1944–5 to May 1949 (in $ millions)

|  | Provincial grants to municipalities (expended) | Provincial grants committed to municipal-ities but not yet spent | Provincial loans for hospital construction | Grants approved by federal government | Federal grants requested by province but not yet approved |
|---|---|---|---|---|---|
| Rural hospitals | $768 | $177 | $179 | $255 | $85 |
| Urban hospital | $13 | $237 | $0 | $237 | $202 |
| Total | $781 | $414 | $179 | $492 | $287 |

Notes: Urban hospitals are defined as hospitals in Regina, Saskatoon, Moose Jaw, and Prince Albert. In the case of urban hospitals, the amount includes intended request but with applications still pending. All amounts are rounded to nearest million.
Source: Provincial Archives of Saskatchewan, C.M. Fines fonds, F119, R-37, I-30, Grants and loans for hospital construction, 1944–5 to 16 May 1949.

already made by the provincial government between 1944 and the implementation of health grants in 1948, T.C. was nonetheless quick to use the program, which allowed him to supercharge his own plans for hospital expansion, as illustrated in table 7.1.[32] By May 1949, his government had spent or committed close to $1.2 billion in grants for hospital construction. Although the National Health Grants Program had only recently been launched, Saskatchewan had already been approved to receive almost $500 million in federal hospital construction grants. In addition, T.C.'s department was in the process of preparing close to $300 worth of additional federal hospital construction grant applications.

This influx of cash resulted not only in the building of new hospitals where none had existed but also the modernization and expansion of standing hospitals. With universal hospital coverage increasing the demand for hospital services, this hothouse growth in the supply of hospital beds was able to meet the demand and ensure adequate access even in the rural areas.[33] Grants were also used to purchase new medical devices and diagnostic equipment. New specialized wings for cancer treatment, acute psychiatric care, and treatment for cerebral palsy were added to the major hospitals in Regina and Saskatoon.[34]

Under a professional training grant, accountants in numerous Saskatchewan hospitals received two-day courses in modern hospital accounting methods. The idea for the course came from the Department of Public Health, with the objective of improving hospital efficiency and lowering costs. Viewing the project as promising, the federal government subsequently developed a similar training project in New Brunswick, with the hope that it would be adopted in other provinces.[35] The national health grants were used to employ, and improve the education and training of, public health nurses working for the Department of Public Health who were providing services in rural Saskatchewan as well as in the health departments of Saskatoon and Regina.[36] Federal health grants were used to hire two nutritionists to work in the newly forming health regions as well as a travelling dietitian to visit hospitals too small to have a dietitian on staff.[37]

Paul Martin also leveraged national health grants for personal and partisan purposes. Every grant offered Martin a potential media announcement, and the opening of every hospital or similar facility offered an in-person ribbon cutting opportunity. Although the province often put up more money than the federal government, T.C. had to accept playing second fiddle to Martin at such official openings.[38] A media hound, Martin kept close track of the press coverage of these announcements and opening ceremonies.[39]

Martin was extremely adept at using such events to further the interests of the Liberal Party during by-elections and general elections. One example was in the by-election for the federal constituency of Rosthern in October 1948. A by-election was needed because the incumbent MP, Walter Tucker, had resigned to become the leader of the Liberal Party of Saskatchewan.[40] The Liberals wanted to slow the CCF's momentum in the province by keeping the seat, so Martin and Jimmy Gardiner were dispatched from Ottawa to tour the constituency. Martin visited at least six towns, with announcements and ribbon cuttings during the day followed by partisan political rallies in the late afternoon or evening.[41] Using the National Health Grants Program as his chief example, Martin argued that his party could be relied upon more than the CCF to actually implement social reform.[42] In one rally, he went further, predicting that, under its new provincial leader, Walter Tucker, the Liberals would rebound and take back Saskatchewan in the next general election.[43]

For his part, T.C. used the National Health Grants Program not only to further his ambitious health reform agenda but to ensure that his achievements could be used by the CCF as political ammunition in provincial and federal elections. A case in point was the June 1949 federal election. Three months before it was called, M.J. Coldwell pressed Martin on why the Liberal government was refusing to proceed with its "promised" plan of national health insurance. After all, Coldwell

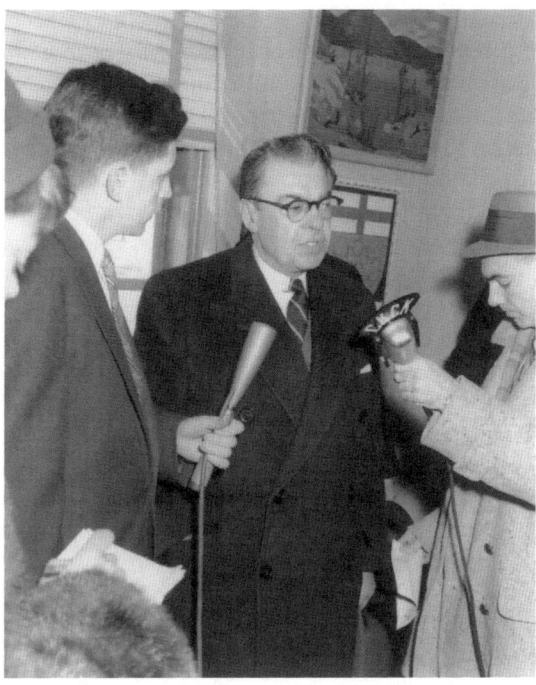

Paul Martin Sr. being interviewed in Regina (PAS R-LP760)

argued, Martin himself said that the purpose of the National Health Grants Program was to establish universal health coverage. When Martin replied that the grants were a prerequisite to national health insurance, Coldwell reminded Martin that the Liberals had already made the promise in the 1945 election campaign and opined that the grants were nothing more than a ploy to continue promising health insurance without delivering on its substance.[44]

In the election campaign in May, the federal CCF circulated a brochure on the Saskatchewan CCF government's achievements over the past four years. Referring to the $30 million earmarked by the Liberals for national health grants as "one-fifth of what the Federal Government promised in 1945," the brochure emphasized that the program provided "nothing for health insurance."[45] In his campaign speeches, Coldwell compared the Liberals' vague promise of national health insurance with the CCF's proposed coverage of hospital, medical, dental, and vision care, to be paid for through social security contributions supplemented by general taxation.[46]

The 1949 federal election was a "resounding" victory for the St-Laurent Liberals, the "greatest sweep" of any party up to that time. The CCF were crushed, losing more seats (fifteen) than the thirteen it was left with. As stated in one scholarly analysis of the election, the CCF was unable to make health insurance – or any other policy – a major issue in the campaign. Without doubt, national health grants insulated the Liberals from their vulnerability on the issue, and that program combined with past and present social security measures, such as unemployment insurance, the baby bonus, and increases to old age pensions, drew at least some potential CCF votes into the Liberal column.[47]

Whatever electoral damage the National Health Grants Program had inflicted on the CCF, there is little question the grants were of enormous assistance to Douglas's health policy ambitions. The balance of this chapter focuses on two key health initiatives in the province that benefited considerably from federal health grants. The first was the one-time grant for a provincial health survey, which provided a foundation for health system planning in Saskatchewan for the remainder of T.C.'s time in office. The second area was Saskatchewan's groundbreaking initiatives in mental health reform and research.

**The Saskatchewan Health Survey**

The purpose of the one-time health survey grant was to allow provincial governments to conduct an intensive study of their respective health systems and thereby provide a more solid foundation to better meet future health needs and services.[48] Douglas and Mott understood immediately that the work and resulting report could be of enormous assistance in their project of building a coordinated and comprehensive health system.

T.C. immediately began to review the possibility of a health survey with stakeholders to obtain their expertise and advise as part of the survey's work. Mott reorganized the HSPC to provide the research and analytic capacity to conduct the survey. He established a Division of Research and Statistics in the HSPC just weeks after the federal announcement of the National Health Grants Program and, as noted above, hired Malcolm Taylor as research director.[49]

The College of Physicians and Surgeons (CPS) expected the survey to be an independent joint initiative of the college and the government. Registering surprise when Mott sent the CPS a preliminary scoping review for the health survey, the college complained about having no input.[50] It confronted Douglas, who stood behind Mott's handling of the matter. While Mott and the HSPC, Douglas explained, would "use appropriate advisory groups to the full possible extent," there could be no debate on the "question of final responsibility and authority for the health survey. These must rest with the government."[51]

Part of the problem was that the federal government had not provided direction on how the surveys were to be administered. Since Saskatchewan already had a dedicated health policy and planning entity, it made sense to Douglas to make the Health Services and Planning Commission responsible for the survey. This clashed with the advice that the Canadian Medical Association was issuing to the provincial medical associations, that they take a very direct role in the surveys. The responses to the pressure exerted by organized medicine varied by province. British Columbia, Quebec, and Nova Scotia eventually vested their health bureaucracies with responsibility for their respective surveys, while other governments established stakeholder-based advisory committees to provide independent reports. Some of these committees were structured to give organized medicine the predominant voice, while others less so: Ontario, for example, gave no voice at all to the Ontario Medical Association.[52]

On 12 December 1948, Douglas and Mott met with college representatives. When the CPS suggested that Saskatchewan was the only province that looked like it was going to rely on a government department to conduct the survey, Douglas finally lost his patience with the doctors. He explained that, "unlike most other provinces," his government "had established an agency with survey and planning functions" well before the National Health Grants Program had been established. From the beginning, he wanted the report ultimately transmitted to Ottawa to "reflect governmental policies," and he stated plainly that, no matter what, "the Health Services Planning Commission must be the agency ultimately responsible for the Health Survey." He then testily added that the HSPC "already had statutory authority to conduct the Health Survey" and that he had already told Ottawa that the HSPC would be responsible for the survey. The meeting ended with the CPS providing a memorandum with suggestions for professional representation on a proposed health survey committee.[53]

Douglas responded two weeks later with a counterproposal. The HSPC would be authorized to appoint a health survey committee on which the HSPC's chair (Fred Mott) and secretary (Malcolm Taylor) would act as chair and secretary, with Taylor also acting as the research director of the survey's full-time staff. The members would include professional representation, as suggested by the college: two CPS representatives and one representative each from the Registered Nurses' Association, the College of Dental Surgeons, and the Saskatchewan

Hospital Association. To these, the government would add members representing other organizations and the general public.[54]

These terms were close enough to what the college had proposed, and the CPS agreed, both sides living with the ambiguous governance structure: the college could say that the Health Survey Committee was an independent body, while the government could say that ultimate responsibility (and perhaps control) lay with the government.[55] Although he felt the college was entirely wrong-headed in its approach, Douglas was willing to countenance some face saving on the part of the CPS so the work could begin. He would trust Mott to stickhandle the doctors.

The whole affair proved less troublesome than Douglas had anticipated. At least one of the college's representatives, Clarence Houston, developed considerable respect for the abilities of Mott and Taylor during the two years the survey committee laboured.[56] Reflecting on Clarence Houston's memories of the Health Survey Committee, his son Stuart Houston said that "Mott's executive abilities as chair, coupled with Taylor's research skills ... persuaded the committee to embrace procedures that emphasized cooperation." When questions arose, they were always "hammered out to the point of agreement."[57]

The committee ultimately produced two major reports, without a doubt the most intensive investigation into the province's health resources and the state of its population's health ever conducted. In the words of a Canadian Medical Association (CMA) spokesperson who wrote a history of medicare on behalf of the CMA, the Saskatchewan health survey "surpassed that for any other province ... It was the classic of such projects."[58] When the reports were tabled in the provincial legislature, Health Minister Tom Bentley made it clear that the government endorsed all 115 of the committee's recommendations.[59] The first recommendation, for the provincial government to implement a comprehensive health insurance program "at the earliest possible date," was especially welcome. Both T.C. and Bentley could only agree with the Health Survey Committee that this program of coverage "should be extended, modified, and coordinated" so that "adequate health care of high quality" can be made "available to all residents of the province on the basis of need and without regard to individual ability to pay."[60]

Given the pitched battle over medicare between Douglas's government and the college less than ten years later, it may seem a wonder that the CPS agreed to such a statement in 1951. Struck by the cooperation of the CPS while he was acting as the committee's secretary and research director, Malcolm Taylor subsequently asserted that if the government had introduced universal medical care coverage at this time, it would have been able to do so with "the profession's approval and cooperation."[61] On this point, surely, Taylor was wrong. While the opposition would not have been as fierce as it proved to be a decade later, the profession was nonetheless opposed to a medical care plan solely financed and administered by the provincial government. Indeed, as discussed in the preceding chapter, this was the reason T.C. focused on universal hospital coverage as his first step towards comprehensive health insurance.

Thus, it was no accident that the Health Survey Committee report refused to specify the model of universal health coverage that should be implemented in the province. The medical profession in Saskatchewan and the rest of Canada was prepared to live with a single-payer plan for hospital care for one simple reason: physicians remained outside the plan. Most of the doctors working in hospitals were independent contractors and, as such, continued to bill patients and insurance companies for their services. In other words, organized medicine drew a major distinction between how hospital services were funded and how their own services should be paid, always insisting that government should never be their sole payer.[62]

By 1950, both the CMA and the CPS were clear that they endorsed a health insurance design in which the poor received public funding to purchase private insurance (especially physician-sponsored medical care insurance) rather than a universal single-payer scheme managed by government. As for any notion of a comprehensive health "system," the report clearly speaks to health insurance alone, as the CPS members on the Health Survey Committee would never have endorsed what they viewed as a "socialized" health system. However, the reality was that health insurance was far from the Douglas government's sole preoccupation.

## Transforming Mental Health Care

Long before he became premier of Saskatchewan, T.C. had been critical of the type of care offered in psychiatric hospitals. Shortly after moving to Weyburn in the early 1930s, he concluded that the two psychiatric hospitals in the province – both in small rural communities, one in Weyburn and the other in North Battleford – were overcrowded holding pens staffed by untrained workers.

Douglas appointed Dr. Clarence Hincks, the founder of the National Committee for Mental Hygiene (renamed the Canadian Mental Health Association in 1950), to review Saskatchewan's mental health services and facilities and deliver recommendations on how they could be transformed. In his report prepared for the government in 1946, Hincks highlighted the problem of overcrowding: the Saskatchewan Hospital North Battleford (opened in 1914) had 1,716 patients in a facility meant for 1,174, while, even more egregiously, the Saskatchewan Hospital Weyburn (opened in 1921) had 2,485 patients in a facility built for 1,040.[63] Hincks argued that the long-term solution to this serious problem was for the government to adopt a more community-oriented system involving regionally based outpatient clinics and psychiatric wards in all the general hospitals. The shorter-term solution was to build a third psychiatric hospital.[64]

In his report, Hincks also argued in favour of the forced sterilization of the "mentally defective," a recommendation immediately rejected by Douglas. By the time he became premier, T.C.'s personal views on sterilization had changed dramatically compared to the position he had taken in his master's thesis in 1933. According to psychiatric historian John A. Mills, this change was clearly reflected in a "set of letters he wrote to concerned members of the public repudiating the use of sterilization."[65] His government's policies on the issue would stand in sharp contrast to those adopted by the Manning Social Credit government in Alberta, which operated a program of sterilization until the 1960s.[66]

To figure out how, precisely, to implement acceptable aspects the Hincks Report, Douglas brought in external expertise in the newly created position of provincial psychiatrist and director of mental services in his Department of Public Health.[67] In November 1946, he recruited Dr. Donald Griffith (Griff) McKerracher, a senior specialist at the Toronto Psychiatric Hospital and resident psychiatrist at the University of Toronto. According to one historian of psychiatry, this would turn out to be "an inspired appointment."[68]

Griff McKerracher had extensive experience at various Ontario mental health institutions and had organized psychiatric treatment for the Canadian Army in Toronto and in England.[69] Douglas expected McKerracher to spearhead a revolution in mental health in the province. In return, he would defer to McKerracher's knowledge and experience by letting him make all the critical decisions on next steps and recruit whomever he chose, and would give him the money needed to carry out an ambitious program of mental health research and treatment in the province's two mental hospitals, as well as introduce outpatient clinics to "pick up cases in their early stages and provide early treatment."[70]

McKerracher moved quickly to change the way in which provincial mental hospitals in Weyburn and North Battleford were caring for their patients as well as to address psychiatric treatment in those long-term facilities and in the acute care psychiatric ward at the Regina General Hospital.[71] At the time he moved to Saskatchewan, most of the staff in

National Health Grants and New Frontiers 191

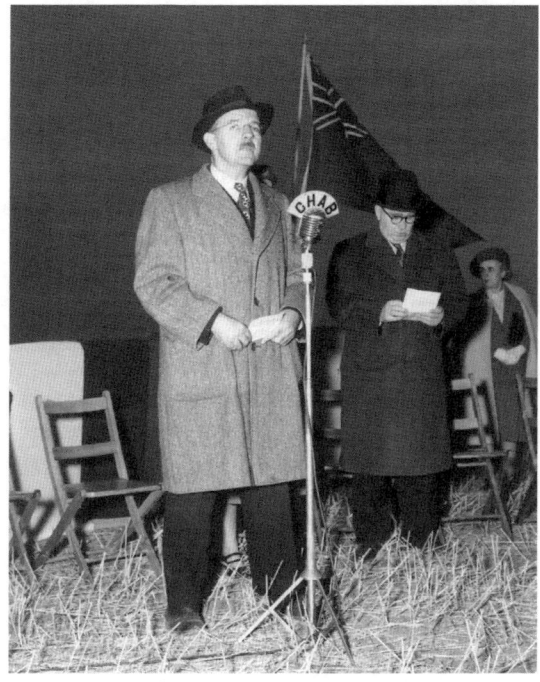

Griff McKerracher making an announcement, 16 October 1950 (PAS R-A2936)

the North Battleford and Weyburn mental hospitals were attendants with limited education and an even more limited understanding of, and sympathy for, mental illness. Their main task was to restrain the "inmates" when necessary. The challenge for McKerracher was that a wholesale change was needed, a move from a model of confinement to one where care and treatment were the focus, and this required a revolution in education, training, and attitudes. He could not replace most of the attendants with existing nurses in the province, because most nurses preferred working in acute care hospitals rather than mental hospitals – the salaries and the working conditions were simply better in the former.[72] With Douglas fully supporting McKerracher, legislation was passed creating a separate profession of psychiatric nursing in 1948.[73]

The first of its type in North America, the full-time three-year program involved courses and a salaried apprenticeship in the province's two mental hospitals. Advertisements were issued and new high school graduates throughout the province were encouraged to apply. Existing attendants were given the opportunity to upgrade their knowledge and skills, and those with sufficient motivation and educational background entered the program knowing that, if they graduated, they would have jobs in this reconfigured model of mental health care. Although there was initially a high exit and failure rate, the program quickly found its feet, and it was soon adopted in the three other western Canadian provinces. One nursing historian described the 1948 legislation and the program as "a watershed moment in the development of psychiatric nursing in Canada."[74]

In 1950, McKerracher set up the Psychiatric Services Branch (PSB) in the Department of Public Health. The PSB would rapidly become a "semi-independent fiefdom" within both the department and the government.[75] Although McKerracher and his successors were expected to report to the deputy minister and minister, they often bypassed these reporting relationships to deal directly with the premier. To generate a pool of new talent, McKerracher established a postgraduate training program for psychiatrists, the first one in Canada accepted by the Royal College of Physicians and Surgeons.[76] This program would become internationally known within a few years. When the celebrated American psychiatrist and mental health reformer Karl Menninger visited Saskatchewan a couple of years after the PSB was established, he concluded that McKerracher's psychiatric program was, in his words, the most "outstanding" public program in North America.[77]

No agency in the Douglas government grew as fast as the PSB. By the mid-1950s, it had more than 1,200 employees, almost 60 of whom were medical staff, including 20 psychiatrists, working at the two provincial mental hospitals, the policy and planning unit in Regina, and a psychiatric research unit in Saskatoon associated with the University of Saskatchewan.[78] By 1964, the year the CCF government left office, the PSB had 2,140 staff members. This represented 17 per cent of the entire public service and about 80 per cent of the Department of Public Health, the single largest department in the provincial government, as measured by the number of employees and expenditures. As the government's golden child, the PSB saw its budget climb almost exponentially from 1950 until 1964.[79] However, the PSB was also a demanding child, insisting that the Douglas government could and should do more for mental health.[80]

The PSB was the "instrument" McKerracher "needed to build a comprehensive programme of community psychiatry" as well as improve care in the two provincial mental hospitals.[81] He began to put together what would become one of the most talented, vibrant, and intriguing collections of psychiatrists and other clinician-researchers ever

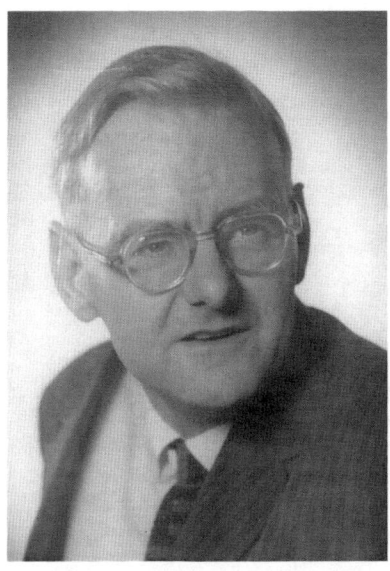

Humphry Osmond, c. 1960
(PAS R-A11559-2)

assembled in one place and at one time in North America.[82] He was also behind the 1950 amendment to the provincial Mental Health Act to change the purpose of mental hospitals from custody to therapy.[83] His PSB psychiatrists would play an important role in transitioning from an emphasis on the permanent custody and periodic pacification of patients to one involving their treatment and potential release.

Humphry Osmond was an example of the high calibre of psychiatrists whom McKerracher drew to Saskatchewan. In 1951, Osmond was senior registrar of the psychiatric unit at St. George's Hospital, one of England's largest teaching hospitals, a position he had held since the end of the war. That year, though, he packed up and moved to Saskatchewan, to become the new clinical director of the Weyburn mental hospital. By 1957, he had turned that backward institution into arguably the most progressive mental hospital in North America. He stayed in Weyburn until 1961, when he left to become the director of research neurology and psychiatry at the New Jersey Psychiatric Institute in Princeton.[84]

In conjunction with other researchers in Saskatchewan, especially the psychiatrist and biochemist Abram Hoffer, who was the PSB's director of research and a faculty member at the University of Saskatchewan, Osmond would become one of the leading researchers in North America on the theory and treatment of schizophrenia.[85] Moreover,

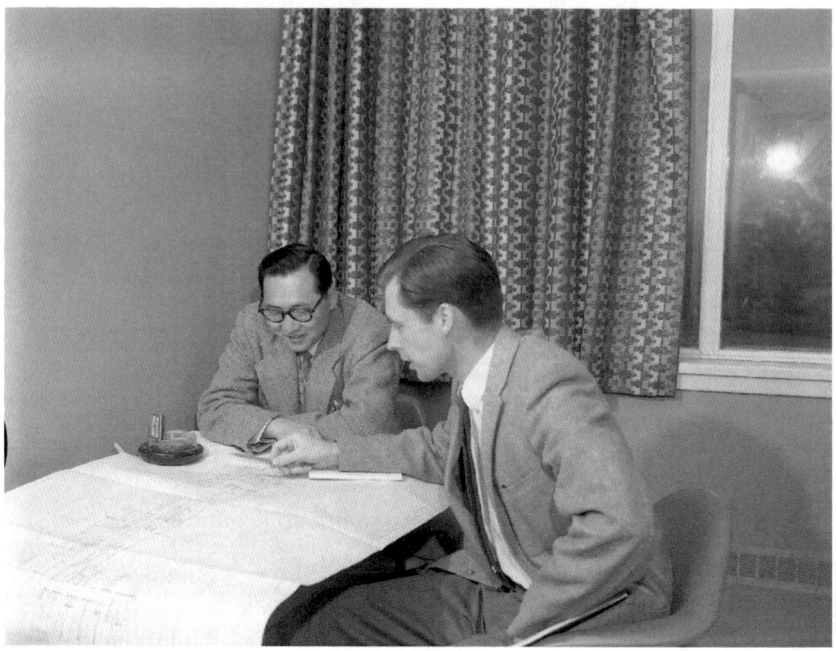

Francis Huxley, on right, with Kiyoshi Isumi, architect for the Saskatchewan Plan for community mental hospitals (PAS R-PS58-056-04)

his work with other PSB psychiatrists on the organic causes of schizophrenia, as well as of severe alcoholism, had impressed and influenced Menninger.[86] Rather incredibly, given their distance from major cities and universities, Osmond and Hoffer would become the leading researchers on the therapeutic use of psychedelics to treat addictions and mental illness, as documented by Erika Dyck in her book *Psychedelic Psychiatry*.[87] Indeed, it was Osmond who, while corresponding with Aldous Huxley, came up with the word "psychedelic" to describe the drug-induced state that brought about "an enlargement and expansion of the mind," quipping in a rhyming couplet: "To plumb the depths or soar angelic/Just take a pinch of psychedelic" – the first time the term was used. In the same series of letters, Osmond described Tommy Douglas to Huxley as "our remarkable and quite brilliant premier."[88]

An English writer and philosopher, Huxley had vaulted into fame with his dystopian novel *Brave New World*, published in 1932. This book's frightening vision was much influenced by the mass depression

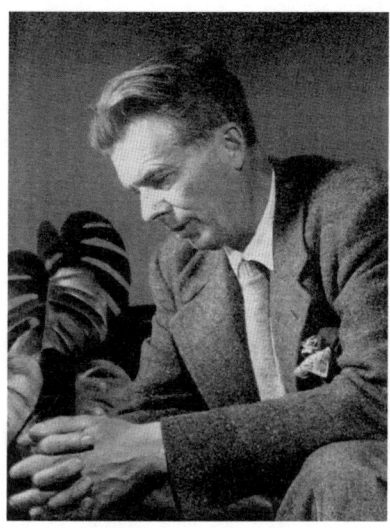

Aldous Huxley in 1954 (Wikimedia Commons)

witnessed by Huxley during the economic and social upheaval of the early 1930s. Based in Los Angeles since 1937, Huxley would go on to publish *The Doors of Perception* (1954) about his experiences with mescaline – an alkaloid derived from the peyote cactus – the year before, a substance already being carefully studied in Saskatchewan for therapeutic purposes. In first few pages of *The Doors of Perception*, Huxley explains the importance of what he saw as major research breakthroughs by Osmond, Hoffer, and their associates.[89] Huxley's nephew Francis Huxley, an anthropologist, was hired by Osmond to undertake an anthropological study of the Weyburn mental hospital. During his time in Saskatchewan, Francis Huxley also participated in research conducted by Osmond and Hoffer on the therapeutic use of LSD in treating alcohol addiction.[90]

In addition to overseeing this groundbreaking work being done in the province's two mental hospitals, McKerracher established full-time and part-time outpatient mental health clinics closely associated with the mental hospitals and the psychiatric unit of the Regina General Hospital. The psychiatrists and other clinical staff were expected to provide consultation and diagnostic services for patients referred to by physicians, social agencies, including the Department of Social Welfare, the organized health regions, and public health nurses working in areas outside the health regions, as well as the two psychiatric hospitals and Regina General Hospital's psychiatric unit.[91]

The second, more novel, function of the outpatient clinics was to educate organizations and individuals on mental health. This was done in a variety of ways, including a one-month training course in mental health for public health nurses and social workers. In its first year of operation, seventy public health nurses and fifteen social workers took the training course under the direction of psychiatrists. After the course, these nurses and social workers were dispatched to carry out community psychiatric duties throughout the province. Since they were in the employ of the provincial government, it was relatively easy to train and redeploy them. In contrast, for teachers, another targeted group, it was necessary to create a very different educational vehicle. Jointly funded by local school boards and the provincial government (through the Departments of Public Health and Education), a teacher with training in psychology visited various schools to educate other teachers on how to create and maintain a classroom environment "conducive to good public health."[92]

To further educational outreach in his campaign to change the public mindset about mental illness, McKerracher was instrumental in the establishment of the Saskatchewan Division of the Canadian Mental Health Association (CMHA), which became the CMHA's first provincial chapter.[93] The other individual who must be given credit was Paul Martin Sr. When Clarence Hincks of the CMHA first approached Martin to obtain federal funding for the establishment of provincial branches, Martin agreed instead to provide funding for a pilot provincial branch in Saskatchewan because of its innovative mental health policies under Douglas and McKerracher. Hincks agreed and dispatched Professor Samuel Laycock, a senior member of his national organization, to Regina to collaborate with McKerracher.[94] Both the federal and Saskatchewan governments provided financial assistance to the new branch. To provide stable funding at the outset, the CMHA (Sask.) was provided an annual grant for three years from the federal government.[95]

Both orders of government had high hopes for the ability of the CMHA (Sask.) to change public perceptions of mental illness. The CCF government supported the CMHA (Sask.), with Douglas and every member of his cabinet becoming subscribing members in the new organization.[96] As for McKerracher, he and the PSB psychiatrists he had hired played a key role in shaping the organization. McKerracher chaired the CMHA (Sask.) Scientific Planning Committee, which advised the board of directors on both policy and program initiatives.[97] In some ways, the relationship between the CCF government and the CMHA was so close that a member of the public could be forgiven for thinking the

CMHA (Sask.) was an agency of the provincial government. Until the late 1950s, the relationship between the two was symbiotic. The CMHA was supportive of the government's reform efforts, while Douglas assisted the CMHA's Saskatchewan branch in its fight against the prejudice faced by those with mental illness and its shift from a regime of permanent custodial care of such patients to one where treatment and release back into the community became the norm.[98]

Yet, changing attitudes in the province would turn out to be more difficult a task than Douglas, McKerracher, and the CMHA anticipated. This became evident in 1951 in an experiment in a small town in southeast Saskatchewan launched by McKerracher with the support of the CMHA and the Commonwealth Fund, a non-profit charity headquartered in New York City, focused on improving access to health care, reducing health disparities, and advocating for health policy reform. The year before, McKerracher had hired John and Elaine Cumming, partners in both marriage and research. John was a resident in a novel postgraduate resident-training program in psychiatry established at the University of Saskatchewan by McKerracher to recruit psychiatrists into the PSB. Elaine had been trained in biology but was drawn to research in mental health.

As proposed by McKerracher, a project was initiated in the town of Indian Head to test attitudes towards mental illness and community psychiatry and the possibility of changing negative attitudes towards the mentally ill. Behind the project lay the idea of moving a large number of patients from large mental institutions – the asylums – to community-based facilities, where they could obtain help when needed while living like everyone else in the local community.[99] Located a hundred kilometres north of the Weyburn mental hospital, Indian Head would provide evidence on the feasibility of deinstitutionalization.[100]

From an operational standpoint, the results from Indian Head were disappointing. Not only did the negative attitudes of the community towards the mentally ill prove difficult to change, but some prominent citizens turned against both the experiment and its two lead researchers. However, from a research perspective, the study contributed much to the existing state of sociological research into mental illness and the potential barriers to change. The book the Cummings wrote on the experiment would launch their academic careers after they migrated to Harvard University to pursue their doctorates.[101] Published in 1957, *Closed Ranks: An Experiment in Mental Health Education* would make the initiative in Indian Head better known and would establish the Cummings' reputations in the field of the sociology of mental health.[102]

## Dr. Sam Lawson and the Saskatchewan Plan

In 1955, Griff McKerracher left the provincial government to become the founding department chair of psychiatry at the University of Saskatchewan. His replacement as director of the PSB was Dr. Sam Lawson. Like McKerracher, Lawson had qualified in medicine at the University of Toronto and specialized in psychiatry in Ontario. McKerracher had recruited Lawson as superintendent of the Weyburn psychiatric hospital in 1947, and, after Humphry Osmond took over as superintendent, he transferred Lawson to North Battleford to become superintendent of the province's other mental hospital.[103]

While Douglas trusted McKerracher to guide the most important details of his government's reform of mental health, his relationship with Lawson would quickly become strained. For his part, Lawson could see his role only as an independent advocate for his own policies rather than as a servant of the government, and he did not hesitate to challenge the premier and his own minister. Even according to Burns Roth, who greatly respected Lawson's knowledge and experience, the PSB director was "proud," "abrasive," and "a little arrogant," and he "loved to brag about what he accomplished" and "loved to prove people wrong."[104]

Unlike McKerracher, who had balanced what the CMHA (Sask.) advocated (which he helped generate in the first place) and what the government was politically and fiscally capable of delivering, Lawson believed only in the rightness of his (and the parent CMHA's) advocacy. A key dispute soon arose over the PSB's recommendation that the provincial government build a network of smaller community mental health facilities that would provide both inpatient and outpatient care – what Lawson and his colleagues called the Saskatchewan Plan.[105]

Although developed collectively by the PSB's senior staff, including McKerracher, Osmond, Lawson, and Abram Hoffer, the Saskatchewan Plan would become most closely associated with Lawson.[106] Almost immediately after his appointment as PSB director, Lawson pressed Public Health Minister Tom Bentley for approval of the Saskatchewan Plan, which would allow the PSB to immediately abandon plans to accommodate more than 1,100 new patients at Weyburn and North Battleford.[107] Though Bentley and T.C. were attracted to the general thrust of the plan, both felt the cost of construction and personnel made it difficult to implement in the foreseeable future.[108] In response to concerns about cost, Lawson simply asserted that the government would save money in the long run, while the immediate cost would be little more than the money needed to refurbish both primary mental hospitals, an assessment with which his old boss disagreed.¹⁰⁹ Indeed, McKerracher told Bentley that the Saskatchewan Plan "will and should cost more" because (finally), "the mentally sick will receive the treatment that sick persons should."¹¹⁰

In response to the PSB's request, Douglas and his cabinet established a subcommittee to examine the potential costs and benefits of the plan. Lawson was infuriated because he thought that cabinet was simply avoiding the difficult decision of downsizing or even closing its two mental hospitals in North Battleford and Weyburn and that the subcommittee was a ploy to delay a decision. After grudgingly providing estimates of cost to the subcommittee, Lawson took great offence when he was cross-examined on the PSB's numbers by Tommy Shoyama, the secretary of the Economic Advisory and Planning Board and one of Douglas's most trusted advisors.¹¹¹

When the costs were finally tabulated, cabinet was astounded: the cost of building eight new regional psychiatric hospitals was estimated to be between $13.2 million and $18.8 million, while annual operating costs were estimated at $11.4 million. This was fully double the $5.7 million the government had budgeted to spend on all the mental health facilities in the province. Even financial aid from Ottawa through the National Health Grants Programs would not be enough, since it was limited at $4.4 million for construction and would not help with the operating costs.¹¹² The government simply could not afford the plan.

Unwilling to take no for an answer, Lawson then used the CMHA in a relentless public campaign to embarrass T.C. into reversing the decision. At the annual Regina branch meeting in January 1957, Lawson unveiled the PSB's architectural plans prepared for the proposed eight community psychiatric hospitals in Regina, Saskatoon, Swift Current, Yorkton, Prince Albert, Melfort, Wadena, and Moosomin.¹¹³ Although he explained that the plan's cost had not yet been approved by the provincial government, he implied government action was imminent. When Lawson's comments were repeated in the media, Douglas unleashed his fury on Walter Erb, the man he had just appointed to take over the health portfolio when Tom Bentley announced his impending retirement from politics:

> Dr. Lawson is an employee of the Saskatchewan Government and any plan which he outlines is assumed by the general public to represent the views of the Government. What Dr. Lawson and other members of the Psychiatric Services Branch are doing is to raise hopes which I see no prospect of the Government being able to satisfy. To speak of eight new hospitals with

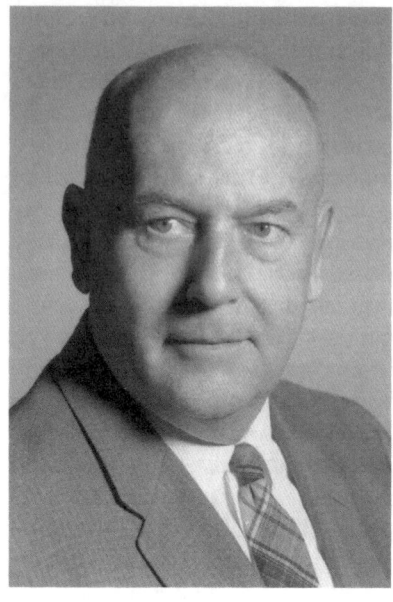

Dr. Sam Lawson in 1962 (PAS R-A11601)

bed capacities ranging from 268 to 448 is to envisage a capital expenditure which the Government has never at any time contemplated.[114]

By mid-March 1957, the dispute became a very public when the executive director of the Saskatchewan Division of the CMHA criticized Douglas and his government for not funding the plan. As a CMHA member, Douglas immediately wrote a letter to the division's president, demanding to know "whether or not the views expressed in the press item" reflected the opinion of and were authorized by "the executive of the Saskatchewan Division of the Canadian Mental Health Association." While he had "no desire to get into a controversy in the press with the officers of the Association," he nonetheless concluded that "some of the statements which were made cannot be allowed to go unchallenged."[115]

Douglas must have been disappointed at the response. Although "very appreciative of all the Government has done and is doing" in terms of mental health, and aware of the "enormous" public investment represented by the Saskatchewan Plan, the president nonetheless felt the building of the regional mental hospitals was still a "reasonable step towards more adequate care." Moreover, in "Canada and in the United States people are looking to Saskatchewan for leadership" and, "even with the progress which has been made in Saskatchewan, the amount of money spent on the care and treatment of the mentally ill is a small percentage of the amount spent to bring health to the physically ill."[116]

Before he wrote back, Douglas sought counsel from McKerracher, who was also disturbed about the "misunderstandings" that had arisen between the government and the CMHA. To McKerracher, it "seemed unfortunate" that the provincial government, which had done more than any other for the mentally ill, and the provincial chapter of the CMHA, which had been more successful than any other provincial CMHA body "in arousing public support," should "be at loggerheads."[117] For this, T.C. blamed the CMHA, which he felt had given his government too little respect for what was the most ambitious and expensive psychiatric program in the country.[118]

Just weeks after the exchange of letters, the president and executive director of the Saskatchewan Section of the CMHA followed up with an open letter to the press that expressed "grave concern about the [government's] apparent disregard for the urgency of immediate action." They insisted that, while the CCF government had once had "the most progressive mental health program in Canada," its current policy of "compromise solutions and half-measures" had allowed it to slip "from its leading position." They then took the government to task for "discriminating against the mentally ill by allocating disproportionate amounts of money for the care of the physically ill." If only the government had "accepted the recommendations of their advisors" – no doubt a reference to Dr. Sam Lawson – to proceed with the Saskatchewan Plan, the government would be spending not much more than the $750,000 it had just approved for an expansion and update to the psychiatric hospital in North Battleford.[119] The CMHA was repeating Lawson's original lowball estimates, not the more careful estimates prepared by Tommy Shoyama on behalf of cabinet.

This dispute would fester for the next five years, reaching a crescendo during the debate over medicare in the early 1960s. Fiercely proud of his government's relationship with civil society interest groups in the province, Douglas could barely believe that an organization whose aims he so shared could turn on him in this way.[120] To an extent, he was a victim of the expectations his government had raised among civil society organizations and pressure groups like the CCMA (Sask.). He was expected to not only take the lead in numerous health policy areas but to continue financing health system changes at a pace and level barely affordable by much wealthier jurisdictions.

Despite the many strong-minded individuals who were drawn to Saskatchewan during the Douglas years, there were surprisingly few clashes between the premier and these figures on the scale of the dispute between Douglas and Dr. Sam Lawson. Most – especially Mott and McKerracher – were creative policy and program inventors and innovators who contributed in major ways to making Saskatchewan a trend setter in health care in the early post-war era. Part of the reason they could succeed was that Douglas, fully aware of the limitations of his own knowledge, gave them the space and resources they needed.

# 8 Next-Year Country

While the previous chapters have focused on the health reforms for which Saskatchewan became well known, the purpose of this chapter is to explore three less visible, though important, health care initiatives. Although not all were successful, these efforts would quietly influence future developments in the province and the rest of Canada for decades. They also raise health policy questions and dilemmas that continue to challenge decision makers in Canada.

First, I return to Douglas's earlier efforts to address the health of residents living in Saskatchewan's enormous and chronically underserviced rural regions through the establishment of health regions. The ongoing effort to regionalize health services posed two perennial questions. The first was how best to reorganize services and providers to improve health outcomes, and the second concerned the appropriate balance between, on one side, central authority and financing and, on the other, local control, innovation, and ownership. These has been the constant questions before provincial decision makers in Canada since the Douglas government's reforms of the 1940s and 1950s, and they remain unresolved.

Next, I turn to the subject of rural, remote, and Indigenous health care. With the most dispersed population in the country in the 1940s, Saskatchewan faced a particularly acute challenge. Almost immediately after taking office, T.C. established the first provincial air ambulance system in Canada. And, in northern areas, the provincial government provided rudimentary health services through nursing stations and a corps of travelling doctors and nurses.

The final subject canvased is oral care, especially dental care for children. In the early post-war decades, Saskatchewan had the worst oral health in the country, a legacy of the impoverishment wrought by the Great Depression and the limited number of dentists. T.C.'s dream was to establish a school-based dental nurse program. Although not achieved during Douglas's tenure, his government's plans were used to create a school-based dental program in Saskatchewan in the 1970s and have remained a reform option for the entire country ever since.

## Building a Better Future

In the decades following the onset of the Great Depression, Saskatchewan was often referred to as "next-year country." The expression means that, although things had not turned out well in the past few years, there was always the hope that they would get better next year. Often used by farmers who had endured years of drought or crop failure, the expression reflected their optimism, however dim or flickering, for the future. Since the provincial economy was dependent on their fortunes, it was a sentiment shared by all.

T.C. wanted Saskatchewan to be much more than next-year country. He was impatient for change. As minister of health, he was at the centre of a whirlwind of reform. These changes required money that had to be drawn from very limited provincial resources. A single large crop failure could, at any time, force the government not only to constrain growth but to make major cuts to spending. Since running a government deficit would only worsen the problem if the province suffered another major crop failure the following year, both Douglas and his provincial treasurer, Clarence Fines, rejected this option.

The only way for Saskatchewan to become more than next-year country was to grow the economy. And the only way to sustain the CCF government's new investments in health services and health insurance, while encouraging new spending in schools, education, road infrastructure, and other public goods, was to diversify the economy beyond agriculture into finance and industry, as well as to encourage the exploration for and extraction and processing of natural resources such as oil, natural gas, potash, and uranium. The sole way his government could sustain its health reform agenda was to increase the size of the economic pie and, along with it, provincial revenues.

In November 1949, a year and a half after the 1948 election, T.C. vacated the health portfolio in favour of a new minister. Satisfied that universal hospital insurance was working seamlessly, Douglas put his plans to expand coverage on hold until the province had the revenue base to support additional programs. It was time to focus on some of the government's other priorities, especially economic development. Due to the centrality of the local cooperative movement in banking and retailing as well as the grain trade, he took on the portfolio of minister of cooperation and cooperative development, a position that did not exist in any other province. Only by being "relieved of the Department of Public Health" would it be "possible" for him "to devote more time to the vital problems of industrial and business expansion."[1] The press release he personally issued the day of the change laid out the reasons:

> Last year I made a public statement, pointing out that during its second term of office the Government proposed to place its major emphasis upon industrial *and agricultural* [inserted in pen by Douglas] development with a view to laying an economic base for a continued expansion of our welfare program. In keeping with the Government's policy of promoting public, private and co-operative enterprise, it is my intention to devote more time to the problem of industrial development, and an organization is being set up for that purpose. It is for this reason that I have assumed the Department of Co-operatives since the co-operative movement has an important part to play along with private and public enterprise in the future development of our province.[2]

In the twelve years after Douglas relinquished the health portfolio, from November 1949 until he left for Ottawa in November 1961, his government attempted to ensure continuity by having only two ministers of health. The first was Thomas J. Bentley, who held the post from 1949 until 1956, when Douglas moved him to social welfare and reconstruction. He was replaced by J. Walter Erb, for reasons that remain obscure. Erb would be minister when relations between the government and organized medicine fell apart in the months before Douglas left the premiership.

Twelve years older than Douglas, Tom Bentley had been a Progressive in the 1920s and had moved to the CCF when it was created in the early 1930s. Bentley was the archetype of the CCF farmer-politician at the time. He moved to Saskatchewan from the Maritimes in 1907 to take up a homestead. Upset with high tariffs and freight rates and low wheat prices, he was active in the Saskatchewan Wheat Pool and the United Farmers of Canada. By the mid-1920s, he had quit farming to become an elevator operator for the Wheat Pool as part of its field staff based out of Swift Current. He was first elected as a CCF MP for Swift Current in 1945 but was defeated in the 1949 election. He then jumped to provincial politics and obtained a seat in a by-election for Gull Lake just west of Swift Current in November 1949, at which time Douglas put him directly into cabinet as the new health minister.[3]

Bentley turned out to be a solid minister who worked well with his two highly knowledgeable deputy ministers, Fred Mott – whose

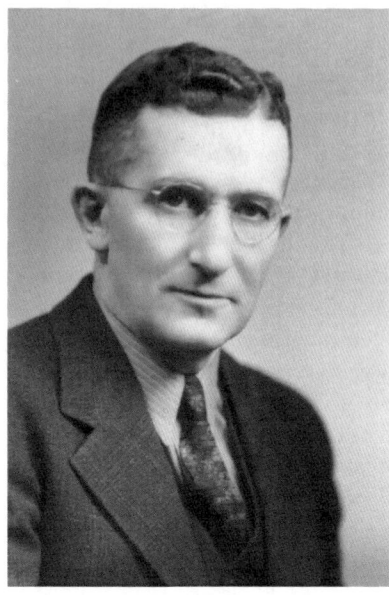

Thomas J. Bentley in 1954, Saskatchewan's minister of public health (1949–56) (PAS R-A5339(2))

pivotal role in the adoption of hospital coverage has already been described – and Burns Roth, Mott's successor.[4] Bentley worked with Mott for slightly more than two years and had immense respect for him. Both Bentley and T.C. deeply regretted Mott's decision to leave Saskatchewan at the end of December 1951. Mott moved back to Washington, DC, to take charge of the United Mine Workers of America's Memorial Hospital Association, which was building hospitals and health centres in underprivileged areas in Kentucky, West Virginia, and Virginia.[5]

Mott's successor, Burns Roth, was a medical doctor with experience in hospital management whom Mott had hired as director of hospital standards and administration the year before. Although less idealistic and, as he himself admitted, not as innovative in terms of health systems and policies as Mott, Roth was nonetheless a talented health administrator who worked well with, and had great respect for, Bentley.[6] Roth would remain the deputy minister for over a decade, until his departure for the University of Toronto in 1962.[7]

Despite facing a rocky relationship with the medical profession, largely due to the frustration of the College of Physicians and Surgeons (CPS) about not being able to deal with the premier directly after having so many years of ready access, Bentley did his best to continue what Douglas had started. At the same time, Bentley did not possess T.C.'s

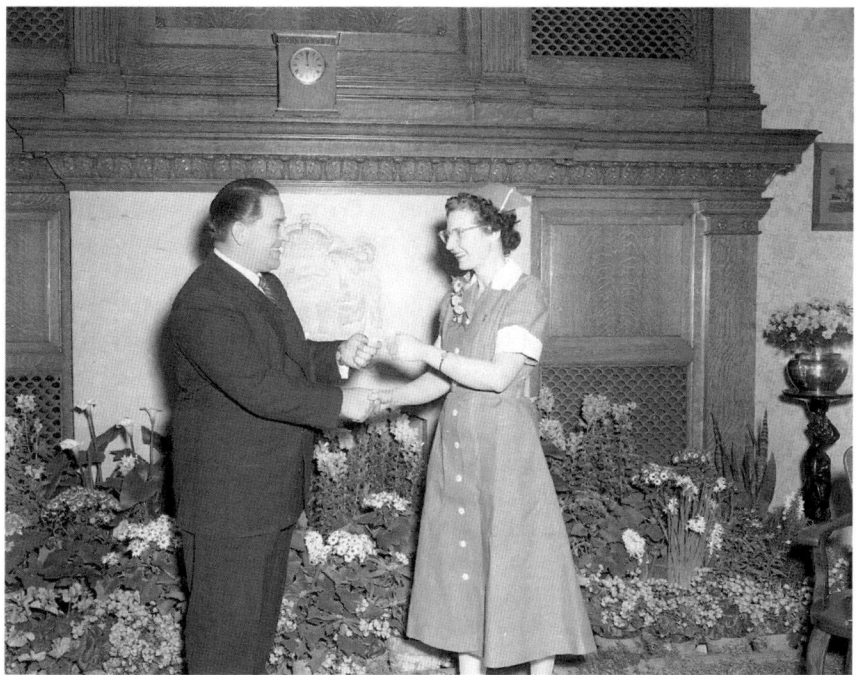

Walter Erb presenting the first nursing assistant certificate in the province, January 1957 (PAS 56-479-02)

sweeping vision and, at first, his extensive knowledge of the health sector. Judging by the regular written communication between Douglas and Bentley, along with Mott and Roth, the new minister was initially reluctant to pursue anything without getting the premier's input and approval. This would soon change. An avid student of the field, Bentley came to know the health field deeply and would ultimately preside over major progress in key areas. This would stand in marked contrast with the uninspired leadership of his successor, Walter Erb, who held the post from 1956 until his controversial resignation and departure from the CCF in 1962, a story that will be told later.[8]

As for Douglas, he felt that his government had hit a fiscal ceiling by the time he "gave up" the health portfolio in 1949. He had long understood that to establish an integrated health system of rural polyclinics and hospitals providing comprehensive health services to most Saskatchewan residents, he needed more money. And to live up to his promise of comprehensive health coverage for all residents, he needed far more public funds than would ever be available through provincial revenue sources. While neighbouring Alberta greatly benefited from a petroleum boom that began in 1947 and would gush money and help pay for public infrastructure and services like health, Saskatchewan's oil and other natural resources were meagre in comparison.[9] And so his government had spread the pain in terms of revenue sources for hospitalization beyond the provincial sales tax (the only tax then available, given the tax rental of income and corporate taxes to the federal government), relying on a flat tax of family and individual contributions. Agriculture was still the province's main source of wealth, but grain prices were fickle and so was the weather, factors that resulted in considerable volatility in public revenues from year to year.

In addition, Douglas could not afford to make spending on health his top priority indefinitely. He had to invest more in economic development, especially in the infrastructure that would attract new industry and wean the province from its almost complete reliance on the production of wheat. Saskatchewan also desperately needed to invest in basic infrastructure like roads and, especially, rural electrification to improve the lives of its many rural residents who were still feeling the aftershocks of the Great Depression.

Rural electrification became Douglas's chief preoccupation in the early 1950s. The Saskatchewan Power Corporation (SaskPower), a provincial Crown corporation, managed the initiative. By 1956, every village and town in Saskatchewan (outside the north) had electricity, and, two years later, SaskPower met the government's target of electrifying 50,000 farms.[10] Why did this matter so much to Douglas? For one simple reason: More than any other single initiative – even more than hospitalization, in some cases – it would fundamentally improve the lives of more than half the population. It is hard to overstate the revolution in modern living brought about by the availability of electricity in rural areas. Aside from universal health coverage, T.C. referred to rural electrification as his proudest achievement.

In an outstanding biography of Lyndon B. Johnson, Robert Caro captures what rural electrification meant to the lives of the hardscrabble farmers and ranchers – especially their wives and children – living in the hill country of western Texas when Johnson was a young member of Congress. In his poignant chapter "The Sad Irons," Caro describes life before the introduction of rural electricity when the daily routines of farm men and especially women were unremittingly gruelling. Among the many chores of farm women was to pump and haul (on average) forty gallons of water to wash, clothe, and feed their families. Another was to haul the wood to feed the wood stove, which was not used only

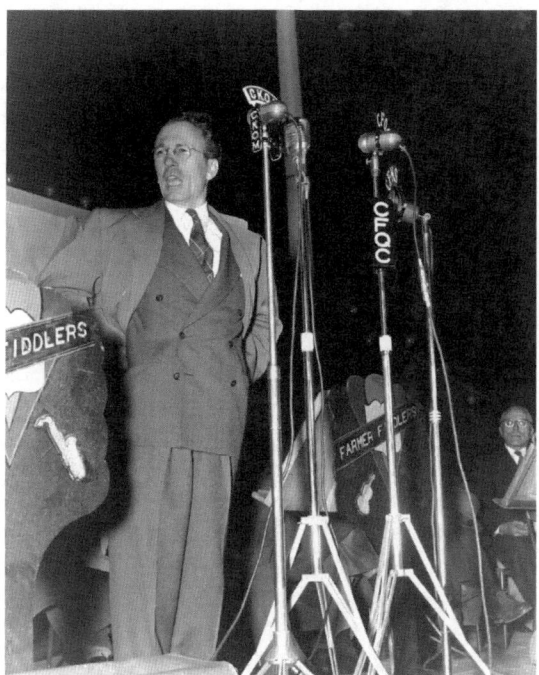

T.C. speaking at the official opening of Saskatchewan Power's natural gas system serving rural residents, 1 October 1953 (SPL B-14767)

for cooking, baking, and canning, but for the backbreaking work of washing and rinsing mounds of clothes in vats of boiling water, and heating the irons, each a six- or seven-pound wedge of solid metal, to press clothes. Of all their chores, West Texas women most hated the full day they devoted to washing and ironing, having to carry the heavy irons back and forth from the stove, constantly cleaning soot from their irons, and periodically burning their fingers and hands on the "sad irons," as they described them.[11] Saskatchewan farm women (and men) faced the same hardships as their West Texas counterparts, a life that T.C. regularly witnessed. Although he was very unlike Lyndon Johnson as a politician and a person, he shared Johnson's understanding of the potential impact of a single effective policy to improve the lives of disadvantaged rural folk.

As late as 1951, long after electricity was extended to the hardscrabble farms and ranches of West Texas, nearly half of Saskatchewan households remained without electricity, compared to a Canadian average of just 12 per cent. While the percentage in Saskatchewan was comparable to that in Alberta (where 43 per cent of residents went without electricity), it was far greater than that in Manitoba, where only 22 per cent of residents lacked electricity by 1951.[12] The reasons were not hard to understand: Saskatchewan was even more rural than its Prairie neighbours, while Regina and Saskatoon were much less populous than Winnipeg, Calgary, and Edmonton.

The fact that the main power producer – the Saskatchewan Power Corporation – was a Crown corporation owned and managed by the provincial government was both an advantage and a disadvantage. On the one hand, the Douglas government had control, but, on the other, Crown corporations were expected to run their operations like a commercial enterprise without taxpayer subsidy.[13] As a consequence, SaskPower used what revenues it could generate in urban areas to subsidize electrification in rural areas. Doing so forced it to move gradually, particularly so in the most rural and remote parts of the province, where the extensions from the main grid were longer and the farms and villages with paying subscribers were few and far between. Public ownership meant the CCF government was held directly responsible for anything done, or not done, by SaskPower. Douglas took much of the brunt of criticism in this regard and was personally attacked in the provincial legislature for SaskPower not providing electricity to rural areas quickly enough.[14]

With a far larger rural geography to serve than Manitoba and less public revenue than Alberta, Saskatchewan was the last province to connect its rural residents to the grid. During the election campaign of 1952, Douglas promised residents that the province would have an additional 40,000 farms electrified within the next four years. To achieve this, his government introduced aerial surveys, rural electrification field days, and a $50 discount for anyone willing to sign up for electrification. The promise was kept, and by 1956 most farms in the province had electricity.[15]

**Health Regions: Frustrated Ambitions and Some Successes**

Even when he was no longer minister of public health, Douglas still expected the Health Services Planning Commission (HSPC) to continue establishing health regions in the province, an essential first step in the establishment of a truly coordinated provincial health system. By the time Fred Mott had taken over as HSPC chair in 1946, four health regions had been organized, with two more established in 1947. However,

Table 8.1. Status of health regions in Saskatchewan, 1945–51

| Health region | Date organized | Area (sq. miles) | Population (1946 census) |
|---|---|---|---|
| Swift Current (No. 1) | 31 Dec. 1945 | 14,805 | 53,218 |
| Weyburn-Estevan (No. 3) | 31 Dec. 1945 | 8,734 | 52,987 |
| Moose Jaw (No. 6) | 15 June 1946 | 5,995 | 47,717 |
| Meadow Lake (No. 14) | 15 Aug. 1946 | 4,958 | 4,598 |
| Assiniboia-Gravelbourg (No. 2) | 31 May 1947 | 6,691 | 31,202 |
| North Battleford (No. 13) | 15 Aug. 1947 | 10,477 | 62,408 |
| Prince Albert (No. 12) | 1 Feb. 1951 | 11,700 | 64,552 |

Source: *Saskatchewan Health Survey Report, vol. 1: Health Programs and Personnel* (Regina: Health Survey Committee, 1951), 35; F. Burns Roth and R.D. Defries, "The Saskatchewan Department of Public Health," *Canadian Journal of Public Health / Revue canadienne de santé publique* 49, no. 7 (1958): 280–2.

one of the unanticipated consequences of provincial hospitalization is that the program reduced local governments' interest in forming health regions, as one of the original attractions of such regions was that opting in would allow the possibility of offering residents hospital coverage, something now provided by the provincial government.

As a result, momentum slowed to the point that only one additional health region was organized in the next four years, when the north-central part of the province around the city of Prince Albert was organized in 1951 (see table 8.1). By this time, Douglas was no longer minister of public health, and the HSPC was incorporated into the Department of Public Health, where Mott became deputy minister while remaining the commission's chair.

As Mott readily admitted, part of the reason it was taking so long to create new health regions was the time and energy the HSPC had to devote to the Saskatchewan Hospital Services Plan. In other words, the government's priority was its new hospital insurance plan. The commission needed to make hundreds of adjustments and refinements after the program's initial implementation. Assigning dozens of staff members to encourage local governments to pursue the steps needed before they could even petition the government to get a health region organized was a luxury that the HSPC could hardly afford. Moreover, Mott's own time and energy had necessarily been focused on hospital insurance. Between 1947 and 1949, for example, the HSPC was getting continual feedback and advice from hospital chief executives on the provincial reimbursement scheme: the result was a complete overhaul of the original funding formula for hospitals a formula that had been constructed in the first place only after months of consultations with the Saskatchewan Hospital Association.[16]

From Douglas's perspective, the main purpose of the health regions was to provide an adequate public health infrastructure and associated personnel for rural Saskatchewan. While he respected the right of local governments to have their respective regions provide health care services beyond public health, he always felt that universal coverage was better provided by the provincial government. Not only was the provincial government in a better position to collect the revenues necessary to fund such expensive obligations, but provincial administration would also ensure that every resident received the same coverage. The last thing he wanted was for every region to provide its own health insurance: doing so was liable to create a patchwork of different standards of care and different conditions concerning coverage, as well as different packages in terms of breadth and depth, something he and the HSPC "were afraid of from the beginning."

> I felt from the very beginning that the only hope of a successful health insurance program is that it would be simplicity itself. That is, when a person is ill, no matter where they are in the province, they are entitled to all of the health services, and if their doctor say they have to be sent outside of the province then the plan should be responsible for taking them outside of the province and getting them whatever care they needed. Above all, there is only one basic principle and that is that inability to pay should never be a factor in preventing people from getting all the health care they needed. You can't do that if you have all of these different restrictions, different qualifications varying from municipality to municipality or from health region to health region.[17]

As T.C. himself explained, the Swift Current Health Region No. 1 had been chosen as a pilot project "not with the idea of it becoming a model to be duplicated around the province, but in order to give us the type of data we needed for a province-wide scheme and for a national scheme." Although initially enjoyed by only a minority of Saskatchewan residents, the benefits of more comprehensive public coverage could be observed by all. While the provincial government would take over the expense of hospital coverage only six months after the Swift Current Health Region implemented its own plan, the region would continue to provide full medical care coverage until it too was eventually absorbed by the provincial medical care plan of the 1960s. Swift Current gave the provincial government a fifteen-year-long pilot project for publicly administered physician coverage on which planners in

Regina could draw when designing a provincial medical care program. This information was also invaluable to the federal government and its Royal Commission on Health Services in the early 1960s. Commission chair Justice Emmett Hall told Douglas that "if it hadn't been for the statistics" collected by the Swift Current health region, "it would have taken much longer to prepare the data" needed to back up a recommendation in favour of a single-payer and universal medical care coverage plan for the country.[18]

Yet the principal reason for the existence of health regions, at least in Douglas's mind, was to "provide an administrative base for full-time public-health services."[19] These services included full-time public health nurses, sanitary officers, and the region's chief medical health officer. In the Swift Current Health Region for example, which was servicing a population of 55,000 residents by 1948, there were nine public health nurses, three sanitary officers, a health educator, and a regional registrar of vital statistics.[20] In the unorganized health regions, these services were provided through part-time municipal medical health officers as well as a corps of public health nurses and sanitary officers assigned to the regions by the provincial Department of Public Health.[21]

Although T.C. was never clear on the overall role of public health in relation to health care services, his planners in the HSPC and the Department of Public Health tried their best to connect the dots between downstream curative treatment and more upstream public health services and interventions. Mott and his successor as deputy minister, Burns Roth, felt that an ideally organized health system would integrate public health into illness diagnosis, treatment, and prevention.

These planners always treated regions as the necessary administrative structures for organizing and integrating acute care with diagnostic services, primary care, and public health. In other words, the health region was much more than the hierarchical integration of hospitals on a continuum from basic secondary care to more specialized tertiary care. It was also much more than the locus of a health centre, whether a polyclinic or a doctor's small rural practice.[22] Although it was extremely challenging to figure out the relationship between, for example, a medical health officer responsible for public health, on the one hand, and the hospitals in each health region, on the other, the question was very much on the minds of Douglas's planners in HSPC and the Department of Public Health.[23]

As previously discussed, Mindel and Cecil Sheps as well as Fred Mott viewed the health regions as the visible hand of management for a new type of health system to be built, piece by piece, by democratically elected local governments but with considerable support and direction from the provincial government. Yet this dimension of the regional project never emerged in a full-blown way. Although the health regions established by 1947 had put components of this organized system together, none had all the ideal elements in place even a decade later. Still, the Swift Current Health Region was close enough to what Henry Sigerist had originally set out in his 1944 report that it is worth reviewing what it accomplished between 1946 and the end of the 1950s.

The "regional health centre" in Swift Current, which included the Swift Current Union Hospital, provided tertiary care, advanced diagnostics, and more specialized physician care for all residents in its catchment, while also providing basic diagnostics and primary care for those living in the immediate area. Secondary care and more basic diagnostic and physician care was provided in the health region's "district health centres" located in the towns of Shaunavon, Maple Creek, and Leader, each the most populous towns in the three districts outside Swift Current itself.[24] The health region with its main hospital in Swift Current and its district health centres constituted the first regionalized hospital and medical care system in Canada, "an early precursor" of the regional health authorities set up in most provinces in the early to mid-1990s.[25] Primary care was provided by physicians on contract with the region, although most were reimbursed on a fee-for-service basis rather than on a salary basis, as originally recommended by Henry Sigerist and Mindel Sheps.

This infrastructure and the associated personnel were accompanied by universal coverage for hospital, diagnostic, physician care, and, as discussed below, targeted coverage for dental care. Hospital and diagnostic coverage within the health region began on 1 July 1946, a benefit it was able to drop six months later with the implementation of the province's hospital insurance program. This program still left the region providing coverage for all medical, surgical, and obstetrical services.[26]

By 1948, the region had contracts with thirty-six doctors, the majority of whom were primary care physicians working in rural areas, closely liaising with the regional and district health centres. These doctors, spread over a population of roughly 55,000 residents, amounted to "a higher ratio of doctors-to-population than any other part of rural Saskatchewan."[27] Almost all the region's physicians were paid on a discounted fee schedule derived from the College of Physicians and Surgeons of Saskatchewan. One important exception was a salaried radiologist based in Swift Current, who also provided services to the other district health centres. Initially, all services were provided free of charge to all residents, but, by 1953, the region had begun to impose user charges on those seeking physician services, mainly to discourage what the region's board viewed as overuse of a free service.[28]

At least initially, one of the most welcome and popular services for those living in the region was dental care.[29] Basic dental services were provided through contracted dentists at the permanent dental clinic in the regional health centre in Swift Current, while travelling dental clinics serviced the rural areas. Initially, all children under sixteen were provided services, but the chronic shortage of dentists forced the health region board to reduce the age for eligibility to fourteen and under in 1953 and then, a couple of years later, to twelve and under. Despite this shrinking of the eligible population, the shortage of dentists remained a chronic challenge such that only 40 per cent of eligible children were actually receiving publicly financed dental services in the health region by the mid-1950s.[30]

Along with these medical and dental services, there were some successes in integrating public health into the region's health system. These were due in part to Dr. Vince Matthews, who assumed the position of the region's medical health officer in 1948 and would remain in this role until 1957. After growing up in rural Saskatchewan, Matthews studied at the University of Saskatchewan and then at the University of Toronto, where he graduated in medicine with a specialization in public health in 1945. Beyond his public health duties, Matthews gathered statistics on both public health and health care in the region.[31]

One example of the way in which Matthews helped integrate public health into a system of early intervention and treatment was how vital statistics were recorded and then used by health region staff. As an experiment, beginning in 1948, "all registrations of births, stillbirths, deaths and marriages occurring in the region" were channelled first to Matthews as medical health officer before being passed on to the provincial director of vital statistics in the Department of Public Health.[32] For each birth, Matthews created a statistical card, which eventually included an infant and preschool record that was then sent to the public health nurse covering the district in which the infant's mother resided. The information enabled the nurse to pinpoint and address potential issues before they grew into major medical problems. In addition, Matthews was able to scrutinize the causes of death recorded by physicians in the region and was able to contact the "physician to obtain additional information" to ensure the death was properly classified.[33] Matthews then forwarded the particulars to the office of the director of vital statistics in Regina. The provincial director, in turn, ensured that his office prepared and forwarded to Matthews's office all relevant statistical details of events outside the region that involved its residents.

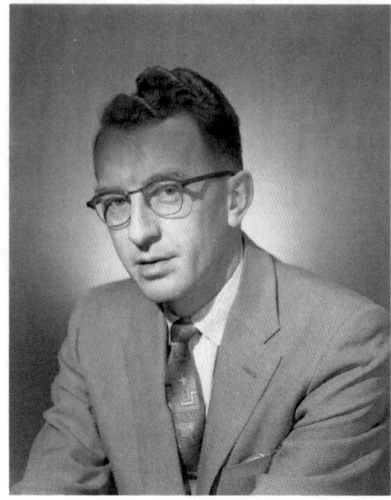

Dr. Vincent L. Matthews, c. 1958 (PAS R-PS56-535-01)

In fact, what Matthews had implemented was a system of public health surveillance that would eventually become the norm in most advanced industrial countries. Two years after Matthews introduced his changes in the Swift Current Health Region, prominent American public health advocate Alexander Langmuir defined public health surveillance as "the continued watchfulness over the distribution and trends of incidence through the systematic collection, consolidation and evaluation of morbidity and mortality reports and other relevant data" and the "regular dissemination of the basic data and interpretations to all who have contributed and to all others who need to know."[34] The concept, already implemented in the southwest corner of Saskatchewan, soon spread. The Swift Current experiment proved so successful that the same reciprocal arrangement for the flow of vital statistics was made for all subsequent organized health regions in the province.[35]

Through his regular contact with medical colleagues and health centres in the region, Matthews encouraged physicians to refer their patients to infant and preschool programs at the health centres. He fostered a close working relationship between public health nurses and physicians throughout the Swift Current Health Region. In Fred Mott's assessment, after less than three years of operation, community and personal health services were being coordinated to the benefit of both and in a manner heartily encouraged by the health planners in Regina.[36] Perhaps the best indicator of the benefits to be derived from integrating public health into a health system was reflected in the decline of infant mortality. When the Swift Current Health Region was first established, it had one of the highest infant death rates in the province, due to a continuing legacy of drought and depression. Two decades later, it had the lowest rate in Saskatchewan.[37]

In the end, however, the health regions – even the much-lauded Swift Current Health Region – frustrated Douglas and his planners.[38] Doctors stubbornly insisted on remaining independent contractors, and those physicians receiving fee-for-service payment operated quite independently of the region's board and salaried health personnel. The health region's insistence on using deterrent fees after 1953 to contain costs irritated Douglas, the HSPC, and the Department of Public Health, all of whom were against user fees in any program of universal coverage. The region's inability to maintain an effective dental service became a major point of concern and contention within the Department of Public Health. But most of all, there was an inherent tension between Douglas's respect for local government autonomy and his strong desire to have uniform terms of coverage.

Douglas leaned, eventually, towards the latter, a tendency fortified by his bureaucratic planners, most of whom preferred a more centralized approach to the financing and administration of health insurance. While this uniformity was immediately achieved when the Swift Current Health Region ceded hospital and diagnostic coverage to the province, it emerged again with the implementation of medical care coverage in the early 1960s. During the legislative debate on the medical care bill in 1961, Douglas tried to resolve the conflict by listing all the reasons the program would have to be centralized in the short run but still expressing his government's "hope and intention" to have the plan eventually administered by the health regions themselves.[39] Despite the special arrangements made for the Swift Current Health Region to administer medical care coverage for a transitional period, it was the sole (and temporary) exception to the rule that the provincial government would administer the program centrally from its inception in 1962.[40]

## Rural, Remote, and Indigenous Health Care

To improve access to health services in rural Saskatchewan, Douglas had to do much more than provide hospital insurance and build new hospitals and health centres. Most residents lived on farms and villages far from towns large enough to have a doctor, much less a district health centre, cottage hospital, regional health centre, or larger hospital. Even in 1955, only 25 per cent of the province's residents lived in the eight communities with a population of more than 5,000. The other 75 per cent lived in rural areas or remote hinterland.[41] To compound the isolation, snowfall rendered the rudimentary dirt or lightly gravelled roads in these regions largely useless from late October until early April; even the paved roads could become impassable during winter blizzards or spring thaws.

Always open to new ideas, Douglas quickly latched on to the possibility of a flying ambulance service, based on the existing Royal Flying Doctor Service in Australia.[42] First proposed to Douglas by Keith Malcolm, a Royal Canadian Air Force (RCAF) veteran, the idea was to have a small aircraft with a registered nurse on board fly to farms and communities some distance from medical facilities and personnel to pick up patients who needed to be transported to a hospital for urgent interventions and specialized treatment.[43] Despite the cost, he approved of the idea, knowing that air transport was the only way to provide timely access to emergency care for most of the population.

In early October 1945, Douglas appointed Malcolm as pilot and supervisor of the Saskatchewan Air Ambulance Service. As a branch of the Department of Public Health, the air ambulance initially reported to Cecil Sheps. By February 1946, it began operating, with a single plane (an RCAF Norseman aircraft in storage purchased at a steep discount), one pilot, and one registered nurse.[44] Malcolm then worked with local governments in rural areas to prepare landing strips, providing extensive direction on how best to construct the landing areas. Understanding that future lives would depend on rapid medical evacuation, municipalities were keen to cooperate with the service.[45]

The service charged $25 per trip regardless of the distance travelled. In cases where the patient's family could not afford the fee, it was waived by the Department of Public Health.[46] Constituting a tiny fraction of the actual cost, the fee was an effort to mitigate against unnecessary use of the service. Beyond transporting patients, the Air Ambulance Service was also used to deliver medical supplies, vaccines, and pharmaceuticals to isolated communities facing epidemics such as tuberculosis, along with needed medical personnel.[47] Although the service covered only the southern "settled" half of the province, the Department of Health contracted with the Department of Northern Resources, which already had a fleet of planes, to provide medical supplies, vaccine, and drugs in more remote northern areas.[48] However, these flights, intended mainly to transport people, equipment, and supplies as part of the economic development of the north, did not have dedicated nursing personnel on board.[49]

By the end of 1946, the air ambulance had flown 173 patient missions and acquired a second airplane. In 1948, the service conducted

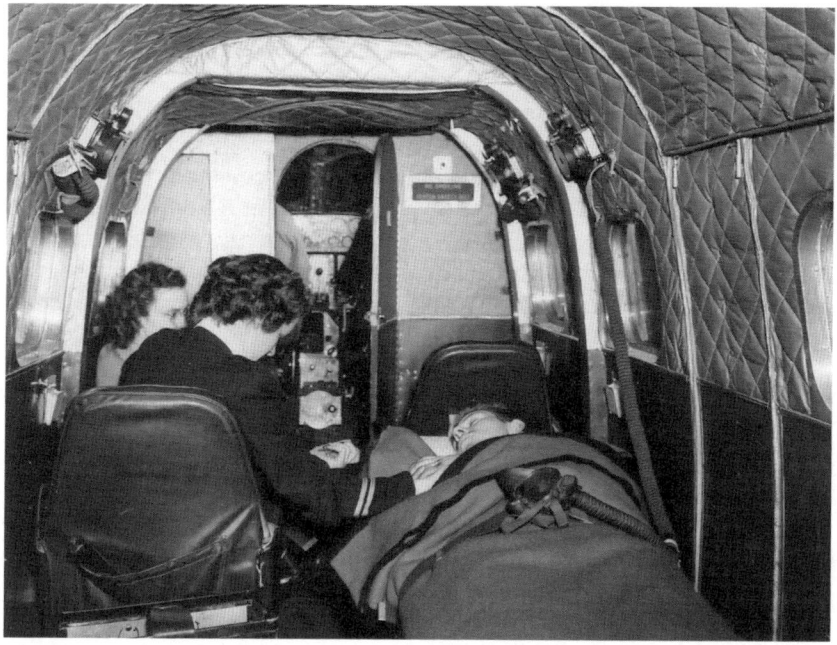
Inside an air ambulance aircraft, c. 1949 (PAS R-A3016)

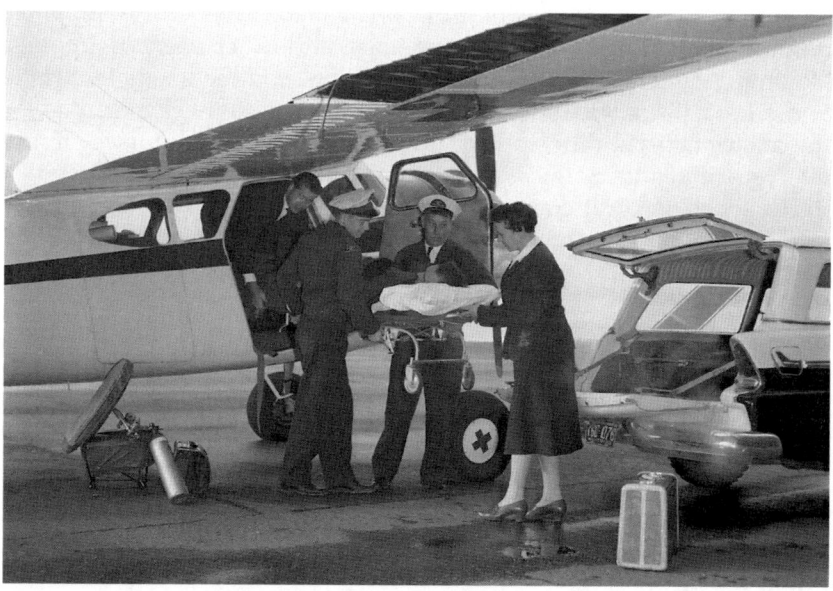
Unloading an air ambulance patient (PAS PS56-256-02)

937 emergency flights. By the end of its first decade in operation, it had flown 7,446 patients over 3.7 million kilometres, with 5 per cent of all flights taking patients to more specialized facilities outside the province, including the Mayo Clinic in Rochester, Minnesota. By 1956, the service had six aircraft – two of which were larger, twin-engine craft used for longer distances – four pilots, and four registered nurses. Peak use of the air ambulance was always in August and September, when farmers were rushing to get their crops harvested and at greater risk of serious injury from farm and grain elevator machinery. Other common conditions necessitating medical evacuation included distressed pregnancies, heart attacks, serious intestinal disorders, strokes, and cancer.[50]

The first service of its type in Canada, the Air Ambulance Service became the subject of a 1948 National Film Board documentary entitled *Wings of Mercy*.[51] As with the Royal Flying Doctor Services (and very much despite the misleading name in the Australian case), registered nurses were the medical core of the Saskatchewan air ambulance service. In addition to taking care of their patients, these flight nurses were responsible for recording the patient's history, including any changes during the flight, supervising the patient's appropriate transfer on and off the plane, medical-level sanitation of the aircraft cabin, and the maintenance of all medical equipment and supplies. By the mid-1950s, the equipment aboard all planes included an incubator for premature babies, a respirator, an electrical aspiration apparatus, a fracture board, an oxygen tank and respirator mask, and a medical crash kit with pharmaceuticals, syringes, clamps, dressings, and other needed supplies. Having completed a specialized course on aviation medicine, Irene Sutherland, the service's senior registered nurse, prepared a manual for the other nurses and personally trained new registered nurses joining the Air Ambulance Service.[52]

The focus on rural communities in the province's southern regions at this time was symptomatic of a separation between northern and southern Saskatchewan that went far beyond the geographical. In the south were the farms, villages, and market towns that made up an agricultural society – a settler society, in contemporary parlance. By contrast, the north was a region of vast boreal forests, thousands of lakes, and a veritable treasure trove of natural resources that had barely been identified, let alone exploited. The relatively sparse population included First Nation and Métis inhabitants who were marginalized due to poverty and limited education, largely provided in residential schools by Roman Catholic and Anglican missions. Northern residents continued to receive only minimal benefits from modern medicine and public health measures.

Douglas saw the problems, but he also recognized the north's opportunity, and he linked the two into a single policy. His government would clear out some of the vestiges of the colonial past by challenging the HBC's monopoly and the influence of missionaries by using the government and cooperatives to develop and market the north's resources. This would generate new wealth for the province in two ways. The co-ops would directly benefit Indigenous producers by ensuring they received their fair share of the profits from their work, while the province would see an increase in taxes and royalties that then could be invested in schools, medical clinics, and small hospitals in these northern regions.[53]

The legacy of the CCF government in northern Saskatchewan has been subject to some historical revisionism, in part driven by a more fundamental reconsideration of settler-Indigenous relations.[54] In his 1997 book *Walking in Indian Moccasins: The Native Policies of Tommy Douglas and the CCF*, Indigenous studies scholar Laurie Barron argued that, despite the many progressive merits of the Douglas government, it "was not a saviour of Native people and in some cases its policies proved to be destructive of Native interests." At the same time, T.C. honestly wanted to improve the living conditions of northerners, especially First Nation and Métis residents. Indeed, according to Barron, fuelled by its "burning sense of social justice," the Douglas government was the first to attempt to "integrate" Indigenous people into the provincial lifeblood, and "it did so with an intensity and sincerity that" made "the CCF's efforts remarkable by any standard."[55]

In his 2004 book *CCF Colonialism in Northern Saskatchewan*, David Quiring presents a consistently negative view of the CCF government's northern policies and programs. When it came to social assistance, education, and health, the Douglas government invested less in the north than in the south for the simple reason that it "did not want to spend much on the north and its people."[56] Although T.C. initially "set out to provide a basic humanitarian level of northern health care through a network of remote outpost hospitals," this effort was flagging by the early 1950s. The result, according to Quiring, was that, after twenty years of CCF government, "the quality of northern health care remained far behind that available in the south."[57] While this assessment is correct due to the huge expansion of hospitals as well as medical and nursing personnel in the south in the early years of the CCF government, it is also true that, proportionately, the Saskatchewan government provided more services and set up more facilities in its provincial north than did other Canadian jurisdictions, which relied more heavily on federally financed and managed nursing stations and "Indian" hospitals.

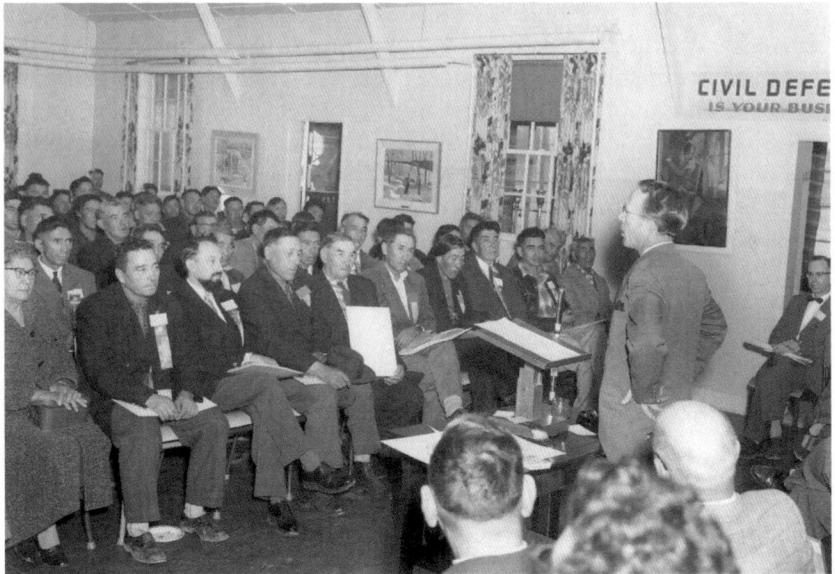

T.C. speaking with First Nation chiefs and councillors at a conference, Fort Qu'Appelle, October 1958 (PAS R-B8435(1))

In the case of health policies in the north, Quiring's assessment ignores critical aspects of the larger policy context of the era. Before Douglas took office, the few health services that existed in northern Saskatchewan – and in the northern regions of western Canada in general – were provided by Roman Catholic and Anglican missions, charities such as the Red Cross, and the government of Canada, which had begun to build and operate outpost hospitals and clinics. Almost nothing was being provided by the provincial government. By 1944, although it encouraged the charities and churches to provide care wherever possible, the federal government was beginning to assume the lion's share of responsibility for health services in northern regions. In the immediate post-war years, the Department of National Health and Welfare's Indian Health Services division accelerated this development and, by the late 1950s, was operating its own health system made up of twenty-two Indian hospitals, thirty-eight nursing stations, and a hundred health centres throughout Canada.[58]

Douglas considered these federal services insufficient and made sure that doctors and nurses, employed by his provincial Department of Public Health, serviced the north. Although the federal government

Table 8.2. Nursing stations in northern Saskatchewan

| Community | Established | Governed and operated by |
|---|---|---|
| Île-a-la-Crosse | 1927 | Roman Catholic Church |
| Cumberland House | 1941 | Provincial government |
| Buffalo Narrows | 1947 | Provincial government |
| Sandy Bay | 1948 | Provincial government |
| Snake Lake* | 1948 | Provincial government |
| Stony Rapids | 1948 | Provincial government |
| La Loche | 1951 | Roman Catholic Church |
| Lac La Ronge | 1951 | Federal and provincial government |
| Uranium City | 1952 | Community |
| Pelican Narrows | 1955 | Federal government |

Notes: This list does not include the mining company nursing outposts at Gunnar and Uranium City on Lake Athabasca.
*Snake Lake was subsequently renamed Pinehouse Lake.
Source: Lesley McBain, "Caring, Curing, and Socialization: The Ambiguities of Nursing in Northern Saskatchewan, 1944–57," in *Caregiving in the Periphery: Historical Perspectives on Nursing and Midwifery in Canada*, edited by Myra Rutherdale (Montreal and Kingston: McGill-Queen's University Press, 2010), 285.

expanded the number of its nursing stations in Indigenous communities in the early post-war years, the CCF government established a network of provincial nursing stations concentrated in northern Métis communities not served by Ottawa.[59] Before T.C. assumed office, only one provincial nursing station had been set up, in the northeastern community of Cumberland House. As table 8.2 shows, the Douglas government established four northern nursing stations between 1947 and 1948; it also worked with the federal government to set up a nursing clinic in the north-central community of Lac La Ronge in 1951. At the same time, the Roman Catholic Church operated two nursing stations, while the federal government was solely responsible for the nursing station in Pelican Narrows, which it began operating in 1955. This pattern was the opposite of developments in other provinces, where the minimal investments in northern Indigenous hospitals and nursing stations were left to the federal government, churches, the Red Cross, and other organizations.

In 1948, the Department of Public Health had three full-time nurses and one part-time nurse working in the north – a contingent that grew to six full-time nurses by 1953. These nurses not only worked in their stations but regularly provided care in the homes of northerners. In 1948, these provincially employed nurses made just over 1,000 home visits, a number that climbed to slightly more than 7,000 by 1953. They were supported by the department's public health nurses, who set up and operated immunization clinics throughout the north in a successful effort to reduce contagious diseases such as measles, smallpox, typhoid, and tuberculosis.[60]

## Children's Dental Care

Douglas always included dental care in his ideal of what constituted comprehensive health coverage. No different than hospital and medical care, basic dental care and oral health were things every citizen needed for a productive life.[61] In the short run, budget constraints meant he was limited to covering the dental costs of public assistance recipients and to his health department's support for the newly established health regions to provide basic dental services. For the longer term, the Department of Public Health worked behind the scenes to develop a plan that would have dental nurses (later called therapists) deliver basic oral treatment and prevention services to schoolchildren throughout the province, based on a similar program in New Zealand.[62]

The challenge was daunting. Henry Sigerist pulled no punches in describing the situation in his 1944 report to Douglas, calling the province's dental situation "appalling": "A large percentage of the population has no dental care whatsoever, and the overwhelming majority of the people has not sufficient dental care." "It is no exaggeration to say," he went on, "that dentistry in its present organization has failed to serve the population, whatever the causes may be."[63]

So, what were the causes of this appalling situation? Without a doubt, the poverty caused by the economic and environmental collapse of the 1930s meant that most families, especially those receiving relief vouchers, had no discretionary cash to spend on anything beyond the essentials needed to survive. Visits to the dentist became a luxury limited to a minority of better-off residents. Then, with the war, came rainfall, considerably higher wheat prices, and new employment, including service in the Canadian military.[64] By that time, though, not only had a generation already missed out on regular dental care, but children – particularly those living in rural and remote regions – continued to go without, due to the lack of access to dentists, whose practices were far away in Saskatchewan's cities and larger towns. In these early post-war years, most of the province's population lived in the vast rural regions, part of an economy and society built on the family farm, with most living far from any available dental services. In an examination of 5,708 children in Weyburn-Estevan Health Region No. 3, the rate of decayed teeth was 2.3 per child. In another, albeit smaller, survey in North Battleford Health Region No. 13, the average was 1.7 decayed teeth per child.[65]

A Department of Public Health survey in 1950 showed the extent of dental decay among school-aged children, describing the issue as "rampant" and noting that 90 per cent of twelve year olds required "immediate dental care to the extent of 3.0 fillings and 0.5 extractions per child."[66] At the same time, Saskatchewan had the lowest dentist-population ratio in the country (until Newfoundland joined the Canadian federation in 1949), with most of its dentists having practices in Saskatoon and Regina. This meant that, even if it were possible to double the number of dentists so that the ratio approached the Canadian average, this would have done little to improve the situation in rural and remote areas.

Public health and prevention services were automatically part of the mandate of the health regions established by municipalities with the encouragement of the Douglas government. Two of these regions also set up community-based dental programs. However, these programs soon failed, due to an inability to recruit and retain salaried dentists.[67] To increase the government's expertise on the subject and provide an ongoing stream of advice, Douglas created the Division of Dental Health in the Department of Public Health in 1948, in part because of the province's ability to access federal money to support dental care initiatives through the National Health Grants program.[68] As its director, he appointed A.E. Chegwin, a dentist with a diploma in public health dentistry who would remain in his position until the early 1960s.[69] Based on his curriculum vitae, Chegwin seemed a logical choice at the time. However, he was very unlike the other individuals, such as Mindel Sheps, Fred Mott, and Griff McKerracher, whom Douglas had hired to launch similarly bold new programs.

Unfortunately for Douglas, Chegwin proved to be a highly risk-averse public servant who always insisted on the need to obtain the support of the dental profession for any government policy change. More importantly, he assumed that organized dentistry's unwillingness to support government proposals to improve dental health stemmed simply from the profession's lack of understanding rather than a protection of its privileges and financial interests. In contrast to Douglas and his successor as health minister, Tom Bentley, Chegwin also accepted the profession's strongly held view that treatment was first and foremost the responsibility of the individual and the family, and that any government intervention should focus solely on prevention.[70]

Chegwin floundered when it came to the larger policy picture and instead found refuge in the smaller details of existing and proposed programs. He was also hands-off, preferring that the government restrict itself to providing education and support to facilitate prevention and dental health promotion rather than providing services directly. In this, he stressed what he perceived as a perennial trade-off between prevention and treatment. In his view, if the government provided treatment services, these would come at the expense of funding and facilitating disease prevention and dental health promotion policies and programs.

Chegwin at least did not block the health regions from establishing their own oral health and prevention programs, and he even provided limited human resource support paid by the department. However, by 1952, senior officials in the Department of Public Health viewed these regionalized efforts to provide dental services, including those buttressed by salaried dental hygienists supplied by Chegwin's division as failures. In response, Bentley and his deputy minister pressured Chegwin to propose bolder change. They were focused on the possibility of a school-based program staffed by dental nurses as an alternative to delivery by private dentists and looked to a program in New Zealand that seemed to fit with the province's needs.

Since 1921, the government of New Zealand had been running a school-based dental service that attracted considerable attention from policy decision makers around the world.[71] The New Zealand plan relied on salaried dental nurses rather than dentists to provide a combination of basic treatment and prevention education. Trained for two years followed by experience in the field, the dental nurses worked in community-based public facilities – generally schools – rather than through private dental clinics, cleaning, filling cavities, and extracting children's teeth. Naturally, most dentists hated the program, arguing that the education and training of the nurses fell far short of what dentists received. The counterargument was two-fold. First, there would never be enough dentists to service so many children, particularly those who did not live close to urban centres, and so some treatment was better than none. Second, their work actually compared well to that done in private dental clinics.[72]

Although the New Zealand program seemed to work well in a largely rural jurisdiction where dentists were scarce, the program was rarely imitated elsewhere, due to the opposition of dentists. In Saskatchewan, Chegwin, not wanting to ruffle dentists' feathers, resisted the idea of dental nurses "invading" the province. In 1952, Chegwin summarized for his minister the province's existing dental programs and their deficiencies but proposed little beyond some highly incremental changes to try to improve the situation in the health regions.[73] Although he referred to the New Zealand plan, he did so only in one short sentence concerning the possibility of eventually attempting a trial project using dental nurses. Given that only the Swift Current Health Region had made any progress at all with dental care (and even this was a mixed success), it was hardly surprising that Douglas and Bentley were very disappointed with Chegwin's memorandum.[74]

In April 1953, when the Department of Public Health met with the College of Dental Surgeons of Saskatchewan, Chegwin and the department's deputy minister, Burns Roth, discovered that the college was entirely opposed to the idea of even a small demonstration project. The college's representatives argued against the feasibility of adapting the New Zealand program to Saskatchewan. As Roth explained to his minister, the dentists "pointed out that these dental nurses are trained for two years and if the rate of withdrawal of these girls is the same as the other health professions," then the government could only "expect five or six years service for each" woman, as they would invariably get married, have children, and leave to become housewives. The college then pointed out that, while the training of a male dentist "takes four years," their "working time" would amount to "35 or 40 years."[75]

While Roth was hardly swayed by the dentists' arguments and viewed the meeting as a temporary setback, Chegwin saw this rejection by those he viewed as professional colleagues as fatal to any plan.[76] Instead, Chegwin insisted on trying a different kind of pilot project, encouraging the health regions, especially the Swift Current region, to use more dental hygienists under the direct control and authority of dentists in order to extend the work being done by salaried dentists there. However, this pilot suffered numerous problems from the beginning, and Chegwin himself was criticized by senior officials in his own department for not providing adequate "on-the-ground assistance" to the regional dentists and hygienists.[77]

The more Chegwin's incremental approach failed, the greater became the demand for more radical action. Roth decided he had to work around Chegwin's division, and he assigned other officials in the Department of Public Health to do a comprehensive review of the New Zealand program to prepare the ground for a major policy shift. When the review was completed in September 1954, Roth's department officially endorsed the New Zealand approach. The report's authors were "of the firm opinion that a new and bold approach must be taken to achieve the objective of a sound preventive dental health program for children," and favoured "organizing the means for training and utilizing a corps of dental auxiliaries on the New Zealand pattern."[78] Only this approach, they argued, would ensure that preventive care became part of the oral habits of the children being served by the program and was transmitted by them to future generations. Increasingly isolated in the department, Chegwin reacted to the report by referring to the plan as "a perfect illustration of an outright socialist approach to the dental problem," seemingly oblivious to the fact that he was working for a government that proudly described itself as socialist.[79]

Despite the strong report, the momentum in favour of a New Zealand–style dental program in Saskatchewan quickly dissipated. The major challenge was money. The government's two powerful cabinet committees and their secretariats, the Economic Advisory and Planning Board and the Treasury Board, felt that the provincial health budget was already crowding out public investment in social services, education, and public infrastructure such as highways. Of course, the idea could be revisited if the federal government would ever come to the table with contributory health funding, but this seemed unlikely. When Roth suggested bringing in a few dental nurses from New Zealand to replace the dental hygienists who were continually quitting their jobs in the health regions due in part to difficult working conditions, the dental profession was implacable in its opposition.[80]

Roth then established a government-professional committee to conduct a study on dental therapists.[81] However, the idea of a children's dental plan would be elbowed out by the urgency and expense of implementing universal medical care coverage, and a premier preparing his government for a confrontation with organized medicine. T.C. hardly wanted to open up a new front in his engagement with dentists, some of whom were supporting the doctors. Instead, he settled for a smaller pilot project in the meantime, one not requiring a major draw on public finances needed to implement medicare.[82]

As a consequence, the blueprint for a province-wide school-based dental therapist program would remain dormant in the filing cabinets of the Department of Public Health until resurrected and implemented by an NDP government under Premier Allan Blakeney in the early 1970s.[83] Dental care stood in stark contrast to mental health, where the Douglas government would set new benchmarks for the care, treatment, and understanding of psychiatric conditions.

# 9 National Influence, 1948–1958

*My dream is for people around the world to look up and to see Canada like a little jewel sitting at the top of the continent.*

Tommy Douglas to his daughter Shirley, 1951[1]

Tommy Douglas always carried the hope that the federal government would reconvene a first ministers' meeting and resurrect the Green Book proposals of 1945. His government desperately needed the money that would come with federal cost sharing. Between providing universal hospital coverage and extensive mental health and cancer care services – the largest items in the provincial budget – his government simply could not afford to do more. Yet almost everyone in his own party expected him to deliver on his earlier promise to establish comprehensive health insurance, while the more left-wing activists were still pushing for a fully socialized health system well beyond hospital insurance.

But Douglas was also motivated by something larger than the money he needed from Ottawa to help finance his ambitious agenda in Saskatchewan. He wanted comprehensive health insurance for the whole country. He saw Canada as lagging behind some other high-income countries, especially Britain, New Zealand, and Sweden, which had enacted far-reaching, progressive social programs, including universal health coverage, under Labour or social democratic governments. He could see no reason why Canada, given its material and intellectual resources, should not match and even surpass those nations and become a model for the rest of the world. As he told his young daughter Shirley, in 1951, he dreamed of a Canada that everyone could admire and emulate.

To this end, Douglas had constantly lobbied Prime Ministers King and St-Laurent while his top officials persistently broached the subject of shared-cost financing for provincial hospital insurance programs with the most influential Ottawa mandarins. It was all to no avail. As already discussed, Douglas felt that the federal Liberals was using the National Health Grants Program as a political defence against his charge that theirs was a do-nothing government. And he was unrelenting in his insistence that the federal government go beyond the health grants and implement a national shared-cost program of health insurance.

As we shall see, the opportunity finally presented itself in 1955, when St-Laurent convened a meeting of first ministers. Although the prime minister wanted the conference to focus on fiscal issues, Douglas worked with a few provincial allies to get hospital insurance onto the agenda. It would take until July 1958 for federal shared-cost money to flow to Saskatchewan for its long-standing hospital insurance program, allowing T.C. to move to the next step of comprehensive health insurance: universal coverage for physician services. Throughout, Douglas played a role in national policy that well exceeded his position as premier of Saskatchewan. His voice carried beyond Saskatchewan, to church groups, trade unions, and other civil society organizations wanting to see a national program of universal health insurance. He became a champion for all Canadians who wanted health care transformed from a commodity bought and sold on the market to a public service to which everyone was entitled, solely on citizenship and medical need.

## The Hospital Plans in British Columbia and Newfoundland

Once successfully on its feet in 1947, the Saskatchewan hospital plan exerted great influence on federal and provincial officials across the country and beyond. Regina became a required stop for interested delegations of experts who wanted to see how the program was set up and its day-to-day operations. These delegations included one in early 1948 from the BC Liberal-Conservative coalition government under Liberal leader John Hart, one of the first governments to study the Saskatchewan plan firsthand.[2]

Although the Liberal-Conservative coalition had been created to keep the CCF out of office, the BC government felt that enacting a program of Douglas-style hospital coverage would further ameliorate the threat posed to the coalition by the CCF. However, the coalition government rushed the planning and design of its plan, with the legislation passed in 1948 for a start date of 1 January 1949.[3] Unlike Douglas's government, British Columbia was not systematic in building up its hospital infrastructure and expanding the needed health workforce in advance of implementing universal hospital coverage. The bigger problem was the government's mistake in trying to finance hospital insurance solely through premiums, which soon produced a program that was chronically short of funds and continually required premium increases.[4]

To the great consternation of many British Columbians, their government then imposed a per diem cost on patients for the first ten days of a hospital stay, to raise further revenue as well as reduce utilization. This user charge seemed to many to break the promise of providing completely prepaid hospital insurance financed solely through premiums and without any cost at the point of service.[5] Unlike hospitalization insurance in Saskatchewan, which had no user charges, the BC program was "plagued by administrative and financial problems."[6] Moreover, lacking the expertise that had been gathered by Douglas to implement hospital coverage in Saskatchewan, the BC government seemed unable to fix the problems and soon faced a storm of criticism from the provincial media and the public.[7]

The BC hospital insurance plan detracted from the otherwise positive results obtained in Saskatchewan. It was to be a short-term problem, as the BC plan would eventually be placed on a more secure footing by a new provincial government, which had promised to fix it. This new government was formed, not by the CCF, which had seemed poised for victory, but in a surprise upset by Social Credit under the leadership of W.A.C. Bennett in 1952.[8]

In Newfoundland, a unique program predated the Saskatchewan and BC hospital plans. Initiated in 1936, Newfoundland's cottage hospital system – a term originally used in the United Kingdom for small rural hospitals with several beds providing very basic emergency and urgent treatment – offered prepaid hospital and medical care to everyone living in the many small harbour communities, a program that covered close to 50 per cent of that province's population. The Highlands and Islands Medical Services in northern Scotland served as the model upon which the system in Newfoundland was based.[9]

Built in isolated outports and staffed by salaried doctors, cottage hospitals allowed Newfoundlanders to avoid the long journey to larger hospitals in St. John's. By 1949, the year that Newfoundland joined the Canadian federation, the provincial government had funded the construction of fifteen cottage hospitals to serve people living on the island (Labrador was already being served by a voluntary organization).[10] The "dispersed population, poverty, and the vagaries of the fishing economy" form a direct parallel to the dispersed population, poverty (during the Great Depression, in any case), and the vagaries of the wheat economy of Saskatchewan, and explain why such challenging environments have the capacity to produce unconventional health programs, whether cottage hospitals or municipal doctor plans.[11]

Housing between ten and thirty beds, the cottage hospitals were staffed by salaried doctors and nurses paid by the Newfoundland's Commission Government. Residents paid an annual premium, $5 per person or $10 per family, plus a user charge of $10 for every baby that was delivered. After 1949, the province's first premier, Joey Smallwood, took full advantage of the National Health Grants Program to construct new hospitals. Yet, even with new hospital construction, Newfoundland in 1956 still had the fewest hospital beds per capita and the lowest ratio of hospital and medical personnel to population in Canada. Indeed, the enormous challenge facing medical staff, especially doctors, working in these isolated areas of Newfoundland limited the cottage hospital system from the beginning.[12] Nonetheless, the system gave the government of Newfoundland "a vested interest in" federal cost sharing for universal hospital and medical care insurance, and therefore generally allied it with Saskatchewan.[13]

## Ottawa and the Alberta Alternative

From 1948 until 1955, the federal government remained silent on the issue of reopening discussions on a comprehensive health insurance program for the entire country. At the same time, Douglas faced a new challenge from Ernest Manning and the Social Credit government of Alberta. While Douglas's efforts were directed to removing health care from the market, Manning believed fervently in the moral and economics benefits of a free market.[14]

In 1950, Manning introduced a model of hospital insurance that was anathema to T.C. Instead of providing universal coverage, the Alberta government subsidized the purchase of private health insurance for those residents who could demonstrate need through a means test. The plans was supported by the insurance industry and by organized medicine, and Douglas feared that it would become the federal government's model for health insurance, when (or if) it finally decided to assume some national leadership on health care.

T.C.'s suspicions about St-Laurent's personal position on the future of universal health coverage soon proved accurate. In the House of Commons in June 1951, the prime minister stated his personal preference for the Alberta approach. Instead of a publicly administered universal plan, St-Laurent wanted to see governments subsidize the purchase of private health insurance, whether provided by private commercial carriers, the non-profit Blue Cross plans for hospital insurance, or the doctor-sponsored plans for physician care coverage.[15] In this statement, he aligned himself with the Canadian Medical Association (CMA), which had come out against state involvement in health insurance – particularly universal plans like hospital coverage in Saskatchewan and British Columbia – except to provide some assistance to those who could not otherwise afford to pay the premiums for private health insurance.

It is often said that history is written by the victors. In the case of universal health coverage in Canada, victory ultimately went to T.C. and his working design. As a result, it has largely been forgotten that an alternative model of medicare, one administered directly by the health insurance industry and offering different levels or tiers of hospital coverage, was a viable contender for national attention in the 1950s, and again for a critical period in the 1960s. In both cases, this alternative model, where the poor received public subsidies to purchase private health insurance, was associated with Premier Manning and his multi-payer hospital insurance program in Alberta.

Unlike T.C.'s hospitalization plan, the Alberta model also imposed patient fees at the point of service to control utilization and cost. And the Alberta plan was not universal. Unlike the Saskatchewan plan, which was compulsory, in the sense that all Saskatchewan residents were expected to enrol, with the objective of attaining as close to 100 per cent coverage as possible, enrolment in the Alberta plan was voluntary in two senses. It was voluntary for municipalities, which, in order to participate, had to co-finance the subsidy plan with the provincial government; and it was voluntary for individuals, who could choose to purchase health insurance, or not.[16]

Douglas and Manning were the most electorally successful Canadian premiers of the twentieth century. T.C. would win five elections in a row, while Manning won seven successive provincial elections.[17] Four years younger than T.C., Manning grew up in rural Saskatchewan but moved to Alberta as a young man to attend William Aberhart's Prophetic Bible Institute in Calgary. Manning became the closest acolyte of "Bible Bill" during the early years of the Great Depression. In 1935, when Aberhart created the Social Credit Party and ran for office, Manning dutifully followed, entering government as a minister and deputy premier.[18] When Premier Aberhart died of liver cancer in 1943, the Social Credit caucus voted in Manning as his successor. At thirty-four years of age, Manning was the youngest premier in Canada at that time.[19]

Douglas and Manning were rivals in terms of religion, political ideology, and partisan politics.[20] In the post-war era, they were the best-known politicians from the two protest parties challenging Liberal and

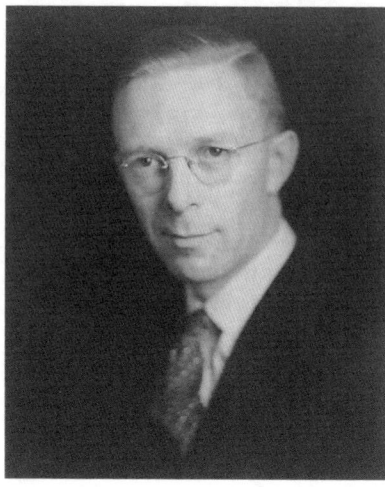

Ernest C. Manning, 1943, the year he succeeded William Aberhart as premier of Alberta (Wikimedia Commons)

Conservative hegemony. They competed to get national attention for their respective party positions and ideas on federalism, economic management, and social policy. In each of these areas, the two men were on opposite sides of the political spectrum. The most striking difference concerned their respective views on the welfare state. For Manning, government aid should be restricted to those who, through no fault of their own, were unable to care for themselves or their families, and he was opposed to universal social programs on principle.[21]

Manning was also a provincialist, who held a strict interpretation of the constitution. In this view, the federal powers enumerated under section 91 of the 1867 British North America Act should be the sole purview of the government of Canada. Likewise, the provincial powers listed under section 92 of that act should be the sole responsibility of the provinces, and the federal government should not use its fiscal spending to interfere in areas of provincial jurisdiction. This "watertight compartment" interpretation of the constitution stood in sharp contrast to T.C.'s flexible and instrumentalist view. Douglas believed strongly in the need for federal direction of the economy as well as national standards for social programs, including public health insurance, consistently arguing that the constitution should not stand in the way of such changes.[22] In the St-Laurent years, he complained of Canada as "a collection of almost little independent nations (a Balkans of North America)," due to the lack of national direction, and he welcomed the federal government using its spending power to set national standards.[23]

When Manning established his hospital insurance program in 1950, his multi-payer voluntary plan posed a major ideological and programmatic challenge to T.C.'s national ambitions for universal health insurance. While Manning recognized the public policy problem posed by the lack of access to hospital care – he estimated that between 15 and 20 per cent of residents could not afford the premiums for private hospital insurance – his solution departed markedly from the Saskatchewan hospitalization plan. Table 9.1 summarized the five main points of policy contention between the two programs.

The first policy difference was the requirement of a means test. The government of Alberta subsidized the purchase of private hospital insurance for those residents who demonstrated their inability to pay the full cost. Manning felt that the "cradle-to-grave" welfare state that was emerging in Canada and was actively promoted by left-wing intellectuals, the labour unions, the CCF, and progressives within the Liberal Party of Canada, would irreparably damage individual choice and initiative.

Like T.C., however, Manning was moved by the suffering of the Great Depression, and his version of hospital insurance reflected his belief that government did have a responsibility "to see that those who were unable to provide for themselves were cared for."[24] At the same time, he insisted that those who could pay for insurance should do so of their own volition, with the state only subsidizing the purchase of health insurance for residents who, through no fault of their own, could not do so. The means test was Manning's way of determining whether an individual really "deserved" the aid of the state. As Manning expressed it, the question was, "Has he the physical capabilities, the training capabilities? If he can, that's his responsibility. If he can't, then by all means, as a group we'll look after him."[25]

The key to Manning's design was the idea of voluntary action – that is, the choice of individuals to purchase hospital insurance. In fact, two years before his hospital coverage law was implemented in 1950, Manning's government sponsored legislation on behalf of Blue Cross to sell hospital insurance on a provincial basis and did the same for medical care insurance offered by a physician-based company, Medical Services Incorporated (MSI).[26] For those who met the means test, the provincial government paid one-half of the subsidy, with the other half provided by participating municipalities.[27]

To reinforce individual responsibility, all participating Albertans were charged a dollar per day spent in hospital. This feature was so important to Manning that he embraced the name "Dollar-a-Day hospitalization" for the program.[28] Unlike Douglas, whose more optimistic

Table 9.1. Competing designs and values for hospital insurance in Saskatchewan and Alberta

| Saskatchewan design | Alberta design | T.C. Douglas's stated values | E.C. Manning's stated values |
|---|---|---|---|
| Right to coverage based on provincial residency; compulsory enrolment with payment of poll tax | Right to coverage based on purchasing insurance coverage, paying premiums, and paying fee for each day in hospital | Access to hospital coverage should be a right of citizenship | Access to hospital care is a benefit that should be paid for |
| Compulsory enrolment, resulting in complete coverage of population | Voluntary enrolment, resulting in partial coverage of population | Universality as defined by uniform terms and conditions | Individual, hospital, and local government choice to opt in |
| Financed by general taxes and fixed premiums (poll taxes); no user charges at point of access | Financed by general taxes, premiums (poll taxes), and hospital user charges to reinforce personal responsibility, restrain demand, and deter abuse | Access without financial barriers | Individual responsibility |
| Single-payer administration managed by a single public authority | Multi-payer administration managed by numerous private insurance carriers, with public subsidy based on means test for poorer residents to help them pay private insurance premiums | Public administration and democratic accountability | Consumer choice through the market |
| Centralized provincial control of financing regulation and administration to ensure consistency of coverage and services | Decentralized local government control for majority of financing and administration to encourage involvement, including voluntary effort, at the local level | Uniform coverage and standards throughout province | Voluntary association and subsidiarity |

Sources: Gregory P. Marchildon, "Douglas versus Manning: The Ideological Battle over Medicare in Postwar Canada," *Journal of Canadian Studies / Revue d'études canadiennes* 50, no. 1 (2016): 134; Provincial Archives of Alberta, Premier's Office fonds, 1969.289, 1718, letter, E.C. Manning to V.A. Newhall, 11 Dec. 1948; Provincial Archives of Saskatchewan, T.C. Douglas fonds, R33.1, file 575b (14-28-2), memorandum, F. Burns Roth to T.C. Douglas, 2 Feb. 1960.

theology led him to the conclusion that human nature was basically good and therefore only an exceptional few would abuse free access to health care, Manning's pessimistic theology led him to believe that it was only natural for the typical individual to try to take advantage of anything provided freely, including hospital care. "In any scheme of this size" he explained to one Alberta resident, "it is necessary to have a small deterrent charge to avoid abuse of the services by many people who, if no charge whatsoever was involved, would quickly take up all the available hospital space simply because they did not have to pay any amount whatsoever."[29] This "abuse" was, in his view, unfair to all the residents paying the full cost of hospital care, whether out of pocket or through insurance.

The remaining differences in the features of the Alberta and Saskatchewan plans – multi-payer administration and decentralized control through the participation of local governments and private insurance companies – naturally flowed from these first features. Assuming that the St-Laurent administration could be coaxed or embarrassed into cost sharing provincial health insurance, the question for Douglas was whether the federal government would endorse his design or the Alberta alternative. Manning viewed health care as the exclusive responsibility of the provinces, and he had no intention of pushing the federal government in this direction. However, if Ottawa wanted to share the costs of his hospital program, he was happy enough to accept, if the federal government did not try to push the single-payer and compulsory registration approach to hospital insurance adopted by Douglas.

**National Health Insurance in the Shadows, 1949–54**

During the election campaign of 1949, the federal Liberals repeated their promise, previously made before the 1945 election, to institute a program of national health insurance. Douglas worked closely with the national CCF office to brand the Liberals as insincere and convince the Canadian public that only the CCF would deliver on such a program.

One of the key pieces of CCF campaign literature was a pamphlet extolling the virtues of Saskatchewan hospital coverage and other health services, with a promise that a CCF government in Ottawa would use what Saskatchewan had accomplished in terms of hospital insurance, cancer care, mental illness, communicable disease control and treatment, and long-term planning as a reference point. After all, if all these things could be accomplished "in a province whose resources" were "among the most limited in Canada," why could the same not be achieved for the entire country?[30] Referring to the National Health

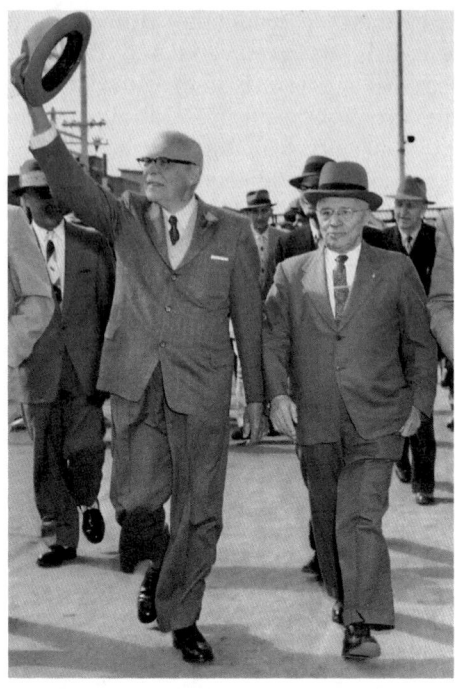

Louis St-Laurent (centre left) campaigning in Saskatchewan with Jimmy Gardiner (centre right), 7 May 1957 (SPL B-7096)

Grants Program as "a start, but no more!" towards a comprehensive health program for Canada, the CCF claimed that it would "complete the job" for the rest of Canada. To make the promise seem as real as possible, Douglas's hospitalization card was reproduced in the pamphlet with the statement that everyone in Saskatchewan had the same access to hospital care and diagnostic services because a CCF government "gave priority to a great human need."[31]

Despite these efforts to brand the Liberal promises as insincere, the party, under Mackenzie King's successor, Louis St-Laurent, won a sizeable majority in 1949. For the CCF, the election was a disaster, worse even than the federal election four years earlier.[32] The Liberals obtained 49.2 per cent of the popular vote (up 9.4 per cent from the 1945 election) and increased their seat count by seventy-three. In stark contrast, the CCF slipped in popularity from 15.5 per cent to 13.4 per cent and plummeted from twenty-eight members to thirteen. In Saskatchewan, where the CCF kept only five seats, compared to the fourteen won by the Liberals, the results were extremely disappointing to Douglas. Whatever the policy merits of his hospital insurance program, it had not become a clear political winner, even though most Canadians – some 80 per cent – in a Gallop poll survey held immediately following the election said they supported a government-funded health plan. This was the same percentage that supported the plan in a similar opinion survey held five years earlier.[33]

Douglas sent St-Laurent the customary note congratulating him "on the overwhelming vote of confidence which the Canadian people gave to you and your government on June 27th." He then stated that it was "now the duty of all of us who believe in democracy and who desire to see our nation progress to co-operate with you and the members of your government to advance the welfare of the people we represent." He reminded St-Laurent of the fact that the Liberals had campaigned on the promises, including comprehensive health insurance, contained in the Green Book proposals, and that the voters "gave very emphatic approval to the principles contained in the Dominion-Provincial proposals of August, 1945, and this was especially true in those provinces [i.e., Ontario and Quebec] where the Federal Government had some reason to entertain doubt in respect of the public mind on these matters."[34] Douglas asked St-Laurent to convene a meeting of first ministers "at the earliest possible date in order to discuss some of the more pressing matters that have been left in abeyance since the first conference nearly four years ago," noting that the "problems which the Federal Government recognized as crying for attention then" were now "even more pressing." Among these issues, Douglas put health insurance at the top of the list, stating that it needed to be "tackled without further delay" due to developments since 1945:

> Saskatchewan, and later the province of British Columbia, have instituted province-wide hospitalization schemes which are placing a very heavy financial burden upon the individual taxpayer and upon the provincial treasury. The widespread acceptance of these hospitalization plans are ample proof, if proof were needed, of the keen desire on the part of the Canadian people to have some system of prepaid health services established in some provinces at least. I believe most of the provinces would welcome an opportunity to discuss a health insurance program and the immediate steps that might be taken toward its implementation.[35]

Douglas circulated a copy of this letter to other premiers to enlist their support in his campaign.[36] St-Laurent took his time to answer. With a commanding majority in the House of Commons and every region of the country, he felt no need to accommodate Douglas or any other premier. In his reply, St-Laurent agreed that it was their duty "to co-operate with each other to advance the welfare of the people whom we represent." However, he disagreed "that the best way" for him "to discharge that duty is to come together at once in a full-dress Dominion-Provincial Conference." In his view, there was simply too high a risk of failure in the face of the continuing demands of some provincial premiers for Ottawa to give up some of its taxation authority to the provinces.[37]

Douglas had seen how the Liberals deployed the Green Book proposals of 1945–6 to convince voters that the party was as progressive as the CCF. To the CCF's detriment, the tactic worked, not only in the 1945 election but again, with even more effectiveness, in 1949, in part because the Liberals could easily point to the concrete benefits generated by the National Health Grants Program. All Douglas could do was to highlight, after the fact, that once the promise of comprehensive health insurance and other social security measures "had served their purpose of getting the Liberals" a huge majority in the 1949 election, the promises "were dropped."[38] Due to the CCF's poor showing in the election, he knew that, nationally, the Liberals felt almost no threat from his party. The only thing left was to try to convince St-Laurent that the CCF was not alone in wanting health insurance and that other provincial governments, including the Liberal-Conservative coalition in British Columbia, calling for federal cost sharing for health insurance. However, Douglas could not hide his annoyance with the prime minister:

> The Saskatchewan Government learned with a great deal of regret that you felt that no good purpose could be served by holding a full-dress Dominion-Provincial Conference. I have reason to believe that our regret is shared by many of the other provinces and indeed by large numbers of people across Canada. May I respectfully suggest that the main reason given in your letter for not holding such a conference is hardly germane.[39]

Douglas told St-Laurent that, since the federal government was responsible for setting the agenda, the risks that the prime minister feared could be avoided very easily by putting health insurance and other social policy issues at the top of the agenda and fiscal matters at the bottom, or by simply not including the issue of taxation in the agenda at all. Given that other premiers shared Douglas's desire to hold a meeting of first ministers, he urged St-Laurent to reconsider.[40]

St-Laurent again dismissed Douglas's arguments. The prime minister could not be moved by his own members of government, much less a political opponent like Douglas on the issue. Indeed, St-Laurent would also reject Paul Martin Sr.'s request to place health insurance on the agenda for the Conference of Federal and Provincial Governments that was held in early December 1950. Whether aware of Martin's efforts or not, Douglas too made a pitch to St-Laurent to include health insurance on the agenda, but the prime minister was adamant to the point that he dismissed the idea in his opening remarks at the conference itself.[41] It would take almost five more years and another federal election before St-Laurent would invite the premiers to a federal-provincial conference. Martin himself described the years following the 1950 first ministers' conference as "dark ones for hospital insurance," given the lack of support from St-Laurent and most members of his cabinet.[42]

A very similar scenario would unfold in the campaign leading up to the federal election of 10 August 1953. Once again, the Liberals trotted out the National Health Grants Program as its down payment on the greater promise of national health insurance. However, this time St-Laurent hedged this promise, stating that the federal government would move ahead only if most premiers agreed to implement provincial programs under the national plan. This added ammunition to the CCF's attack on the Liberals and the argument that only the CCF could be trusted to implement comprehensive and universal health coverage.[43]

No matter. Canadian voters gave the St-Laurent Liberals a convincing majority and the CCF saw its share of the national vote drop even further, to 11.2 per cent. However, due to slipping support for Social Credit, the CCF was able to increase its seat count to twenty-three, making it the third party in Parliament. Still, with the Liberals holding a huge majority of 191 seats in the 265-seat Parliament, the election result gave the CCF almost no political leverage. T.C. gained some small comfort from the provincial result in Saskatchewan. There, the CCF was able to win eleven seats, close to half the CCF total in Parliament, compared to the five seats eked out by the Liberals.

After the election, Douglas tried to put pressure on the prime minister to drop the majority province requirement for health insurance. As he explained in an address to the National Old Age Pensioners' Federation in March 1954, even if just two provincial governments "set up a complete system of health insurance it would only be a comparatively short period of time until the other provinces came into the plan." He expressed the "wish" that "the Federal Government would exercise as much ingenuity in implementing health insurance as they do in conjuring up excuses for further delay."[44]

Fortunately for Douglas, Paul Martin Sr. was reappointed minister of national health and welfare following the election, and he remained very supportive of national health insurance. However, it was obvious that Martin was an isolated figure in the St-Laurent cabinet. Alone, he was not able to change the prime minister's mind on the issue of pursuing national health insurance in the foreseeable future. Likewise, Martin needed premiers like Douglas to put external pressure on a cautious St-Laurent and his largely "small c" conservative cabinet.

**Getting National Health Insurance on the Federal Agenda: April 1955**

As it turned out, it was a decision by the premier of Quebec that would offer Douglas another opportunity to get national health insurance on the agenda of the federal government. Refusing to continue with a tax-rental agreement with Ottawa, Maurice Duplessis's government decided to levy a provincial income tax. When St-Laurent determined that it was time for all provincial governments to move beyond the wartime tax agreements, he organized a federal-provincial conference on fiscal arrangements. In January 1955, he wrote to the premiers to let them know that he was intending to amend the federal Income Tax Act to grant a reduction of 10 per cent in federal income tax for all provinces to make room for them to introduce their own provincial income tax. Moreover, he wanted to host a federal-provincial conference to discuss fiscal arrangements more generally, given the expiry of the tax-rental agreements at the end of 1956.[45]

A preliminary meeting of first ministers was held in Ottawa on 26–27 April 1955, to flesh out an agenda for a full meeting in the fall of that year. While the speeches and interventions of the first day of the meeting were public, the second day was slated to be in camera. T.C. arrived in Ottawa a few days in advance of the meeting to spend time preparing his strategy. With him were Clarence Fines, as well as their top civil servants and policy advisors: A.W. (Al) Johnson, the deputy provincial treasurer; T.K. (Tommy) Shoyama, the secretary of the Economic Advisory and Planning Board; and Tim Lee, T.C.'s cabinet secretary.[46] Although considerably smaller than the federal and Ontario delegations, the Saskatchewan delegation more than made up for its size with its intellectual firepower, especially that of Johnson and Shoyama.

First joining the Douglas government in 1945, Al Johnson played an important role in helping establish the administrative machinery for universal hospital insurance. Although only in his late twenties, he was appointed deputy treasurer in 1952. A recognized expert in federal-provincial fiscal relations, Johnson was also a keen advocate of the

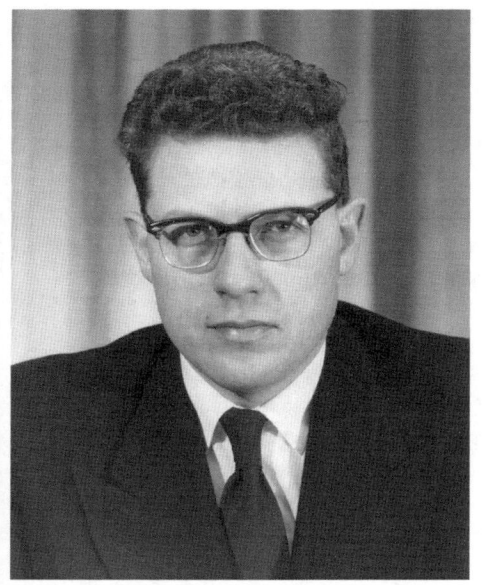
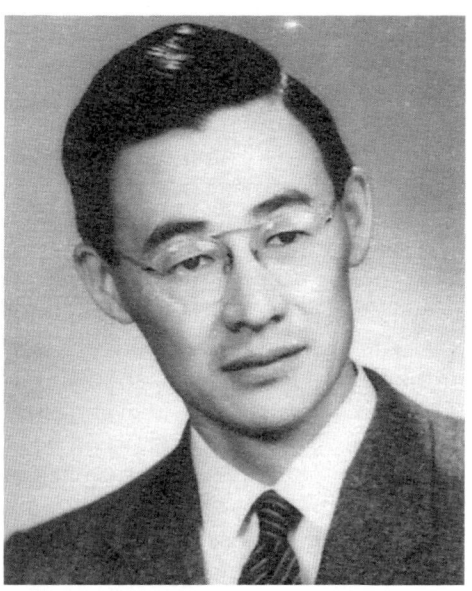

A.W. (Al) Johnson in 1957 (PAS R-B6094)   T.K. (Tommy) Shoyama, c. 1950s
(PAS R-PS59-293-05)

welfare state.[47] Tommy Shoyama's career in the Saskatchewan government was similarly impressive. When George Cadbury departed Saskatchewan in the early 1950s, Shoyama quickly filled the vacuum, replacing Cadbury as Douglas's most trusted advisor. Like Johnson, Shoyama believed fervently in Douglas's brand of social democracy and in the desirability of universal health coverage.[48]

The conference was scheduled to begin on Tuesday. Johnson and Shoyama spent Sunday with Douglas, Fines, and Lee in the premier's hotel room, working on his opening presentation. On Monday evening, Johnson, Shoyama, Fines, and Douglas joined Douglas Campbell, the premier of Manitoba, and his delegation for dinner and a discussion about their respective positions. A fiscal and social conservative, Campbell had never been supportive of health insurance, but the Saskatchewan delegation hoped they could convince him to change his position.

Only days before, in Toronto, Fines and Johnson had had a meeting with Fines's counterpart at Queen's Park. They knew not only that Ontario premier Leslie Frost was going to support placing health insurance on the federal-provincial agenda, but also that T.C. and Frost would "coordinate their efforts" to press St-Laurent "to the wall." Still, they would need other provincial allies to get the PM to change his government's long-standing position.[49]

On the first morning of the conference, Douglas and Frost joined the eight other provincial delegations as well as St-Laurent's sizeable team at the Railway Committee Rooms of the Parliament buildings to have their photographs taken. In a private letter to his parents, in which he gave a fulsome description of the first ministers and their respective jockeying, Johnson described St-Laurent as a "very quiet" and "able" man who "showed up very well" despite his seventy-three years. But "what he said," according to Johnson, "was disappointing."[50]

The prime minister made it clear that the meeting should focus on the fiscal question of taxation and not stray into other matters. Indeed, there was no point in revisiting social policy because, in his view, "a large proportion of" the Green Book proposals had already "been carried out" and "those that have not been implemented have been reconsidered from time to time and found to be either inappropriate at the time, or impractical in the light of the further study" they have been given.[51] According to St-Laurent, national health insurance was a perfect example of the latter. The program, he argued, had not been implemented beyond "the planning stage" because "the federal and most provincial governments" had "given higher priority to other programs, including the increasing of the basic services and facilities which would be necessary to carry the load of a health insurance system" – the main point of the National Health Grants Program. He therefore concluded that "the proposals of 1945" were "no longer suitable for our agenda in 1955."[52] St-Laurent urged the premiers to focus the agenda on two items: 1) federal-provincial fiscal relations, especially what would replace the tax-rental agreements, and 2) federal willingness to financially assist provinces to provide unemployment insurance.[53]

In Johnson's mind, St-Laurent's opening statement amounted to a repudiation of the original Green Book proposals and evidence that the federal government was not "prepared to pioneer, change, or recognize public insistence on social progress." Moreover, he felt that the PM and his government were "complacently ignoring the problems of any Province but Ontario and Quebec." Since "the Premiers spoke in the order in which their provinces joined Confederation," the Progressive Conservative premier of Ontario, Leslie Frost, spoke first.[54] He proposed that national health insurance be inserted in the agenda in the hope that the first ministers would recommend a study that would address such a program's details.[55]

Again, Johnson had his own assessment. As a "very effective politician," Frost was motivated by the fact that he faced an election later that year and wanted to make hospital insurance a plank in his electoral platform.[56] At the same time, Frost wanted control over program design, insisting that the "provinces cannot be put into one mould."[57]

Although St-Laurent was made "visibly uncomfortable" by this unexpected gambit from Frost, he knew exactly what the premier of Quebec, the next speaker, would say.[58] Although he was against any national (or even Quebec) hospital insurance plan, Duplessis chose to be brief at this point. In Johnson's view, Duplessis, "no fool," would save his arguments for the real conference in the fall, when decisions would actually be made. Next came Henry Hicks, the young Liberal premier of Nova Scotia, "an interesting person," a Rhodes scholar, and a potential Saskatchewan ally, according to Johnson. However, Hicks did not second Frost's suggestion in the public meeting.[59] Then came Hugh John Flemming, the premier of New Brunswick. Johnson described his long and tedious speech as a "wet firecracker" that gave little indication of his position on health insurance. During the in camera meeting the next day, though, Flemming would favour at least including health insurance on the agenda for the fall meeting.[60]

Like Hicks, Manitoba's Douglas Campbell did not support having health insurance as an independent agenda item.[61] "An ineffective little man" according to Johnson, Campbell preferred to have "a very general agenda for the fall Conference."[62] Clearly, the Saskatchewan delegation's discussion with Campbell and his people had not been successful. Campbell was followed by BC premier W.A.C. Bennett, who argued that the "proposals of Canada for health insurance embodying medical, hospital, dental and pharmaceutical services" constituted "a major and integral part of an effective social security program for the people of Canada." As such, "and insofar as possible, the proposals of Canada of August 1945, should again be considered."[63]

After some perfunctory comments by the premier of Prince Edward Island, it was finally Douglas's turn to speak. He forcibly stated the need for the conference to "go beyond" the issue of federal-provincial tax arrangements and "return to the broad perspective which marked the Federal-Provincial discussions of the immediate postwar period" captured in the Green Book proposals. He reminded everyone in the room "of the Federal Government's long-standing commitment to meet up to 60 per cent of the cost of approved provincial health plans" and argued "that a comprehensive scheme of health care must remain as a major national goal."[64]

Drawing on his own decade-long experience in government, T.C. urged Ottawa's return to its position a decade earlier, "which visualized the development of an adequate health program in well-planned successive stages." National health grants alone were inadequate, and the "time for further major advance is long overdue." Now that the country had a sufficient infrastructure of hospitals, universal hospital coverage was the "most logical" next step. Four provinces, Douglas added, already had hospital plans in place, "which could be integrated rapidly into a framework of national assistance."[65] He purposely did not comment on the position of provinces beyond British Columbia, Alberta, and Newfoundland, for he knew, based on his own government's survey of provincial positions months before, that those premiers were opposed, for differing reasons.[66] He also did not address the profound differences between the single-payer hospital plans in Saskatchewan and British Columbia, the multi-payer plan in Alberta, and the publicly owned and operated cottage hospital system serving the isolated outport communities of Newfoundland.[67]

For T.C., the real problem lay with the Alberta plan. If the national standards accompanying any proposed federal cost-sharing scheme were lax enough to allow such plans to be eligible, other provinces such as Ontario might adopt some version of the voluntary Alberta plan. This would result in a patchwork quilt, in which some Canadians remain uninsured in provinces endorsing a voluntary plan. Such schemes would also encourage multiple tiers of coverage and, with that, different standards of care, depending on the insurance policy. The worst feature for Douglas was the fact that the subsidy approach imposed a means test on the poor.[68] While T.C. was confident of Paul Martin's commitment to universal coverage and would never recommend a federal investment in plans that resulted in piecemeal coverage, he knew these design issues were precisely those that would divide the premiers. Worse, as already mentioned, St-Laurent seemed to prefer the Alberta-style model.

After Douglas was done speaking, it was Ernest Manning's turn. While he too agreed "that the subject of health and welfare" should be included in the agenda, contrary to St-Laurent's wishes, he also made it clear that the federal government should provide unconditional rather than conditional transfers for such programs. Conditional transfers were, in his view, "unwarranted and impractical in their application."[69] In other words, he wanted shared-cost financing for his provincial-municipal dollar-a-day hospital plan, but this should not give Ottawa the right to dictate any of the features of that program. After all, hospitals had been placed under provincial powers in section 92 of the British North America Act, and, according to Manning's watertight interpretation of the division of powers, setting national standards or conditions was contrary to the letter and spirit of the constitution. Describing

Manning as an "efficient little man," Johnson admitted that the premier "spoke well and impressively," even if the speech merely amounted to little more than an "appeal for free enterprise, free enterprise and more free enterprise."[70]

Joey Smallwood of Newfoundland was the last premier to speak that day. First, he made fun of the fact that "virtually every Premier who has spoken has suggested other things to go on the agenda." But then he elicited the first laugh of the day by stating that he was "agreeable to all of them – I think they should be put on." Why not, he asked, and then added his own agenda item, the "question of the costs of exploring and measuring and blueprinting, and finally developing the natural resources of Canada."[71] Flippancy aside, Smallwood could only benefit from federal cost sharing for health insurance, given his government's extensive spending on the cottage hospital system, so Douglas knew he could rely on the Newfoundland premier. Al Johnson's own reaction to Smallwood was overwhelming positive: "a delightful man – a vitality, humor, and intensity that is quite refreshing." His speech "was almost messianic – there should not be too classes of citizens in Canada based on the regions from which they come."[72]

Thus, St-Laurent faced a common front of four premiers, representing four political brands, in favour of national hospital insurance. After Smallwood, St-Laurent closed the public portion of the meeting. Still trying to avoid broadening the agenda to include health insurance and numerous other matters raised by the premiers, the PM suggested that the first ministers should discuss whether some issues could be dealt with in a forum outside the main federal-provincial conference. This suggestion was rejected in the in camera meeting the next day. The charge for including health insurance was predictably led by Douglas and Frost, supported in full by Bennett. Only the premier of Quebec remained entirely opposed to the idea. Privately, Manning indicated that he would support health insurance being placed on the fall agenda, perhaps searching for federal cost sharing for his own hospital program.[73] The rest agreed "that the time was ripe for detailed studies to be undertaken" on the question of health insurance so that they could eventually make a more informed decision on federal cost sharing.[74]

In the in camera meeting the next day, Douglas, with the support of the premiers of Ontario, British Columbia, and Newfoundland, led the charge again to have health insurance formally inserted into the agenda. St-Laurent and Duplessis continued to resist. In the late afternoon, a compromise was put forward. Rather than placing "health insurance" as a separate agenda item for the October conference, why not use a more general heading of "Health and Social Services." Exhausted with the debate, the other first ministers, including the PM, agreed to the compromise.[75] The door was now open more than a crack for national health insurance although what shape such a program would take was unknown.

This question of design had been bubbling in the background for years. In 1951, for example, the CMA had issued a formal statement rejecting universal health coverage. Instead, it believed that prepaid hospital and medical care coverage should be provided through private insurance carriers, and the role of government should be limited to subsidizing those unable to afford the premiums. At the time, commercial carriers as well as non-profit hospital insurers such as Blue Cross were expanding, while insurance for medical care provided by physicians was also increasing, thanks largely to the rapid expansion of doctor-sponsored insurance plans in the provinces.[76] When St-Laurent was asked in the House of Commons if he agreed with the CMA's position, he enthused that "it would be a most happy solution if the medical profession would assume the administration of, and the responsibility for, a scheme that would provide prepaid medical attendance to any Canadian who needed it."[77]

Martin, for one, "did not like this backsliding" by his boss, but he could hardly contest him in public. Instead, it was left to Stanley Knowles, at the time the federal CCF's critic on social security issues, to challenge the PM on welcoming "the idea of a form of health insurance being administered, not by the government but by the medical profession under its own autonomous powers." Referring to numerous previous policy statements by Liberals, Knowles argued that, prior to this, the Liberal Party had always assumed that national health insurance required government direction on a federal-provincial basis, and had never suggested – as St-Laurent was now doing – that it was in favour of a system administered by the CMA. Perhaps Liberal MPs, Knowles argued, should be at least as concerned as CCF MPs about this shocking reversal of what had been a long-standing Liberal policy.[78] For reasons of population size and political clout, Ontario held greater sway than any other province in Ottawa, and the question of federal shared-cost eligibility requirements for hospital insurance could easily be determined by that province rather than Saskatchewan or Alberta.

## Malcolm G. Taylor and Ontario

Malcolm G. Taylor, a veteran of Saskatchewan's Health Services Planning Commission (HSPC), attended the conference as a member of the Ontario delegation. In his detailed account, which was made a prominent part of his book on the history of the development of Canadian Medicare, Taylor noted how Paul Martin Sr. viewed the provincial interventions with "quiet satisfaction" underneath his outwardly "calm countenance."[79] However, Martin's optimism soon dissipated when he found it impossible to get his boss to review the question of health insurance. Worse, he discovered that the prime minister was once again intending to try to dismiss health insurance from the agenda. In complete frustration, Martin had to threaten his resignation in order to keep the issue on the agenda and allow his department to prepare a federal position on health insurance for the October meeting.[80]

Throughout his tussle with the PM, Martin could rely on Frost's steady pressure on the federal government. Even in the face of some internal opposition – influential members of his own party continued to maintain that the private, voluntary plans were enough – Frost very much felt his government needed hospital insurance if it was to win the next election.[81] With an Ontario election looming that year, both the Liberals and CCF put forth platforms on public hospital insurance, reflecting the favourable public mood towards such a step. In the Ontario Legislature, the leader of the provincial CCF constantly reminded Frost of the success of the Saskatchewan hospital plan and "that a much less wealthy province had introduced its program without federal subsidy."[82] Yet, unlike Douglas, Frost would not consider a provincial hospital insurance plan without federal cost sharing to support it.[83] Hence, Frost's insistence on Ottawa adding the question of hospital insurance to its federal-provincial agenda for the 1955 conference.[84]

An unlikely proponent of hospital insurance, Frost had opposed the idea in the earlier part of the decade as being too expensive and, potentially, creating too much pressure for hospital beds that were just not available. He saw his job as encouraging business development in Canada's most populous and industrial province and keeping tax rates down (including the taxes he had rented to Ottawa) as a critical part of his stewardship. When he first became premier in 1949, he was encouraged by the rapid expansion of private health insurance, including the Blue Cross plan sponsored by the Ontario Hospital Association, and saw no need for government intervention. His attitude changed a few years later, first in response to his personal experience of having his own health insurance terminated by an insurance company due to his age, but also because of the growing public support for government-administered health coverage for those unable to get insurance due to age, pre-existing conditions, or inability to afford the premiums. With federal cost sharing thrown into the mix and an election around the corner, Frost wanted change.[85]

To help him work through his government's options on health insurance before the 1955 federal-provincial conferences, Frost had hired Malcolm Taylor as his government's principal advisor early in 1954. As noted earlier, Taylor had left Saskatchewan in 1951 to become a professor at the University of Toronto. He was among only a handful of individuals in the world who was intimately familiar with the mechanics of the Saskatchewan hospital plan and had the knowledge and analytical ability to compare it to programs in British Columbia and Alberta.[86]

On 31 August 1954, Taylor delivered his 186-page report to Frost, which was then distributed to all cabinet members as well as senior health, welfare, and treasury officials.[87] In addition to comparing the hospital coverage programs in the three western provinces, the Taylor Report, as described by Taylor himself over two decades later in his influential 1978 book *Health Insurance and Canadian Public Policy*, "analyzed the economics of hospital and medical care in Ontario, reviewed the services desirable in a comprehensive system, and the effects of introducing them in stages," as well as "the costs of providing each stage of a health service to all residents." Presenting "six different ways of providing health coverage, ranging from full government administration to various forms of government subsidy," Taylor's report, strangely enough, made no firm recommendation as to which design the Ontario government should adopt.[88]

At the same time, the report made it clear that relying on the expansion of private insurance was insufficient. Roughly two-thirds of Ontario residents were covered through private insurers, many as part of employment-based plans. This left one-third of the population – the chronically ill, the working poor, and the aged – without coverage, as private carriers deemed them too risky to be insured or they were unable to pay private insurance premiums. Only government intervention of some type could ensure that this substantial segment of the population would get coverage for hospital care.[89] Drawing heavily on his Saskatchewan experience, Taylor's transmittal letter urged the creation of a health services planning agency like Saskatchewan's HSPC, as well as provincial grants to expand the hospital infrastructure and human resources required to support a universal hospital insurance plan.[90]

As expected, Frost used the promise of health insurance as part of his provincial electoral campaign two months after the April meeting in Ottawa. The campaign succeeded, and his Progressive Conservatives (PCs) received an overwhelming majority of eighty-three seats (its fifth consecutive victory) compared to eleven for the Liberals and a measly three for the CCF.[91] Clearly, however much people in his party as well as the business community were hostile to publicly financed health insurance, his political instincts about what the public expected from his Red Tory government were amply rewarded. With his election victory behind him, Frost decided that he would have Taylor lead his team in drafting a detailed proposal on health insurance for the October conference.

While the leader of the Ontario CCF, Donald C. MacDonald, had "grave doubts as to whether Frost" was "really serious," he knew that the gambit might work. Consequently, he called upon the national executive of the CCF "to salvage as much of the credit" as it could "for leading the battle for health insurance" over the past decade. He also urged Douglas "to call Frost's bluff" by suggesting that the province proceed on its own as a first step "as Saskatchewan and British Columbia have."[92] The following months would determine whether the fraught provincial coalition in favour of national hospital insurance would not only hold but grow in size and strength.

## Negotiating the Terms of National Hospital Insurance

In the months leading to the federal-provincial conference set for 3 October 1955, the Saskatchewan government worked out its position for the first stage of a national health plan. Burns Roth, Saskatchewan's deputy minister of health, conducted a survey of provincial health deputies and found that most were more interested in first covering hospital services rather than physician services. In contrast, in his discussions with federal health officials, he found a strong sentiment in favour of prioritizing medical care over hospital care. But such a position was a non-starter among many provincial officials, who feared that it might precipitate open warfare with their respective provincial medical associations. Douglas had always wanted mental hospitals included in any federal cost-sharing scheme, so Roth tried to convince his counterparts that they should push the federal government in this direction. In this, he utterly failed. His colleagues simply felt that the subject was too difficult to grapple with, and could, in any event, be postponed to a future phase. Trying to include mental hospitals at this point would simply muddy the waters.[93]

Whatever these officials thought, the decisions would ultimately be made by their political masters, and matters remained very unclear in Ottawa. By July, in his internal discussions with cabinet and officials, St-Laurent decided that if – still a major "if" in his mind – a health insurance program was to proceed, there would be some national requirements. These were, in St-Laurent's view, a matter of accountability. When the federal government raises and then spends money through

Table 9.2. Public coverage of hospital, diagnostics, and medical services, Canada, estimated costs, 1956

| Category of service coverage | Overall cost ($ millions) | Per capita cost |
|---|---|---|
| Hospital services | $330 | $20.50 |
| Diagnostics, inpatient and outpatient | $30 | $2.00 |
| Medical (physician) services | $260 | $16.50 |
| Total | $620 | $39.00 |

Source: Public Archives of Saskatchewan, C.M. Fines fonds, F119, R-37, file IV-3, Dominion Government Health Plan, correspondence with Ottawa, memorandum, Burns Roth to A.W. Johnson, 8 July 1955.

"health grants to the provinces, it is its responsibility to exercise some control and to make sure that the money is spent for useful purposes."[94] However, the question of design remained open, with Paul Martin supporting a Saskatchewan-style approach and the PM preferring the Manning-CMA formulation.

On 4–5 July, the provincial deputy ministers of health met with the federal deputy minister and his key officials in the Department of National Health and Welfare to do some advance work on national health insurance before the October conference. These officials painstakingly estimated the individual cost of coverage for hospital, diagnostics, and medical care costs in Canada for 1956 (see table 9.2). Although hospital coverage was more expensive than physician insurance, the former was tried and proven in Saskatchewan and faced no powerful opposition while the latter was opposed by a powerful lobby of organized medicine and the insurance carriers they sponsored.

While the officials were working out these numbers, St-Laurent was more than a little uneasy about the potential cost of a national health program. He also knew that the premier of Ontario, despite his positioning at the April federal-provincial meeting, shared his concerns. Frost believed that higher tax rates would dampen economic growth in his province. More importantly, the promise of health insurance had just helped Frost win the provincial election, undercutting similar Liberal and CCF promises. It was safe for him to retreat to a more cautious (and less expensive) position. Knowing this, St-Laurent asked Frost to provide him with a memorandum on his views concerning a national health insurance scheme, which would support his own position within cabinet. Understanding the game afoot, T.C. asked Tommy Shoyama to dig up as much information as he could find on the confidential Frost memorandum. Despite these efforts, it would take until the first ministers met in October before the Saskatchewan delegation knew fully what Frost had recommended.[95]

When the premiers reconvened on 3 October 1955, they faced a prime minister reluctant to pursue the medicare issue. St-Laurent opened the discussion by reminding everyone that health insurance fell "squarely within provincial jurisdiction." The federal government, he said, did not "wish to see this position altered; nor would it wish to be a party to a plan for health insurance which would require a constitutional change or federal interference in matters which are essentially of provincial concern." At the same time, he recognized "that there may be circumstances in which it would be justified in offering to assist provincial governments in implementing health insurance plans designed and administered by provinces."[96] However, the PM encouraged the premiers to focus as a first step on the least expensive option, that of diagnostic (laboratory and radiological) services. If that worked out well for everyone in the next few years, they could then consider an incremental expansion of public coverage. And he insisted that Ottawa could not cost share at any stage until a majority of provinces with a majority of the population agreed to implement – the double-majority rule.[97]

Just as Douglas and Frost had coordinated their efforts for the earlier meeting in April, St-Laurent had prepared in advance with Frost for the October meeting. The notion of restricting health insurance to diagnostic services as a first stage had been proposed in a memorandum the PM had received from Frost just weeks earlier. Prepared by Taylor and his team, Frost's memorandum emphasized the "administrative problems" concerning hospital coverage, and instead suggested an implementation strategy involving five discrete stages: 1) diagnostic care, 2) home care, 3) extraordinary costs for prolonged illness, 4) maternal hospital care, and, only at the end of all that, 5) comprehensive hospital coverage.[98] The great advantage of the first step was that it would cost less than one-tenth of a hospital insurance program (see table 9.2).

As T.C. saw it, the Frost memorandum was just the excuse the prime minister needed to put off hospital insurance indefinitely. He had to wait until later in the evening before he could take his turn to speak. Rejecting the idea that federal cost sharing be limited to diagnostic services, Douglas accepted but inverted the incremental strategy, arguing that the first step should include both hospital and diagnostic services. This would be followed by medical services in a subsequent phase, and then, eventually, home care, outpatient drugs, and dental care for a fully comprehensive package of health coverage for all Canadians. He vehemently disagreed with the PM's double-majority rule, urging the federal government to provide cost sharing for any province (i.e., Saskatchewan) ready to insure medical care services.[99]

In T.C.'s view, the politicians had forgotten the national purpose embraced by most in the 1945 Dominion-Provincial Reconstruction Conference: implementing a "comprehensive plan for the well-being and security of the Canadian people." Since that time, it seemed to Douglas, too many first ministers, "blurred by sectionalism," had become "preoccupied with fragments of a National programme" and had lost sight of their purpose as leaders of the country.[100] He stopped short of singling out Frost, refusing to goad the premier of Ontario, despite the recommendation to do so by the leader of the Ontario CCF. Ontario was the one province essential to meet St-Laurent's double-majority requirement because there was no possibility that the province of Quebec under Duplessis would ever agree to a hospital insurance scheme.

Still, T.C. questioned Frost's intentions and his tactics. The detailed proposal that had been circulated by Frost was overflowing with administrative and financial details of interest to experts in the field (like its principal author, Malcolm Taylor) but lacked any clear recommendations or sense of direction concerning a final decision. Even more unhelpful was Frost's suggestion that the first ministers establish a working committee of officials "to study some of the details regarding health insurance." Douglas said he was willing to set up such a committee made up of ministers and deputy ministers of health, but first it was essential for the federal government to lay out its conditions for federal cost sharing of hospital insurance and then for the premiers to formally agree, or not, on their respective participation.[101]

Douglas would not get what he requested. Even though the first ministers talked about health insurance in camera for three more days, no commitments were made. Instead, they established a committee of health ministers to work through the issues and adjourned on the understanding that they would meet later.[102] For its part, the federal government felt it was premature to lay out its conditions for cost sharing.

Shortly after the meeting, in mid-October, Douglas met with his conference delegation to strategize. Douglas, along with Tom Bentley and Clarence Fines, debated the written analyses and recommendations from Tommy Shoyama, Al Johnson, and Burns Roth. At the time, it seemed clear that they were far from getting enough provincial support to meet the double-majority rule. The only sure ally was Bennett's Socred government of British Columbia. Even though

Newfoundland should have been highly supportive, given the fact that it was underwriting the hospital and medical care coverage for almost half of its residents through its cottage hospital system, even Smallwood expressed concern that the limited number of hospital beds and doctors would not be sufficient to cope with patient demand following the introduction of free access. Alberta would agree only if Manning received some assurance that no strings would be attached and that the federal cost-sharing formula would be purely per capita so that it would not penalize a province growing richer by the day from oil. Manitoba and the Maritime provinces feared that they could not afford hospital coverage, even with half the money coming from Ottawa. The key remained Ontario, but there was no hope of getting a national hospital insurance program if the Frost government continued to insist on a limited diagnostic services program in the first phase. T.C. and his team concluded that they needed to focus their attention on convincing Ontario to once against support hospital and diagnostic coverage, rather than diagnostics services alone, as the first stage of a national plan.[103]

Burns Roth suggested the logic. Although the smaller step was one that most provinces and Ottawa were prepared to take, Roth felt that "we should argue very strongly that this step is not enough." Hospital services need to accompany diagnostic services because they are "a component part of the total hospital service and should not be set up as a separate program."[104] On this issue, T.C. continued to have an ally in Paul Martin, who, unlike his boss, also wanted hospital services included in the first step. Martin continued to meet with the provincial health ministers and, quietly, with his officials, continued to lay the groundwork for universal hospital coverage. Tom Bentley supported Martin in almost every way that he could. Before the end of the year, Roth, Johnson, Shoyama, and their respective ministers had managed to convince Alberta and Newfoundland to join the BC-Saskatchewan coalition in favour of universal hospital and diagnostic services coverage.[105]

In early December, just days before Martin's scheduled meeting with provincial ministers of health, Al Johnson was in Ottawa negotiating fiscal arrangements. He had already received a favourable impression from Ontario finance minister George Gaithercole that the province had shifted its position. To get further intelligence, he looked up his old colleague Malcolm Taylor, who "confirmed (in a whisper)" that Ontario would agree to hospital services being included with diagnostics as a first step.[106] St-Laurent's earlier effort to use Ontario as a stalking horse for a very limited first step had failed.

## The Federal Offer to Cost Share Hospital Insurance

On 26 January 1956, the prime minister made his long-awaited statement on the federal conditions for cost sharing. St-Laurent spoke in the House of Commons. Simultaneously, in a room adjoining the Commons chamber, Martin provided the details of the federal offer to the provincial ministers of health.[107]

St-Laurent announced that Ottawa agreed to pay 50 per cent of the provincial cost of standard ward care plus diagnostic services when a "majority of provincial governments, representing a majority of the people of Canada," were ready to implement their coverage plans. To encourage cost containment by the provincial governments, only 25 per cent of the actual provincial costs would be shared, while the other 25 per cent would be based on the national average of the per capita costs. Despite the arguments made by T.C. concerning the need to integrate mental health and contagious diseases into the basket of coverage, federal cost sharing would exclude care for psychiatric patients and tuberculosis patients being cared for in TB facilities.

When St-Laurent sat down, Stanley Knowles jumped to his feet and asked him when in the coming days the members could expect to see hospital insurance legislation. St-Laurent dismissed the question by stating that his government would bring in legislation when the time was right.[108] While little more was said about federal conditionality in the House of Commons, Paul Martin was providing more detail next door to the provincial health ministers. Only provincial plans that made "coverage universally available to all persons in the province" would be eligible.[109] While Martin avoided the term "compulsory," this would make it difficult, if not impossible, for voluntary multi-payer plans, such as the scheme in Alberta, to meet this standard.

In addition, provinces were expected to place a limit "on co-insurance or deterrent charges so as to ensure that an excessive financial burden" not be placed on patients at the point of service.[110] In other words, while user charges such as the dollar-a-day deterrent fee in the Alberta plan would not make it ineligible for federal cost sharing, the onus was presumably on the provincial government to demonstrate that the fee was modest enough not to block access.

T.C. was in full agreement with such conditions. However, he remained highly aggrieved that St-Laurent had made the federal offer contingent on double-majority agreement. In his mind, this requirement allowed St-Laurent to assert that the federal government was ready to implement universal hospital coverage if a majority of Canadians (as represented by their provincial governments) desired the

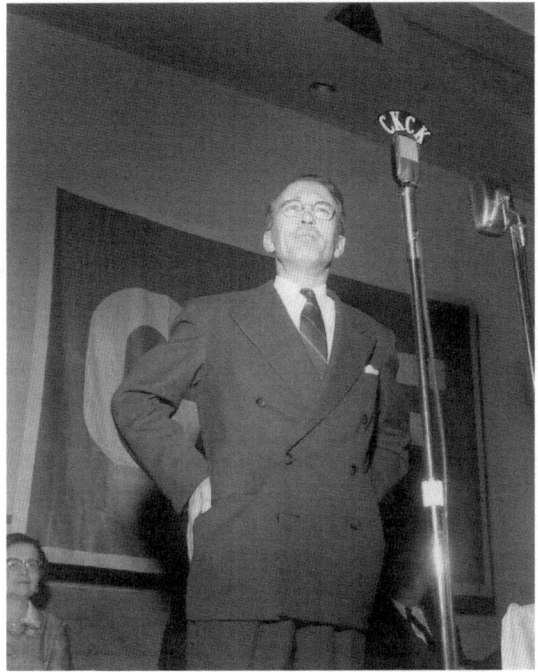

T.C. speaking to the media, 1956 (PAS R-LP1234)

program, knowing full well the double-majority rule could prevent implementation for years to come in light of the opposition of Ontario and Alberta (and some other provinces) to the design requirements set out by Paul Martin.

Moreover, during the discussions at the federal-provincial conference in October, the federal government had doubled down by suggesting that it would not be enough for a majority of the more populous provinces to agree to the principle of national hospital insurance and any federal conditions: they would also have to be in a position to actually implement the program. As Douglas explained to one constituent, "the Government of Canada has inserted a proviso in their proposal which seems to have escaped public notice. The proviso is that the contribution to hospital care and diagnostic services will only be made available when six provinces, representing a majority of the people of Canada, have assented to the plan *and have it in operation*."[111]

In the House of Commons, in response to needling on the issue by Stanley Knowles, Martin justified his government's insistence on the need for a majority of provinces with a majority of the national population to have a plan in place by claiming that it would be wrong of Ottawa "to use the money of the majority of the people of Canada to assist a province or group of provinces which represent a minority of the total population."[112] While there was merit to the argument, both Douglas and the federal CCF felt that the real reason for the double-majority rule was that it allowed the St-Laurent government to delay implementation, potentially forever. St-Laurent and almost everyone in his cabinet, except Martin, preferred taking the political credit for appearing to be in favour of universal health insurance while delaying for as long as possible the financial burden of such a program.

There were other areas where Douglas disagreed with the federal government. First, Ottawa insisted on excluding mental hospitals, and area of particular concern to Douglas: when it came to mental health care, no other provincial government had expended more of its budget or devoted as much effort and expertise to improve the state of care for patients.[113] As Douglas explained to a representative of the Saskatchewan Psychiatric Nurses Association, Ottawa's decision to exclude psychiatric patients from the national plan was "a serious and regrettable omission," given that 50 per cent "of the hospital beds in Canada are occupied by mental patients."[114] In the House of Commons, the CCF's health and social security critic, Sandy Nicholson, stated that the exclusion of mental hospitals was a major blemish on what was otherwise "an epoch-making step in the field of health."[115]

A further area of contention was that provincial governments could not include the cost of administering hospital insurance.[116] Intimately familiar with the critical importance and the sheer challenge of putting the necessary administrative machinery together for an effective single-payer insurance system, T.C. viewed this as unnecessary penny pinching. From Ottawa's perspective, however, this restriction provided maximum incentive to provincial governments to minimize administrative costs.

Another question was whether the federal government would continue to provide hospital care for First Nations as well as continue to own and operate its network of "Indian hospitals."[117] The motives of the St-Laurent government were two-fold: to devolve the responsibility for and cost of hospital care for First Nations onto the provinces; and to ensure that First Nation residents in any given province received the same health insurance benefits as all other provincial residents. Although it is difficult to determine the relative weight of each motive with respect to the key actors, the result was the same.[118] The federal government insisted that the provinces include hospital care for all "registered Indians" and therefore that the definition of "provincial resident" needed to include all Indigenous residents, including "registered Indians" living on reserves.[119] On this, T.C. agreed with Ottawa. Indigenous residents should be treated no differently than anyone else. The only question was whether the federal government would pay the provincial hospital premiums for "registered Indians," given that most did not have the means to pay. The federal government readily agreed to do so.[120]

This issue as well as other questions would be the subject of multiple discussions between Saskatchewan officials, other provincial governments, and the federal Department of Health and Welfare.[121] For his part, Paul Martin Sr. had almost no manoeuvrability. He had pushed his cabinet colleagues and the PM as far as he could: they were simply unwilling to countenance any changes that would increase the government's financial exposure.[122] These restrictions would be reflected faithfully in the federal legislation that would eventually be presented to the House of Commons in 1957.

## The Hospital Insurance and Diagnostic Services Act

An engrossed observer with a stake in the outcome, given his advisory role to Premier Frost and the minister of health at Queen's Park, Malcolm Taylor described the period between January 1956 and the passage of federal hospitalization legislation in April 1957 as never "ceasing to arouse" controversy:

> Like a smoldering brush-fire there was always some smoke and some heat, and intermittently it flared up in brilliant flames of rhetoric, argument, charge, and counter-charge. Political parties, provincial ministers, hospital, medical, and insurance associations, the labour unions, and every newspaper editor and commentator in Canada defended, praised, criticized, or denounced some or all of it. It was too much, it was too little, it was too soon, it was overdue, it drained the federal treasury, it did not offer enough to the provinces, it was the road to socialism, it was the beginning of a new day, it would not represent any additional expenditure, it would bankrupt the nation, it would jam the hospitals, it was the only way to get more hospital beds.[123]

At the left end of this polarized spectrum, Douglas and his officials did everything they could to get the federal government to be less restrictive. Despite their differences, two months after the federal proposal had been announced, he let Paul Martin Sr. know that his government would enter an agreement in principle on cost sharing but emphasized the two problems that would need to get sorted out before signing a final agreement: 1) the precise extent of coverage, especially as it pertained to care in psychiatric hospitals; and 2) "the problem of hospital care of Indians and the relationship of existing Indian Hospitals operated by the Government of Canada."[124]

On these issues, Martin would yield little to Douglas and the CCF. Instead, he used his limited flexibility to appease the PC government of Ontario, since he viewed that province as critical to clearing the double-majority hurdle. Unlike St-Laurent and perhaps a majority of his cabinet colleagues, Martin wanted to see a national hospital plan implemented sooner rather than later. Consequently, he watered down the requirement on universal coverage. After months of protracted and sometimes tense negotiations, Martin agreed that if Ontario could guarantee an initial registration of the population above 85 per cent, then Ottawa would agree to a partial voluntary plan. Frost's solution – accepted by Martin – was that his premium-based plan would be mandatory for all employers having fifteen or more employees but would be voluntary for everyone else.[125]

To emphasize his commitment to the double-majority rule, St-Laurent informed the premiers that the federal government felt under no obligation to prepare federal legislation until at least six provinces representing over 50 per cent of the country's population signed on to the deal. This position further confirmed T.C.'s suspicion that the federal Liberals were trying to do everything possible to avoid a final commitment on hospital insurance. However, on 5 March 1957, St-Laurent reversed course and announced that legislation would be introduced before the spring adjournment of the House of Commons.[126] The new haste was driven by the Liberals' decision to hold an election in June and the usefulness of legislation to demonstrate their commitment to a national hospital plan and refute CCF allegations of insincerity during the coming campaign.

Less than three weeks later, a beaming Martin introduced Bill 320, the government's hospital insurance legislation. On 4 April, the bill went to second reading. During the ensuing debate, the CCF again raised the issue of the exclusion of psychiatric hospital beds and the imposition of the double-majority rule, as well as other restrictions. However, with no leverage, Douglas and his party grudgingly swallowed the limitations in the law. On the third and final vote on 10 April, MPs, including the CCF MPs, voted unanimously in favour and gave the passage of the bill "a tumultuous applause." On 1 May 1957, the Hospital Insurance and Diagnostic Services Act (HIDSA) was proclaimed into law.[127]

## Federal Election of 1957

After the national hospital insurance law had passed, the country was plunged into an election campaign, one that would produce a major surprise. The PCs under John G. Diefenbaker, its new populist leader from Saskatchewan, unexpectedly beat the Liberals, which had been the governing party since 1935.[128] It is almost impossible to know the impact of St-Laurent's position on national hospital coverage on the electorate in the 1957 election, but it does not appear to have played an important role. Based on John Courtney's careful analysis of that election, the top policy issues were the TransCanada Pipeline controversy, the Liberal government's response to the Suez Crisis, the question of old age pensions, and agricultural supports.[129]

These items marginalized hospital insurance as an election issue, despite the best efforts of the CCF. In mid-May, in a radio speech recorded in Toronto, T.C. blamed the Liberal's double-majority rule for forcing Canadians "to wait at least two more years before national hospital insurance becomes a reality" – an unconscionable delay from the party that "first promised health insurance in 1919."[130] After outlining how his CCF government had implemented and managed universal hospital coverage in Saskatchewan for a decade, he urged all Canadians who desired hospital insurance in their own province as soon as possible to vote CCF, even if they party could not form the next government.

Douglas noted that, as "the constant advocate" of the plan that had been proven to work in Saskatchewan, the CCF had pressured "an unwilling Liberal Government" to act "against its own wishes and inclinations." Only "the CCF group in Ottawa can rightly claim to have exerted a decisive influence in this belated advance." And only the CCF could force the Liberals to expand coverage for the chronic care of those suffering from tuberculosis and mental illness. Moreover, only

> the CCF is pledged to work unceasingly for the improvement of the present inadequate hospital legislation until it is expanded into a full-fledged national health service plan. Only the CCF will speak for this objective in Parliament with power and sincerity of purpose. Why? Because the CCF stand alone among the political parties of Canada with its belief in the ultimate co-operative nature of human society – with its conviction that our nation can only achieve real progress as we learn more and more to share each other's burdens.[131]

While campaigning in Regina, Paul Martin took great exception to Douglas's claim about the CCF's pivotal role. Martin contested "CCF claims that there would be no social welfare program but for them" by describing the benefits of the National Health Grants Program and the federal contribution that would be made to Saskatchewan once shared-cost financing kicked in under the Hospital Insurance and Diagnostic Services Act.[132]

However, realizing that hospital insurance was not a wedge issue in the campaign, given the position of the two main political parties, T.C. emphasized other issues such as agricultural supports in his speeches in support of federal CCF candidates.[133] Nonetheless, even in Saskatchewan, both the Liberals and the CCF saw their respective parties begin to lose ground to the Diefenbaker Conservatives over the course of the campaign.[134] Still, almost everyone assumed that the St-Laurent Liberals would win: indeed, *Maclean's* magazine "went to print before the votes were counted with an editorial that declared: 'For better or worse ... Canadians have once more elected one of the most powerful governments ever created.'"[135]

When the votes were counted on 10 June 1957, the results were a shock. The Progressive Conservatives under their populist leader Diefenbaker had defeated the Liberals by the thinnest margin. Although surprised by the result, Douglas saw the defeat of the Liberals and the new minority government as presenting "the CCF with the opportunity to exercise an influence on the social and economic life of this country out of all proportion to its numerical strength in Parliament." He celebrated the end of a "stagnant" Liberal regime, which had held power continuously for almost a quarter century. In contrast, the minority Diefenbaker government would have to perform or would be brought down.[136]

**Diefenbaker and the Removal of the Double-Majority Rule**

Under Diefenbaker, the new PC government had positioned itself as the visionary and activist alternative to the Liberals. In terms of his attitude towards the welfare state, Diefenbaker – to the great consternation of some in his party – had moved somewhat to the left of the Liberals under St-Laurent. In a speech in Parliament as early as 1944, Diefenbaker had upset some Conservatives with his ringing endorsement of a modern welfare state, arguing that the "state must guarantee and underwrite equal access to security, to education, to nutrition and to health for all," and that this was a "recognition of all men of their responsibilities for the welfare of all other men."[137] During the 1957 campaign, he had promised to call a first ministers' meeting to settle outstanding matters, including the question of hospital insurance.[138]

Although political rivals, Douglas and Diefenbaker had warm personal relations, due in part to their common fealty to the province of Saskatchewan. Most of all, they shared a common enemy – the Liberals. They also shared voters, with some provincial CCF support moving to the PCs in every federal election once Diefenbaker became leader, and some PC voters supporting the Douglas government in provincial elections, all in opposition to the Liberal Party. The provincial PCs posed little threat to the Saskatchewan CCF, while the federal CCF posed only a minor threat to Diefenbaker's Conservatives. On both fronts, the Liberals posed the major challenge.[139]

In mid-July, before Diefenbaker had fully settled into the PM's residence at 24 Sussex, Douglas phoned him to request a meeting. Douglas followed up with a letter stating that, if the double-majority rule were followed, then, in a best-case scenario, he and the other premiers with universal hospital insurance plans would have to wait until the beginning of 1959 for federal cost sharing. Some provinces, he noted, were keen to start before that date, and Saskatchewan was ready immediately and could cost share under HIDSA at the beginning of 1958. He could see no reason why Ottawa shouldn't "contribute financially to the plan as it became operative in each province."[140]

In response to Douglas, Diefenbaker bought some time by stating that he was not prepared to make any major policy announcements until Parliament resumed. By the end of the summer, however, a sixth province – Prince Edward Island – indicated that it was prepared to establish universal hospital coverage that would meet the requirements of HIDSA. This prompted yet another letter from Douglas beseeching Diefenbaker:

> Now that a majority of the provinces representing a majority of the people of Canada have indicated their willingness to proceed with hospital insurance and out-patient diagnostic services we are hopeful that the Government of Canada will be prepared to proceed with this program commencing January 1st, 1958. The Provinces of British Columbia, Alberta and Saskatchewan could have plans in operation by that date. It seems most unfair to deny these provinces the benefits of Federal participation until 1959 merely because other provinces who have indicated their willingness to participate are not ready to proceed at the present time. I would therefore urge that consideration be given to Federal participation in a hospital insurance program at the beginning of the calendar year 1958.[141]

Although Diefenbaker would not give an immediate response, he did invite the premiers to a first ministers' conference slated to start on

25 November 1957. In a radio broadcast weeks before the conference, Douglas appealed to the public:

> You will remember that the government of Mr. St-Laurent agreed to pay approximately half the cost of a hospital insurance program providing six provinces agreed and providing that one of these provinces was either Ontario or Quebec. That looked like a pretty large order but this year six provinces, including Ontario, finally agreed to institute a plan for hospital insurance and diagnostic services. At this point, however, we ran into a snag. The Federal Government [under St-Laurent] stated that not only must six provinces agree but all six provinces must have plans approved and in operation before they would contribute their share of the cost. This would mean that no financial contribution would be available to the provinces before January 1st, 1959.
>
> There are three provinces, namely Saskatchewan, Alberta and British Columbia, which have plans ready to go into effect next January. It seems most unfair that these provinces should be required to wait until 1959 merely because some of the other provinces are not ready to proceed ...
>
> I have written Prime Minister Diefenbaker urging that the National Hospital Insurance Plan becomes effective January 1st, 1958. I shall renew these representations when we meet in Ottawa in November. I am convinced that our request is reasonable and that our claim is just.[142]

As it turned out, T.C. had little to worry about. At the opening of the conference, Diefenbaker announced his intention to get rid of the double-majority requirement.[143] This change would allow provinces with a smaller population, such as Saskatchewan, to get shared cost dollars for a program it had been running for a decade and thereby give it the fiscal room to expand its coverage to medical care. Douglas was convinced "that if Mr. Diefenbaker hadn't taken that clause out, it [wasn't] likely that we would have had hospital insurance for many years, if ever."[144]

As Douglas recollected years later, Diefenbaker's approach to federalism "was not only much more flexible, but it was much more in touch with the political situation" and with the "mood" of the general public at the time than St-Laurent's had been. Douglas was even more pointed in his judgment that Diefenbaker, unlike St-Laurent, was very aware of the danger of a country that continued to be little more than a collection of "little independent states," and that the new PM saw universal hospital insurance as a national unifier.[145]

By default, the single-payer and single-tier hospital coverage that Douglas as premier and minister of public health had first implemented in 1947 was the design adopted by all other provincial governments. Despite the efforts of both Ontario and Alberta to get their voluntary plans accepted as eligible for federal cost sharing under the Hospital Insurance and Diagnostic Services Act, they both ended up establishing single-payer, single-tier plans. Without a single insurance contract, it was impossible to meet the federal universality condition that demanded that coverage be provided on "uniform terms and conditions." This effectively prevented a plan based on the subsidizing of private health insurance premiums for lower-income individuals as was then being promoted by the insurance lobby and organized medicine, even though such a plan had been operating in Alberta since 1950 and had been under active consideration in Ontario.[146]

On 26 June 1958, HIDSA was amended to allow provinces to begin accepting shared-cost financing for eligible hospital insurance plans on 1 July. On that date, Saskatchewan along with British Columbia, Newfoundland, and Manitoba all had plans that met federal eligibility.[147] The fifth province to join them was Alberta, where Premier Manning had moved early in 1957 to replace his multi-payer plan with a provincially administered single-payer insurance program that would meet the federal criteria.[148] As Manning himself admitted, 25 per cent of the Alberta population had remained without health insurance under his municipal plan, and his new single-payer plan now covered that gap. However, he continued to insist on his dollar-a-day deterrence fee as part of the new plan.[149]

Permitting user charges was the price grudgingly accepted by Paul Martin and his Department of National Health and Welfare officials to get Alberta into the national program. As for Ontario, that province, along with Nova Scotia and New Brunswick, needed an extra six months to get its administrative machinery in place. It would take Prince Edward Island a little longer – until 1 October 1959 – to implement an eligible plan. As for Quebec, Premier Duplessis and his Union Nationale government simply refused to introduce hospital insurance. It would take a new government with a very different view of the welfare state to enable an eligible plan to take shape.[150] However, when Quebec's plan began on 1 January 1961, Liberal premier Jean Lesage made it clear that this would be the last cost-shared federal initiative that his government would accept.

With federal cost sharing in place for Saskatchewan starting on 1 July 1958, T.C. was able to use his new fiscal flexibility to, at long last, extend his hospital insurance program to medical care coverage. At the same time, he understood the dangers ahead. There were many signs that the position of organized medicine both in Saskatchewan and the rest of the country had hardened against government-administered medical care coverage. He knew this next stage would be trickier to navigate than hospital insurance. He would soon find out how difficult.

# 10 Setting the Political Agenda Once More

*The problem of politics is [that it is always] a double program. It is a program of carrying on certain measures which you believe because of your political philosophy but at the same time it is a program of public education telling people why you are doing it.*

Tommy Douglas, 1981[1]

With a population of slightly fewer than a thousand souls in 1959, the farm town of Birch Hills lies in the parkland region of Saskatchewan slightly southeast of Prince Albert.[2] Its name refers to the hills in the area, once marked by the trees used to make birch bark canoes during the high point of the fur trade in the late nineteenth century. In the early twentieth century, the many farms in the area attracted merchants, blacksmiths, millers, and grain buyers, who incorporated the village in 1907. The village grew slowly over the decades, and, in 1951, the sixteen-bed Birch Hills Memorial Union Hospital was established, offering X-rays and basic surgery, to serve the community and surrounding area.[3]

On 29 April 1959, Birch Hills was selected by T.C. as the location to announce that his government intended to introduce universal medical care coverage.[4] He chose to do this at a nominating meeting to select the candidate who would run for the CCF in a provincial by-election. While he did not provide much detail, he did reveal that the program would follow the lines of the Saskatchewan Hospital Services Plan.[5]

Days before, Douglas had come out of a cabinet planning conference with a clear consensus to proceed with a medical care plan.[6] He and his cabinet well knew that it would be far more contentious than hospital insurance had ever been, due to organized medicine's growing hostility towards a universal program and the need to raise taxes to finance it, but it was a long-held promise that every member of cabinet felt had to be kept.[7]

## Medical Care Coverage: Pie in the Sky or Viable Option?

Douglas had been trying to add medical care coverage to hospital insurance since 1947. Over these years, he had done everything possible to convince the federal government to cost share a more comprehensive package of health coverage. In the face of Ottawa's reluctance and lack of decisiveness – what he often perceived as bad faith, given the Liberal Party's penchant for promising universal health coverage during elections – he examined the option of going it alone.

Starting in 1950, in response to T.C.'s request, the Health Services Planning Commission (HSPC) worked on a preliminary plan for universal medical care coverage to be introduced "over a five-year period, either with or without federal assistance," along with draft legislation that could be presented to cabinet.[8] The premier made it clear to the HSPC that he wanted to see options that involved either full coverage from the beginning or the phasing in of medical care services over time. He also wanted to see options that explored both centralized administration and a decentralized alternative in which the health regions would provide coverage based on a provincially determined package of coverage.[9] The HSPC dutifully submitted four alternatives to T.C in 1951.[10] After discussing these alternatives with his health minister, Tom Bentley, Douglas asked for a refined version to be prepared for submission to an all-party legislative committee as a public sounding board, but Bentley and his officials felt that "the setting up of a legislative committee might involve certain undesirable risks," including proposals that might resemble the multi-payer, voluntary hospital plan in Alberta.[11]

They had a point. By this time, organized medicine throughout the country had hardened its stance against government-administered medical care insurance. Aware of the government's planning – and Douglas's strong preference for a single-payer and single-tier design – the province's doctors, supported by the Canadian Medical Association (CMA) were proposing an alternative that resembled the Alberta hospital plan, which had been in operation since 1950. They were fortified in this position by the growth of their own non-profit plans in Saskatoon (Medical Services Incorporated, MSI) and Regina (Group Medical Services, GMS). As T.C. himself explained to a local supporter in 1952:

> During the past few years the medical profession has decided that if it is going to prevent a complete health insurance plan being put into

Table 10.1. Enrolment in doctor-sponsored medical care insurance plans versus number of municipal doctor contracts, Saskatchewan, 1951–61

| Year | Medical Services Incorporated (MSI) | Group Medical Services (GMS) | Municipal doctor contracts |
|---|---|---|---|
| 1951 | 48,893 | 17,186 | 173 |
| 1953 | 92,530 | 26,768 | 157 |
| 1955 | 122,191 | 38,348 | 160 |
| 1957 | 164,573 | 62,173 | 154 |
| 1959 | 211,514 | 69,305 | 136 |
| 1961 | 217,795 | 78,787 | 126 |

Source: C. David Naylor, *Private Practice, Public Payment: Canadian Medicare and the Politics of Health Insurance, 1911–1966* (Montreal and Kingston: McGill-Queen's University Press, 1986), 179.

operation it can only do so by setting up some alternative of its own. This is why [physician-owned] Medical Services Incorporated was organized and why they are now seeking to persuade municipalities to discontinue their municipal doctor plans and to enter into an agreement with them."[12]

After 1952, the position of the College of Physicians and Surgeons of Saskatchewan (CPS) only hardened as enrolment in MSI and GMS grew by leaps and bounds (see table 10.1). By the time of T.C.'s speech in Birch Hills, MSI and GMS enrollees constituted slightly more than 30 per cent of the provincial population. The influence of these two plans was, however, much greater than this statistic reflects. In fact, many insurance subscribers were breadwinners whose family members were included in the policies – thus, the two plans likely covered well over half the provincial population. In addition, some residents in southern Saskatchewan were receiving medical care coverage under GMS's contracts with municipalities.[13] Beyond this, MSI and GMS were the college's most effective weapons in slowing the expansion of municipal doctor plans by having their physician-based carriers offer the municipalities insurance contracts in their stead. Between 1951 and 1959, the number of municipal doctor contracts fell from 173 to 136, a decline of 21 per cent.[14]

Immediately following the Birch Hills announcement, CPS registrar George Peacock sent a letter to Douglas stating that doctors in the province should have been consulted well in advance rather than finding out after the fact through a newspaper article.[15] "As you realize," Peacock wrote, "your planning could have considerable impact on the practice of medicine in the Province, and as such, we would be most appreciative if you would favor us with some indication of what your proposed plan consists."[16] Immediately after his Birch Hills speech, Douglas told the press it was his "Government's intention to have the fullest possible consultations with those most vitally concerned" with medical care, especially the doctors themselves.[17] T.C. assured the CPS that he would call upon it for advice before any final decisions. However, it would be months before the government would be ready to discuss alternative ways to implement the plan:

> As you know, this is a matter which the Government has been studying for a considerable period of time. Up to the present our research has been mainly concerned with gathering statistical data in order to give us information regarding possible costs and anticipated growth of expenditures. Just as soon as these studies have reached a point where concrete proposals can be considered, it is the Government's intention to call in representatives of those giving the services and of the general public in order that we may have the benefit of their advice before any policy decisions are made.[18]

In fact, the work already conducted within his government dealt with issues of central importance to the CPS. Just days before the Birch Hills announcement, Douglas had been locked in an intense cabinet planning meeting that reviewed alternate approaches to providing medical care insurance as well as methods of paying physicians that ranged from salary and capitation to the traditional fee-for-service remuneration endorsed by organized medicine. The discussion was based on a twenty-three-page report prepared by Dr. Vince Matthews, the former medical health officer for the Swift Current Health Region, and now the director of the Medical and Hospital Services Branch in the Department of Public Health.[19] Matthews avoided any recommendations beyond suggesting that a more comprehensive study taking from six to eight months be undertaken.[20]

T.C. agreed.[21] He wanted an interdepartmental team of his most competent officials to dig down into the implementation details and make concrete assessments on a range of issues, including the position of organized medicine and how best to deal with the college. Once this was done, then a more consultative process – a public advisory committee made up of key stakeholders including the CPS – could be launched that would study the various options, but within a framework established by cabinet based on the advice provided by the swat team of officials. Since representatives of the CPS would form part of the public committee, its most important task would be to devise implementation options acceptable to most doctors in the province.[22]

## The Internal Review of Medicare: April–November 1959

To conduct the internal government research, the Douglas cabinet called upon eight of the government's most knowledgeable and experienced public servants, almost all of whom were deputy ministers or of a similar rank. The chair this Interdepartmental Committee to Study the Medical Care Insurance Program was deputy minister of health Burns Roth, who was joined by his senior departmental colleagues Vince Matthews and Murray Acker. Al Johnson, the government's deputy treasurer, along with Tommy Shoyama and David Levin from the powerful Economic Advisory and Planning Board, and local government experts Meyer Brownstone and William Harding, rounded out this high-powered group.[23]

T.C. knew that the province's doctors would propose targeted rather universal coverage of physician services, one in which the government's role would be limited to paying the premiums of those unable to afford private health insurance premiums. As a consequence, he needed the interdepartmental committee to construct as strong a case as possible to ensure that the public committee's terms of reference were firm on the issues of public administration and universality even if flexible on other implementation details, including the ways in which doctors would practise and the manner of their payment.[24]

In October 1959, one month before the interdepartmental committee submitted its seventy-five-page report at a cabinet planning meeting, the CPS issued a resolution at its annual general meeting, declaring that, while it was "in favour of the extension" of health insurance benefits though existing plans (such as MSI and GMS), it opposed any "government-controlled, province-wide medical care plan."[25] This set the doctors on a collision course with the government as, in its final report delivered in early November, the interdepartmental committee rejected anything other than a universal medical care program administered by the government. The committee concluded that "true" universality – in the sense of covering all residents on uniform terms and conditions – could be achieved only through "statutory compulsory coverage" and not by subsidizing the purchase of private health insurance premiums for residents who met a threshold means test. At the same time, the interdepartmental committee informed T.C. and his cabinet that the doctors had in practice "accepted the principle of compulsory, universal coverage" because GMS was offering physician insurance contracts to municipalities and health regions.²⁶ This would turn out to be an entirely erroneous assumption – a surprising mistake in judgment, given that the political purpose of the GMS contracts was to prevent municipalities and health regions from running their own health coverage programs.²⁷

Douglas and his ministers were willing to yield on details beyond the essential universal and compulsory features and felt that a year – from appointment to the final report – should be sufficient for the advisory committee to find a suitable compromise. This timing was critical. After the 1960 provincial election, assuming his government won what T.C. intuited would become a de facto plebiscite on medicare, the plan needed to be delivering benefits well before the 1964 election.²⁸ Moreover, it might take a year for the government to set up its machinery and at least as much time for the CPS to wind up its existing insurance plans. After reviewing the interdepartmental committee's report, cabinet set a target date for implementation between July 1961 and January 1962.²⁹

As for step two, the interdepartmental committee recommended the creation of a ten-person Advisory Planning Committee on Medical Care (APC), at least four members of which would come from the medical profession – three nominated by the CPS and one Faculty of Medicine representative from the University of Saskatchewan. These numbers translated into significant influence for the doctors, given that, at least as recommended by the interdepartmental group, the government's representation would be limited to three (two advisors from the health department and one cabinet member, former health minister Tom Bentley), while only three more members would represent all other stakeholders, including the public.³⁰ Only through such a public consultative body would these groups become "educated as to the total picture" and therefore accept some compromises, or so it was assumed by the interdepartmental committee:³¹

> Recognizing that each [interest group] has an understandable tendency to see its own problems from its own special point of view, it becomes imperative for some mechanism to be developed which will force each agency to examine its premises and arguments. Having to defend these premises can be a most useful experience which may lead to substantial modification of false assumptions. It is suggested that a public committee would be an excellent forum for this critical examination and compel a thorough self-examination.³²

The soundness of the decision to give the CPS such a central position in the APC was questioned by more leftist CCF activists who felt this gave the chief "enemy" of the plan far too much say in its ultimate design. T.C.'s position was clear, however: the government could not, ultimately, conscript the profession into a medical care insurance plan, as doctors always had the option of leaving Saskatchewan to practise in another province or the United States. Douglas fully understood the danger the CPS posed to the plan. In the words used by President Lyndon B. Johnson in 1963 to explain why he did not fire J. Edgar Hoover, the Federal Bureau of Investigation's untrustworthy head, T.C. wanted organized medicine inside his "tent pissing out, rather than outside" his "tent pissing in."[33]

As for the CPS, its position against a universal plan had hardened not simply because of its desire to protect its two physician-sponsored plans in the province but also because of the growing influence of newly emigrated British doctors in organized medicine. These physicians had fled what they viewed as the constraints and low salaries imposed by the National Health Service (NHS), moving to what they expected to be a laissez-faire environment.[34] By 1959, 200 of Saskatchewan's slightly fewer than 1,000 physicians – that is, 20 per cent of all doctors – were recent graduates of British medical schools, most of whom saw themselves as "refugees" from the NHS who had moved to Canada to get away from socialized medicine.[35]

The interdepartmental committee carefully reviewed all the options, from salary and capitation to fee-for-service models and blended forms of physician remuneration. It then stated the central conflict of choosing a payment form: "The idea of a salaried service is most attractive to all but the practising profession where it is strongly resisted."[36] Salary remained the strong preference of left-wing activists within the CCF, who had been pushing Douglas for years to make this part of his health reforms. Douglas agreed in principle but knew that, if he forced the doctors to accept the design of a compulsory single-payer plan, he would have to be more flexible on remuneration to retain any hope of getting them to help his government with implementing and managing the plan for the long haul. Thus, he was in complete agreement with the interdepartmental committee's recommendation that the proposed APC further study the question and make the final decision on physician payment.[37] On this question, the Douglas cabinet firmly believed that it had no option but to start the plan with the method of payment the doctors preferred, and any changes to payment would have to evolve over time as physician attitudes (hopefully) changed.[38]

T.C. and his cabinet also received guidance from the interdepartmental committee on other issues. One was the basket of coverage the provincial government could afford, including knowing in advance what medical care services might have to be excluded for cost reasons. Such recommendations were necessary to dampen expectations among those within his own party and pressure groups closely aligned with the CCF, many of whom felt that the government should go further. The interdepartmental committee focused on the coverage of medically necessary physician services, in particular the preventive, diagnostic, and treatment services provided by physicians in the immediate term. The committee recommended against the inclusion of optical services, eyeglasses, dental services, prescription drug therapies, home-care services, and chiropody services, largely for cost reasons, and suggested that they "be added in phases" as fiscal resources permitted. Moreover, medical care was the one area most likely to be cost shared by the federal government in the future, prompting the committee to suggest that the provincial government should keep as many diagnostic services within hospitals rather than allow them to migrate to physician outpatient offices in order to keep the benefit of federal cost sharing.[39]

**Centralization versus Decentralization**

There was one further subject that Douglas hoped the interdepartmental committee would provide clear guidance on: the decentralized administration of medical care coverage through the health regions. The terms of reference for the committee mentioned the fact that Vince Matthews's report reviewed at the cabinet planning board conference in April had pointed out the popularity of the pilot medical care insurance program in the Swift Current Health Region.[40] Given Matthews's work in the health region, as discussed earlier, this inclusion was hardly surprising. Moreover, many in the CCF's grassroots – especially the more left-wing activists –still clung to the original Sigerist-Sheps vision of a comprehensive system of publicly owned and managed hospitals, polyclinics, and health centres staffed by salaried doctors and other professionals.[41] In the interdepartmental committee, Matthews's view was shared by two others, Meyer Brownstone and William M. Harding. Although public servants, Brownstone and Harding were also members of a left-wing group within the CCF that was at times quite critical of the party – and Douglas – and what they considered the government's bias towards bureaucratic centralization. Both were strong proponents of local government democracy.

Brownstone was the more intellectually imposing of the two. Like Mindel Sheps, he had grown up in the hotbed of Jewish socialism in Winnipeg's North End. In 1947, at the age of twenty-five, having just completed a master's degree in economics at the University of Minnesota, he joined the Saskatchewan government as a research economist

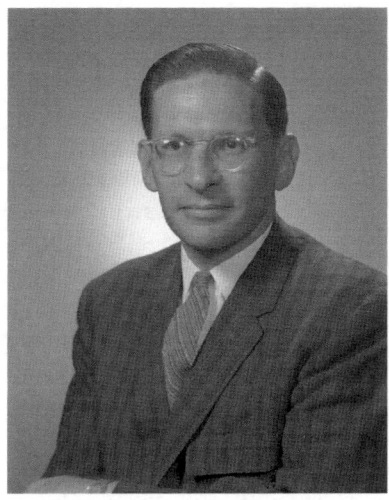

Meyer Brownstone in 1961 as deputy minister of Saskatchewan's Department of Municipal Affairs (PAS 61-258-01)

with the Economic Advisory and Planning Board under George Cadbury. Subsequently, he became the director of research for the province's Royal Commission on Agriculture and Rural Life (1952–7). He would later become the deputy minister of municipal affairs (1961–4).[42]

In 1959, both Brownstone and Harding were leading the Local Government Continuing Committee, which had been established by the Douglas government to figure out how a new county system of local government could be introduced. The 296 rural municipalities – established decades earlier when farms were smaller and the population more concentrated in rural areas – were the core of local government in the province, but they did not have the professional staff, resources, or capacity to deliver the range and quality of services being demanded by their respective taxpayers.[43]

Brownstone and Harding were both convinced that the county system would rejuvenate local government democracy in the province and "reverse" what they saw as a troubling "trend to centralization of services" in the provincial government.[44] A consistent champion of local government democracy and community-based organizations, Brownstone took great pains to point out the danger of the trend towards the centralization of service delivery and the supplanting of local activity by the provincial government.[45] Strengthened local government would, in their view, be capable of administering a coverage program for hospital and medical care, and they pointed to the danger of a provincial scheme being "too remote from the people."[46]

Whatever the merits of this argument for the future, the fact remained that the county system of government did not exist. Moreover, it seemed a pipe dream to the other members of the interdepartmental committee because of the consistent resistance to, and even outright rejection of, the county idea by most local government leaders.[47] In other words, the foundation of existing and planned health regions was a rickety structure of roughly nine hundred separate rural and urban (town, village, and hamlet) municipalities. Moreover, in areas where health regions were not yet organized – including those in which a majority of municipal voters rejected the creation of the proposed health region, as had occurred in 1955 – the provincial government could not delegate the administration of the medical care plan. As a result, the majority of the interdepartmental committee of deputy ministers recommended "a centrally-administered and controlled program," with the provincial government alone deciding the package of coverage, raising the revenues necessary to finance the program, and paying the doctors under the terms of medicare. At the same time, the regions could, if they so desired, "develop additional ancillary programs" beyond medical care coverage, such as home-care services.[48]

The Douglas government digested the contents of the interdepartmental committee's report in late November 1959. Most cabinet members expressed the view that medical care coverage in the health regions should be relatively centralized "in order to develop reasonably uniform patterns according to provincially established standards." In particular, the government must not create a structure in which health regions would compete against each other in terms of physician remuneration.[49] This position prompted Brownstone to fire off a letter to Douglas, outlining what he thought were some of the political advantages of regionalizing medical care coverage, advantages he clearly felt that Douglas and his cabinet were not fully appreciating. He argued that "the assurance of a strong interest by the government in decentralization would do much to counteract arguments opposing the scheme."[50]

Upset about what he viewed as the dismissal of a more decentralized option, Meyer Brownstone appealed to T.C. directly, citing what he viewed as both the political and administrative advantages of "some spreading of public responsibility" to local governments and health regions. In Brownstone's view, local organizations, including health region boards, regional hospital councils, and "perhaps" even local medical societies, might become supporters of the plan. Further, he contended that "regional responsibility should weaken the case, if any, for a provincial plebiscite on medical care coverage."[51] On this question, however, the Douglas cabinet felt that the scheme needed to be centrally administered to ensure provincial standards of care and "reasonably uniform" patterns of service.[52]

While T.C. himself was torn on the issue, he consistently leaned in favour of a more centralized scheme. He always thought that only the provincial government could ensure that everyone in the province received uniform coverage. If left up to the regions to administer, they might develop coverage terms that varied from each other. While Douglas admired the moxie of the municipal leaders in the Swift Current Heath Region in going beyond public health to provide hospital and medical care insurance for its residents, he felt that the province should take over from the region and provide coverage for everyone living in the health region on the same terms and conditions as everyone else in the province. This is exactly what had happened in the case of hospital insurance. As he put it, "Swift Current wasn't chosen to have a curative program of health insurance with the idea that eventually every region in the province would have [its own program of] health insurance." The "last thing we wanted" was "to start carving" medical care coverage "up into areas."[53]

While the question of decentralization was being actively debated within the Douglas government, the proposed medical insurance scheme came under concerted attack. Organized medicine said that the province's "doctors would not work under a scheme that was brought in without a referendum," a position soon adopted by the provincial Liberals.[54] When asked by the media whether he agreed with the position of the CPS and the Liberal Party, T.C. said that the coming provincial election would itself act as a referendum on the issue.[55] At the same time, he recognized that the time had come to explain his position to the public and not let his enemies define the issue.

**The Douglas Radio Broadcast of 16 December 1959**

Since the mid-1930s, Tommy Douglas had used radio broadcasts as a way of communicating directly to the people of Saskatchewan. Not only did the medium allow him to bypass the Sifton press and its predictably negative editorial opinion on the CCF and its policies, but it played to his strength as a populist communicator. Radio also reached people living on the scattered farms and hamlets far from the province's cities and their daily newspapers and was a critical source of information and entertainment until television became more common in the 1960s. On 16 December 1959, T.C. would give one of the most significant radio addresses of his career. Entitled "Prepaid Medical Care," his

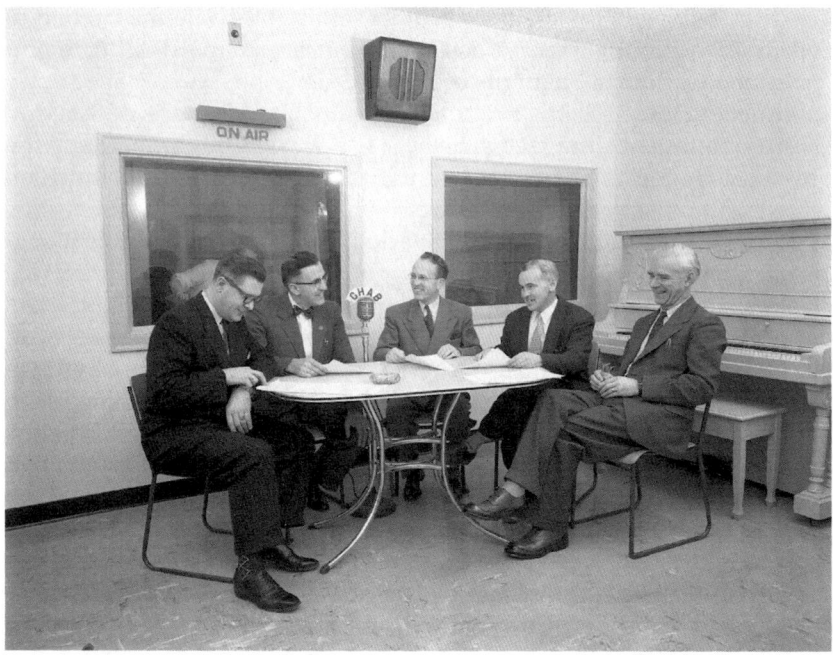

T.C. in the radio room of the Legislative Building, for a government broadcast, 1956 (PAS R-PS6-455-01)

fifteen-minute speech was broadcast throughout Saskatchewan as part of the government's own Provincial Affairs series.

He began by stating that, all his life, he had "dreamed of the day when we would have in Canada a program by which health services would be available to all, irrespective of their individual ability to pay." He quoted the World Health Organization's proclamation that health care should be "the inalienable right of every individual." This meant "not merely the absence of disease" but "the achievement of the highest standard of physical, social and emotional well-being" that could be attained. He pointed to the progress in Western Europe, citing evidence from a recent trip he had made to Britain and Israel. While he admitted that "many aspects of their programs" were "not applicable" to Saskatchewan conditions, in T.C.'s mind, they nonetheless proved "the advisability of having a plan which makes health services available to all."[56] The time had come, he argued, for medical care coverage "as the next logical step" in the "march toward a comprehensive health insurance program."[57]

Setting the Political Agenda Once More 279

He waved away the college's arguments that "a government-sponsored program" was "unnecessary" by demonstrating, through the results of the federal government's Canadian Sickness Survey, that low-income Canadians were receiving much less care than high-income Canadians, even though they had much higher health care needs. The simple reason for the discrepancy was cost.[58] T.C. began his speech by acknowledging the growth of prepaid health coverage through private health insurance and his government's public assistance medical program:

> It is a significant fact that in 1957 only 45.8% of the money paid to Saskatchewan doctors for medical care was paid directly by the patients. This means that 54.2% of the doctors' income in 1957 was paid from public programs or through voluntary and commercial medical care plans. This would indicate that a large number of people are already seeking to insure themselves against costly illnesses by availing themselves of the protections offered by public or voluntary medical care programs.
>
> Unfortunately, however, there are many people who cannot avail themselves of the voluntary plans, either because they cannot afford the premiums or because they have congenital conditions which are not covered by them. It is for these reasons that the Government has come to the conclusion that it should embark upon a comprehensive medical care program that will cover all our people and will ensure a high standard of medical care to every citizen of Saskatchewan.[59]

In pursuing medicare, T.C. committed his government to adhere to five principles: 1) prepayment; 2) universal coverage; 3) high quality; 4) public administration; and 5) acceptability both to those providing the service and those receiving it. The first principle, "prepayment," simply meant that residents would pay in advance for medical care services out of taxes. This would allow all medically necessary physician services to be provided free at the point of access.

Universal coverage through a compulsory program was needed, T.C. argued, because otherwise "there would be a tendency for those who are more prone to sickness to come into the plan while the healthier age groups would tend to stay out." A compulsory plan would spread the cost of good risks and bad risks over the entire population and thereby keep costs down for everyone. Moreover, a population-wide plan would have much lower administrative costs than private health insurance. There would be no need for risk assessment, advertising, marketing, and other expenses that were associated with private insurance carriers. He then compared the administrative cost of private hospital insurance programs in the rest of Canada (16 per cent) to the

Saskatchewan Hospital Services Plan (4 per cent).[60] T.C. had a point: the single-payer coverage model would save Canadians a fortune in administrative costs in the years following the implementation of national medicare.[61]

As for the principle of high quality, this covered a ragbag of factors, the key elements of which could be traced back to the original objectives of "socialized medicine" propounded in the province by Henry Sigerist, Mindel Sheps, Cecil Sheps, and Fred Mott. T.C. never wavered in his belief in the desirability of this principle, even if the manner of its attainment in practical policies and programs was never obvious:

> We believe that a medical care program must have as its major objective the improvement of the quality of care as well as a better distribution and availability of care. This implies the introduction of incentives to assure a better distribution of medical personnel as between the urban and rural areas. It means encouraging group practice where doctors are desirous of doing so and making provision for medical practitioners to take post-graduate work and refresher courses. It also involves fostering medical research and the development of facilities and techniques designed to improve the quality of service.
>
> Most important of all, such a plan will permit the integration of curative and preventive services. A medical program must not only be concerned with curing disease but also with the much more desirable objective of keeping people well.[62]

As T.C. explained, public administration meant public regulation and public accountability. As he had demonstrated through hospitalization, it did not mean public ownership of health care facilities or the public employment of all health care providers, a distinction he made once again in his radio address:

> The fourth principle we have accepted is that this [plan] must be a government-sponsored program administered by a public body responsible to the Legislature and through it to the entire population. If the Government is going to spend the taxpayers' money to provide medical care, then we feel that it must be accountable to the Legislature and the public for the expenditures made and for the administration of the program. For that reason, it is our intention to have this plan administered by the Department of Public Health and responsible to the Legislature through the Minister of that Department in the same manner as we do now with the Saskatchewan Hospital Services Plan. In fact these two plans can be integrated for the purpose of collecting the per capita [health premium] tax, thereby effecting considerable savings in administrative costs.

An additional advantage is that in a government-sponsored plan part of the cost can be borne out of general revenue, thereby keeping the per capita tax at a figure which every family in the province can afford to pay. This is the principle we adopted when we set up the hospital insurance program. When you pay $35 for your family hospital card you are paying only about 30% of the hospital bills. The balance comes from other taxes which have a better relationship to the ability of the individual to pay.[63]

The fifth principle – acceptability to both doctors and patients – was already weighed down with considerable baggage by 1959. As discussed previously, organized medicine in Saskatchewan opposed the extension of the single-payer design of hospitalization to medical care when the former plan was first presented by Douglas in 1946. By the mid-1950s, the CMA and the provincial medical associations had become implacably opposed to a government-administered single-payer system. Douglas underestimated the extent of organized medicine's opposition, initially viewing it as mainly a bargaining ploy to prevent governments from forcing doctors to become salaried employees, to protect their clinical autonomy, and to protect and potentially increase their fee-for-service tariff.

T.C. was more than ready to accede to such demands if the doctors accepted the government's single-payer design and its insistence on universal coverage, even if some in his party were dead set against such a compromise, and even if he personally did not think fee-for-service arrangements produced good care for patients. He felt that these concessions were essential to avoid a mass exodus of doctors. As for patients, unlike the situation in the NHS, the Saskatchewan plan would place no restrictions on the choice of doctor, thereby eliminating this contentious issue from the debate. On this point, he was trying to address the fears that emigré British doctors had instilled among Canadian doctors.[64] He did this by distancing his own plan from the NHS.

In emphasizing that the plan would "be in a form that is acceptable both to those providing the service and those receiving it," T.C. intended to give doctors some comfort about the government's intentions, and he aimed his remarks at physicians throughout the province:

> It has been said in some quarters that the Government is going to make all the doctors civil servants and in consequence we will see an exodus of doctors from Saskatchewan. In the first place I would point out that there is nothing wrong with doctors being on salary. The President of the Canadian Medical Association has stated that 20–25% of the doctors in Canada are now on salary. Of the 930 doctors in Saskatchewan 181 of them are on salary at the present time. The doctors in our cancer clinics, T.B. Sanatoria,

Health Regions, Mental Hospitals and Medical College are all on salary and provide a high quality of service.

The Government, however, has never suggested that all doctors ought to be on salary. The medical care program in the Swift Current Health Region has been in operation for over ten years and the doctors there are on a fee-for-service basis and the doctor-patient relationship has been scrupulously maintained. When we were setting up the Swift Current Plan I was warned by a number of groups that the result would be a loss of doctors from the area. Well, when we started the plan we had 19 doctors in the Region and today we have 41.

The Government believes that we must retain the principle of free choice of doctor so that the doctor-patient relationship will be maintained to the fullest possible extent. To recognize that no plan will operate successfully unless those giving the service and those receiving it are fully satisfied with it, we have no intention of pushing some pre-conceived plan down the doctors' throats. We want their co-operation and from our experience with other health programs I am convinced we will get it.[65]

While Douglas remained confident that most rank-and-file doctors would eventually accept his plan, he would still have to deal with their CPS representatives and reach some kind of compromise. This was best done, he had already decided, through the Advisory Planning Committee on Medical Care, where the representatives of the college, government, and civil society would work to find "the best method of developing a medical care program in keeping with the [five] basic principles."[66]

He ended his address on an optimistic note that played upon provincial pride in setting the direction for the rest of the country:

If we can do this – and I feel sure we can – then I would like to hazard a prophecy that before 1970 almost every other province in Canada will have followed the lead of Saskatchewan and we shall have a national health insurance program from the Atlantic to the Pacific. Once more Saskatchewan has the opportunity to lead the way. Let us therefore have the vision and the courage to take this forward step, believing that it is another advance toward a more just and humane society.[67]

Following his address, Douglas was flooded by questions and concerns. These were carefully tallied and then addressed in a television appearance in January 1960. The format involved Marjorie Cooper, a CCF backbencher, interviewing Douglas with a series of carefully prepared questions. When asked if access could be addressed by expanding the currently existing private plans, Douglas's answer was simply "No. Private plans like Group Medical Services and Medical Services Incorporated have served a very useful purpose, but there are a great many people who cannot afford to pay the premiums and there are others who would not be covered by such plans." However, on the question of whether these private plans would be eliminated, Douglas deftly sidestepped, saying that his government had asked the APC "to study how all existing plans, whether regional, municipal or private can be integrated into a provincial plan."[68]

**Preparing for an Election**

To counter the powerful voices of opposition to medicare, Douglas needed a demonstration of the general public's support. In his mind, the most convincing evidence of this could be obtained only through his government's winning the next provincial election, as medicare would be the principal plank in his party's platform.

The impending provincial election preoccupied parties and interest groups well in advance of the writ being dropped. Moreover, anyone interested in provincial politics knew when the date would be. Douglas had always insisted on having elections every four years and always preferred a time just after the crops were seeded but before summer had set in. This meant sometime in June, like all previous elections that had been held since 1944. As a result of the predictable timing, the parties were preparing months before the official campaign, for an election which they knew would be dominated by the CCF's proposed medical care plan.

Douglas's main challenger was Ross Thatcher, a new and much more dangerous Liberal leader than any he had faced in the past. A former CCF member of Parliament for many years, Thatcher had broken with the party and joined the Liberals with the intent of eventually displacing Douglas as premier. In September 1959, he won the provincial Liberal leadership on the first ballot. Douglas and fellow party members naturally viewed Thatcher as a self-seeking traitor. Having underestimated him once – over two years before in a debate over the province's public corporations that resulted in a draw at best – Douglas knew better than to do so again.[69]

While the other parties had far less of a chance of dethroning Douglas, they nonetheless hoped they could make some gains at the expense of the CCF. In the federal election of 1959, the Progressive Conservatives under Diefenbaker had just about wiped out the CCF in the province, leaving it with only one federal seat. This was a humiliating defeat

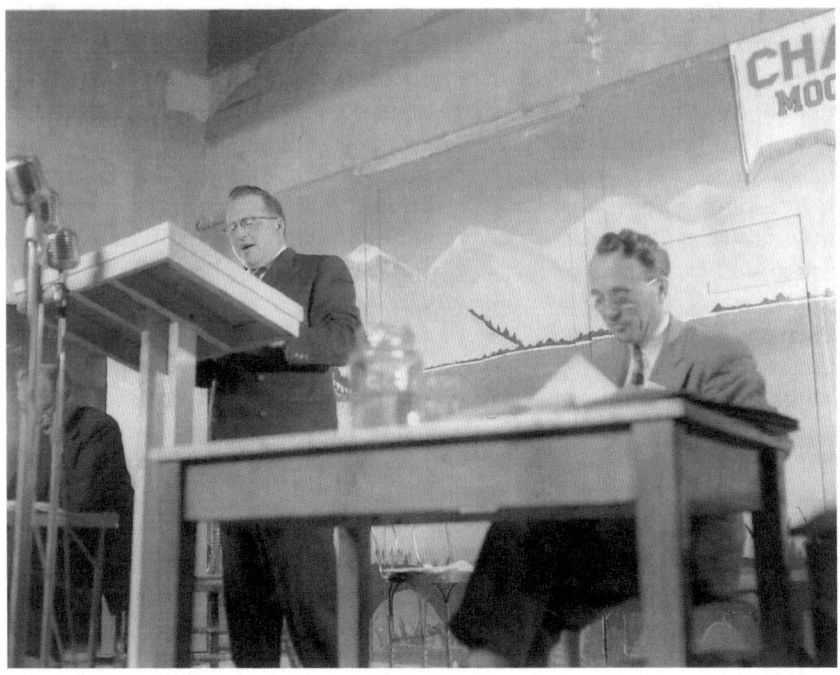

Ross Thatcher in debate with Douglas at Mossbank, Saskatchewan, 20 May 1957 (PAS R-LP1231)

for a party that viewed the province as its stronghold. Provincially, the leader of the PCs, Martin Pederson, hoped to ride on Diefenbaker's coattails to official opposition if not outright victory. Sidestepping the issue of medical care, Pederson called for a royal commission to examine the issue in order to keep it from being used "as a political football."[70] As for Social Credit, it was openly opposed to a government-sponsored medical care program and hoped that it could reap the votes of the growing number of those opposed to (or even uneasy about) the proposed scheme.

As the leader of the only party other than the CCF that could realistically form the government, Thatcher took a more strategic position. Not wanting to alienate the members of the public who supported a medical care plan, he stated that his party was, in principle, in favour of the change. However, if elected, he would conduct a study on the most cost-effective way to achieve better coverage, and afterwards would hold a general referendum so that the public could make a final decision once it understood the costs and the trade-offs.[71]

Wanting to better understand the political environment he was facing in the coming election, T.C. felt he needed an outside opinion, one relatively free of the fixed views held by members of his own party. He asked Graham Spry, his agent general in London, to spend a few weeks travelling in Saskatchewan and, after careful study, provide some suggestions on how best to frame the CCF's position for the electorate. Douglas trusted Spry's political savvy.

Six years older than Douglas, Spry had worked for the *Winnipeg Free Press* while pursuing his BA at the University of Manitoba.[72] In the early 1920s, he went to Oxford as a Rhodes scholar and there became part of a Canadian group that included Lester B. Pearson, Arnold Heeney, and King Gordon. After three years at Oxford, he moved to Geneva for one year to work for the League of Nations. In the 1930s, he played a key role in the establishment of what would become the Canadian Broadcasting Corporation.[73] Radicalized by the Great Depression, Spry was a founding member of the League for Social Reconstruction and worked extensively, both in the backrooms and openly as a candidate, for the CCF. Supporting the Republican cause in Spain, he established the Spanish Hospital and Medical Aid Committee and personally arranged to get Dr. Norman Bethune, despite his communist affiliation, transported to Spain to aid the Republican cause. Bethune would become notable in medical circles by creating and managing the first mobile blood transfusion service.[74] He would become even more famous for his medical work for Mao Zedong's communist forces in China, where he contracted septicaemia and died in 1939.[75]

By 1937, Spry was not only penniless but found, when he sought a permanent position in the federal public service, that he had become a political pariah in the eyes of the government of Canada. Consequently, he left the country, moving to London to work for Standard Oil and its interests in the Persian Gulf region. He took a leave of absence in 1942 to work for Sir Stafford Cripps, a leading UK Labour Party figure and member of the war cabinet. When the war ended, Douglas tried to hire Spry to promote Saskatchewan's interests in London, particularly its wheat exports to Britain and the rest of Europe. Spry turned him down initially but, two years later, in 1947, he accepted the position of agent general for Saskatchewan in London, a position he would hold for the next twenty years.[76]

Spry was much more than the province's representative in London. He was Douglas's political confident, and the two men had a regular chatty exchange, with Spry satisfying Douglas's immense interest in British politics, including any inside gossip on the leading Labour and Conservative personalities of the day.[77] As part of his job, Spry would make an annual trip to Saskatchewan to review the province's economic

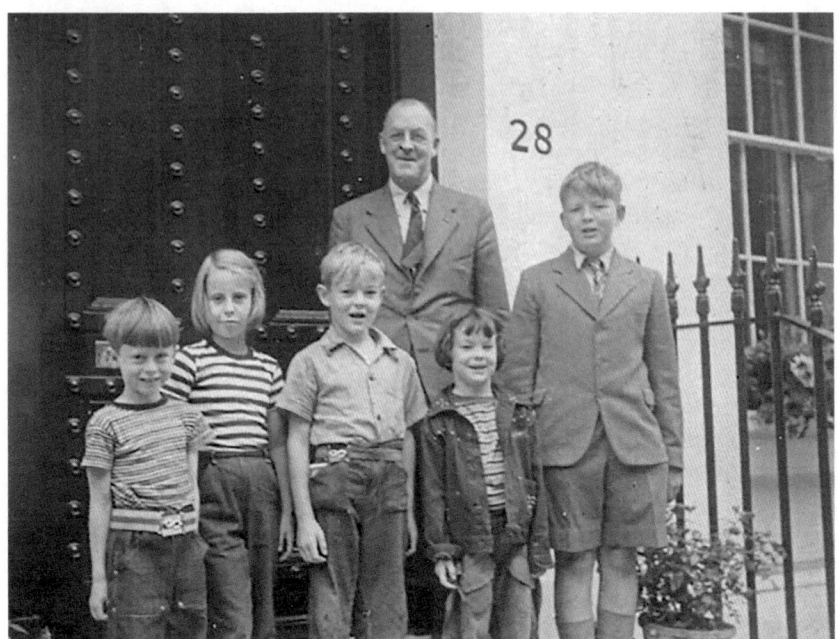

Graham Spry, agent general for Saskatchewan in London posing with his five children, c. 1951 (LAC, Graham Spry fonds, box 5825, item 4939130)

and trade needs, but in 1960, Douglas gave Spry the distinctly more partisan task of analysing the political landscape in preparation for the June election.

In mid-April, Spry delivered a twenty-one-page report to Douglas. To Spry's mind, there was no question that medicare was the best single issue upon which the CCF could campaign and win. Medicare had the "wide appeal" that would help "reduce the pettiness, the inevitable disgruntlement, disappointments, irritations, etc." of those "who waver between supporting or not supporting the Government after a long term of office." The promise of medicare would advance "a successful proven policy of the Government" and attest that the Douglas administration – despite the passage of sixteen years in office – was "decisive, firm, uncompromising and unafraid." In response to the expected opposition slogans that it was "time for a change," Spry urged Douglas to adopt the mantra (derived from Churchill) "Give us the tools and we'll finish the job."[78]

The issue of medicare, if driven hard enough, would also reveal the Liberal opposition as "unclear, vague and uncertain."[79] It was evident to Spry that Thatcher was trying to have it both ways. When pushed, Thatcher stated that he was in favour of the basic concept but against the way Douglas was going about it. The Liberal leader tried to enlist the support of the CPS by adopting its idea of a referendum on medicare, arguing that such a momentous decision "with such far-reaching consequences and involving such huge expenditures" should not be made "by a few socialist planners without direct consultation with all citizens."[80] Still, this was not enough for some members of the CPS executive, who wanted Thatcher to commit to implementing their proposed multi-payer program based on physician-sponsored health insurance. As an MSI form letter to all its subscribers pointed out:

> Government-controlled medical care already is a political issue in Saskatchewan. It seems now that in the 1960 provincial election campaign one party and perhaps two will seek office by promising to introduce compulsory medical insurance. This promise will look inviting to the naïve. Examine it closely, however, and grave objections appear – objections that concern your medical welfare.
>
> In the first place, what would happen to Medical Services Incorporated if a government medical plan came into operation in Saskatchewan? What would happen to contracts giving medical coverage to one-third of the province's citizens, including yourself? Make no mistake, these contracts would be affected. Chances are that they would be rendered null and void, with compulsory laws and regulations replacing them. In that event, M.S.I. would soon disappear.[81]

The college and its insurance carriers were not the only interest groups engaged in the pre-election campaign. Organized labour too joined the fray, in large part to try to countervail the influence of organized medicine and the insurance carriers. For years, the CPS had warned the government that it would not support its single-payer medical care while, at the same time, the Saskatchewan Federation of Labour had urged the provincial government to carry out its promise. Although the college had shown little obvious preference for any one of the three opposition parties in the past, it now aimed to defeat the Douglas government.

In response, trade union leaders in Saskatchewan threw their support behind the Douglas government. The CPS's support of physician-based insurance carriers was openly attacked by organized labour, which passed local motions in support of the government's proposed plan.

The Regina Labor Council, for example, described all private health insurers, including MSI and GMS, as "more interested in dollars than in service to people." More importantly, such plans could never "achieve universal coverage," since they excluded those with "pre-existing conditions." The council added that the "unemployed, the underprivileged, the chronically ill and the underpaid" simply could not afford the premiums for private health insurance and that these individuals could "only be taken care of by a comprehensive, government-sponsored and administered medical care program."[82]

In this increasingly polarized environment, Douglas's ministers and backbenchers rallied around the principles laid out by Douglas in his radio speech before the cabinet planning session. However, to achieve the principle that the plan must be acceptable to both those providing and receiving medical care services they had to be prepared to compromise with the CPS on some issues. After a long planning discussion of alternate methods of payment, including salary and capitation, cabinet decided that, to get "the co-operation" of doctors, the "government must start where it can" – by accommodating the fee-for-service system that the CPS insisted on. Collectively, the members of cabinet felt that this was one area where the government could be flexible, with the goal of getting the CPS to live with a compulsory, single-payer plan.[83]

At the same time, they knew that their activist allies within the CCF (as well as few backbenchers) and the labour movement were adamant that they should replace a fee-for-service schedule with a salaried service. To avoid a rupture within the party, T.C. tried to avoid any statements beyond what he had already said in the December radio broadcast, and instead focused on making it clear that such matters would be dealt with by the Advisory Planning Committee on Medicare (APC), which he hoped to appoint as quickly as possible.

**Appointing the Thompson Committee**

With the CCF government insisting on a publicly funded universal program and the doctors insisting on targeted subsidies for private health insurance, Douglas needed to find the right chair for the APC, someone sympathetic to the government's ultimate objectives yet capable of bringing the doctors on board by being flexible on other points, including physician remuneration.

The individual T.C. thought might be ideal for the job was Walter P. Thompson, the recently retired president of the University of Saskatchewan. For one thing, Thompson seemed to fully understand the challenge the doctors posed to medicare. But, like Douglas, he was confident that the doctors, once they understood that the government would be proceeding, would accept the medical plan and simply want the college to negotiate the best deal possible on their behalf – a view he set out in detail to Douglas after asking about the premier's intentions in dealing with the doctors.[84] Douglas replied immediately and set out his objectives for the Advisory Planning Committee:

> You may be sure that the Government has no intention of preparing a plan and then forcing it either upon the profession or the public. I have always taken the position that any plan, if it is to operate successfully, will have to be acceptable to both those giving the service and those receiving it. Therefore, what I have in mind is setting up a committee or commission of which one-third of the representatives would be from the medical profession, one-third from the general public and one-third from the Government, the latter being mainly technical people, and giving this group the responsibility for working out the details of the plan in order that the various viewpoints might be reconciled before the plan is put into operation.[85]

Thompson responded positively to Douglas's request, despite anticipating "many difficulties and much criticism for the committee."[86] For his part, Douglas promised that his government would "do everything possible to protect" Thompson's "committee from criticism." He reminded Thompson that the government alone was responsible "for the decision to proceed with the medical care program" and that the APC's responsibility was restricted to "working out the details in order that the interests of those receiving the service and those providing the service will be adequately safeguarded." In Douglas's typical style, he ended his letter on an optimistic note: "I know it will entail a great deal of work but I feel that it provides a wonderful opportunity for some social pioneering. I am convinced that if we can make such a program operate successfully in Saskatchewan, within ten years it will be copied in almost every other province in Canada."[87]

After Thompson met with Douglas, Minister of Health Walter Erb, and health deputy Burns Roth, the arrangements were finalized, with Roth acting as deputy chair, an appointment very much desired by Thompson.[88] Almost immediately, the CPS went on the attack. Just one week after Douglas's broadcast, at the behest of the CPS, MSI sent a form letter to all its subscribers stating that the future of the doctor-sponsored insurance carrier was "in danger" and that "unless you and 300,000 other subscribers make known your opposition, M.S.I. may be forced out of existence by a compulsory government-operated medical scheme."[89] A few weeks later, the doctors stated that they would

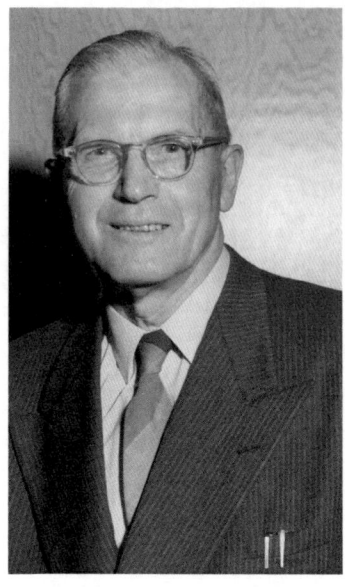

Photograph of Walter P. Thompson while president of the University of Saskatchewan, 1956 (SPL QC-578)

be willing to appoint their members to the APC only if they could substitute their proposal for what they perceived as the overly restrictive terms of reference provided by the government.[90]

Explicitly rejecting that a universal, tax-funded program be the starting point for discussions, the doctors wanted the Thompson Committee to address the desirability of co-insurance or user fees, ways to improve the quality of services, the adequacy and distribution of health human resources, how prevention might best be integrated into existing services, and ways in which existing private insurance programs and municipal doctor programs could be integrated into a new medical care program.[91] The CPS also demanded what it termed "sufficient time, without arbitrary limit," to complete the study. Of course, as the college well knew, this demand directly threatened the government's timetable. More ominously, the doctors insisted on the right to issue a minority report if a unanimous report could not be achieved, and that this report be made public along with the majority report.[92]

Although the CPS had not yet criticized Douglas's choice of chair, it would have seen the other two "public" representatives as CCF activists and therefore inimical to organized medicine's interests. One was Beatrice Trew, a former CCF farm activist who had served as MLA in the first term of the Douglas government; the other was Cliff Whiting, a local government politician and CCF member representing the province's cooperative movement. While the CPS had no objection to former health minister (and now social welfare minister) Tom Bentley's appointment, it did object to Douglas's appointment of Burns Roth and Vince Matthews from the Department of Public Health. Douglas quickly rejected the CPS's argument that Roth and Matthews, as the plan's "potential" administrators, were in a conflict of interest.[93]

T.C.'s expectation that the Thompson Committee complete its work by the latter part of 1960 might have been realistic if the doctors were willing to assist the government to meet this deadline. But it was obvious from the beginning that they had no intention of doing so. Worse, the election meant that the CPS had the incentive to drag its feet until at least June in the hope that the CCF would be defeated. In the meantime, it would do its best to force concessions on the committee's mandate. After weeks of getting no response from the CPS to the government's request for names of doctors who might serve on the committee, Douglas finally met with the executive of the college on 3 February.

Based on the notes from the meeting prepared by the CPS, Douglas was at his most conciliatory in explaining that he needed the "wholehearted support of the Medical Profession," wanting the government and the doctors to work together, "hand in glove" on the plan. Since the plan was always limited to securing "a premium payment for all citizens," he had "not originally considered there would be anything but co-operation from the Profession." Despite this charm offensive, the doctors raised their two main points of contention. The first was their very different perspective on how universality could best be achieved. The CPS argued that universality had largely been achieved, between the medical care insurance provided to 300,000 MSI and GMS subscribers and the 300,000 residents covered under municipal doctor plans, the Swift Current Health Region's medical care plan, and the coverage provided by the province to those receiving public assistance. According to the CPS's estimate, the remaining provincial residents could easily be taken care of by the government subsidizing the purchase of premiums.

The second point was that the CPS did not want a plan run by the government. T.C. tried to explain that the plan would be administered *under*, but not *by*, the Department of Health, and that the scheme had to be governed by a public body responsible to the legislature. When asked what functions the department would perform, Douglas said its role would be limited to establishing the premiums and tax rates required to fund the plan and negotiating the rate of payment to doctors. He insisted that the Thompson Committee would have complete latitude to decide the type of contract and payment and the level of physician remuneration. He then went further, stating that, if the committee recommended against any type of "Government Plan," then this would have to be accepted, and if it recommended in favour of a public plan, then "it could only be implemented" by his government upon "a clear mandate of the people and unanimous co-operation by the Profession." Rejecting Douglas's assurances, the CPS described the Thompson Committee as a "loaded rubber stamp" for a publicly administered plan, and protested that any appointment of CPS members to the committee "would be tantamount to an acquiescence to Government Medicine."[94]

The extent to which each side was miscalculating the other was becoming obvious. T.C. mistakenly thought the APC's broader terms of reference provided the college with adequate incentive to participate and reach a deal the doctors could live with. For the doctors, however, Douglas's efforts to be flexible concerning the details of any implementation plan devised by the APC was simply a reflection of the fact that he was "running scared" and could be forced to retreat from the entire plan.[95]

The CPS then moved to the question of timing. The premier was wrong, the college argued, to insist on the appointment of a committee just prior to an election. Douglas defended his decision as "reasonable due to the length of time required" to formulate a plan so that it could be implemented no later than 1962. As reflected in the cabinet planning discussion months before, this was indeed a major preoccupation of his entire cabinet. However, the CPS saw the APC strictly as a political ploy, that T.C.'s "*real anxiety* is that he have this Committee appointed early in the Session to silence criticism from the opposition i.e. he can pass off any criticism by notifying the House that the Government and their *good friends* – the Doctors – have mutually agreed to sit down together and discuss the whole question."[96]

Douglas's became less conciliatory when the CPS admitted to him that it would work to prevent the plan from being implemented in 1962. In response, he "threatened to proceed, if need be, without College of Physicians and Surgeons appointees." He then added that "the Profession would be ill advised not to participate in the hearings and assist in preparing a Plan which might not necessarily be a Government Plan" in the form he originally anticipated.[97]

Was Douglas serious in potentially conceding on a government-administered medicare plan? There are at least three reasons for believing so. He was desperate to demonstrate to the public that he was doing everything possible to consult with the doctors. He needed most of the doctors to continue to practise medicine in Saskatchewan if any plan was to work. And he might have been confident that the government and public representatives on the Thompson Committee were not likely to recommend a multi-payer plan, even if administered by an arms-length commission agreeable to the college.

While the CPS had many reasons to continue to obstruct Douglas, its executive wanted the public to believe that the profession was not being unreasonable. At the same time, Douglas wanted to public to know that he was consulting with the doctors – and it was true that, at this point, Douglas needed the doctors' eventual agreement far more than they needed to compromise with the government. So, he again offered an olive branch, something that had not been contemplated in the interdepartmental committee recommendations or in the cabinet planning discussion. Douglas told the CPS that, if recommended by the Thompson Committee, he would be willing to contemplate the government contracting out the administration of medical care insurance to one of the physician-based carriers as long as the plan was under the supervision of the Department of Public Health and accountable to the people through the legislature. He even encouraged the CPS to have its two insurance carriers present evidence to the APC on how such an arrangement might work.

The offer was a pleasant surprise to the college, and, privately, the doctors decided to have MSI and GMS prepare a proposal for the government, including the idea of considering a merger into one physician-operated plan.[98] But the premier's offer would have shocked the members of his own party. Those CCF activists who had long been calling for socialized medicine already viewed the government's health insurance plan as far too limited. They would have perceived this arrangement as putting the fox in charge of the hen house.

Was Douglas's offer serious or an effort to test whether the college had the willingness to compromise? It was more likely the latter. T.C. knew that most of the committee – the three public members and the three government members – would never agree to such an arrangement, so he felt safe in encouraging the doctors to think that, by participating in the process, they might be able to convince the committee to recommend the use of MSI or GMS as a contracted agency. By the end of the long and difficult meeting, Douglas acceded to the broader mandate insisted on by the CPS. He then got cabinet to approve a revised terms of reference adopting the CPS's language in the hope that the doctors would immediately forward the names of its three representatives on the APC.[99] It was not to be.

When the revised mandate was sent back to the CPS for approval, the doctors dragged their heels, and the quibbling over the wording continued for weeks. During this time, Douglas accepted an invitation to explain his position on Regina's CKCK-TV's one-hour program *Opinions*

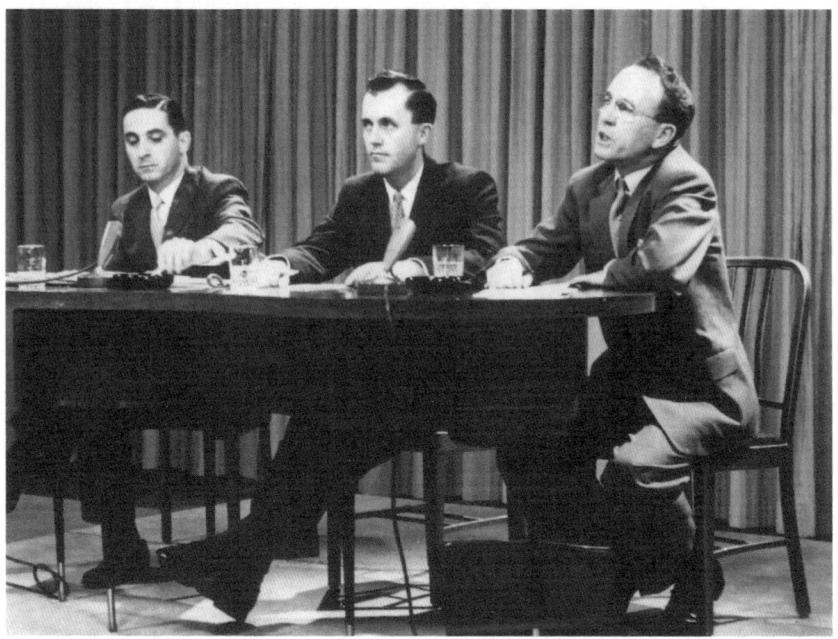

T.C. (right), Dr. E.W. (Staff) Barootes (left), with moderator (centre) on CKCK-TV's *Opinions Unlimited*, 20 March 1960 (PAS R-B2871(1))

*Unlimited*, on 20 March 1960. The debate format allowed Douglas twelve minutes to present the case in favour, and Dr. E.W. "Staff" Barootes, a Regina specialist and one of the CPS's chief spokespersons, the same amount of time to present his case against a government-administered medical care plan.[100] This was followed by moderated questions from the studio audience, which was normally about seventy-five individuals but, because of the topic, had ballooned to about 120. To end the program, Douglas and Barootes were each allotted three minutes to sum up.[101]

In his carefully prepared opening remarks, Douglas was at pains to explain that the government's objective to make health services, like education, "available to every citizen irrespective of their financial status" was hardly a "shocking" idea. The plan proposed to build upon the universal hospital plan and the province's targeted programs for tuberculosis, cancer, and mental illness. As for doctors, "the only difference under a medical care program from what we have at the present time is that at the end of the month the doctor would send his bill to the agency responsible for paying medical bills under the proposed plan."[102]

If the scheme was to be universal, T.C. emphasized, it had to be government-sponsored. Moreover, and in tension with the impression he had left the CPS the month before, he argued that he could not simply extend either the voluntary plans or the Swift Current plan. Explaining that, since the government-sponsored plan would rely for two-thirds of its financing on general tax revenues and only one-third on a direct premium tax on individuals and families, the government-sponsored plan would be affordable for everyone. In contrast, in the doctor-sponsored and health region plan, "the cost of paying doctor bills must be borne by the members of the plan on a per capita basis. This amounts to anywhere from $75 to $90 per family per year," an amount that might be "a comparatively minor item" for some families "but for others" was "almost prohibitive." In contrast, he hoped to keep the per capita direct tax down to $35 per family, the same amount as was then being charged under the provincial hospitalization plan.[103]

In response to the common argument by the CPS that doctors never (or rarely) turned down patients due to an inability to pay, Douglas pointed out that there were "thousands of people who cannot afford to belong to private plans who are fearful of incurring medical bills" and therefore avoid seeing doctors. "It's all very well to say that no one is ever refused medical care because they haven't any money," but "there are great numbers of people on low incomes who do not go to the doctor because they know they can't pay them unless they go into debt." These people "don't want charity. They want to be able to contribute a sum of money each year which they can afford," so that they know they can get medical help when they need it "without a loss of dignity and without the worry of unpaid debts hanging over their heads." Only a government-sponsored program could lift the "standard of care" by persuading people to "visit their doctor regularly for periodic checkups."[104]

One of the most articulate members of the CPS, Dr. Staff Barootes vigorously put the college's case. He took aim at two of T.C.'s five principles, universal coverage and public administration, arguing that they would lead to a lowering of the standard of medical services and were therefore inconsistent with his principle of ensuring "high quality" medical care. Still not willing to commit the college to participating in the Thompson Committee, Barootes did say the CPS was prepared to support a "competent and non-political committee representative of the people" if the mandate was suitable expanded so that it would "not be confined to studying problems and solutions within the narrow field of five principles outlined by Mr. Douglas."[105]

A little more than a week after the Barootes-Douglas television debate, the CPS agreed to participate on the Thompson Committee. In return, the doctors obtained two major concessions. The first was that the terms of reference were broadened, and, with them, the implicit right of the doctors to not accept Douglas's principles was understood. This concession was reflected in the doctors' explicit right to submit a minority report. The second major concession was on timing. The committee would not face a forced deadline for its final report, although T.C. made it clear that the government retained the right to request an interim report based on its own schedule.[106] When asked by the press whether the government's five principles still held, the premier responded in a way that must have given pause to both his supporters and detractors: "The government has expressed its opinion through these principles about the form a medical plan should take, but the committee is free to make any recommendations it likes, and the government is bound to give them very careful and thorough consideration, whether they come within those principles or not."[107]

In April 1960, the college put forward the three names of its representatives on the APC.[108] Dr. Barootes of Regina and Dr. Jack Anderson of Saskatoon were the college's resident hardliners, while Dr. Clarence J. Houston, based on his long and generally constructive relationship with the Douglas government, was perceived by both sides to be more flexible. Although the Douglas government originally wanted a nine-person advisory committee with three members representing the CPS, three members representing the government, and three drawn from the public, T.C. acceded to the CPS's demand for three additional members, one representing the Faculty of Medicine at the University of Saskatchewan (Dr. Ivin Hilliard), one representing business (Donald McPherson), and the third representing the Saskatchewan Federation of Labour (Walter Smishek), bringing the total to twelve appointments. At this point, the Thompson Committee should have been ready to start its work, but the college representatives insisted that there was no point in commencing until the after the provincial election (which everyone assumed was coming in June, given Douglas's past proclivity for June elections dates), clearly hoping that the CCF government would be defeated.

**The Medicare Election of 1960**

In early May, to no one's surprise, the writ was issued for an election to be held on 8 June. Having levied a fee of $100 on each of its members to fund a public relations campaign, the CPS had a war chest that rivalled, and even exceeded, those of the province's political parties.

The dual role of the college as a licensing and disciplinary body (of which all doctors had to be members) and the doctors' political representative (a voluntary association) raised the question of whether the levy was compulsory. CPS officials justified it on the grounds that it would be used to inform the public of the doctors' position on the government's medical care plan and not to take a partisan political stand. In the end, about six hundred doctors – roughly two-thirds of the CPS membership – paid the levy.[109]

Without doubt, the CPS had the support of the province's private practice doctors, 90 per cent of whom, based on a CMA survey, said they opposed a compulsory and publicly administered medical care insurance plan.[110] The CMA fully supported the position taken by its Saskatchewan division and added a further $35,000 to the $60,000 already raised through the CPS's levy. The Ontario Medical Association had already provided in-kind resources by sending its public relations coordinator to Saskatchewan in late February to direct the information campaign. Entitled Political Medicine Is Bad Medicine, the CPS's information campaign paid for radio and newspaper advertisements as well as the writing and printing of information kits that were disseminated to Saskatchewan physicians, with pamphlets that could be given to patients.[111]

The tenor of the information was perhaps best summarized in one CPS handout that stated that "the concept of universal medical coverage is not new and the approach by government to seek support is just the same as it was when first enunciated by Karl Marx in his Communistic Theories of the last century." Arguing against any compulsory scheme of health insurance, another handout stated that compulsion "carries with it the aroma of medieval times when slavery was an accepted standard of living; when a minority group dictated its will upon the masses and used every means of cruelty known to men – the whip and the rod – to make sure slaves toed the line." Catholic women were warned that the proposed "government controlled plan offers a latent but potential threat to certain dogmas and views of the Catholic Church relating to maternity, birth control, and the state."[112]

Adopting the techniques of the American Medical Association, the CPS relied on a "key man" responsible for a small cell of doctors, acting as a facilitator between the CPS and rank-and-file doctors.[113] Patients as well as nurses and others who worked with doctors were warned about the many dangers of the government's medical care plan, as represented in the information kits. Some took their message out to public meetings, where they repeated key messages from the kits or confronted CCF politicians at their campaign events. While a few undecided voters may have been swayed by the doctors, the reality was that the messages they conveyed using the kits as speaking points were so over the top that they worked in the CCF's favour. Running as a CCF candidate in his first election, Allan Blakeney used the kits to great advantage, taking them to, for example, the Hungarian Centre in Regina, and repeating some of the more racist statements about how foreign (i.e., non-Canadian and non-British) doctors – "the garbage of Europe" as suggested by some local physicians – would move in to replace the doctors leaving the province because of the medical care plan.[114]

Blakeney, who would serve as premier of Saskatchewan from 1971 until 1982, later remembered the 1960 election as the most "bitterly fought campaign" he had ever experienced in Saskatchewan either as an observer of previous campaigns or as a participant and eventually party leader in several subsequent campaigns.[115] For this part, T.C. publicly feigned shock at the CPS's tactics, but he had not only anticipated its moves but knew its actions would make medical care the critical issue in the campaign, reinvigorate CCF supporters, and bring around at least some undecided voters who would be put off by the doctors' tactics. In other words, he believed that the college's excesses would help him win an election that he might otherwise lose after being in office for sixteen consecutive years.

As election day approached, Douglas was increasingly confident. One week before the vote, he proclaimed that information in the CPS information kits was among "the most scurrilous trash that ever was printed in the province" and condemned the college for its unscrupulous attack on the government's proposal. Since the literature was unsigned, he suggested that it was contrary to the provincial Elections Act. Unlike the PCs and the Liberals, his CCF government would "not hide behind royal commissions and plebiscites" and "would rather lose fighting for a cause that will ultimately win than win fighting for a cause that will ultimately lose."[116]

The doctors' interventions were so extreme that even the Liberals and PCs kept a healthy distance. The only party that seemed comfortable with the red baiting and exaggerated language of the CPS was Social Credit. Hopeful of finally making a breakthrough in the province, its local organizers brought in big names from the Socred governments in British Columbia and Alberta to help in the campaign, including Alberta premier Ernest Manning, who did a provincial tour. Addressing a huge crowd of over 1,300 supporters in Regina, Manning said that the defining issue was whether Saskatchewan residents were really prepared to accept this new form of state intervention as well as pay an extra $25 million a year for the CCF's plan.[117] As was the case for hospital insurance a decade earlier, Manning opposed universal health coverage on religious and moral, not merely fiscal, grounds.[118]

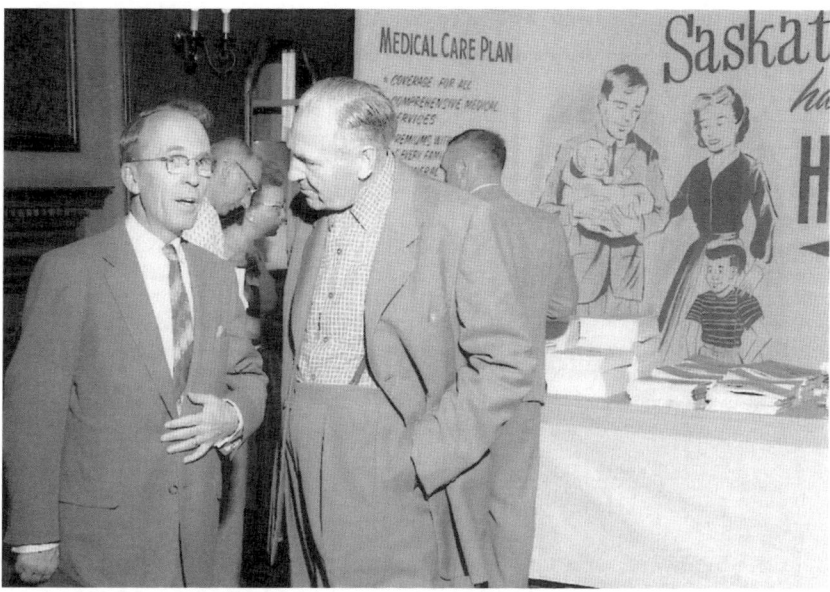

T.C. talking to a supporter in front of a medical care plan promotional booth, 1960 (PAS R-LP1247)

Douglas also brought in external help, including his old friend and close ally from Ottawa, M.J. Coldwell. Like Manning, the national leader of the CCF toured the province. Coldwell made medical care the central issue in his speeches, arguing that its opponents were misrepresenting both the Saskatchewan plan and the NHS in Britain. In some respects, he argued, the Saskatchewan approach should be more acceptable than the NHS because, under the plan, everyone would be given a choice of general practitioner, and doctors could continue to practise on a fee-for-service basis – the latter an interesting claim, given the fact that the APC had not even begun its hearings much less issued its recommendations on remuneration.[119] However, Coldwell knew Douglas's oft-stated position that his government was quite willing to compromise on renumeration in exchange for the CPS's participation, however grudging, in the plan.[120]

### Electoral Mandate for Medicare?

The election outcome vindicated Douglas's political conviction that universal medical care would mobilize his core voters and deliver another CCF majority. Despite the complacency associated with sixteen years in office, his supporters came out and voted because of the debate

Table 10.2. Results of Saskatchewan elections, 1956 and 1960

|  | CCF | Liberal | Social Credit | Progressive Conservative |
|---|---|---|---|---|
| Seats – 1956 | 36 | 14 | 3 | 0 |
| Seats – 1960 | 37 | 17 | 0 | 0 |
| Change in seats | +1 | +3 | –3 | 0 |
| Per cent vote – 1956 | 45.25 | 30.34 | 21.48 | 1.98 |
| Per cent vote – 1960 | 40.76 | 32.67 | 12.35 | 13.95 |
| Change in per cent vote | –4.5 | +2.3 | –9.1 | +12.0 |

Note: "Per cent vote" does not add up to 100 per cent due to the votes cast for independent candidates and Labour Progressive/Communist candidates.
Source: Elections Saskatchewan online data for election results in 1956 and 1960: https://www.elections.sk.ca/reports-data/election-results/1956-2/; and https://www.elections.sk.ca/reports-data/election-results/1960-2/.

over medical care: a remarkable 84.1 per cent of eligible voters cast their ballot.[121] As shown in table 10.1, the CCF gained one seat, despite a 4.5 per cent decline in popular support compared to the 1956 election. In Douglas's mind, he had won the referendum on medical care, and his government would proceed immediately after the Thompson Committee delivered its report.

The leading doctors in the CPS came to the opposite conclusion. In their mind, the drop in CCF support could be directly linked to the medicare issue, and some believed that the result meant that less than half of the population had voted in favour of the government plan. They may have lost the first battle in the war over medical care, but they vowed to be better prepared in future skirmishes, and this time without the public relations advice that had ultimately proved so ineffective.[122] Above all, they intended, more than ever, to block a universal, publicly administered plan from being implemented in the province.

Douglas felt he had his mandate from the people to proceed. However, if he thought that the election result would convince the college to come to the negotiating table and work out a compromise, he was dead wrong. Instead, his struggle with the CPS would intensify over the coming months.

# 11 The Thompson Committee and the New Party

*I am afraid there is little likelihood of my opportunity for relaxation for the next few months, since as you know I am to carry on as Premier here [in Saskatchewan] until November and at the same time I am trying to do the work of Leader of the New Democratic Party.*[1]

Tommy Douglas, August 1961

Following the medicare election of 1960, the Thompson Committee could finally begin its deliberations. As we shall see, however, T.C.'s desire for a rapid report along with the ongoing delay tactics of the College of Physicians and Surgeons of Saskatchewan (CPS) put the government on a collision course with organized medicine. Matters became further complicated when Douglas decided to become a candidate for the national leadership of what would soon become the New Democratic Party.

Although T.C. was ultimately successful in his leadership bid, the campaign and the immediate demands of the new post made it exceedingly difficult for him to manage the growing controversy over medicare in Saskatchewan. This pressure cooker of events contributed to missteps and major bumps on the road to implementation and would hound Douglas for years to come.

## The Trials and Tribulations of the Thompson Committee, 1960–1

Although the Thompson Committee met once before the election, it was not able to conduct its work until afterwards, in large part because of the doctors' campaign against the government. After the CCF's election victory, it would have been reasonable to assume the CPS would alter its strategy and work with the other committee members to devise a plan suited to its members' interests. However, it was obvious within days following the election that the college was taking a position on the government's proposed medical care plan that was even more hostile than that of its national organization, the Canadian Medical Association (CMA).

The day after the election, CMA general secretary Dr. A.D. Kelly said the election result in Saskatchewan removed all doubt that the people of Saskatchewan endorsed a government-sponsored medical care plan. As Kelly put it, "This is democracy," and the CMA "accepts the decision in this light." Kelly went on to suggest that the CMA would drop its opposition and instead cooperate with the government, "bent on avoiding the defects we see in government plans" in other countries like the United Kingdom.[2] This last point was particularly important to former UK-based physicians who had moved to Canada because of their dissatisfaction with the National Health Service.

The CMA's Saskatchewan division immediately took issue with Kelly's statement. Speaking on behalf of the college, Dr. Alan Davies said that Kelly could not be speaking for the CMA, since Kelly had been told by his "confreres in other provinces that they oppose state medicine just as strongly as" Saskatchewan doctors did. Not surprisingly, Douglas welcomed Kelly's statement and expressed the hope that the CPS would take a similar position and help – through the Thompson Committee – to formulate the implementation details. "It is hoped," Douglas said, "that they will use their long experience for this purpose rather than trying to obstruct the introduction of a medical care plan."[3]

One week later, in Banff, at the CMA's annual meeting, the divergence between the uncompromising CPS (doing double duty as the Saskatchewan Division of the CMA) and its national organization became clearer. While the CMA was not prepared to "rule out" a compulsory, tax-supported scheme as long as it remained consistent with the association's previously enunciated principles, the CMA's Saskatchewan Division insisted that any acceptable plan would have to be voluntary and non-governmental in design.[4] After a long and heated discussion, the doctors did agree on one point, in language proposed by a doctor from Moose Jaw: a single-payer and "government-controlled scheme is not the answer to our health problems." In the end, the CMA passed a resolution that "a tax-supported comprehensive program, compulsory for all, is neither necessary nor desirable."[5]

For the CPS, the Thompson Committee was simply another front in the war against the Douglas plan. While it was impossible for T.C. not to know this, he still assumed that the CPS appointees' continual interaction with the other committee members, as well as the public hearings, would eventually take some of the hard edges off the college's position. While Thompson himself initially shared T.C.'s optimism, he soon became convinced that at least two of the three CPS doctors were doing everything in their power to delay the commission's work by insisting it focus on every health care problem and issue other than medical care. In Thompson's words, Staff Barootes and Jack Anderson insisted on "going over as much ground, not related to the Medical Care Plan," as possible, to undermine the government's timeline.[6]

Without doubt, timing was Douglas's Achilles heel. The Thompson Committee's originally proposed terms of reference had a clear timeline inserted that fit with the government's own agenda, but this clause had been dropped at the insistence of the CPS. In a letter to the college, T.C. grudgingly agreed that "no arbitrary time limit" would be placed on the Thompson Committee and that it would "have the sole right to determine the amount of time" required to complete its studies and public consultations and make its recommendations. "It would seem fair to assume, however, that the people of the province will expect the committee to make reasonable progress and to submit their recommendations as expeditiously as possible," even with enlarged terms of reference that went beyond the question of the best way to implement universal medical care coverage.[7] T.C. could say what he wanted, but the reality remained that, far from agreeing to a commitment on timing, the CPS was determined to delay, if not scuttle, deliberations.

That summer, over a month after the provincial election, Douglas attended a conference of first ministers called by Prime Minister Diefenbaker. Convinced that his program was imminent, Douglas made a major pitch for the federal government to cost share universal medical care.[8] Diefenbaker delayed making any commitments, having already decided to establish a royal commission on health services to study the matter.

By early October, the Thompson Committee had held its first half dozen meetings. It was now blindingly obvious to Thompson that his committee had no possible chance of meeting the government's preferred timeline – one that Douglas and his minister of health, Walter Erb, were in the habit of repeating in their public statements. Every time this happened, Barootes and Anderson would disrupt the committee's work by alleging bad faith on the part of the government. This made Thompson's job of keeping the peace almost impossible, and he asked that both Douglas and Erb refrain from discussing dates, given that the committee had been assured by the premier that it "would not be pressed for time."[9] The tactics of the two doctors – joined on occasion by Dr. Clarence Houston, the third CPS physician, and Donald

McPherson, the representative of the Saskatchewan Chamber of Commerce – drove Thompson to consider resignation.[10] In early November, he wrote the premier to tell him that the committee had become dysfunctional in the extreme:

> I think I should inform you that I told the Advisory Planning Committee on Medical Care at our meeting on Saturday last that I was considering very seriously submitting my resignation because of our lack of progress. We have scarcely touched our main task and then only incidentally. Nearly all our time has been devoted to an examination of present health services and health conditions, for the most part considering matters which have no connection with a medical care program or only a very tenuous connection, and many of them quite trivial.[11]

Douglas wrote back immediately, stating that he understood Thompson's "feelings of impatience" and his "natural desire to have the Committee tackle the main purpose for which it was set up." He more than anyone wanted the committee to get on with its main task, but many years of political experience had shown him "how long it takes to reconcile various viewpoints and to disseminate sufficient information so that some common understanding can be reached." In other words, T.C., unlike Thompson, still believed that some reconciliation between the CPS and the government was possible. While he hoped the committee would "not take anything like three years to complete its task," he nonetheless understood that it would take a bit more time for it "to assimilate all the information available regarding existing programs and to analyse the basic principles upon which these have been established," especially those of the province's hospital insurance plan. Moreover, "it is only by understanding these basic principles," such as universality and single-payer financing, "that the Committee can hope to formulate a medical care plan which is soundly based and administratively feasible."[12]

Expressing the hope that Thompson's threat to resign had "a very salutary effect" on the committee members, Douglas begged him to carry on chairing the commission, even offering to drive from Regina to Saskatoon to discuss the matter with him in person. Thompson, he felt, was "more likely than anyone else" to be "able to bring together the conflicting points of view on the Committee and to reconcile some of the basic differences" of opinion. Douglas was "determined to proceed with a medical care program," but he still wanted the committee "to canvass every conceivable possibility of getting the co-operation of the medical profession."[13]

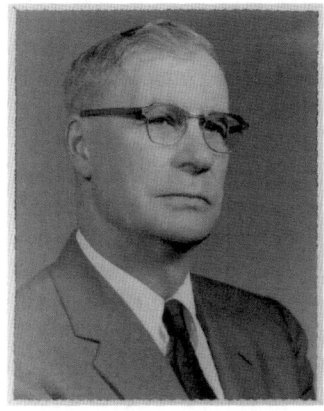

Walter P. Thompson, chair of the Advisory Planning Committee on Medicare, 1960–2 (PAS R-LP1142)

Douglas's reply had the desired effect. Thompson agreed to continue, despite his "deep discouragement." However, he warned Douglas that, given that the CPS members and McPherson were "strongly and unalterably committed to opposition to our main function and repeatedly show that their purpose is to block it, one can't help but question whether the approach is sound." Given the fact that the CPS members were not sincere in trying "to reach the best solution," the doctors and the business representative on the Thompson Committee were not prepared to compromise and instead would end up writing a minority report "with all that will mean in this case."[14]

Douglas's exchange with Thompson is revealing about the premier's state of mind at the time. Despite the attitudes and actions of the College of Physicians and Surgeons, he still believed there was at least the hope of a deal being reached. And even if that hope was rapidly diminishing, he knew he needed to be seen to be doing everything possible to get the profession to accede to his plan. He had made a firm promise to introduce a plan acceptable to both doctors and the public. The public might be fearful and confused due to the (at times) effective campaign of the CPS and its allies, but he had, in his mind, nonetheless been given a mandate by the public in the June election. He needed to convince the population, including as many doctors as possible who were not executive members of the college, that he had done everything he could to live up to his promise of a plan acceptable to doctors, and that it was only the unreasonable intransigence and bad faith of the CPS leaders that had prevented him from doing so.

The very real possibility of a dissenting report from the CPS concerned Douglas much less than it did Thompson. "It may be," Douglas told Thompson, "that we shall end up with a minority report from some members of the committee. However, a lot will depend on who signs the minority report. If the public representatives, and particularly those from labour and business, agree with the majority we shall have gone a long way toward establishing a foundation upon which to build a medical care program." At the same time, the emotional load of chairing a committee that, in the end, would not produce a consensus report, was not lost on Douglas. "I must confess," he went on, "that sometimes I have a guilty feeling about having placed such a heavy burden upon you. On the other hand, I felt certain that this was the kind of assignment for which you were admirably suited and that you would probably welcome the opportunity to make another lasting contribution to the province for which you have already done so much. Believe me, we are all deeply grateful for your efforts."[15]

Douglas may or may not have been correct in his calculation that a polarized report from the committee, one that pitted the majority report against a strong dissent by a minority, was still better at this point than no report at all. However, he was wrong in thinking that the Thompson Committee members would, minority report and all, be able to reach, in his words, "some definite conclusions as expeditiously as possible."[16]

**The New Party**

The Diefenbaker sweep in the federal election of 1958 was, in David Lewis's words, an "unmitigated disaster" for the CCF. The party lost two-thirds of its seats, including that of its national leader, M.J. Coldwell.[17] These losses forced a major reappraisal within the CCF, which led directly to a "New Party" proposal. At its heart, the New Party initiative was an effort by the CCF to expand beyond its rural prairie populist base to urban voters, especially unionized workers.

For Douglas, the initiative was an effort to "to bring together in one movement all those progressive elements who are desirous of extending the principle of social democracy in Canada."[18] Key to this was a formal link with organized labour, similar to the relationship that had been forged between the British Labour Party and the trade unions in Britain.[19] The challenge lay in the historic tension between farm organizations and trade unions, with the farm leaders distrusting what they viewed as the more conservative position of organized labour and the fact that the big union leaders and union money would displace the influence of farmers within the CCF.

With his old friend Stanley Knowles and the central Canadian brains trust of Lewis and Frank Scott, Douglas supported the New Party movement from the beginning. He had played an important role in the Winnipeg Declaration of 1956, adapting and refitting the Regina Manifesto for the post-war Keynesian welfare state.[20] The Winnipeg Declaration was the first step towards making the party more relevant to urban workers and professionals. The second step was the New Party movement, an effort to change the organization of the national CCF so that it would be more appealing to industrial (and some public sector) workers by providing trade unions with an institutional voice at party conventions.

Due to his obligations as premier and the enormous task of keeping medical care coverage at the top of his government's political and policy agenda, Douglas was not able to attend all the New Party meetings, which had begun in 1958.[21] However, in 1960, unhappy at the direction of the movement and what he felt was its inability to keep the farm organizations onside, he devoted precious time on New Party national business, despite the growing campaign against medicare in his province.

To broaden its base beyond its origins as a party of protest supported by prairie farmers, the New Party needed to be seen as a more organic coming together of farm groups, labour unions, cooperatives, and progressive professionals. Douglas anticipated that doing so would squeeze out the Liberal Party, which he felt was – ideologically – a spent force that should shrink into oblivion, as it had in Britain. He decried the conservatism of the Liberal Party, claiming that it had "forced me to the conclusion that in some respects they have become more Tory than the Conservatives." He felt it was only a matter of time before "the right wing of the Liberal party and the great bulk of Conservatives will amalgamate leaving all the left-of-centre groups no alternative but to coalesce," at which point Canada would once again have a "two party system," but one "in which political affiliations will have some real meaning."[22] But if the New Party could not fill this natural vacuum, then the country would simply slip back into the status quo, with power being traded back and forth between the two old parties.[23]

He thus wanted a New Party that would attract social democrats who tended to drift to the Liberals in central Canada and the Atlantic region. When asked by the *Toronto Daily Sar* how he felt about Mike Pearson and Paul Martin Sr., he quickly responded that they were "fine progressive men" whom he could easily work with on many policy and program issues. In fact, they saw immediate things "pretty much the same way," but "eventually they start chiding me for 'Socialist planning' and I start chiding them for 'laissez faire Liberalism.' When that happens, the gulf between us gets pretty wide."[24]

At the same time, he felt that some central Canadians – David Lewis was not mentioned by name, but this was who he really meant – had made a major misstep in describing the New Party as a CCF–Canadian Labour Congress (CLC) merger. That characterization was doubly galling because the reality was that the CLC did not intend to provide direct support to the CCF but, in Douglas's words, would "merely ... make it possible for its affiliates to do so." In his view, Lewis's claim had given "the farmers and white-collar groups the idea that the CCF is going to sink its identity in the Canadian Labour Congress."[25] He wrote Knowles about his grave concern and sent a copy of the same letter to Lewis:

> For some time I have been intending to write you regarding the strategy which is being employed in connection with the formation of a new political party. Frankly, I am very disturbed by the way in which the whole thing has been handled and I am becoming increasingly convinced that we started at the wrong end. The original idea was to bring farmer and labour groups together at a grass roots level so that gradually the pressure for some new political alignment would become evident. Instead of that, most of the discussions have been at a top level and very little seems to have been done on a provincial or constituency basis.
>
> Most alarming of all is the fact that the C.L.C. and C.C.F. seem to be pushing ahead without waiting for the farm groups who, in my opinion, are indispensable in such an alignment. I know it will not be easy to bring the farm groups in, but I think we have to wait until we can, even if it means setting up some special organization such as a farmers' committee for political action.
>
> I don't want to add to your worries or frustrations, but I think you should know that the public relations boys for Big Business have done a very effective job of poisoning the minds of the farmers and white collared class regarding trade unions.[26]

In fact, Douglas was fighting a war inside his own provincial party at the very time he was trying to marshal his forces to combat the powerful and growing coalition against medicare. As the New Party movement grew, relations between the grassroots leadership of the Saskatchewan CCF and the national CCF soured, and Douglas was increasingly squeezed between the two. While the whole purpose of a New Party was to get beyond the CCF's base in Saskatchewan, any successful launch depended – as Knowles admitted – "very largely on the Saskatchewan section of the CCF going along."[27] However, the truth was that many rank-and-file CCFers in Saskatchewan were opposed to what they saw as a shotgun marriage between the CCF and the CLC. Consequently, Douglas had to spend much of his precious time swatting away such perceptions before party members in Saskatchewan would give the idea of the New Party a fair chance.[28]

The legacy of this struggle would continue for years, exemplified by the simple fact that the Saskatchewan CCF refused to abandon its name until 1967, five years after the New Democratic Party's founding.[29] A similar negative reaction had set in among the CCF grassroots in Manitoba, who also felt that the New Party idea "was an imposition" by national party figures, especially David Lewis and Stanley Knowles, on the federal CCF. As if he did not already have too much on his plate, Douglas was asked by the CCF's national office to contact the presumed leader of the "dissidents" in Manitoba and calm the waters next door.[30]

Adding to the demands on his time, Douglas became the subject of a major campaign to enlist him as leader of the New Party by October 1960, just as Thompson was threatening to resign as chair of the Advisory Planning Committee on Medical Care (APC). Part of the problem was that other candidates had been ruled out, especially the two individuals most responsible for promoting and organizing the New Party – his old friend Stanley Knowles and his national ally of many years, David Lewis.[31] Knowles was seen as too close to labour, given that he had taken the position of vice-president of the CLC after his defeat in the 1958 Diefenbaker election.[32] Unknown to those around him, Knowles had multiple sclerosis and privately felt that this condition prevented him from meeting the rigours of leadership.[33]

Douglas thought that Lewis should become the New Party's leader, favouring him even over his old friend. The national president of the CCF and the leading proponent of the New Party, Lewis was also a Toronto labour lawyer whose clients included the CLC and its affiliates. Not surprisingly, many within the CCF perceived Lewis as too close to the unions to act as a neutral link between organized labour and supportive farm organizations. He was also seen by some rank-and-file party members as too much of a backroom operator, someone who had never been a politician, much less an MP. Moreover, Lewis had ruled himself out, believing that the Canadian public was not yet ready to elect a Jewish leader. Although Douglas emphatically rejected this assessment of the public, Lewis nonetheless insisted that Douglas was "the only realistic choice," and he used his considerable influence and power to pressure Douglas to take the job.[34]

The only other leadership candidate was Hazen Argue, the lone CCF MP from Saskatchewan to survive the devastation of the 1958 election. However, according to the leaders of the National Committee for the

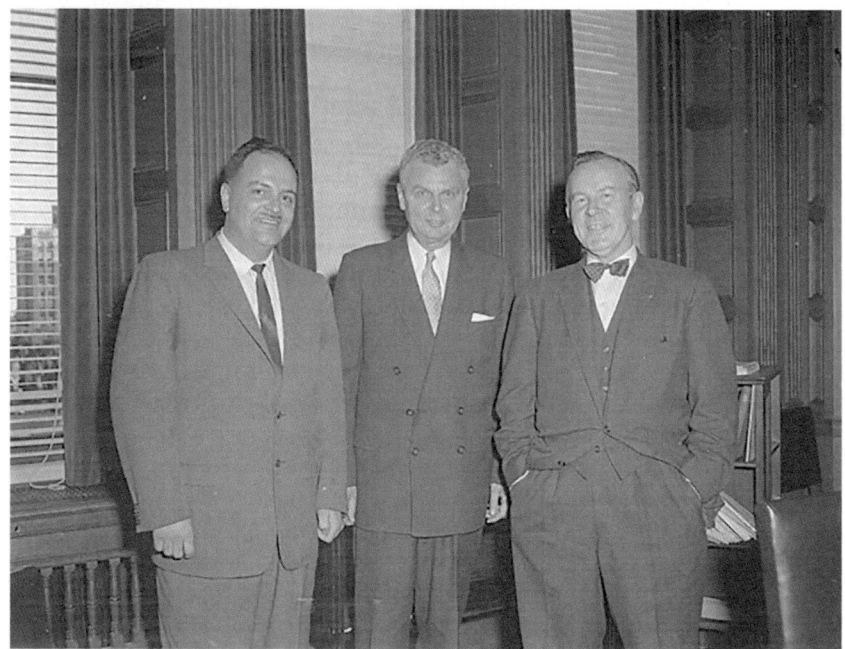

Three federal parliamentary leaders pose on 5 September 1959. From left to right, Hazen Argue, John G. Diefenbaker, and Lester B. Pearson (LAC, Duncan Cameron, e007150491)

New Party who were close to Knowles and Lewis, Argue lacked "the strength and character required" for the job and, as a prairie farmer, could not bridge the gap between farmers and organized labour and urban voters. Only Douglas, they felt, was capable of appealing to all three. In a straw poll in October 1960, fifteen of the sixteen members of the National Committee voted for Douglas as leader. Moreover, this group believed that the vast majority of "the rank and file" of the CCF and the unions "would feel the same way." But the clincher was their assessment of "the impact that your [Douglas's] selection" as leader of the New Party would have on undecided voters and what they saw as his unique ability "to appeal to this group throughout Canada."[35]

At this point, Douglas rejected the entreaty of the National Committee, stating bluntly that he would under no circumstances consider leaving his premiership for the national leadership.[36] He still loved his job as premier and derived "a good deal of personal satisfaction from being able to see some practical results from my efforts." In contrast, the idea of being an opposition leader in Ottawa reminded him of his nine years as MP, when "at times I was almost overcome with the frustration and futility of being 'a voice crying in the wilderness,'" and the prospect "of putting in six or seven months a year listening to endless debate which never gets anywhere" held scant appeal.[37] However, the most important reasons were his existing obligations, especially the finesse, judgment, and focus needed to implement medicare in Saskatchewan. As T.C. explained to a prominent CCFer from Toronto:

> The doctors have not by any means given up their tactics of obstruction against the medical care plan. It is going to take a good deal of forcefulness and determination to put the plan into operation. If we are unable to establish a medical care plan in Saskatchewan, the whole idea will be set back for a quarter of a century in Canada. I feel that my first duty is to stay here and get this plan operating on a sound basis. There are a number of other programs such as the reorganization of local government which will tax our ingenuity to the limit and, while no one is indispensable, I think the situation requires me to stay here until we have passed the critical stage in which we find ourselves.[38]

Douglas insisted on Lewis, with his bilingualism, "intellectual capacity," and "gift of leadership," as the most "logical person to head the New Party. Douglas was also certain that if the committee members would show Lewis as much "willingness to support him" as they had Douglas himself, then the CCF president "might be persuaded to let his name stand."[39] Yet Lewis continued to feel that Douglas was exactly the leader the New Party required to be successful, and he joined the press gang intent on conscripting him. In response, Douglas continued to contend that Lewis was the best person for the job. Moreover, the more he thought about the national leadership, "the less inclined" he was to allow his name to be put forward as a candidate. But then he opened the door a crack by stating that, if he did end up as leader, the National Committee could be sure he "would give it everything" he had.[40]

This crack noticeably widened after late January 1961, when Knowles travelled to Regina to spend some time alone with Douglas. From this point on, while Douglas continued to proclaim his preference to stay in Saskatchewan, he became increasingly open to the blandishments of the draft-Douglas-for-Ottawa movement. Gradually, he began to prepare his people in Saskatchewan for a decision that many would not like.

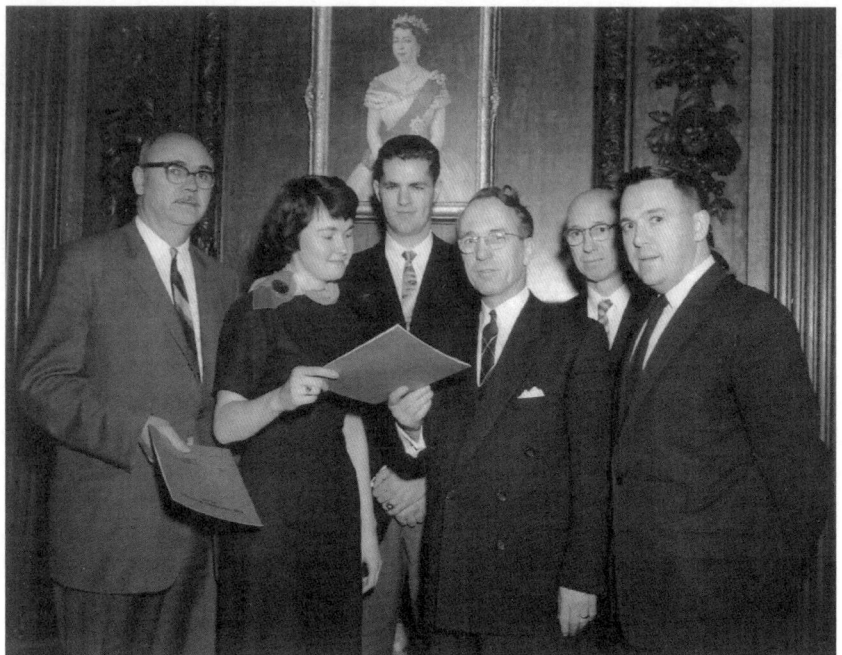

T.C. with Woodrow Lloyd (far left) and Allan Blakeney (far right) at an event at the University of Saskatchewan, 1961 (PAS R-A10657)

Less than a month after begging Thompson to remain chair of the Advisory Planning Committee on Medical Care, Douglas gave the keynote speech at one of the New Party's policy seminars in Calgary. Joining him were two key members of his cabinet, Woodrow Lloyd and Allan Blakeney, as well as Walter Smishek, the labour member of the Thompson Committee.[41] Although Douglas was warming up to the idea of becoming the New Party's first leader, he found himself returning to Regina only to witness an attack on Walter Thompson's integrity.

**Public Attack on Thompson**

In March 1961, a Dr. Leishman, a Regina-based physician, gave a speech condemning Thompson as "prejudiced and biased" and alleged he had been made chair of the APC to ensure that the government's intentions on medicare were implemented in exactly the way it wanted. He described the Thompson Committee as merely "window dressing," intended to "whitewash the policy of the politicians" rather than investigate the real "problems and needs of the people." He then went on to defend the position of the CPS, stating that the medical profession was "opposed to a government-controlled, compulsory scheme because we know it will lead to deterioration of services, government bureaucracy, uncontrolled spiralling costs, loss of privacy for the patient and loss of freedom for patient and doctor alike."[42] When his speech was quoted in the *Regina Leader-Post*, it became a political football.

The next day in the legislature, T.C. hit back hard. First, he defended Thompson as a scientist who had devoted his life to research and university administration and whose "fairness and impartiality has commended itself to the great majority of the people of the province." Then he pointed out that, beyond the three government members of the committee and the chair, the other members were nominated by the groups they represented, including the CPS, the University of Saskatchewan, farm organizations, trade unions, and the business community. Douglas sent a letter to Thompson enclosing his statement to the legislature and pointed out that, in his opinion, Leishman was speaking "for an infinitesimally small section of the people of Saskatchewan."[43]

Although, as chair of the APC, Thompson felt the brunt of the attack, he told Douglas that "anyone who did not express agreement" with the CPS members of the committee "on all points" could also be attacked. Moreover, it seemed to him that Leishman was expressing a view "held by quite a number of doctors" beyond the CPS executive, and that this boded ill "for the success of any [future] medical care plan."[44] T.C. felt he needed to respond to Thompson's pessimistic assessment that the entire medical profession had turned against both him and the committee. Most of all, he wanted to stiffen Thompson's resolve to see the job through:

> The public have complete confidence in your impartiality and so have a great many of the doctors. There are a few of them like Dr. Leishman who have become extremely interested in the business world and have tended to bring a commercial approach to the whole question of medical care. These men do not represent the profession at its best and I find that large numbers of general practitioners in the country are appalled at the statements which have been made by their colleagues.
>
> It seems to me that this is the time for all of us to stand firm. If this small but powerful group ever become convinced that by vilification and newspapers advertisements they can frighten decent people away from much needed changes, then progress will come to an end. Every forward step which humanity has taken has been opposed by a wilful group of

men who have a vested interest in maintaining the status quo. While one must be careful to protect the interests of all groups who are affected, nevertheless it is the welfare of society as a whole which must be the major consideration.[45]

To T.C.'s relief, Thompson did not resign after the attack, as he felt that he needed to salvage his own reputation. However, the next few months would see strains between the two men as both faced an openly hostile college.

**Waiting for the Report**

In April, just as T.C. was beginning the process of having the provincial CCF approve his decision to run for the leadership of the New Party, he and the rest of cabinet noted with some concern that a report would be needed from the Thompson Committee sooner rather than later. Douglas and the cabinet had expected some direction from the committee early in the year so that they could introduce a bill in the house before the end of the session. Upon being informed of the government's expectation by Walter Erb, the province's minister of health, Thompson rejected the timetable as impossible.[46] Rather than engaging Thompson and convincing him of the government's need for an earlier report, Erb simply accepted Thompson's statement without informing Douglas or cabinet.

Just weeks before the New Party's founding convention in Ottawa, T.C. decided that he needed to get something soon from the Thompson Committee so that a medical care bill could be introduced in the provincial legislature early in the special autumn session. To get the bill into the legislature, Douglas felt he needed to demonstrate that it reflected the recommendations of the committee, which, after all, had been set up to forge a consensus across the province on medicare. Of course, the problem was that the committee members representing the CPS were doing everything possible to paralyze the work, block any possible consensus, and delay the final report for as long as possible.

Although T.C. had previously been in direct contact with Thompson, he insisted on all future communication between the government and the committee being done through Erb. As a result, it was Erb who finally sent a letter in early June 1961 asking the committee for an "interim" report before the special fall sitting, one that would "enable the Government to prepare the legislative provisions which will be required" to implement "medical care insurance in Saskatchewan in 1962." As for the myriad other issues being examined by the committee, these could be addressed in its final report.[47]

Sensitive to the concessions the CPS had received regarding the time that the committee would be permitted to complete its work, Erb explained that, while he realized "that no time limit was set on the deliberations of the Committee, it seems reasonable to suggest that the Committee may be able to establish the broad outlines of a desirable insurance program for physicians' services" by early September. By restricting itself to recommendations on "coverage, extent of benefits, financial provincial and general administrative responsibilities concerning physicians' services only," the committee would later have time to work on "needed improvement" in other areas and programs, and the recommendations on these could wait for a final report.[48]

Something strange then happened. Commission secretary John Sparkes prepared a letter on behalf of Thompson stating that it was "the intention of the Committee to prepare the interim report as requested," but Thompson refused to sign the letter.[49] Instead, he verbally informed Erb that there was little hope of producing a report, much less a unanimous set of recommendations, by the date put forward by the government. Even in the last week of August, according to Thompson, the attempts at generating a single report had completely failed. The committee's staff, under the direction of Sparkes, produced an incomplete draft, but, as Thompson emphasized, "not a single word of the report" had "been approved." To help the government, Thompson suggested that the committee's deliberations, published as formal motions, be used as a basis for drafting legislation.[50]

Thompson felt so sandwiched between the committee's inability to make progress and the government's continuing demand for an interim report that he let Sparkes speak to the media on his behalf. In contrast to Thompson's pessimism, Sparkes presented a more optimistic picture, stating that a report would be ready sometime in September.[51] When he was asked about his reaction to the news, Douglas simply said that he hoped the report would have enough substance on which to base enabling legislation.[52] The truth was that Douglas was in the midst of preparing for the founding convention of the New Party and its national leadership and was forced to put his worries about the Thompson Committee to one side.

## Assuming Leadership of the New Democratic Party

Douglas may have been more than a little ambivalent about leading the New Party, but once decided and backed up by the support of provincial CCF constituency associations, he never revisited the decision as he and his rival, Hazen Argue, vied for the leadership.

Both of the New Party leadership candidates were steeped in the politics of Saskatchewan, but they had strikingly different dispositions. Argue was almost a generation younger than Douglas: he was only twenty-four years old when he won a seat in Parliament, the province's youngest ever MP. As the representative of the rural constituency of Wood Mountain, Argue spoke to issues of great concern to prairie farmers and was quick on his feet in parliamentary debates. His nickname "Blazen Hazen" said it all. He was so effective as a constituency politician that he was the only CCF MP from Saskatchewan to survive the Diefenbaker sweep of 1958.[53] With the federal CCF leader, M.J. Coldwell, defeated in the same election, Argue ran for the position of house leader and was elected by a bare margin. In August 1960, despite powerful opposition from the national party's executive, especially David Lewis and Stanley Knowles, Argue became the CCF's temporary national leader, a placeholder position until the New Party could hold its convention to choose both a new name and a new leader.[54]

The reason Lewis, Knowles, and the other members of the national CCF executive were dismissive of Argue was that they saw him as representing the agrarian wing of the old party and knowing little outside of the business of farming. He was hardly the person to appeal to union members and middle-class urbanites living in Toronto, Montreal, and Vancouver. These stalwart CCFers just did not think Argue could be a credible leader of the New Party. In their view, only Douglas, a proven governmental leader, someone who had dealt with national issues long before he had become premier, and a name known to many Canadians, could keep the original base of the CCF in western Canada while reaching out to workers and their unions in central and eastern Canada.[55] However, their open support of Douglas backfired when Argue used it as part of his campaign against what he framed as the anti-democratic instincts of the party's unelected bigshots.[56]

By mid-June, forty-five days before the convention, the bitterness between the executive and Argue had grown to the point where T.C. himself feared that the damage being done to the CCF, not to mention the New Party, might be irreparable.[57] Lewis would later admit he and the other members of the CCF national executive had made a strategic error in so obviously supporting Douglas from the beginning. Argue took advantage of the error by painting Douglas as the candidate of the party's establishment, an assessment that would contribute to a small but growing anti-Douglas movement within the party and make T.C.'s life difficult in the months ahead.[58]

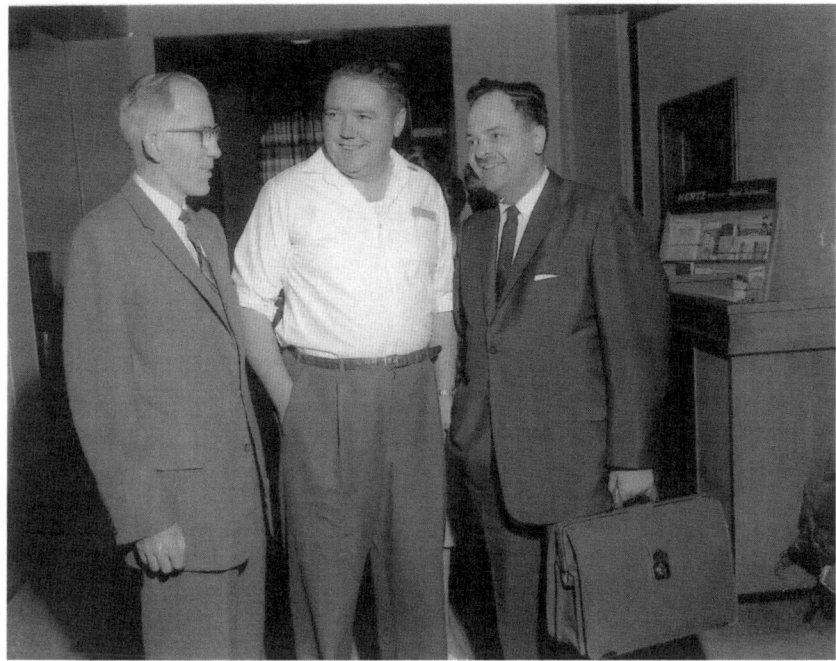

Stanley Knowles (left) and Hazen Argue (right) in 1961 (PAS R-LP1251)

At the time, Douglas refused to respond to Argue's criticisms that he was little more than a creature of the backroom party establishment. Waiting until the end of June to formally announce his candidature (although everyone already knew he had decided to run), T.C. then declared that, while he would let his name stand, he would "not campaign for the office." Moreover, if he was elected leader, he insisted that he would "not start his full-time duties" until he had introduced "legislation for Saskatchewan's medical care program at a special legislative session expected in October" so that the program could be launched early in 1962. He would therefore step down as provincial leader only at the Saskatchewan CCF convention scheduled for the beginning of November.[59] Although the decision to do both jobs at the same time for a few months may have appeared logical to Douglas at the time, it would give the province's growing anti-medicare coalition additional ammunition with which to fight the provincial government and delay the program's implementation.

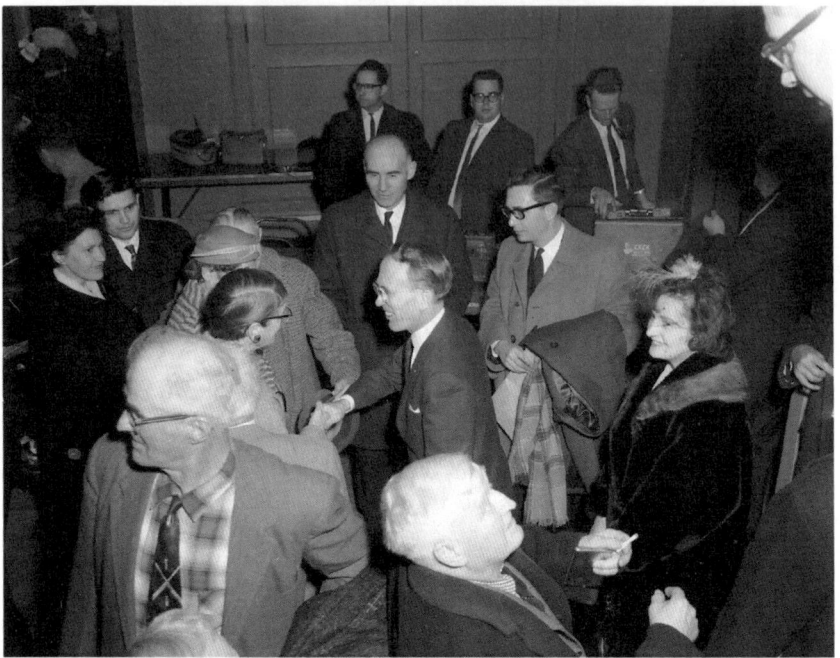

T.C. arriving at the New Party's founding convention, Ottawa, 31 July 1961 (PAS, *Regina Leader-Post*, T.C. Douglas negative no. 2)

Douglas saw no reason to run a campaign, in part because he was confident that he would win the leadership. In addition, he wanted to know how much support he had in the party without having to campaign for it.[60] This attitude frightened some of his supporters, who were convinced that Argue's campaign "as the poor innocent little David who dares oppose the Goliath of the labour and C.C.F. bosses" would prevent Douglas from winning the 80 per cent plurality he was seeking.[61] Whatever his rationale, the fact was that Douglas simply did not have the time to sustain a national campaign, considering all that was on his plate in Saskatchewan, especially medicare. And, given the fact that Blazen Hazen *was* actively campaigning, Argue was particularly annoyed with the final sentence in Douglas's press release announcing that, while he was "free and willing to serve as Leader of the New Party if the majority of the Founding Convention delegates so decide," he would "definitely not campaign for the office nor seek it in any other way."[62]

## The 1961 New Party Convention

Held during a five-day heat wave in Ottawa between 31 July and 4 August 1961, the founding convention of the New Party was in many respects the first modern political convention of the television age in Canada. Also, for the first time, the 2,083 delegates had the benefit of simultaneous translation into both official languages, one of the New Party's many efforts to reach into Quebec. For some, however, the convention smacked of American style "show biz," with its "banners, flags, hats, buttons, music," a striking contrast with past conventions "of CCF people poring over books of resolutions and warding off temptations to enjoy themselves."[63]

In contrast to the convention hoopla, the New Party's declaration was a 168-paragraph tome that harked back to the CCF past. For some of the delegates, the New Party declaration was simply too long and detailed to be read in full, and it never became part of the party's folklore like the Regina Manifesto (1933), or even the Winnipeg Declaration (1956) that had toned down the anti-capitalist language of the original manifesto.[64] Under the heading "A Health Plan for Canada," three paragraphs rejected the pro-centralist stance of the party decades before, a change necessitated by the desire to make the CCF more appealing in Quebec and, to some extent, because of Saskatchewan's proven leadership role in implementing universal hospital coverage. Emphasis was placed on the need to consult all the health professions, in part a rejection of the privileged position of doctors relative to other health professionals. The "National Health Plan" of the New Party began with the assertion "that a country's most precious possession is the health of its citizens." Building on national hospital insurance, a New Party federal administration would work with the provincial governments and all health professions to "cover a full range of services: medical, surgical, dental and optical treatment, as well as prescribed drugs and appliances." Knowing that universal coverage would increase the demand for health services, the National Health Plan included grants to governments and postsecondary institutions to increase the supply of health providers.[65]

The statement was fine as far as it went, but it did little to differentiate the New Party from its main competitor, the Liberal Party of Canada, which had begun to move to the left under Lester B. Pearson's leadership. Indeed, at their own national convention in January 1961, the Liberals had already stated their intention to cost share provincial coverage for medical care as well as outpatient prescription drugs. The mechanism differed from hospital coverage in that the fees paid by governments on behalf of patients would be included as taxable income, a

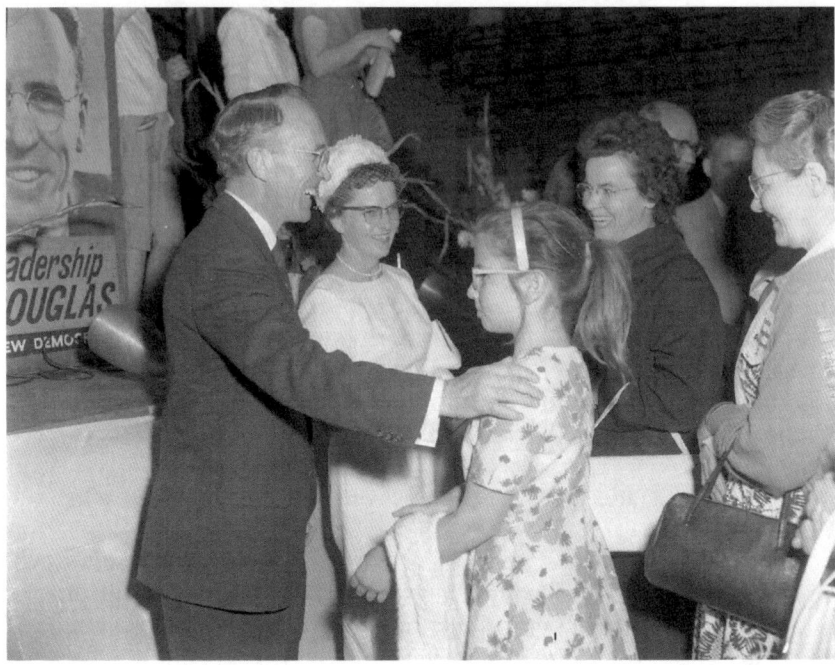

T.C. with Irma talking to delegates and supporters at the New Party's founding convention (PAS, *Regina Leader-Post*, T.C. Douglas negative no. 1(1))

policy justified on the basis that this would ensure the rich paid more than the poor, while ensuring free access at the point of service.[66]

At the New Party's convention, a preferential balloting system was used to select the name from among four choices: New Party, Social Democratic Party, Canadian Democratic Party, and New Democratic Party. In the end, the last name – NDP for short – was selected.[67] The name was Douglas's personal favourite because, as he explained to one of his backbenchers, Marjorie Cooper, some three weeks before the convention, "it implies the building of a 'new democracy.'" He suggested to Cooper that, while taking the train from Saskatchewan to Ottawa, she test out the name on "some of the other delegates."[68] He also thought the name offered the basis for what he felt would be a great slogan: "Vote for the New Democracy." The new name would make it easier, Douglas felt, to "get the idea over to the public that the new democracy is one which adds social and economic democracy to our present political democracy."[69]

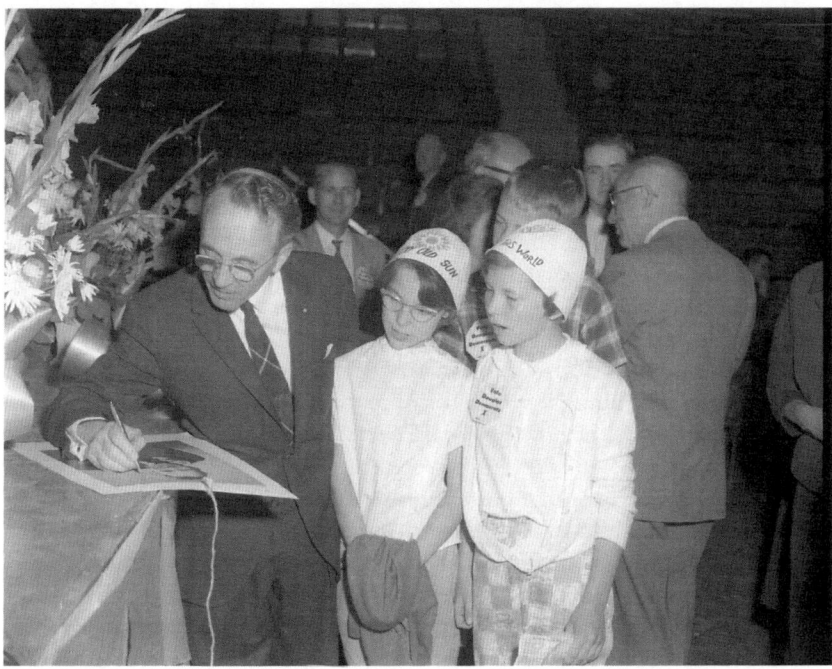

T.C. signing posters for youthful "Douglas for Democrats" supporters (PAS, *Regina Leader-Post*, T.C. Douglas negative no. 1(3))

For sure, Douglas hated the idea of making the transitional name of "New Party" the permanent name. As he explained to Cooper, "it is easily laughed at. It means absolutely nothing," and it did "nothing to convey the philosophy or the platform or the type of organization of the party. To me it is negative, suggesting only something new, whatever that may mean."[70] He also seemed to agree with Cooper's own assessment that names such as Social Democratic Party or Democratic Socialist Party had "too much of a European flavor, and are too easily confused with National Socialists, or Soviet Socialists," and she could "see no point in frightening people away by such names."[71]

On Friday night (1 August), Hazen Argue came close to pulling out of the race; at least one of his key advisors realized that most of the delegates intended to elect Douglas and suggested that Argue's post-convention influence in the party would be greater if the exact margin of his support remained unknown. Argue saw the logic of this but was talked out of withdrawing by his wife, Eugenia. She reminded her husband of Douglas's remark that "the job should seek the man rather than the man seeking the job" as proof that T.C. always felt he was entitled to the federal party's leadership, and it was therefore Argue's duty to make sure he was not anointed as leader.[72]

In the end, Argue held firm, and both he and T.C. gave their respective leadership pitches to the delegates. In his speech, Douglas emphasized the importance of coming together and, in a direct attack on Argue's contention that T.C. represented a right-wing tendency in the party, maintained that he had not "talked as glibly as some others about our devotion to socialism" because he had "been too busy putting into practice" socialist policies, including "public ownership and development of our basic resources in the interests of all our people." He pleaded with the delegates to avoid the factionalism that had emerged during the establishing of the New Party:

> This is not a time to argue about right-wing and left-wing; this is the time to unite all our forces for the task which lies before us – that of creating a society which will make the wealth potential of this country available to all who work with hand and brain. Leadership does not consist of accentuating or exploiting our differences but rather in finding those areas of agreement within which we can work together for common objectives. More social democratic parties have been ruined by dissention from within than have ever been destroyed by attacks from without. Any party which expects to win the confidence of the Canadian electorate must demonstrate its ability to manage its own affairs. And with dignity and unity, we must learn to work together as a team, each of us with a part to play, but always remembering that our individual contribution will only be valuable if it contributes to the victory of the team as a whole.[73]

When the ballots were counted, T.C. received 1,391 votes compared to 380 for Argue, a convincing margin. Although slightly less than the 80 per cent Douglas had hoped for, he and the party executive were nonetheless satisfied by the expression of confidence, and he was thrust into the middle of a "wildly cheering, singing, banner-waving melee of joy."[74] Photographs were taken of the two men arm in arm, looking reconciled. Argue told the delegates, "No matter what my role in the years ahead, I shall speak for you, I shall work for you. I shall never let you down."[75] Argue did not mean a word of it, but, for a few months at least, Douglas could bask in the optimism that rang out from what he and some in the media described as "the largest and most enthusiastic convention in the political history of Canada."[76]

The Thompson Committee and the New Party 323

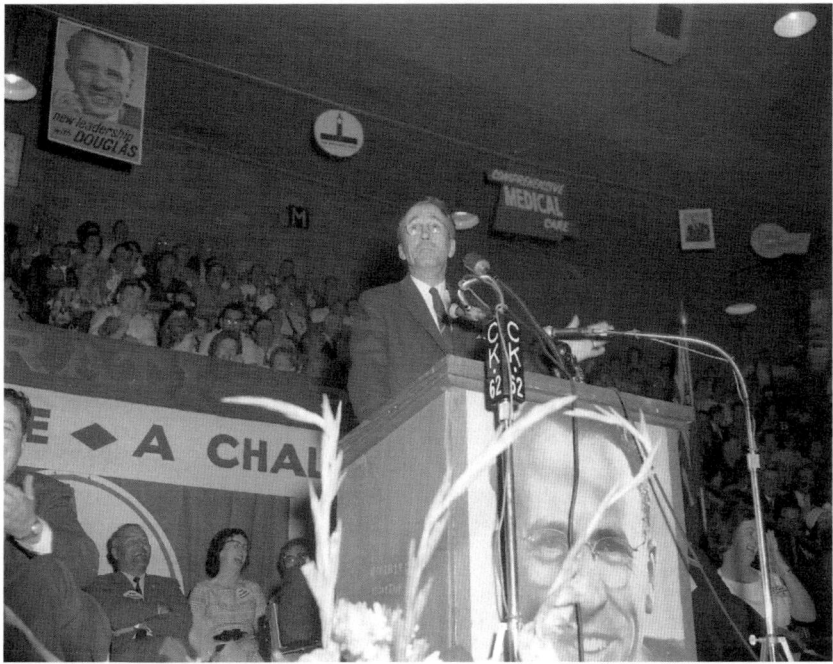

T.C. giving his leadership speech at the NDP's founding convention in Ottawa (PAS, *Regina Leader-Post*, negative no. 1(2))

Douglas began his victory speech in French.[77] Given his inability to pronounce the words, these were the most painful two minutes of the convention. In response to one supporter who described his French as "horrible," Douglas readily agreed, and pledged to do his "best to improve it." As he explained, he hadn't studied French since he "was a boy in Scotland during the First World War," so it would be "quite a struggle to get back to it again."[78] This moment revealed one of Douglas's critical weaknesses as NDP leader, the other being his understanding of the Quiet Revolution then unfolding in Quebec.

Identifying the need for "national purpose" through programs such as universal health coverage, Douglas argued that government should be seen as an "instrument by which we provide for ourselves collectively the kind of security which we cannot attain individually." He went on to suggest two major objectives leading up to Canada's centenary in 1967. First on his wish list was the establishment of "a comprehensive national health insurance program which will provide every citizen of Canada with the right to all the health services they need in the same manner that education is now available to every child." Douglas's second wish was for "a national system of retirement allowances on a contributory basis."[79] His speech ended with a slightly altered verse from a poem by William Blake, which had become a hymn for the Labour Party in Britain: "I shall not cease from mental strife / Nor shall my sword sleep in my hand / Till we have built Jerusalem / In this green and pleasant land."[80]

The founding convention of the NDP appeared at the time to be a great victory for both Douglas and his party. Despite the scepticism of some that little had changed, most commentators felt the "new" party, with its emphasis on a growing middle class and urban blue- and white-collar workers, was better suited for the 1960s than was the old CCF.[81] To have a proven winner at its helm seemed to be the icing on the cake. But problems continued to brew in his home province, and Douglas had to return to Regina as quickly as possible. Time was running out on his clock for the introduction and implementation of medicare.

## The Thompson Committee "Interim" Report

For four months, between August and November 1961, T.C. would be both premier of Saskatchewan and leader of the federal New Democratic Party. Each was more than a full-time job, and it was close to impossible for him to do well at both. The file that suffered most was medicare, in part because its opponents took full advantage of the premier's focus being elsewhere. In September, when the Thompson interim report was finally conveyed to the government and decisions needed to be made on how best to prepare and then steer the medical care bill through the house, Douglas was in Ontario and Alberta giving speeches on the dangers of nuclear proliferation and the need of economic planning at the national level.[82]

T.C.'s frequent absences from the province were seized upon by his political opponents. Declaring that Douglas should either tend to his job as premier or resign, Ross Thatcher claimed that the province could ill "afford the luxury of absentee leadership."[83] In an editorial in the *Saskatoon Star Phoenix*, Douglas's out-of-province speeches were parsed, and his "radical" rhetoric as a national leader was deemed by the newspaper's editors to come from a different man, not the one "who had become mellowed by the political facts of life in Saskatchewan."[84]

By early September, T.C. had reluctantly accepted that the most he could get from the Thompson Committee was an interim report and that even this would be marred by a minority report from the CPS representatives. Although this was a flimsy basis on which to present a bill in the legislature, it was the best he could expect in the circumstances. At least he would be able to say, based on the public hearings and the deliberations of the committee, that the people of Saskatchewan, not just the government, had some influence over the basic architecture of the program. Surely the public – including, he hoped, at least some rank-and-file physicians – would view his government as having done everything possible to meet the college halfway.

On 27 September, Thompson submitted his committee's interim report to the provincial government. It included a minority dissent in a separate chapter signed by all three CPS representatives and the Chamber of Commerce representative. This dissent reiterated the long-held position of organized medicine rejecting the single-payer design, including single-tier universality, endorsed in the majority report. As set out in the dissenting report, only a system financed through the private payment of premiums to non-governmental insurance companies, supplemented by government subsidies for the residents who could demonstrate need, could protect the freedoms of both doctors and patients. Instead of the "monopolistic plan" endorsed by the majority, the minority continued to extol the virtues of the subsidy-based multi-payer plan favoured by both the CPS and the Canadian Medical Association.[85]

The fact that eight majority members of the Thompson Committee recommended a government-financed universal medical care insurance plan met Douglas's minimum requirement. However, one member, the Saskatchewan Federation of Labour (SFL) secretary, Walter Smishek, disagreed with the majority on three recommendations it made as concessions to the medical profession. A seasoned labour negotiator, Smishek refused to go along with the three recommendations, given the fact they did not produce any quid pro quo by the college.[86] Smishek's points of departure are worth reviewing, as they reflected the views of organized labour at the time, views that were at the opposite ends of the spectrum from the CPS and faithfully reflected the views of T.C.'s more left-wing critics.

The first item was that doctors should continue to be paid mainly on a fee-for-service basis but on the understanding that, on some occasions, other modes of remuneration such as salary or capitation could be used if the doctors agreed. The majority came to this conclusion, not on the basis that they felt it was the best way to pay doctors, but simply because it was the only form of remuneration that most doctors in the province would accept. Smishek considered this too damaging a compromise, arguing that fee-for-service would undermine the key objectives of medical care coverage, which he enumerated as promoting "the prevention of illness and disability," providing "comprehensive care," and achieving "a high quality of care." From his perspective, fee-for-service was "the *least desirable* system of payment and would simply "encourage the growth of a purely sickness insurance program rather than a health service in the best sense."[87]

The second flashpoint was the committee's recommendation that the government impose user fees on patients to reduce unnecessary demand and control costs: $1 for an office visit, $2 for a home visit, and $3 for a night consultation, with specialist visits exempted. In contrast, Smishek argued that "deterrent charges" followed "directly from the recommendation for a fee-for-service method of payment," were "characteristic devices of the private insurance industry," and should "have no place in a public program of health insurance." User fees violate "the principles and objectives of a health service – which are to promote health, to prevent illness, to provide early diagnosis and treatment of disease, and to promote rehabilitation." In his opinion, the majority's view that some sort of deterrent fee was required to contain the growth in the cost of the program simply underlined "the inherent weaknesses of such a system. Deterrent charges have to be entertained solely because the fee-for-service system encourages *quantity medical care* under conditions of competitive solo practice, rather than *quality medical care* with physicians working co-operatively in groups."[88]

The third difference concerned the majority recommendation that the plan be administered by a public commission separate from the Department of Public Health. In this recommendation, seven committee members still adhered to the principle of public administration, since such a commission would still be "responsible to the government, through the Minister of Public Health."[89] Smishek, however, felt such a public commission would prove to be an unworkable arrangement. Since universal medical coverage entailed "the expenditure of large sums of public funds," the government needed to "be answerable to the Legislative Assembly for questions relating to the program." Having sat in dozens of meetings with the CPS representatives, Smishek knew that they wanted a commission entirely independent of the provincial government, violating the basic principle of democratic accountability.

While these concessions were unacceptable to Smishek, he was also worried about the majority's rationale that a limited degree of independence would somehow protect the program from political interference. Elected officials were chosen by the people to govern such programs, and the public had the tools to hold them to account in a

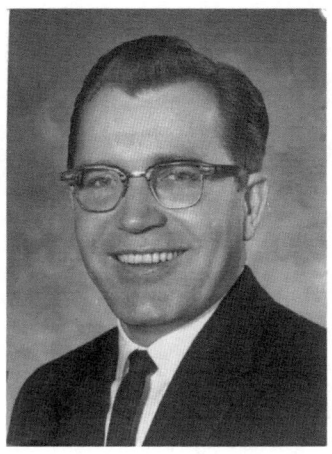

Walter Smishek left the labour movement to become a politician. First elected in 1964 and re-elected in 1967 (when this photograph was taken), Smishek would become the minister of health in the Saskatchewan NDP government in the early 1970s (SPL QC-4286-3)

way they could not hold an independent commission to account for the how the program was being run. He could not "see why a medical care program should be 'safeguarded against political interference' to any greater extent than other" public "services such as education and social welfare." Moreover, to separate "physicians' services from the hospital program, the preventive services, the programs for special diseases (cancer, mental illness, etc.) and from the rehabilitation program" in the Department of Public Health could only "lead to fragmentation and work against effective planning and operation."[90]

Smishek spoke for many CCF activists who had been calling for socialized medicine for decades. They wanted to see the entire system of delivery revamped, starting with getting doctors out of the small physician practices they operated like businesses and into larger group practices focused on clinical care, illness prevention, and health promotion rather than individual fee-based piecework. In their view, health insurance was not enough: it should be treated only as the opening salvo in the creation of a joined-up health system. Simply introducing health insurance on top of existing approaches would lock in the worst features of what they viewed as a failing system. They were impatient with the CCF government's willingness to compromise with the doctors and with the willingness of the public representatives on the Thompson Committee to try to satisfy the doctors when it was clear that the CPS was doing everything it could to sabotage medicare.[91]

Thompson explained to Douglas that the only reason he supported fee-for-service payment and a non-governmental commission to administer the plan was his judgment that these compromises "were necessary in order to secure the minimum of cooperation from the doctors" and therefore were "essential for the operation of the plan."[92] T.C. unburdened himself in a particularly candid response to Thompson:

> Like yourself, I agree with some of the views expressed by Walter Smishek but I have learned over the years that "politics is the art of the possible." It is not, therefore, a matter of formulating a perfect plan but rather devising one which will be acceptable and then hoping that it will be improved in the light of experience.
>
> Personally, I can understand the fear which some doctors have of bureaucratic red tape and the possibility of political interference. If the commission form of administration will help to remove these fears, then I do not think this is too great a price to pay for getting acceptance by the medical profession. The same is true of the method which will be used for paying the providers of service. The fee-for-service system of paying doctors has already been established in the Swift Current region and in the private plans. It has some disadvantages but I think it would be too much to expect that the doctors would accept a salary system of payment. [But] I am glad the Advisory Planning Committee on Medical Care left the door open so that arrangements could be entered into with doctors who are willing to work on some method of remuneration other than the fee-for-service.[93]

## A Divided Report

As noted in chapter 1, the debate on the medical care bill in October 1961 was a pivotal event in Douglas's life and a truly historic moment in the political history of the province. Getting the bill into the Saskatchewan Legislative Assembly, however, had proved exceedingly difficult in such a short timeframe.

The problem lay less in the content of the Thompson Committee report than in the process. In early September, the government decided to begin the special fall session of the Legislative Assembly on 11 October so that it would end in time for the provincial CCF convention beginning November 1, at which time Douglas intended to resign as party leader and premier. Given that he did not receive the interim report from the Thompson Committee until the dying days of September, a bill needed to be prepared, finalized, and introduced in less than two weeks. This meant the ink was barely dry on the bill when it was introduced in the assembly by Douglas.

Even if Douglas had wanted to, he had no time to consult with anyone in advance, especially the CPA executive, who had become masters at dragging out any consultation. So the college was not given an advance copy of the bill, an omission very effectively used by the CPS and its allies to argue that the Douglas government had acted in bad faith. Such criticism may have been a price that Douglas was willing to pay – after all, he very well knew that nothing positive could come out of such consultations, given the unyielding position held by the CPS representatives on the Thompson Committee. Nonetheless, it made him vulnerable to the charge that he was not upholding his earlier promise that his medical care program had to be acceptable to those delivering the services.

Originally, Douglas thought that the position of the college's representatives, once revealed to the public in the form of the minority report, would be enough to demonstrate the unreasonableness of the CPS leadership and release him from his obligation to have a plan that was satisfactory to the doctors as represented by the CPS. However, the lack of advance consultation on the medicare bill was a major strike against the government in the eyes of the average general practitioner working in Saskatchewan, and even more among the wealthier and more anti-medicare specialists clustered in the cities. And the main purpose for which Douglas had set up the Thompson Committee – to implement a program after due consultation with the medical profession that would ensure its willingness to work with the government – had failed miserably. The committee had done nothing to improve the government's relationship with the CPS. If anything, the committee process had exacerbated the tensions between the two.

At the same time, the committee may have protected Douglas's left flank. As already noted, T.C. felt some concessions were essential – concessions rejected by many left-wing activists in his party – the most significant of which was the acceptance of fee-for-service remuneration and, with it, the business model of medical practice as opposed to a salaried service. The other concession was the setting up of an arm's length medical care commission, with representation from the CPS, to administer the plan. T.C. could point to the Thompson Committee's public consultations and final recommendations as to why his government eventually accepted these two design features. Introduced in the Legislative Assembly on 13 October, the government's medicare bill, while rejecting the committee's majority recommendation for deterrent fees, did accept an independent business model of fee-for-service physician practice as well as a medical care commission, rather than the Department of Public Health, to administer the medical care plan.[94]

Douglas had always disliked user fees at the point of service, as these were likely to deter only those who most needed medical care and would undermine the goal of having individuals see physicians before serious illnesses could develop into life-threatening conditions. Premiums were another matter. Adopting the same procedure as he instituted in the hospital insurance plan, he thought at least some of the revenues should still be collected through individual and family premiums. For the medical care plan, this would amount to roughly one-third of the total revenues needed to administer it, the other two-thirds being raised through general revenues. While he knew that many in the party, as well as organized labour (including Smishek, in his own minority report), argued in favour of medicare being paid entirely out of general taxes, he was concerned about raising either income or consumption taxes too high if there was no premium. And he had a second reason. In an interview conducted twenty years later, he argued a premium could be useful for psychological reasons:

> My argument ... was that if you are going to have something like health insurance at least in the preliminary period you had to make people realize that you can't get something for nothing. And if the thing is just paid out of general revenue, well where does general revenue come? Well who cares where general revenue comes? The fact that it comes from them doesn't even occur to them. But if they had to pay, go and pay $10 a head with a maximum of $30 per family or whatever it might be, then they know they are paying for it. They get that [provincial health] card in the Fall and it says "Mr. So and So and the following members of his family are entitled to medical care, surgical care" and so on and so on. He has paid for that. Now he doesn't pay the whole cost and never did, we still had to pay out of the general revenue of the province a good part; but it gave them a sense that I am paying for this, this is part of a program.[95]

This was an argument that Douglas knew was shared by few within his own party, but he argued that this psychological factor was most important when implementing a new and very expensive program as a way of reminding residents "that there is no pipe line to the mint." The trade-offs in a less wealthy province like Saskatchewan were such that it was essential to be fiscally vigilant, always keeping in mind that numerous other meritorious programs needed to be financed, and the premium helped individuals think about those trade-offs. As for the regressive nature of premiums, Douglas felt this was best managed by ensuring that most of the financing – two-thirds in this case – came from more progressive general tax sources, such as personal and corporate income tax, and by ensuring that the poorest and most dependent residents received coverage without paying premiums.[96] In fact, medicare premiums would eventually be eliminated in Saskatchewan: in 1973, the NDP government under Allan Blakeney and his health minister, the same Walter Smishek who had argued so eloquently against user fees in the Thompson Committee, finally did what many in the CCF-NDP had always urged.[97]

Douglas agreed with the Thompson Committee that an arm's-length commission rather than the Department of Public Health administer the plan, and the government's medicare bill stipulated the creation of the Saskatchewan Medical Care Insurance Commission (MCIC). To try and satisfy the CPS, of the six to eight commission members, at least two had to be physicians. The MCIC was also to be supported by a Medical Advisory Committee, the members of whom had to be approved by the CPS. While the MCIC operated separately from the government, it would nonetheless report to the minister of health through the deputy minister, who would be a non-voting MCIC member.[98]

On the issue of the form of physician payment, the medical care insurance bill was mute, simply stating that it would be up to the MCIC to administer payment. However, Douglas knew that he would have to keep fee-for-service remuneration to prevent an overnight exodus of doctors from the province. Still, he hoped to see salary and other payment methods introduced by the MCIC, but this would be done gingerly over time.

The sharp debate on medicare dominated the fall sitting of the Legislative Assembly. The high drama in the legislature during the second reading of the bill was mirrored in the growing polarization of the population throughout Saskatchewan. There was no place to hide: almost everyone took a side either for or against what the government was doing. Even families were divided. The atmosphere everywhere, from coffee row and fall suppers in countless villages and towns to the gatherings and lecture halls in the cities, was heated and became increasingly toxic.

Naturally, the insistence on a fall session combined with the short time between the Thompson Report and the presentation of the medicare bill and T.C.'s previously announced departure in early November made it easy for Thatcher to argue that Douglas was trying to "steam-roller" the medicare bill through the house without enough discussion.[99] To this charge, T.C. could simply respond that he had been talking about more comprehensive health coverage, including medical care, since 1944. Moreover, the Thompson Committee had been working and consulting on the issue since 1960, the same year he had fought and won the election on the issue. The time to act had come, and Douglas had repeatedly stated to the press and in speeches that medicare would begin on 1 April 1962. When Thatcher suggested the province should wait on a national cost-sharing plan like hospital insurance, Douglas derided the notion and argued that such delay tactics were nothing more than a thinly disguised effort to derail the plan altogether. Indeed, since the only medical care plan supported by the Thatcher Liberals was one that "could be done without hardship to the taxpayer," he really had no plan in mind at all.[100]

The question of Douglas's highly publicized departure continued to fan much debate. On the pro-medicare side, many saw him as leaving when he was most needed, while a few others felt he had always been a little too accommodating, and thus saw his leaving as an opportunity to bring in a leader who might be a little tougher with the doctors. Within the CCF itself, although the constituency associations had voted in favour of releasing Douglas the previous spring, a number of rank-and-file members felt that the decision was wrong and, further, that the closer relationship with organized labour in the NDP was a major mistake.[101] Those on the anti-medicare side saw Douglas's departure as a major opportunity to stop the government from implementing its bill, now that the gifted political magician who had, so often in the past, persuaded the unsure and disarmed the naysayers, was finally leaving.[102] No one else in the CCF, his opponents believed, had his political or persuasive skills, and no one else had the fortitude to see the plan through. On this, they would soon be proven wrong, as the medicare bill was presented and debated in the Legislative Assembly.

# 12  Political Repudiation

I felt a Funeral, in my Brain,
And Mourners to and fro
Kept treading – treading – till it seemed
That Sense was breaking through –
And when they all were seated,
A service, like a Drum –
Kept beating – beating – till I thought
My mind was going numb –
>   *I Felt a Funeral, in My* Brain, Emily Dickinson, 1861

Many enemies, much honour.
>   Proverb often quoted by German chancellor Otto von Bismarck

In the year that followed his election as national leader of the New Democratic Party (NDP), T.C. was forced to endure a rapid succession of political embarrassments and defeats. The defection of prominent members of his party to the Liberals damaged him, but his election defeat in the federal election of June that year would forever diminish his reputation as a winner. It would also cause a chain of problems for him in managing the NDP. He would never again enjoy the unquestioned position of leadership he enjoyed as premier of Saskatchewan or the capacity to set the policy agenda in terms of health care.

At the root of T.C.'s problems was the growing opposition to his proposed medical care plan and his insistence that the Thompson Committee continue despite its sabotage by organized medicine. The Douglas government's demand that the Thompson Committee provide an interim report after promising that it would not impose a deadline made T.C. vulnerable to accusations of rushing the legislation through without adequate consideration or consultation. Prior to this, Douglas's political judgment, as reflected in his proven ability to adeptly manage powerful interest groups, had been consistently spot on. However, in this case, he miscalculated how far the College of Physicians and Surgeons of Saskatchewan (CPS) was prepared to go to block medicare after the 1960 election as well as the combination of sticks and carrots needed to get the profession to accept his medical care plan, however grudgingly.

Part of the reason for his miscalculation was that T.C. needed to devote ever more time and focus to the NDP and national issues. The question of the creation of the party and its leadership occupied Douglas continually from 1960 until the NDP's founding convention in the summer of 1961. And, for months following the convention, Douglas continued as premier of the province while performing the role of national leader. It was impossible to do both jobs equally well, and the pressure of both had a deleterious impact on T.C.'s management of medicare at the very time when his political acumen was most needed. Swept into the maelstrom of national politics, he was less able to do what he had always done best in the past – inspire supporters, neutralize opponents, and convince the ambivalent.

This chapter describes the political price T.C. would pay for his missteps on the Thompson Committee and for dividing of his time and attention between provincial and federal politics. Although he and the colleagues he left behind in the provincial government would eventually win the war on medicare, the bitterness engendered during the years of struggle would contribute to the party's loss of office to the Liberals in Saskatchewan in 1964. As for Douglas, medicare in Saskatchewan was not enough of a policy achievement for the NDP to become a contender for national office or even the official opposition.

**The Medicare Bill**

On 11 October 1961, after the first day of the Legislative Assembly's special fall session on medicare, Douglas appeared on a provincial affairs television broadcast to convince the public of the merits of his government's medical care plan, the main subject in the Speech from the Throne and its reply.[1] The bill itself would be presented for first reading two days later, launching a polarized debate in Saskatchewan and the rest of Canada.

In the broadcast, T.C. first thanked the viewers for all their "kindness" for the many advances made over the past seventeen years, giving credit to the "people of Saskatchewan who have always been willing to tackle their problems in a spirit of co-operation."² His summary of accomplishments included building an electric power and natural gas infrastructure that improved the lives of rural residents, passing the country's first Bill of Rights, providing more and better education, ensuring greater farm security, and increasing social assistance. But it was his government's spearheading of major changes in health care that he expressed his greatest pride:

> Health services have improved tremendously since a CCF government was elected seventeen years ago. Free health services have been provided for needy citizens. Our cancer program cannot be equalled anywhere in Canada. Our psychiatric program has been greatly expanded and the cost is now borne entirely by all the people of the province rather than falling on the families of those who are mentally ill. Physical restoration centers provide care and treatment to the physically disabled. Most important of all Saskatchewan pioneered in the field of hospital insurance – and did it so successfully that today the rest of Canada has followed our example.³

T.C. then devoted the rest of the broadcast to medicare, arguing that the subsidy of private health insurance was an inadequate alternative to the universal plan under debate in the provincial assembly. He did not believe "that people should be required to go through the humiliation" of a means test. As he had stated many times in the past, all citizens "in a humane society should be entitled to medical care without the stigma of having to prove that they are in destitute circumstances." The time had surely come "when people should be entitled to all the medical care they need without having to worry about how they can pay the bill." Proud Saskatchewan was leading "the way," he felt "certain" that the province's "example will be followed by other provinces," supported by federal cost sharing."⁴

The following week, T.C. spoke on national television about the need for a comprehensive pan-Canadian health insurance plan, one that not only adopted the Saskatchewan universal approach for hospital coverage and medical care but would, over time, add further health services. He assured Canadians that, if elected, "a New Democratic government would contribute generously" to those provinces introducing medical care coverage and "would extend it to include dental care, optical care and essential drugs."⁵

By the time of his national broadcast, T.C. realized Bill No. 1, the Saskatchewan Medical Care Insurance Act, would not get passed in the Legislative Assembly before the CCF provincial convention, when he was scheduled to resign as party leader and premier.⁶ Originally, he hoped that, after first reading on Friday, 13 October, the bill would go through second reading the following Tuesday and then to third and final reading and passage by the end of that week.[7] However, the opposition Liberals were determined to prevent this, doing everything possible to prevent the bill from being passed on Douglas's watch.[8]

Instead, first reading continued for weeks. Then, despite the acrimonious debates of the previous two weeks, the second reading vote, a vote on the principle of the bill, was unanimous. The Liberals justified their vote in favour at this stage by citing their support for the value of prepaid medical care. But Liberal leader Ross Thatcher made it clear that, unless the CCF was prepared to change critical aspects of the bill, his party would vote against it on third reading.[9] The Legislative Assembly adjourned immediately after the bill passed second reading on 27 October, with the intention of resuming the special fall session on 13 November for debate on the medicare bill before third reading and passage. In the meantime, T.C. would exit the provincial scene, and another leader would take over as premier.

**Farewell to the Saskatchewan CCF**

The CCF provincial convention began on Wednesday, 1 November, at the Trianon ballroom in Regina. The first order of business was the problematic question of the new federal party's name. Many provincial members, loyal to the old CCF identity and its farm movement history, did not want to give up the old name, so the provincial party found a compromise. The CCF (Sask.) was renamed the Co-operative Commonwealth Federation: The Saskatchewan Section of the New Democratic Party, or CCF-NDP for short.[10] This awkward name reflected the ambivalence of party members squeezed between those who continued to oppose the change and those who supported a new direction for the CCF.

The next evening, the party held a banquet to say goodbye to Douglas as it leader. M.J. Coldwell, the former national leader of the CCF and T.C.'s close friend and ally, appeared as the guest of honour. He thanked T.C. for laying the foundation of "a great revolution" in Saskatchewan upon which the new national leader and the NDP would build a program of social justice nationally.[11] When presented with a brand new 1962 Pontiac as a parting gift, a car he would use in the federal election campaign the following year, Douglas was, according to the *Regina Leader-Post*, "overwhelmed" by the gesture and, for "one of the few times in his political career, ... at a loss for words."[12] Telling the crowd that the "greatest days of this movement" lay ahead and not behind, he reached out to those who were dubious about what the NDP

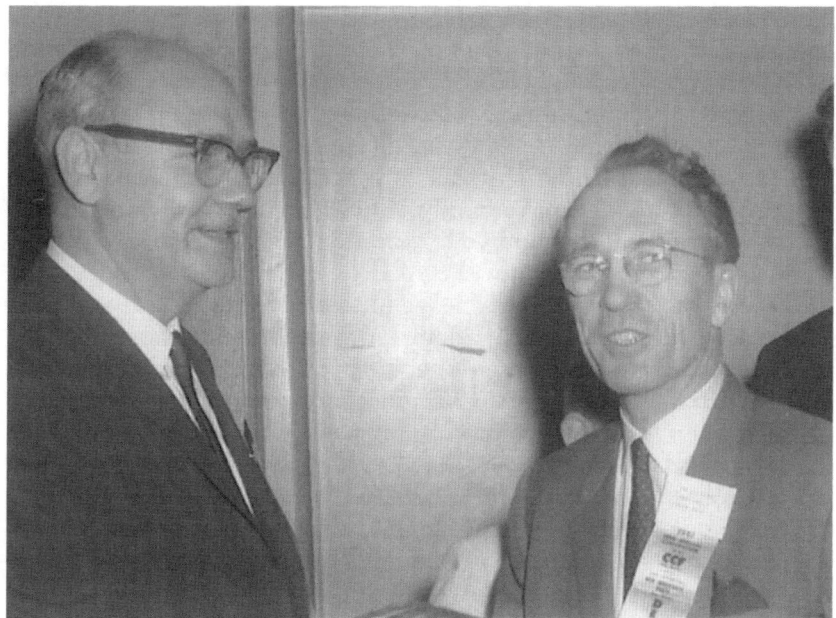

Woodrow Lloyd and T.C. greeting each other at a CCF convention in 1961 (PAS R-LP1252)

really meant by saying he would, as national leader, never let them down by departing from the policies originally established by the CCF. These were, after all, policies that he had been instrumental in setting in the first place.[13]

Before the convention, many assumed there would be a contest between the veteran cabinet ministers John Brockelbank and Woodrow Lloyd. However, when Brockelbank told everyone he would support Lloyd for premier rather than put his own name forward, many thought that Lloyd would simply be acclaimed leader. This changed during the convention, when one of the party's MLAs, Olaf Turnbull, decided to contest the leadership, despite his lack of political experience (he was first elected in 1960), in order to give party delegates some choice.[14] When the ballots were counted, Lloyd won 425 votes to Turnbull's 109 – a margin of over 75 per cent.[15] Douglas stood up and led the cheers that followed the announcement.[16] Taking the stage with his wife and son, Turnbull, and Douglas, Lloyd reminded everyone of the difficulties that lay ahead and that his first job after appointing his cabinet was "to complete the passage of the most important and greatest piece of legislation this province has ever seen."[17]

The new premier had been one of the stalwarts of Douglas's successive cabinets. When Clarence Fines retired from politics in 1960, there was really only one person Douglas felt could fill the vacuum, and that was Lloyd, whom he appointed as provincial treasurer. Born in 1913, Lloyd was the youngest in a family of twelve and the only one born in Saskatchewan after the family emigrated from Wisconsin. He entered engineering at the University of Saskatchewan in September 1929. Although he was at the top of his class at the end of his first year, the Great Depression forced him to abandon his studies and return home to assist his family. He then trained as a teacher and became increasingly involved with the CCF. After being promoted to school principal, he used his salary to pay for university correspondence courses and received a bachelor of arts degree in 1940, the same year he was elected president of the Saskatchewan Teachers' Federation.[18]

Now premier of the province, Lloyd was sworn in by Saskatchewan's lieutenant governor on the Tuesday following the provincial convention, with T.C. in attendance.[19] The new premier was tentative at first. Other than shifting Allan Blakeney from the post of education to the provincial treasury and appointing Turnbull as minister of education, he made no other changes to the cabinet.[20] However, Lloyd had been among those cabinet ministers who felt that Walter Erb's lack of spine in dealing with the college had contributed to the CCF's problems. Lloyd also had concerns about Erb's efforts to convince cabinet to agree to the college's alternative plan in order to end the controversy and staunch the CCF's declining popularity.[21] Needless to say, this made Erb less than popular among his cabinet colleagues. However, as the minister who had introduced Bill No. 1, Erb needed to remain in place until the it was passed in the Legislative Assembly.

**The Demotion of Walter Erb**

The week following the provincial CCF-NDP convention, the legislature resumed. Although the government was also passing a major income tax bill in the special fall session, due to the expiry of the federal-provincial tax-rental agreements at the end of the fiscal year, it was the medical care bill that remained at the centre of everyone's attention. For five days, debate descended into heated invective and name calling.

Although Douglas was not physically in the chamber, he might as well have been, given his close association with the bill. In the event, he was referred to by one Liberal MLA as "that former, smiling, two-faced premier" who had deceived everyone into believing the medicare bill was unproblematic.[22] Thatcher claimed the government had pulled a bait and switch – that, instead of health insurance, the CCF-NDP was in fact introducing a regimented system of socialized medicine. The bill, according to him, was nothing less than the "conscription of the medical profession" designed to "put doctors into slave camps."[23]

Organized medicine used similar language, saying that while it was prepared to accept health insurance, the current bill amounted to the state control of medicine. Concurrent with the bill's second reading, the CPS passed a resolution at its annual convention stating that it would never agree to, or compromise with, the government's medical care plan. On the first day of the college's week-long session in November, CPS president Harold Dalgleish reminded everyone that doctors had "no intention" of negotiating with the CCF government on the bill or its implementation.[24]

The statement triggered an immediate riposte from the Saskatchewan Federation of Labour (SFL). In a news release, SFL president F.W. McClelland stated that the CPS "has apparently decided to revive the campaign of fear they started in 1960 (when) Premier T.C. Douglas announced that if his party was re-elected, they would establish a public medical insurance program." McClelland went on to say that, in effect, the doctors were "challenging democracy and [a] democratically elected government by saying they have no intention of negotiating with the government, and that they will not co-operate with the government to establish a medical insurance program." Although McClelland said that (consistent with the dissenting views lodged by federation's secretary Walter Smishek in the Thompson Committee's interim report) the SFL did not like some aspects of the bill, it would nonetheless support it in order to see medical care coverage finally implemented. The SFL then appealed "to all doctors of good will to take a stand and declare themselves against the obstructive tactics" of the college.[25]

Divisions were also evident within the ranks of the CCF and its supporters, some of whom were influenced by anti-medicare advocates. As discussed previously, mental health activists, including a number of psychiatrists and others working in the Psychiatric Services Branch of the Department of Public Health, had for years been advocating in favour of building a network of cottage-style psychiatric hospitals to replace the large mental hospitals in Weyburn and North Battleford, a program known as the Saskatchewan Plan.[26] Its strongest advocates were members of the Saskatchewan branch of the Canadian Mental Health Association, many of whom had strongly supported the Douglas government's improvements to mental health in the late 1940s and

1950s. However, when the provincial government decided to delay the construction of the first such facility in Yorkton in order to have enough revenue to finance the first year of the medical care plan, some of the association's most prominent spokespersons argued that it would be better for the CCF to focus on more pressing mental health needs before instituting any new health insurance program.[27] This prompted a *Leader-Post* editorial urging the government to "take time out from the frantic endeavor to push through the medical care plan" and instead "implement the Saskatchewan Plan and resume building the Yorkton facility."[28]

Meanwhile, another source of tension was developing within the cabinet, one that Douglas had managed effectively – by placing himself in the middle – until the national leadership of the NDP diverted his attention. On the question of medical care, the cabinet was divided between hawks and doves. The hawks felt that attempting to compromise with the CPS was fundamentally impossible and that Douglas had been too patient with the Thompson Committee, contaminated as it was with the college representatives. The doves felt that more time was needed for the committee to issue its final report and for the doctors to come to their senses.

Minister of Public Health Walter Erb was the most conspicuous dove, and the hawks perceived him as not being forceful enough with the college.[29] Douglas had given Erb considerable latitude in dealing with the CPS and the Thompson Committee, in part because he was so absorbed with getting the new party off the ground and making his personal decision on its leadership. However, by the late spring of 1961, Douglas and other members of cabinet had lost patience with Erb for giving the college the impression the government was willing to endure further delays.[30]

Since leaving the post of health minister in 1949, Douglas largely (but not entirely) had left the management of relations between the college and the government in the hands of his health ministers. Naturally, the doctors always preferred to deal with Douglas directly and, predictably, complained about his first successor in the position, Tom Bentley. After Douglas replaced Bentley with Erb in 1956, the relationship between the minister and the college improved, for the simple reason that Erb, unlike Bentley, wanted to be liked by the doctors and bent over backward to be agreeable.[31] This became a serious problem after Douglas's Birch Hills speech in 1959, when he first publicly conveyed the government's intention to implement medicare. As the conflict between the college and the government worsened, Erb became a weak link at best, and dangerous at worst, as he "always gave both the government

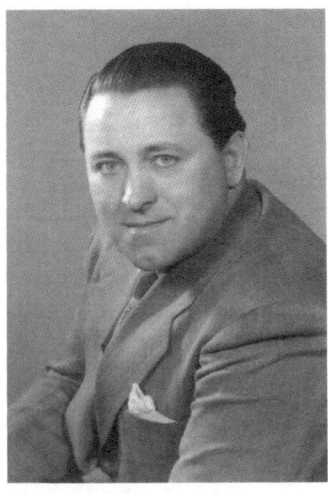

J. Walter Erb, Saskatchewan minister of the Department of Public Health (1956–62) (PAS R-A7933)

and the doctors the impression that the other side was ready to make concessions."[32]

Douglas's more hawkish ministers felt that Erb's spineless behaviour posed a danger to the government.[33] But Douglas would not consider firing any minister. His style was to keep ministers in place for as long as possible and let their deputy ministers – also generally long-serving – make up for their deficiencies. As Blakeney described it, "Douglas was never the heavy."[34] Woodrow Lloyd, however, had no intention of letting Erb continue in such a sensitive position.

Lloyd waited until after Erb had "piloted the bill" through the Legislative Assembly. The precipitating event was Erb's statement immediately following the third reading, where he raised the possibility of delaying the implementation date from 1 April 1962.[35] The statement appeared to reflect a government wavering in its resolve. To counteract that impression, the very next day, Lloyd moved Erb from public health to public works and the public works minister, Bill Davies, to health. Davies was the former executive secretary of the SFL, and his promotion was welcomed by organized labour as well as the hawks in cabinet but was condemned by the college.[36]

Despite Lloyd's efforts to avoid characterizing Erb's new position as a downgrade, public works had always been viewed as the bottom of the heap in terms of cabinet posts, and the daily newspapers characterized the move as a demotion.[37] However overdue and justified this decision might have been, it would set in motion a chain of events that would embarrass the provincial government and hinder Douglas in his capacity as federal NDP leader.

## The Weyburn By-election: December 1961

Douglas had been in political control of Weyburn and the surrounding rural area for over twenty-five years, first as an MP and subsequently as an MLA and premier of the province. Before his decision to leave the provincial scene in 1961, his position seemed unassailable. With his departure came a provincial by-election in Weyburn, which was set for 13 December 1961. It must have felt like a very safe riding for the newly nominated CCF candidate, Oran Reiman.

A small-town school principal, Reiman had also worked as an assistant in Douglas's office during three summers in the late 1950s, and the former premier spoke on his behalf during the by-election, the kind of support that, ordinarily, no amount of money could buy.[38] The Liberal candidate, the former mayor of Weyburn, J.H. "Jun" Staveley, had been defeated twice by Douglas but was heavily supported by Liberals, especially Ross Thatcher.[39] Upon his nomination, Staveley said his real target was Douglas, whose "influence has poisoned the province for too long," and the Liberals would, in this by-election, finish off "socialism in Saskatchewan" in the very place it had started.[40]

Three new factors appeared to suddenly change what should have been a sure thing for the CCF-NDP. The first was the ongoing struggle to implement medicare and the fact that the provincial government was losing the war of words with the powerful anti-medicare lobby of the doctors, the business establishment, and most of the provincial media. The second was the continuing dissatisfaction among older rural CCFers about what they saw as the NDP's unholy alliance with the unions and the downgrading of the influence of farm organizations. The final factor was Ross Thatcher and his diamond-hard focus on using the Weyburn by-election to hurt Douglas federally and damage the CCF-NDP brand in Saskatchewan. Portraying the Liberals as a broad anti-CCF movement, he managed to convince the Conservatives and Socreds not to run their own candidates in the riding.

At first, Thatcher tried to prevent the CCF-NDP from turning the by-election into yet another plebiscite on the medical care plan, a repeat of that party's successful strategy in the provincial election eighteen months earlier.[41] However, early in the campaign, Thatcher realized that sentiment was turning against the plan because of a threatened exodus of doctors from the province, and so he and the Liberal candidate soon began to use the fear and uncertainty that existed in many

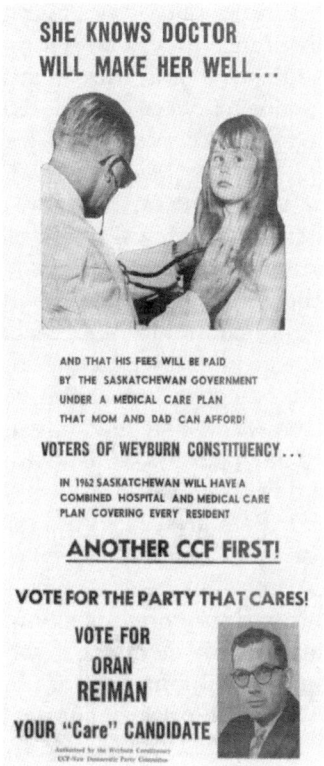

1961 by-election ad for CCF candidate Oran Reiman (*Regina Leader-Post*, 9 December 1961, 5)

minds about medicare to their advantage. Other prominent Liberals joined Thatcher to speak on behalf of Staveley, pointing to the growing discontent over the dictatorial manner in which "the socialisits" were implementing medicare.[42]

Even if he also sensed a shift, T.C. nonetheless continued to make the by-election a mini-referendum on medicare.[43] In a message filmed and then broadcast in the constituency in late November, Douglas stated that the by-election would "be watched with great interest by people all over Canada" because it would "be the first time that any group of Saskatchewan citizens" expressed "their opinion of the medical care insurance plan since" the provincial election eighteen months before. Moreover, since Canadians were "tremendously interested in the proposed medical care insurance program" and "anxious to see it copied in other parts of the country," they will want to know whether "voters in the Weyburn constituency" support the plan.[44] He urged voters not to support the Liberals, who were misleading the public by not being explicit about the type of prepaid medical insurance they would support. The fact that they voted against the medicare bill on third reading meant they really supported the college's alternative of subsidized private insurance. A vote for Reiman and the CCF-NDP was a vote for universal medicare.[45]

Speaking in the village of Creelman in the Weyburn constituency a week before election day, T.C. repeated his argument that Canadians across the country were ready to proceed with medical care coverage and were looking to Saskatchewan to lead the way.[46] The next day, in another tiny village in the constituency, Douglas said that the medical care plan was the only issue in the by-election, and he spent ninety minutes discussing its many features. He demonstrated its redistributive nature using a graph, explaining that 80 per cent of Saskatchewan residents would pay less than they were currently paying for private health insurance covering fewer services.[47] The next day, the CCF-NDP placed an ad in the newspapers stating that a vote for Reiman was a vote for the party that "will have a combined hospital and medical care plan covering every resident" in 1962.[48] Hazen Argue, the federal NDP's house leader (T.C. was not yet an MP), also toured the constituency to help Reiman. Argue too could not help wading into the medicare issue, stating that the province's doctors were watching the outcome of the by-election and that a vote for the CCF-NDP would be a vote of support for the medical care plan's implementation.[49]

Describing cafés, hotels, and motels crammed with MLAs, strategists, and workers from both parties, one veteran CCF politician and cabinet minister claimed that the Weyburn campaign was the most intense he had seen since 1935.[50] In an editorial criticizing the CCF-NDP campaign, with barely a mention of Liberal efforts, the *Regina Leader-Post* declared it "the most costly byelection campaign ever waged on behalf of a government in Saskatchewan's history." The newspaper's editors expressed their "hope the voters will not be bedazzled by the flamboyant CCF-NDP campaign in electing Mr. Reiman."[51]

In the end, the Sifton press need not have worried. Thatcher had been accurate in sensing a shift of sentiment during the campaign. When the votes were counted, Staveley won by a comfortable margin, 5,187 votes to Reiman's 4,317. T.C.'s mini-referendum had failed. With a front-page headline trumpeting "Staveley Captures Douglas' Old Seat," the *Regina Leader-Post* stated that the Liberals had finally ended "a reign of 17 years during which T.C. Douglas held the seat for the CCF."[52] The election result was less the product of a two-party fight than the fact that the CCF-NDP did poorly in the rural polls relative to the past. It is impossible to know the reason, but this may have reflected dissatisfaction among some about the direction of the provincial CCF-NDP without Douglas at the helm, concerns about medicare, or (as speculated in the *Leader-Post*) hostility towards the New Party project.[53]

The editors of the *Leader-Post* called upon the CCF-NDP to pay "heed to the voice of the electors and take a second look at its medicare plan," given the results of the by-election.[54] At home in Regina sick with the flu, T.C. shifted ground in an interview with the *Leader-Post*. Now downplaying the by-election as a mini-referendum on medicare, he referred to the 1960 provincial election as giving the provincial government the legitimacy to proceed, and he had "no doubt" that Lloyd would soon implement the plan.[55]

If the defeat had embarrassed Douglas or diminished his confidence in the public's desire to see medicare implemented, he did not let on. And if his faith in the CCF makeover and his ability to lead the new party was shaken – this was, after all, the first by-election since the inaugural NDP convention the summer before – he did not show it. However, as one editorialist put it, the by-election result had removed the NDP leader's "halo of invincibility."[56]

Mindful that a federal election was only months away, T.C. thought the Diefenbaker government weak and ready to fall. Until the by-election, he felt that the NDP was in the best position to pick up disaffected Diefenbaker voters, particularly in western Canada, and he must have been concerned about the possibility of a resurgent Liberal Party under Lester B. Pearson snatching away this possibility. Overjoyed with the victory, Pearson sent Staveley a telegram congratulating him on his "magnificent victory," a portent, he hoped, of a Liberal victory in the upcoming federal election.[57]

**More By-election Defeats in Ontario: January 1961**

If anyone thought that the Weyburn by-election was an anomaly due to the special circumstances of Saskatchewan, especially the perception of many farmers that the NDP was turning the CCF into an "eastern" trade union party, this was put to rest in the five provincial by-elections held in Ontario on 18 January 1962, in which not one NDP member was elected or managed second place. Even in the constituency where the majority of breadwinners were trade union members, with one of their own as a candidate, the NDP came in third.[58]

As in the Weyburn by-election, Douglas was directly involved in the Ontario by-elections, appearing in photo ops with the provincial leader and the local NDP candidates.[59] He used his experience in Saskatchewan to fortify the federal NDP's provincial election promise that coverage for physician services should be added to existing hospital coverage in Ontario. Douglas stubbornly thought that medicare was the NDP's political ace in the Ontario by-elections, despite the result in Saskatchewan. As he travelled through the by-election constituencies in Ontario, he asserted that the adoption of universal medical care was "the most important issue facing voters at this time." As the results demonstrated, however, the issue did not seem as salient to voters in Ontario.[60]

Just months after its founding, the NDP seemed stuck. As one editorial put it, the party's "bid failed all along the line, its representatives placing third in each case."[61] Hazen Argue spoke for many NDP supporters who were beginning to realize that formal union support for the party had not translated into votes when he noted that "even in Canada's largest industrial province, labor has shown little inclination to support a labor party."[62] This statement was the prelude to Argue's own defection to the Liberals.

Given the results of the by-elections, it is hard to understand why Douglas insisted on using medicare as the main plank in his national campaign to convince Canadians to elect an NDP government or at least to make it the official opposition in Ottawa. It would have been different if the medical care plan had already been implemented in Saskatchewan and he could point to its obvious benefits as well as demonstrate how so many fears about it had been mere phantoms. However, in the midst of a titanic struggle in the province over implementation, where hatred and panic were rampant, the timing was all wrong. In the Weyburn by-election, medicare had worked against both the provincial party and Douglas; in the Ontario by-elections, medicare could not be transformed into a salient issue, largely because it had not yet been implemented in Saskatchewan. Still, in part because of his considerable investment in the policy since 1959, Douglas insisted on continuing to use medicare as the NDP's principal calling card.

On Valentine's Day, T.C. used a free national party telecast to once again explain why Canada needed comprehensive health insurance. Arguing that if the federal government contributed 60 per cent of the provincial cost of universal health coverage, it would enable the addition of medical care, dental care, optical care, and prescription drugs to hospital care. Speaking to those Canadians who feared socialized medicine, he pointed out that the only difference between private insurance plans and the Saskatchewan plan was that everyone would have access to needed care under the latter, without "interference with the doctor-patient relationship." Moreover, doctors would be in exactly the same position as they currently were, given the retention of physician independence and fee-for-service payment. In other words, there was nothing to fear and much to gain.⁶³

## Hazen Argue's Defection

On the eve of Weyburn's December 1961 by-election, rumours were already rampant that Hazen Argue was about to quit the NDP and join the Liberals, rumours that he batted away by speaking in support of the CCF-NDP's candidate.⁶⁴ However, Argue had likely made up his mind to bolt from the party by the time he expressed his disappointment with the outcome of the Ontario by-elections the following January.

Tensions had mounted between Argue and Douglas on numerous fronts, including the question of Canada's remaining in the North Atlantic Treaty Organization (NATO). As he had argued at the NDP founding convention, Argue wanted Canada to pull out of its NATO membership. Douglas's position was more nuanced. While he agreed that Canada should exit the bilateral North American Air Defense Command (NORAD), T.C. still felt Canada required the collective security offered by NATO, given the ongoing threat posed by the USSR. The rumours of bad blood between the two got to the point that the National Council of the NDP tried to quell the talk by announcing that Argue would continue as house leader for the duration of the current parliamentary session. This statement hardly helped the situation, given the leaks from MPs and NDP party officials quietly telling the media that, if the differences between Argue and Douglas persisted, Argue would have no choice but to resign his position.⁶⁵

Argue did not bother waiting until the end of the session to bolt. On Sunday, 18 February 1962, he resigned from the NDP. Despite their history, the announcement came as a surprise to Douglas. Two days before, Argue had joined Douglas at a CCF-NDP Provincial Council meeting in Regina to map out the party's strategy in the impending federal election campaign. He sat between Douglas and Premier Lloyd at the head table at the banquet that evening. The next morning, the meetings continued, and he even went over to Douglas's home in the afternoon to work with him on how best to divide up their respective itineraries in the coming weeks. Argue and his wife then drove to Moose Jaw, where they spent the evening and night with Ross Thatcher. Argue and Thatcher knew each other well, from the time they were roommates at university and office mates on Parliament Hill when Thatcher was still in the CCF, although Argue had joined the rest of his party in condemning Thatcher's decision to quit the CCF and join the Liberals. Who better than Thatcher, then, to guide Argue through the divorce? The next day, Argue and Thatcher drove to Regina together for the pre-arranged press conference.[66]

Argue's departure was billed as a shock to the NDP by newspapers at the time.[67] For his part, Douglas was convinced that, during their meetings on Friday and Saturday in Regina, he and Argue had finally managed to reconcile and they were ready to work in tandem moving forward. He could not believe that behind the smokescreen of newfound friendliness and joint political strategizing, Argue had been working out the logistics of his exit.[68] When a journalist reached out to David Lewis in Ottawa to give him a head's up that Argue had arranged a news conference, an incredulous Lewis immediately phoned Douglas, who told him that, given the last two days of working with Argue in Regina, the rumour simply could not be true.[69] But, disastrously for Douglas and his NDP leadership, it was not only true, but the break was designed to cause maximum damage to the party's future prospects.

In his statement, Argue claimed that the "NDP has now become the tool of a small labor clique" that had put the revamped party under its "domination and control." He then described how the three most influential men in the party were the leaders of the United Auto Workers Union, the United Steelworkers of America, and the United Packhouse Workers of America, all affiliates of the Canadian Labour Congress.[70] At the press conference, Argue rejected any notion that he was disgruntled with Douglas personally, other than saying that if he had been leader he would have prevented control of the party falling into organized labour's hands, thus portraying his departure as a matter of high principle.[71]

The leaders of the main federal parties took some delight in the political chaos unleashed by Argue. Pearson solemnly declared that Argue had made very important points about the nature of the NDP, while Diefenbaker poked fun at the confusion among "the socialists."[72]

That Sunday, T.C. was forced to share a flight with Argue from Regina to Ottawa. According to one press report, they "sat 20 feet apart" in complete silence, neither one acknowledging the other, for more than four hours. When they arrived in Toronto, they "refused to pose together for photographers, and engaged in a bitter slinging match in interviews at opposite ends of the airport waiting room."[73] Douglas characterized Argue's rationale for quitting the NDP as "nothing more than a smoke screen to cover up his abject betrayal of his friends and his political party." In fact, "Mr. Argue saw no labor bogey-men in the NDP organization and administration until he was beaten by me in the leadership contest."[74] But in a subsequent statement, Argue would double-down on his critique of the NDP by stating that the "announced policies of the Liberal party contained as much reform as those of the New Democratic party," a view calculated to infuriate Douglas.[75]

Based on the editorials in all the major newspapers, Argue was winning the war over the narrative. Even the *Toronto Daily Star*, a left-Liberal organ read by the very people the NDP was trying to recruit, and a newspaper that regularly provided positive coverage on Douglas's policy efforts in Saskatchewan as premier, was overwhelmingly negative:

> Hazen Argue has dealt a severe blow to the New Democratic Party by resigning from it on the ground that it has become a party dominated by organized labor.
>
> Mr. Argue believes – and many Canadians, including this newspaper, agree – that the New Democratic Party is based on too narrow an appeal. It is, in effect, a class party, relying on trade unions for most of its financial strength. Canadians may fairly ask whether the new party will be free to adopt policies which labor leaders may regard as being against the best interests of organized labor.
>
> … The leadership of the New Democratic Party ought to ponder long and hard over Mr. Argue's indictment, for it reflects the views of many Canadians who are generally sympathetic to many of the aims of the party.[76]

When the NDP Constituency Association in Argue's Assiniboia riding in southeastern Saskatchewan demanded that the MP resign his seat immediately, Douglas was asked by the constituency to take his place. But by this time, he felt he needed to run in an urban seat.[77] He told the press that looking after a national party while attending to the needs of dispersed constituents in a rural seat would simply be too challenging, remembering the months he used to spend visiting his constituents while a federal MP before he became premier.[78] Argue then announced in the House of Commons that he wanted to run for the Liberal Party in his home constituency of Assiniboia. This ended the matter for T.C., as any direct contest between the two would simply have attracted more national attention to a candidate portraying the NDP and its leader as tools of organized labour.[79]

In the first months of 1962, every party was running a perpetual campaign while waiting for Prime Minister Diefenbaker to set an election date. Douglas had even announced to the press the previous November that he was reasonably certain that Diefenbaker would choose a date in June, a prediction that turned out to be correct.[80] Aside from a lack of resources – the financial support of the unions did not live up to its initial promise – Douglas was also having to justify the existence of a more labour- and urban-oriented NDP to the media and voters outside the party as well as to long-time CCF supporters on the prairies.

Given the bitter struggle in Saskatchewan over medicare, it was challenging in the extreme for T.C. to use the program to lure the uncommitted or the disaffected to his party. In this sense, the 3 May resignation of Walter Erb, his former minister of health who had introduced the medical care bill in the provincial legislature, did him more harm than even Argue's departure to the federal Liberals. The roots of Erb's departure lay in his demotion by Premier Lloyd months earlier. But also, like Argue, Erb had resumed an old friendship with Ross Thatcher, whom he had assisted during Thatcher's days as a young CCF MP.[81]

**Delayed Implementation**

The timing of Erb's departure could not have been worse for both Douglas and the NDP nationally and for Lloyd and his government provincially. At the heart of Erb's decision was a medicare controversy that soon attracted attention well beyond Saskatchewan. As the struggle between the government and the doctors intensified in the first half of 1962, media in the other provinces began to provide regular reports.[82] To understand Erb's resignation, we need to review the deteriorating relationship between the Lloyd government and the CPS in the weeks and months following Lloyd's assumption of the premiership.

Shortly after his appointment as minister of health in November 1961, Bill Davies phoned CPS president Harold Dalgleish, asking for a meeting to review how the medicare plan would be administered. Dalgleish said that unless the government was willing to replace its plan with another "within our principles," the doctors would not meet with Davies. As to Dalgleish's charge that the government had never consulted the profession on the bill before it was passed, Davies responded that the CPS was "well aware from past statements of the Government what the shape of the legislation would be and ... had in fact been provided with copies of the legislation at the time it was introduced in the Legislature."[83]

In early December, Davies followed up with a formal letter to Dalgleish, again proposing a meeting and pointing out that the government "would be glad to receive co-operation from the College on these matters and that we would prefer not to proceed unilaterally" in setting up the Medical Care Insurance Commission (MCIC), the agency that would administer the plan on behalf of the government.[84] Receiving no response, Davies went to Dalgleish's office in Saskatoon on 21 December, only to be told that the CPS's reply was in the mail.[85] Dalgleish then prepared and sent a letter, which, although dated 22 December, was not mailed until a week later.[86] The message was clear: the college had "decided it would be pointless to meet with the Government."[87]

Given the CPS's lack of cooperation, Davies "personally contacted several leading physicians" who "could not be accused of being supporters of the Government" to serve on the MCIC. While some showed interest and "even sympathy of the Government's desire to have an impartial commission," they refused.[88] To accept would be to incur the wrath of their colleagues. Some even told Davies that the college would come down on them "like a ton of bricks" if they agreed to work with the government.[89]

Consequently, Davies established the MCIC without college agreement or representation. For chair, he selected Donald Tansley, the head of the government's Budget Bureau, who had a known ability to deal with difficult situations and people. When asked if he would take on the thankless job, Tansley jokingly asked if it came with "danger pay."[90] To get doctors on the MCIC board, Davies had to reach out to two physicians with known ties to the government: Dr. Samuel Wolfe, an assistant professor of social and preventive medicine at the University of Saskatchewan, who had been consulted on the bill shortly after its introduction, and Dr. Oville Hjertaas, who had worked for the Health Services Planning Commission in the 1940s.[91] Both were staunch believers in what the government was doing and were prepared to be treated as traitors by the college.[92]

Shortly after the MCIC opened its doors, Tansley sent a letter to Dalgleish requesting a meeting with the college to work out an implementation plan.[93] When the request was rejected, Tansley sent a letter to all doctors in the province asking for input on the medicare care plan, explaining what the MCIC was trying to do and how the CPS had refused to meet. Very few doctors responded, and those who did said that the college spoke on their behalf. In the meantime, the MCIC continued to work on the administrative structure, but by late February, Tansley and his team realized they could not be ready for a 1 April start date. Though not happy, Premier Lloyd and his cabinet decided to delay implementation until 1 July and use the extra time to reach out one more time to the CPS.

Thus, on 2 March, Davies sent another letter to the college, indicating that the government would consider some changes to the bill.[94] Davies and Lloyd were "willing to discuss the Act and to consider specific changes" if the CPS could demonstrate "that they are required to protect the medical profession's legitimate interests."[95] Davies then announced the postponement in the Legislative Assembly. The news made headlines in the major provincial newspapers.[96] Davies's statement came only one day after Jun Staveley, in his maiden speech in the house on 1 March 1962, lambasted the medical care bill and the former premier "who was prepared to gamble with the health of the people of his province in the hope that he might stay alive politically."[97] The Liberals were on a roll, and, in response to Davies's announcement of the delay, Liberal leader Thatcher asked if the minister of public health could give the Legislative Assembly "any assurance that even on July 1st, you will get the co-operation of the medical profession to make the plan work." Davies assured the MLAs that he had "confidence that some arrangement" with the college could be made by that date, but nothing came from the CPS to indicate any willingness to compromise.[98]

In T.C.'s judgment, the delay was a major tactical error that could only serve to encourage the college to believe it could block the bill from being passed and thus reinforce its strategy of non-cooperation.[99] Reflecting on the episode years later, he felt the three-month delay gave the doctors "the idea that they could get it postponed a year or two years or three years." He admitted that, if the decision had been his, he would not have "budged" on the timeline.[100]

In hindsight, we can see that Douglas was probably correct. But the delay of three months pales in comparison to the earlier delays caused by the paralysis within the Thompson Committee purposely engineered by organized medicine. This strategy was evident when the committee was established early in 1960, at a time when Douglas presumably would have had the justification to abort the process due to the refusal of the CPS to participate. In other words, it was Douglas's insistence on the Thompson Committee that was at the heart of the timing problem. As Thomas and Ian McLeod point out in their Douglas biography, T.C.'s strategy to wait for a divided Thompson Report, just to show that he had consulted with the doctors, set the stage for the mess.[101] He could have relied on his interdepartmental committee report alone to prepare a bill by the end of 1960, which would have allowed it to be passed in the house early in 1961, with implementation as early as April or May of that year.

Perhaps Douglas thought Lloyd and Davies could have pushed back at Tansley and the MCIC the way he had pushed back at Fred Mott, the HSPC, and the Saskatchewan Hospital Association when they had begged for a delay in the implementation of the hospital insurance plan in the fall of 1946. However, the situations were different. The MCIC had even less time than the HSPC to get the administrative apparatus in place and had to do so without CPS support, while Mott and the

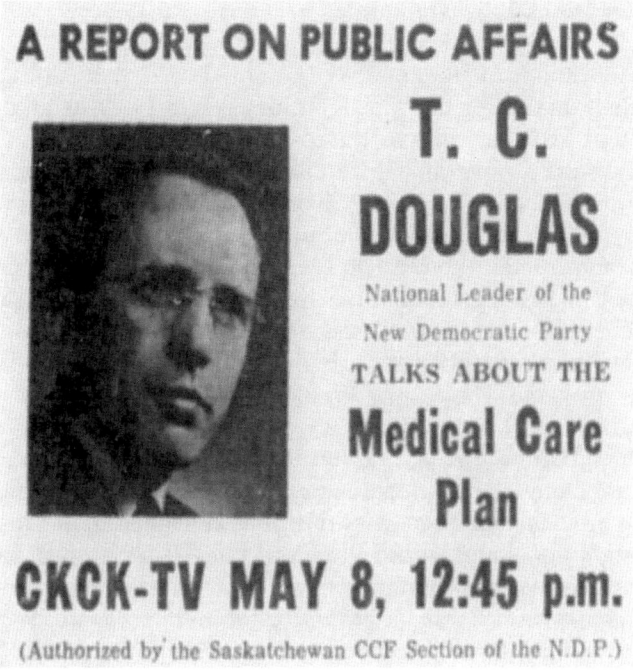

Newspaper ad for a Douglas television talk about the province's medical care plan, May 1962 (*Regina Leader-Post*, 7 May 1962, 2)

HSPC had dealt with a much more compliant and constructive Saskatchewan Hospital Association.

Without question, postponing the implementation date three months threw a monkey wrench into Douglas's strategy for the federal election. With an election likely in June 1962, he had hoped that medicare could be, by the time he was campaigning, a concrete illustration of what his party could achieve for all of Canada if the NDP were elected or at least given the balance of power in a minority government. Instead, he was left with a unimplemented plan that was being viciously attacked by organized medicine and business interests, and a confrontation that generated fear among ordinary Canadians. He spoke on the issue in dozens of speeches and public broadcasts, but his dream of universal medicare was being undermined by a mood that turned uglier by the day in Saskatchewan, exacerbated by Erb's resignation and ultimate defection to the Liberals.

## Erb's Allegations against Douglas

The delay in the implementation of the medicare plan is directly relevant to the reasons for Erb's resignation. While Douglas and the CCF claimed that Erb's action was the result of his dissatisfaction with his loss of the health portfolio, Erb maintained that, in fact, he could no longer countenance what he felt was the government's intransigence in dealing with the college, combined with his discomfort with the new pro-labour federal NDP. Erb's version of events, which spilled out gradually through the media after his resignation, put Douglas centre stage in the drama, and it was used by Douglas's many enemies to hold the former premier to blame for the doctors' strike that would soon shake the province.

According to Erb, Lloyd had asked him to the premier's office on 11 March. When he arrived, he found Douglas with the premier. The day before, Douglas had been in Regina to appear in a televised talk about the medical care plan as part of the NDP's national campaign.[102] In his resignation statement to Premier Lloyd, Erb claimed that, at this meeting as well as a subsequent one on 12 March involving the premier, Allan Blakeney, and a third member of cabinet, it was made clear that the government intended to proceed with the implementation of the medical care bill, even if doing so meant proceeding without the cooperation of the college. Given Douglas's earlier promise that no program would be implemented without the acceptance of those providing the services and Erb's belief that the province could "ill afford the loss of any doctors from the province," Erb felt it "necessary to abandon the Act" and come up with legislation "that would be acceptable to the doctors."[103] What was unsaid in his statement is that Erb was probably at both meetings due to the fact that he was the cabinet's leading dove in dealing with the CPS and there were likely fears of his breaking with cabinet solidarity, given the persistent rumours – denied by both Erb and the college – that he was privately meeting with the doctors.[104]

Immediately following the second meeting, Erb met with his constituency association and raised the issue of his resignation. However, according to the riding executive, "his attitude" that day "was one of self-pity" at the loss of the health portfolio rather than anything that Douglas or Lloyd might have communicated about their handling of the doctors.[105] What was most galling to Erb was the fact that Lloyd had replaced him with Bill Davies, a former union leader, confirming in his mind that the CCF had been taken over by organized labour. According to Erb, the riding executive pleaded with him not to resign and, after a unanimous vote of confidence, he agreed not to step down at that time.

What followed was a series of meetings between the college and the government, beginning on 28 March and 11 April, which seemed to signal to the college that Lloyd was willing to make major concessions. Yet, when the amendments to the act were offered in writing, the CPS rejected the proposals because it felt the government had preserved the essence of a single-payer plan, even if it had changed other key provisions to satisfy the profession. For its part, the government had, in its view, gone as far as it could in giving the doctors commitments concerning their continuing independence, additional influence over the MCIC, and new mechanisms and appeal procedures in determining "fair and equitable" physician remuneration, and even the possibility of direct patient payment to doctors with subsequent reimbursement by the MCIC.[106] The college's reply with its multi-payer counter-proposal – the "final concession," in the words of the CPS – launched a discussion within the cabinet.

According to Erb, Lloyd and the cabinet were on the threshold of accepting a deal when Douglas again entered the scene. He and Lloyd conferred privately. Immediately following the meeting, the premier announced that there would be no further compromises with the college and that the government would proceed with or without its support. While Erb's rendition of events does not match the documentary record or the recollections of any of the other members of cabinet, what is undisputable is that he resigned without notice at possibly the most embarrassing – and politically damaging – moment imaginable.

In the immediate aftermath of a failed meeting with the college on 11 April, Lloyd issued a press release stating that the plan would be implemented whether or not the doctors accepted the MCIC as the sole payer of their bills. However, to deal with the college's insistence that doctors would continue to bill their patients directly, amendments were introduced to the bill on 13 April.[107] One provision – the so-called agency clause – stipulated that if a resident were charged more than the MCIC-accepted fee schedule, the patient could make a complaint to the MCIC, which could take action against the offending doctor on behalf of the patient. From the government's perspective, the agency clause was needed to prevent extra-billing, but from the doctors' already paranoid perspective, the government intended to use the clause to "conscript" them into the plan against their will.[108]

At the time, Lloyd thought most doctors would ultimately accept payment from the MCIC, so he was concerned only about the minority of doctors who intended to continue billing patients directly.[109] For its part, the college responded to the government's proposed amendments with a more aggressive strategy of threatening a province-wide doctors' strike. To lay the groundwork for a withdrawal of services, it called its members together for a special general meeting in Regina on 3–4 May. Offices were closed to facilitate attendance, and approximately two-thirds of the province's nine hundred doctors made it to the meeting despite the short notice.[110]

Recognizing the importance of the meeting, the premier asked for an opportunity to address the doctors at the special meeting. The CPS agreed, aware that it had a golden opportunity to embarrass Woodrow Lloyd and his government. On the morning of 3 May, Dr. E.W. Barootes gave a "rousing exposition of the College's case," to loud applause. An even more thunderous reception was given to the announcement of Erb's resignation.[111] Lloyd had just walked into the hall only to learn the news himself. The resignation of first Argue and then Erb – two long-time CCF politicians – damaged both the federal and the provincial parties and raised some doubts about the leadership and perhaps judgment of both Douglas and Lloyd. To add insult to injury, these men would "cross the floor" to the Liberals in Ottawa and Regina and use their new positions to attack the Saskatchewan medical care plan. It must have been painful for Douglas to recall that, only six years earlier, he and Argue had shared a podium to support Erb in the 1956 election and, immediately following that election, he had made Erb his minister of health.

Woodrow Lloyd now had to face an audience that was not only hostile to his message but revelling in the personal and political setback caused by Erb's sudden resignation. Lloyd took his place on the podium and, in an hour-long address, urged the doctors to reconsider their position. The resident philosopher in the Douglas cabinet, Lloyd was no less so as premier, and he began his address with thoughts about the role of the state and its obligations:

> Basically the issue at stake is a very simple one. A common overriding objective is to promote and protect the health of our people. In meeting this objective a great responsibility rests on both government and the medical profession.
>
> I must say that I find disconcerting some suggestions that governments do not have such a responsibility and moreover are not to be trusted when they attempt to discharge it. Attacks on the integrity of government as an institution can undermine the foundations of the very liberties we prize so much – and can prevent the extension of those liberties.[112]

Lloyd asked the doctors assembled to question the tactics being used by their college:

I do not question your right to quit the practice of medicine or leave the province of Saskatchewan any time you see fit. I do contend that there is no need to make that decision a cause of anxiety to your patients.

If there are any here, and quite frankly I believe there are some, who have contributed to this anxiety in the hope that the government might then be forced to repeal the Medicare Care Insurance Act, I urge them to abandon that notion and the activities that stem from it.[113]

The premier then dealt with the crux of the issue, the distinct roles and responsibilities of the profession versus those of the government, in words that approximated those used by Douglas for almost two decades: "As patients" he explained, "we are perfectly willing to place matters involving medical judgments entirely in the hands of a highly-skilled group." However, "as consumers of medical services, and as taxpayers, have a right to a say in how we pay our medical bills," and we "have a right to construct an administrative agency, responsible to us, to arrange for such payment." This right exists because health care "is not an optional commodity – it is a necessity," and when "medical services are needed they should not, in the interests of each of us, be denied to any of us."[114]

Facing hisses, jeers, and boos, this moment exemplified Lloyd's courage and steely determination. Dalgleish then jumped to his feet to further embarrass the premier. Pointing out that certain (unnamed) members of the government did not believe that the college represented the views of the province's doctors, he asked the doctors in the audience to express their opinion concerning the government's medical care plan.[115] This brought almost all the doctors to their feet, applauding wildly to show their support for the college's position. In response, Lloyd simply suggested it might have been better for the vote of support to be taken after the doctors assembled had more time to consider what he had said. The government would proceed anyway, and those doctors who did not want to be reimbursed by the plan could always practise privately, as long as their patients agreed.[116]

**Preparing for a Federal Election**

In this dismal atmosphere, T.C. had to prepare his party for a national election, which he believed would be held before summer. Beyond the NDP's policy platform, in which comprehensive national health insurance figured prominently, Douglas had to sell his own image and style as a leader, made more important by the advent of television. The two

358   Tommy Douglas and the Quest for Medicare in Canada

establishment parties focused on promoting their leaders, contrasting their styles as much as their respective policy and program platforms.

The NDP and, before it, the CCF had always been a party of policy. Party members worked assiduously on comprehensive policy platforms months, even years, before elections, a process T.C. continued to encourage. The NDP was not immune from the political trends of the time, however, and the new party made Douglas central to the coming campaign. Its main slogan was "New Leadership with Douglas," a phrase "evocative" of the party's name. The PC team went a similar route with their slogan "The Man for all Seasons," while the Liberals were less focused solely on Pearson, with their "Vote the Pearson Team."[117] Whatever the differences in emphasis, all the parties tried to enhance their leaders' images through national tours with extensive television coverage.

T.C. was supported throughout by a tiny team made up of two of his most trusted people from Regina and one from the NDP's national office in Ottawa. Tommy Shoyama took leave as secretary of the Economic Advisory and Planning Board to become, as Shoyama described it, Douglas's research assistant, policy advisor, and, during the campaign, chief luggage carrier. In effect, he became the fledgling NDP's research department in preparing the details of the party's policy proposals and then the speaking points used by Douglas at every engagement.[118] Similarly, Eleanor McKinnon left the Saskatchewan Premier's Office to become Douglas's itinerary and correspondence organizer. Shoyama and McKinnon were joined by Cliff Scotton from the national office to manage the media. The fact that Douglas still relied so heavily on his former Saskatchewan employees reveals what he viewed as a lack of experienced personnel in Ottawa. According to Shoyama, Douglas felt there was more strength to be drawn on in Saskatchewan, so he did not hesitate to use it.[119]

Unlike Diefenbaker and Pearson, whose parties could afford to charter aircraft, Douglas had to travel economy class on commercial flights due to the poor state of the party's finances.[120] Elections always impose hectic schedules on party leaders, but Douglas and his team went beyond the usual craziness.[121] This is best illustrated by describing one week of his campaign, from 28 May until 4 June. On Monday (28 May), Douglas travelled 400 kilometres westwards by car from Regina (where he had flown just two days before to speak at events) to the town of Leader, near the Alberta border, where he spoke at a public meeting and a noon Rotary Club meeting. He and his team then drove 462 kilometres northeast to Melfort, where he spoke at a number of candidate events. The next day, he travelled to Flin Flon, Manitoba, where he

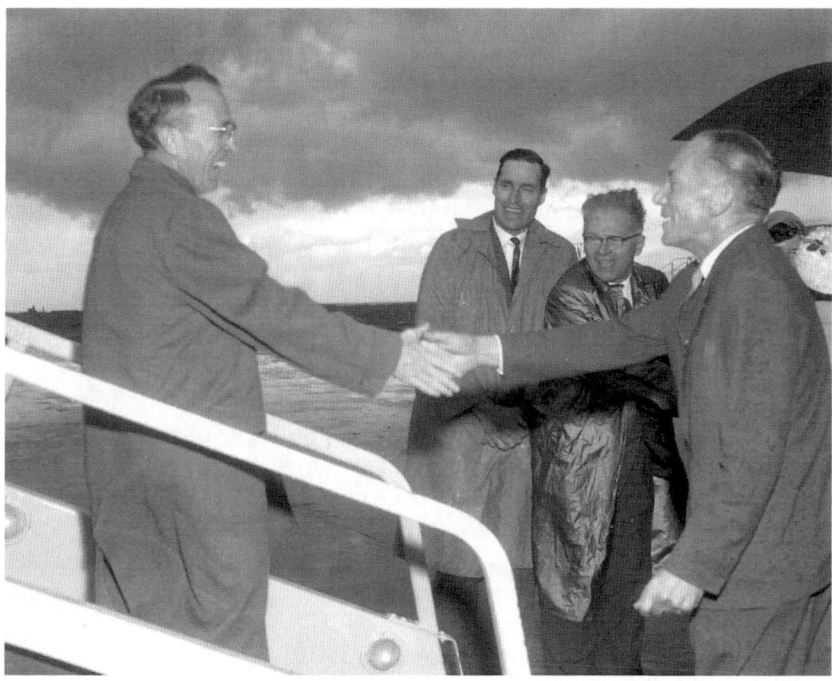

T.C. disembarking from a commercial aircraft during the 1962 federal election campaign (PAS S-SP-B733(2))

entered the city in a motorcade, and had an afternoon reception followed by a public meeting in the evening. Thursday afternoon he spoke in Dauphin, Manitoba, and by evening was back in Saskatchewan campaigning in the town of Kamsack. By Friday, he was back in Regina, to give the keynote at a Co-operative Commonwealth Youth Movement (CCYM) banquet. He had been prepared to rush off for his 8:30 p.m. all-candidate debate on the issue of nuclear proliferation at the provincial museum, hosted by the Regina Voice of Women, but the event was cancelled when the PC, Liberal, and Socred candidates turned down the invitation to attend.[122] Douglas's team still made their way back to the provincial capital, as the next days were filled with events in Regina, which T.C. felt he had to fit in before flying east to begin a speaking tour of the Maritime provinces beginning in Sydney, Nova Scotia.[123]

When his campaign team expressed dismay about what they felt was the growing opposition to the medicare plan within Saskatchewan and the impact this was having on their federal campaign, Douglas remained outwardly optimistic. To Shoyama's question of whether the provincial government might retreat from its commitment to implement medicare, T.C. said he was confident of the implementation plan because "Woodrow is there and Woodrow is like a rock. He's never going to get pushed around or going to give in."[124] In a television address on 9 May, Douglas promised that the Lloyd government would "stand firm" for as "long as we know that the people want a health insurance plan" in Saskatchewan.[125]

In all his campaign stops, Douglas retold the story of how health insurance had developed in Saskatchewan and how the battle for the next step of comprehensive medical care insurance was presently being waged there. He then expressed his complete confidence in the Lloyd government's ability to implement the plan, despite the doctors' resistance. He would end every speech with his optimistic prediction that, five or ten years after medicare was implemented in Saskatchewan, "there will be national medicare from sea to sea."[126] Federal NDP candidates faithfully relied on the campaign literature distributed by the national office, which also highlighted the promise of medicare.[127]

The NDP campaign brochure entitled "The Right to Health" included prescription drugs, dental care, optical treatment, and eyeglasses, in addition to physician care. An NDP government would contribute 60 per cent of the total provincial cost, a percentage that harkened back to the federal Green Book proposals of 1945. Addressing the controversy in Saskatchewan, the brochure explained why an extension of private insurance as promoted by organized medicine could never guarantee Canadians equitable access to needed health services. At the same time, the NDP vowed it would maintain freedom of choice for both doctors and patients and promised that medicare would never interfere with doctors' clinical autonomy.[128] The brochure ended with a smiling photograph of T.C., accompanied by a personal statement:

> There is in Canada today growing recognition that health care should not be a commercial commodity available only to those who are able to pay for it. The New Democratic party believes the time has come when doctors, patients and society generally must make the benefits of medical science available to all who need them, regardless of their income.
>
> The New Democratic plan for health care is designed to guarantee to every Canadian the right to health. With your support and co-operation the plan and the right can become a reality.[129]

With long-time CCF supporters, this consistently hopeful message went over well. On 17 May, Douglas told six hundred supporters in Regina to thunderous applause that the provincial government would never back down. He followed this up with a stinging indictment of the doctors leading the provincial CPS and the CMA, who, he said, "are not only a disgrace to the medical profession but also a disgrace to the human race." He then poked fun at the college about a rumoured purchase of another building immediately beside its existing headquarters, asking "What are they going to use it for?" and then offering his trademark humour: "A museum to display stuffed politicians' heads.'"[130]

## The KOD

Not surprisingly, the words and associated theatrics did not strike quite the same chord with undecided voters. As the campaign rolled on, the doctors and the anti-medicare lobby picked up considerable oxygen, especially after the provincial government announced the three-month delay of implementation. A movement known as Keep Our Doctors (KOD), with various local chapters and committees, had sprung up and was actively campaigning against the implementation of medicare.

The KOD campaign started as a series of petitions organized by mothers sympathetic to the arguments of their own physicians. These petitions demanded that the government "delay the start of the Medical Care program until an agreement can be made which is fully acceptable to the doctors of Saskatchewan."[131] There was a close connection between the KOD and the Liberal Party of Saskatchewan, especially with Ross Thatcher, who would figure prominently in all three of the KOD cavalcades to Regina.[132]

Some KOD representatives were CPS doctors or their spouses. For example, Dr. Noel Doig, a family physician who had emigrated to Saskatchewan from Britain because of his opposition to the NHS, flew back to Britain as the official KOD representative to "set the record straight" and to discourage the recruitment of British doctors by the Medical Care Insurance Commission.[133] The KOD movement took a page from the playbook of the American Medical Association (AMA), which offered assistance to the women's auxiliaries of physician and pro-market organizations in the United States campaigning against civil society groups supporting universal health coverage. The AMA's "Operation Coffee Cup" provided information kits to these women's groups, including posters and a "recording by actor Ronald Reagan speaking against the spectre of Medicare in all its forms."[134]

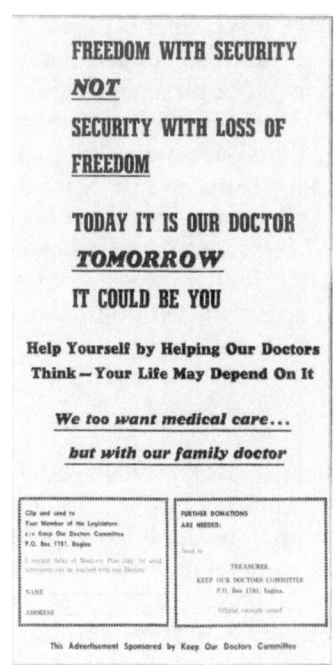

Keep Our Doctors ad attacking the Saskatchewan medical care plan, 9 June 1962 (*Regina Leader-Post*, 11 June 1962, 9)

After the CPS publicly announced that the physicians intended to withdraw their services if the government went ahead with implementation, the KOD gained membership. Everywhere Douglas appeared in Saskatchewan during the campaign, he was challenged not only by male doctors but, increasingly, by female members of the KOD. In the last week of May, when a Douglas motorcade drove through Regina for the benefit of NDP supporters waving from the sidewalks, KOD supporters booed Douglas and embarrassed him. Some put coffins on their front lawns while others, spurred on by the KOD, dashed towards the motorcade "to hammer at, spit at, or throw stones at the Douglas car."[135]

On 30 May, the same day Douglas was campaigning in Melfort, a KOD motorcade carrying banners for the repeal of the medical care bill travelled from Saskatoon, Prince Albert, Moose Jaw, Weyburn, and other centres to Regina. Once in the capital, the KOD held a protest in front of the Legislative Assembly building, one placard stating that "A Douglas Talk a Day Keeps the Doctor Away."[136] Although the ultimate crowd of 1,000 was significantly less than the 3,000 to 5,000 the KOD

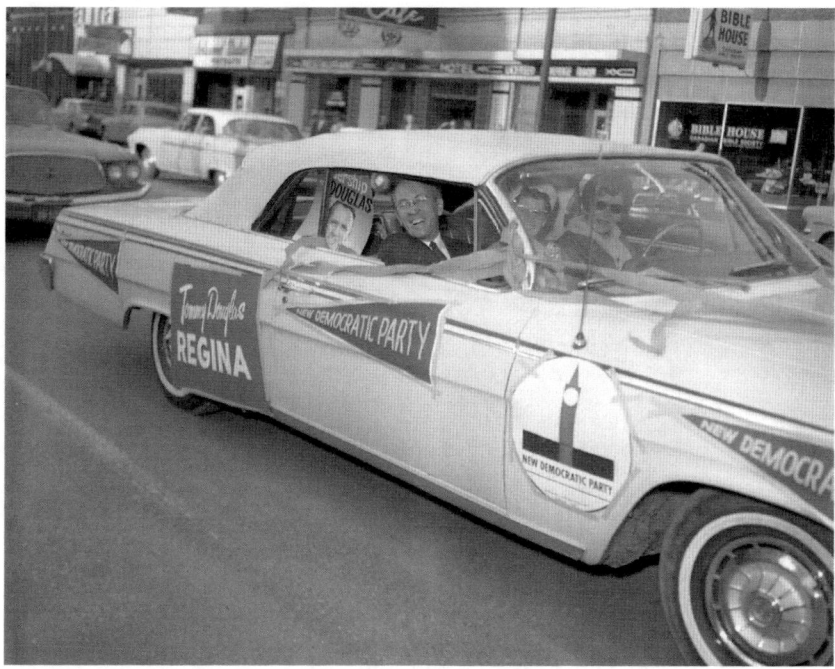

T.C. in a motorcade in Regina during the 1962 federal election campaign (PAS S-SP-B5228(4))

expected to show up, it drew significant press attention.[137] The KOD executive also secured an official meeting with Lloyd and some of his cabinet members. Both sides read prepared statements setting out their respective positions.[138] The battle lines were clearly drawn, with many in the KOD not simply demanding a repeal or delay of the act but a "change of government."[139]

After 30 May, the KOD set its sights on defeating Douglas and other Saskatchewan NDP candidates in the federal election. Advertisements in the Sifton press were headed "Tyranny or Integrity," pointing out that Douglas had not kept his original promise to make the plan acceptable to doctors.[140] Still, Douglas and his NDP candidates in Saskatchewan continued to push medicare, including Ed Mahood, the NDP candidate in Saskatoon whose 15 June advertisement in the *Star-Phoenix* stated that "only a Douglas government in Ottawa will give Canada a national prepaid medical care plan."[141]

> **Here Is Conservative Action on**
> # Medical Care
>
> (FROM THE "STAR-PHOENIX" JUNE 11)
>
> Toronto (CP)—Margaret Aitken, Conservative candidate in York Humber confirmed Saturday, June 9, that SHE HAS ASKED DOCTORS IN HER RIDING FOR MONEY "TO HELP DEFEAT SOCIALIZED MEDICAL CARE."
>
> Her finance chairman sent the following letter, June 1, to every doctor in the riding: "There is good reason to believe that OUR MAIN OPPONENT WILL BE THE NEW DEMOCRATIC CANDIDATE. New Democratic policies, including prepaid medical care, are not in the public interest."
>
> **A Vote for Conservatives Is a Vote AGAINST Prepaid Medical Care**
>
> **A Vote for Dr. Mahood Is a Vote FOR Prepaid Medical Care**
>
> Authorized by the Saskatoon New Democratic Party

Ad for Dr. Ed Mahood, NDP Saskatoon candidate in the federal election of 1962 (*Saskatoon Star Phoenix*, 15 June 1962, 2)

### Federal Party Platforms on Medicare in the 1962 Election

The PCs and Liberals put as much distance as possible between themselves and the controversy in Saskatchewan. Diefenbaker had satisfied the CMA by establishing the Royal Commission on Health Services, allowing the PCs to sidestep the issue in the campaign. In Saskatchewan, where, federally, the Conservatives were the NDP's main opponent, Mahood used a statement by a Conservative candidate in the Toronto area, who said that NDP policies, "including prepaid medical care, are not in the public interest," to argue that a vote for the PCs would be a vote against national medicare. While Diefenbaker was sympathetic to the idea of some form of government-sponsored medicare, many in his party were wary about, if not outright against, the idea. Even Diefenbaker's health minister, Waldo Monteith, told a convention of optometrists in April that there was no consensus among members of the public concerning the desirability of a national medicare plan.[142]

Diefenbaker focused more on attacking Pearson and Douglas as tax-and-spend socialists who must be blocked from gaining government.[143] On 24 May, at a PC rally in Regina that drew 3,000 supporters, the prime minister humorously queried why Hazen Argue, with his "strongly socialist views," had found a new "home so fast"? If Douglas ever became prime minister, he proclaimed, "he'd have the people of Canada paying almost as many taxes as those in Saskatchewan," and he posited that "the main issue before Regina voters is Ken More [the PC candidate] for responsible private enterprise versus Tommy Douglas and irresponsible socialism."[144] This was not the kind of rhetoric Diefenbaker used in more non-partisan events, especially in Saskatchewan. However, in a bid to continue attracting switch-hitters – those who voted CCF in provincial elections but strategically went with Diefenbaker in past federal elections – the prime minister preferred to emphasize the fact that he had implemented national hospital insurance.[145]

Pearson also played both sides, hoping to attract unattached voters who wanted health insurance. The Liberals were in favour of a targeted medical care insurance program that would be free for the unemployed, the retired, and children under the age of seventeen. Everyone else would pay a deductible amount, with public insurance covering everything above the deductible. In addition, a deterrent fee for each service would act as "a safeguard against unreasonable demands for attention." The Liberals stressed that their plan would only "be carried out in co-operation with the provincial governments and the doctors' organizations in each province," thereby avoiding the drama in Saskatchewan.[146] At a campaign event in Regina on 2 May, Pearson said that Liberal medicare would be fiscally responsible because of its targeting of the individuals who most needed it. Moreover, it would be a plan supported by the CMA and its provincial divisions. "I can't think," Pearson added, "of a more difficult project that the one in which the government of Saskatchewan has now got itself engaged – how to provide medical services without doctors."[147]

Ostensibly, the Liberal platform was based on the "Plan for Health" proposal initially conceived by Pearson's chief policy advisor, Tom Kent, and adopted by the party at a 1961 rally. The design involved free medical care, including outpatient prescription drugs, for all Canadians, but the cost of the actual services used would then be included as a taxable benefit, and individuals would pay based on their level of income, with the exception of children, the unemployed, and retirees.[148] The platform was vague – no doubt, purposely so – and emphasized that a Liberal government would discuss the plan with and get the cooperation of both the provincial governments and the medical profession.[149]

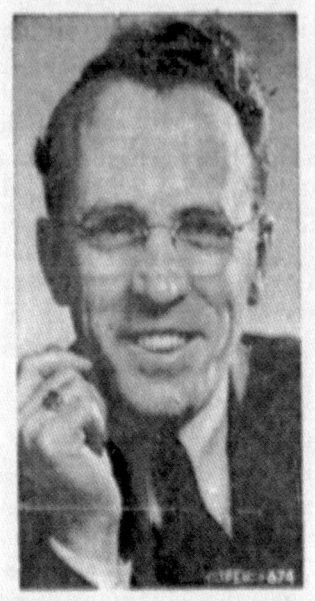

1962 NDP election ad (*Regina Leader-Post*, 9 June 1962, 8)

1962 Liberal election ad (*Regina Leader-Post*, 9 June 1962, 12)

Towards the end of May, Douglas urged voters to send at least 150 NDP members to Parliament so that they could establish a national medicare plan. He argued that neither the Conservatives nor the Liberals had "any serious intention" of setting up a comprehensive and universal medical care program.[150] In a column entitled "Medicare – Tory Obstacle," the well-known national journalist Charles Lynch repeated the Diefenbaker campaign team's gossip that "the little cuss" Douglas was trying to commit "political arson" with the medicare issue, but, if he could be stopped, then the PCs would carry all the seats in Saskatchewan.[151]

In an election television program entitled "The Right to Health: Medical Care and the Doctor," with the arresting byline "A Choice – A Change – A Challenge," Douglas did his best to keep the issue front and centre.[152] While he made it clear that there were other issues, he kept returning to medicare. At the same time, the PCs and Liberals were turning the increasing turmoil in Saskatchewan against him.[153] One journalist put it this way: "Mr. Douglas succeeded in making medicare his fighting ground, but in so doing he may be assured the removal of himself and his party – federal and provincial – from Saskatchewan political life."[154]

In Saskatchewan, where medicare was a major issue because of the ongoing conflict between the doctors and the government, it worked against Douglas and the other NDP candidates. In the rest of the country, medicare seemed unimportant compared to issues such as unemployment. The question remains, then, why did Douglas persist in his election strategy? In his reflection on the election, Shoyama could say only that Douglas did so because medicare encapsulated "the principles for which the New Democratic Party stood." Medicare embodied the idea that Canadians "who were well could help to look after people who had these needs and who were sick and no one should be denied access and that there shouldn't be profit in the health care system and that it should be publicly administered and therefore alive to the needs of people."[155] Yet the problem with this approach was that it was counterproductive in Saskatchewan and of little assistance in the rest of the country. Everyone, including Shoyama, could see that Douglas faced a backlash in Saskatchewan that grew with every day of the campaign. At the same time, Douglas could hardly have changed the channel, even if he had wanted to. He was the principal author of medicare in the province, so it was only natural that the fear and hatred would be directed at him. The fact that it had not been implemented yet made things far worse, in the sense that no criticism or fear, however unreasonable, could be disproven by the facts on the ground, as would have been the case had the program actually been operating by the time of the federal election.

By early June, the Lloyd government began recruiting UK doctors in earnest to replace the services of those expected to go on strike at the beginning of July. According to *Ottawa Citizen* columnist Don McGillivray, Saskatchewan was "meeting the federal election in a state of medical shock." He went on to describe the polarized atmosphere, where "you're either for the provincial government's medical care plan, or you're against it." There had not "been such a bitterly divisive issue in decades. Families are divided. Lifelong friends are no longer speaking to each other. Insults are hurled daily by both sides."[156]

McGillivray included T.C.'s edgy response that the doctors would settle down the moment the federal election was over and "go to the government and say: 'We've had our fun. We've done all the damage we can. Now let's sit down and negotiate.'" But in McGillivray's view, Douglas was responsible for the discord himself, by conducting a campaign in which he recited the opposition of organized medicine in the United States and Canada to every "advance in social medicine." By doing this, McGillivray claimed, Douglas was hoping to repeat the success of his party in the 1960 Saskatchewan election.[157]

And, in fact, Douglas regularly attacked organized medicine, whether the AMA, the CMA, or the CPS, during the campaign. He made it clear that his beef was with those who ran the professional associations, not the doctors daily toiling in their family practices, clinics, and hospitals. No matter, the headlines kept referring to his attacks on doctors in general.[158] As one of Douglas's most sympathetic biographers put it, his constant attack on organized medicine "may have given no comfort" to Lloyd, who was doing his best to find some kind of accommodation with the CPS as well as to lower the temperature in the debate.[159]

One of Lloyd's strongest ministers, Allan Blakeney, exclaimed publicly that organized medicine had become a "fifth political party dedicated to the defeat of Tommy Douglas."[160] For his part, T.C. decided there was only one course open to him and that was to strike back with all his force at organized medicine. The problem was that the fight with the "professional doctors," as Douglas labelled them, had spilled out into the general population. As Mary Batten, a well-known Liberal MLA, said while speaking on behalf of the federal Liberal candidate in Moose Jaw, Douglas had "brought the province to the brink of revolution and rebellion, and civil disobedience by its citizens." She also accused him of fomenting "class hatred" by attacking physicians as a group.[161]

The CPS and the KOD also directed their anger at Douglas, the man they saw as responsible for medicare. As a result, Douglas, even more

Political Repudiation 369

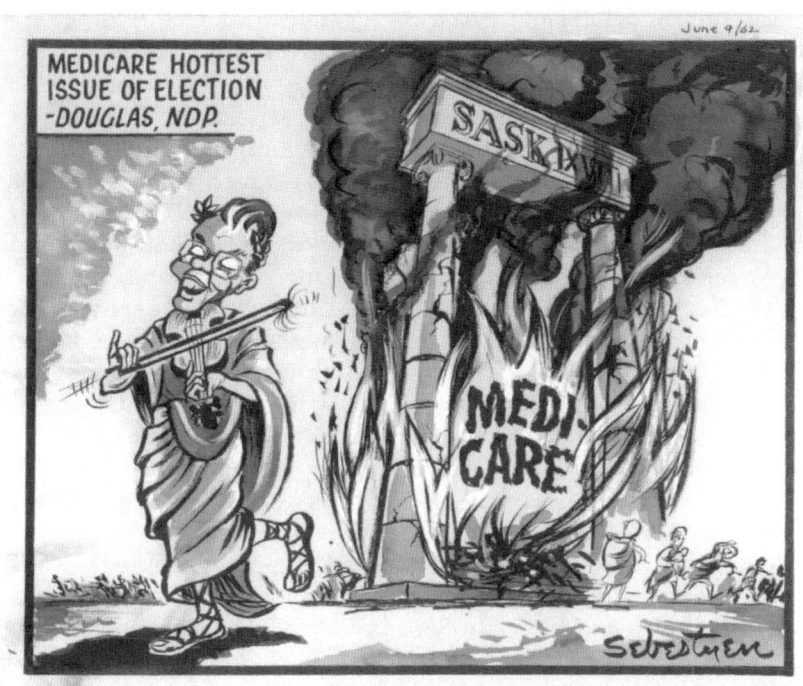

1962 political cartoon in the *Saskatoon Star Phoenix* showing Douglas as Nero purposely allowing Saskatchewan to burn while he makes medicare a key issue in the federal election (SPL IL-95-19)

than Lloyd, was the principal target for all those who were against the policy or feared the loss of their doctors. He received threatening messages on a daily basis. At home, Irma was subjected to menacing phone calls. Managing the office at Douglas's campaign headquarters in a shopping strip in Regina, Eleanor McKinnon recalled the climate of "hate and hostility" she encountered. In the evening, teenagers walked up to campaign headquarters and hissed at McKinnon and anyone inside through the glass. At the calvacades, people "shout awful things and throw things." When McKinnon was going home in a taxi later that evening, the driver, with five children and a sick wife, "blasted" medicare and Tommy.[162]

Ten days before the election, which was set for 18 June, in a campaign event to support a federal candidate in Moose Jaw, Allan Blakeney (unlike Douglas) kept his remarks on medicare to a minimum. He then admitted to the NDP supporters that Douglas was facing the fight of his life in Regina due to the well-orchestrated efforts of the other parties.[163] A husband-and-wife team distributing NDP literature on behalf of Douglas in one of the wealthier neighbourhoods of Regina were, after an anonymous complaint, accosted by a police patrol, who took their names and warned them they could be charged with "trespassing at night."[164]

Some NDP supporters decided to take matters into their own hands. When a member of the audience was not content with merely interrupting Douglas but began to yell profanities at him as he was speaking at a Saskatoon arena, the heckler was punched in the face by a Douglas supporter.[165] Three days before polling day, the words "Doctors Get Out" was painted on a prominent downtown wall, an image that made the front page of the next day's newspapers.[166]

After speaking to 7,000 people in Vancouver at the Pacific National Exhibition Forum mid-week, Douglas returned for the last campaign weekend to Saskatchewan, where he hoped he could prop up his provincial candidates and win his own seat.[167] The same day that the KOD ran a half-page attack ad against Douglas in the *Regina Leader-Post* entitled "Principles and Integrity Both Forsaken," his constituency executive released a statement charging that the Regina KOD was being manipulated "by some individuals behind the scenes with political motives," a statement that did not clarify whether this meant the Tories or the Liberals.[168] That Friday night, Douglas spoke to 3,000 NDP supporters at Exhibition Auditorium in Regina, where the "KOD staged a counter rally."[169] He received a standing ovation when he defended the provincial medical care plan and stated that the payment of doctors was the government's business and alleged that Ross Thatcher's Liberals in cahoots with the Sifton press were behind the "vicious and scurrilous" anti-medicare campaign.[170] The next and final night of the campaign, in front of a crowd of 1,300 supporters in Weyburn, he repeated his defence of medicare and attacks on the Liberal Party as well as Hazen Argue.[171] This event ended the campaign, and Douglas could do little more than recover from the exhausting months of travelling the country and the stress of contending with doctors, KOD protesters, and anonymous death threats.

His campaign team could not admit out loud what they knew in their hearts, that Douglas was going to lose. His media manager, Cliff Scotton, had a "strong premonition that Tommy was going to get clobbered." Unable to stand the thought of being with Douglas and the team in Regina on election night, Scotton flew back east the day before "on the excuse" that he needed to vote at home.[172] A veteran politician,

Douglas also knew the fate that awaited him but could not admit it to anyone, as part of the job of leader was to buttress the morale of everyone else. It was just too obvious that the fear and loathing unleashed by the medicare conflict would defeat him in Regina.[173]

## "I'll Rise and Fight Again"

When the election results rolled in on Monday evening, 18 June, they were disappointing for the NDP nationally, dismal for the Saskatchewan NDP candidates, and disastrous for Douglas and his leadership of the party. Winning just ten more seats nationally than what the CCF had been reduced to in the 1958 Diefenbaker sweep, the NDP gained slightly less than 4 percentage points in the popular vote, considerably less than the breakthrough it expected with urban and trade-union voters beyond Saskatchewan.

Even the Social Credit Party of Canada – resurgent in Quebec under dynamic deputy leader Réal Caouette – ended up with 30 seats, 11 more than the NDP, which had to accept its position as the fourth party in Parliament.[174] The NDP's 19 seats were far below the 40 to 50 that Douglas thought his party could and should have gained.[175] Diefenbaker pulled off another victory, although his PCs were whittled down to a minority of 116 seats, compared to 99 seats for the Liberals, double what they had won in 1958. The Liberals gained almost all their new members in Ontario, where the PC's popularity had plummeted, while in the Maritimes and on the prairies, Diefenbaker's Tories "buried the NDP, just as they had decimated the CCF in 1958."[176]

The NDP picked up 10 of its 19 seats in British Columbia but only 6 in Ontario, despite targeting the urban and union votes in that province. Not only had the union chiefs not come through with the campaign money needed to challenge the two establishment parties, but they could not deliver the votes of their rank-and-file members. The NDP share of the union vote was only 23 per cent, 2 per cent less than the PCs obtained, and 15 per cent less than the Liberals.[177]

The result seemed obvious, even to observers across the Atlantic. The British tabloid the *Mirror* celebrated the defeat of Douglas as a "victory for the doctors" against universal health coverage.[178] According to the *Times* in London, the NDP's difficult alliance between western agrarian socialism and trade unionists had not delivered at the ballot box.[179] A more accurate analysis is that, to some extent, the NDP traded in its agricultural base on the prairies for an urban, industrial base. The urban union vote in British Columbia and Ontario at least allowed the NDP to double its standing in the House of Commons.[180]

In Saskatchewan, the heartland of the old CCF, the NDP was completely shut out. The Diefenbaker PCs swept every seat, except one: Hazen Argue won for the Liberals in Assiniboia, despite a concerted effort by the NDP to make his duplicity a major issue.[181] Argue won because he was able to attract some long-time CCF rural voters in a constituency unhappy with the refashioned party and its links to organized labour.[182] By popular vote, the NDP was the third party, at 22.1 per cent, within spitting distance of the 22.8 per cent the Liberals won but considerably less than the 50.4 per cent the Tories enjoyed. In contrast to every other province, where the NDP saw increases in its popular vote relative to what the CCF had obtained four years before, in Saskatchewan the NDP experienced a painful 6 per cent drop in the popular vote, compared to an increase of 7 per cent in Ontario and 5.5 per cent in British Columbia.[183] It was clear that medicare as an election issue and Douglas as leader had worked against the NDP in Saskatchewan, even while the new party was making gains in more urban provinces.

In Regina, PC incumbent Ken More obtained an absolute majority of 22,164 votes, compared to Douglas's 12,736, while the Liberal (7,569) and Social Credit (1,583) candidates were left even further behind.[184] Fixated as much on defeating Douglas as on electing their own candidate, Liberal Party workers in their Regina headquarters on election night cheered as much for the re-election of More as they did for their own candidate.[185] More said that while he had tried not to campaign on medicare, he felt the issue was partly responsible for Douglas's defeat.[186] A more interesting comment on the election came from David Lewis, who had managed to take the Toronto constituency of York South from the Tory incumbent. When asked if he was pleased, Lewis said his pleasure was "marred by the fact that Canada has lost one of the greatest parliamentarians in T.C. Douglas." Although privately disappointed that the formal union connection had not paid off as much as he had hoped, Lewis publicly stated that the NDP had done "very well" everywhere, "except in Saskatchewan, where the doctors' campaign against medical care appears to have frightened the people."[187]

Douglas attributed his own defeat to the campaign waged against him in Regina by the anti-medicare coalition of doctors and the hostile coverage of the *Leader-Post*. For Blakeney, the minister in the Lloyd government who would be assigned the job of managing the press conferences during the looming doctors' strike, the fact that Douglas received only 29 per cent of the vote meant that the CCF-NDP "were losing the war of public opinion" on medicare in Saskatchewan.[188] When Douglas gave his concession speech on Monday night, he said he had no regrets, despite losing the election, and he told reporters he would "rather be defeated fighting for something I believe in than in winning fighting for something that doesn't matter."[189] To his grieving supporters, he quoted from Corinthians in the Bible: "We are troubled on every side, yet not distressed: we are perplexed, but not in despair; persecuted but not forsaken; cut down but not destroyed."[190] As for himself, he quoted the words of Irish poet Thomas Moore:[191]

> "Fight on my men," says Sir Andre Barton,
> I am hurt, but I am not slain;
> I will lay me down and bleed a-while,
> And then I'll rise and fight again.

As he had not lost an election since 1934, the defeat left – as Lewis observed – "a permanent scar" on Douglas, from which he "never quite recovered."[192] To go from a position of power, in which he was able to make substantive change as the key decision-maker, to the defeated leader of a fourth party in just a few months knocked the wind out of him.[193]

The pain of losing political office is a little like the death of, or divorce from, a loved one. No matter how much Douglas knew that defeat was part of the democratic process, no matter how much he prepared himself for the inevitability of losing, and no matter the extent to which he felt defeat was likely during the 1962 campaign, he nonetheless experienced it as a supreme rejection and saw his inability to truly launch the NDP as a personal failure.[194] However, as the leader of the NDP, T.C. could not afford to let bitterness and self-pity overwhelm him, nor could he admit these darker feelings to the party faithful. Irma felt differently. After all, the very people her husband had devoted his life to serving in the very city they had lived in since he first became premier in 1944 had rejected him. She wanted to leave the province, and Douglas announced that his family intended to move to Ottawa in August.[195]

In an interview shortly after the election, T.C. said he had "no thoughts at present" about his future in politics but added, "I will continue fighting for medical care. I will do so whether in or out of Parliament."[196] Both Douglas and Lloyd emphasized that the election defeat in Regina would have no bearing whatsoever on the provincial government's determination to implement the medical care plan.[197] When asked by the *Leader-Post* to comment on post-election demands by the president of the college for a complete overhaul of the medical care legislation, Douglas "exploded," according to the *Regina Leader-Post*.[198]

The college leaders who believed that the provincial government would back down after seeing the scale of its federal election defeat in Saskatchewan were soon proven wrong. As for Douglas's belief that the few men heading up the CPS would come to their senses after the election once they realized that the government was proceeding with its plan, he was also proven quite wrong. This respective steadfastness and miscalculation of intentions by both sides led directly to a three-week strike by doctors in the province.

# 13 The Doctors' Strike and the Cost of Peace

*This province has been sick. It has had a major operation. It is just convalescent. I prescribe for it absolute rest.*[1]
    Lord Stephen Taylor, after the signing of the Saskatoon Agreement, July 1962

Much has already been written about the twenty-three-day Saskatchewan doctors' strike in July 1962, an event well publicized in Canada and beyond, at the time and afterwards. The actions of the main actors – the provincial government, the College of Physicians and Surgeons of Saskatchewan (CPS), and the colourful mediator, Lord Stephen Taylor from Britain, have been well documented. However, the words and actions of the individual most responsible for the bill precipitating the strike were given much less attention at the time.

As a defeated candidate without a seat in the House of Commons, Douglas had little direct impact on the course of the strike and its resolution. But T.C. was still based in Regina, and he observed the fateful events swirling around him, a little like Banquo's ghost during the banquet in Shakespeare's *Macbeth*. Chiefly responsible for the bill and the design of the medical care plan, he was asked by the media to comment from time to time during the crisis. For Woodrow Lloyd and his ministers grappling with the explosive situation, however, T.C.'s occasional intervention may have seemed less than helpful. Lloyd's greatest challenge was managing rapidly growing polarization during the strike. He wanted to dampen the growing hatred of hard-core partisans by both sides, but this did not stop Douglas from attacking organized medicine when the press asked for his opinion.

The emotional tumult of the strike seemed to force everyone to take sides, and some wondered whether people in the province would ever, or could ever, return to normal. In his sermon at Lakeview United

Church in Regina during the strike, Reverend Reid Vipond told his congregation that he had "never known an issue that so divided people, or where cleavages were so deep, or where people were so certain they were right – on whichever side they" had taken. "Nor," he continued, did he know of "an issue where the consequences could be so grave, for the health and welfare – indeed the very lives of people." In closing, he reiterated a statement that had been issued by the provincial leaders of the Anglican, Roman Catholic, and United Church, calling for "the voluntary withdrawal of all inflammatory propaganda and demonstrations being directed at both the government and the college" and for "all our citizens to exercise steadiness and restraint."[2]

Another clergyman, a well-known Catholic priest and college rector, Father Athol Murray, had done the very opposite just weeks before. At a Keep Our Doctors (KOD) meeting held at St. Paul's High School in Saskatoon, he held railed against medicare and the CCF-NDP. Tearing off his priest's collar, his eyes scanning the audience for "Reds" (government supporters), Murray growled, "I can't see them" but "I can smell them."[3] He urged people to "get off the fence and make our views known. This thing may break into violence and bloodshed any day now, and God help us if it doesn't, or something else is done to stop the government."[4]

**The Strike Begins**

As the province was hurtling towards the 1 July deadline the doctors had set for the government to repeal of its medical care legislation, the NDP's national office was scrambling to find its leader a new seat in the House of Commons. Exhausted, Douglas let the rest of the party figure out a solution and instead went with Irma to their cottage at Carlyle Lake, a two-hour drive east of Regina, rather than fly to Toronto to attend the NDP post-election strategy meeting.[5] Within a week, the party had proposed at least three possibilities, but the one that appealed most was a relatively safe riding in Burnaby, British Columbia, where NDP MP Erhart Regier offered to resign to force a by-election in which Douglas would take Regier's place as the NDP candidate.[6] While Douglas, in his temporary office in Regina, decided whether this would be his best entry point to Parliament, he watched the doctors' strike unfold around him.

At the eleventh hour, the Lloyd government and the college made one more attempt to avert a strike. Between 22 and 25 June, there were four meetings between the two sides. Although Lloyd proposed detailed amendments to the Medical Care Insurance Act in a last-ditch

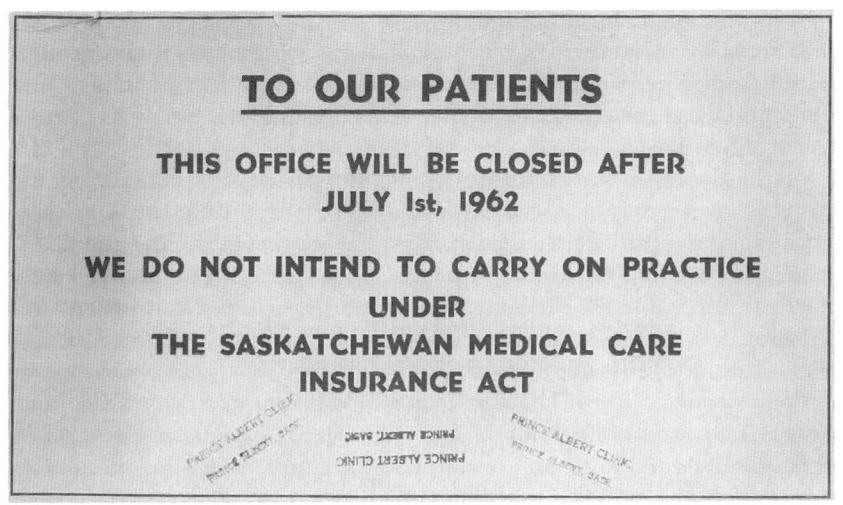

Notice by doctors of withdrawal of medical services (PAS, George and Tilly Taylor fonds, S(A998), file 496)

effort to address the profession's concerns, the only response was a written rejection and a lengthy critique of the government's entire plan, in turn eliciting a lengthy response from Lloyd.[7]

The provincial government, through its proposed amendments, was bending over backward to meet the doctors' demands, but the CPS, led by its president, Harold Dalgleish, and its registrar, George Peacock, simply would not accept any government assurances and instead demanded a new bill. The rigidity of the college was well reflected in Dalgleish's statement to the press at the start of the meetings: "We will tell the cabinet the present act must be substantially changed. This does not mean slight variations in the text of various sections ... but a complete rewriting of the act from the title right through the amendments."[8]

Despite the failed effort to appease the CPS, the Lloyd government nonetheless passed an order in council on 27 June allowing doctors to practise outside the plan, which required patients to seek reimbursement from the Medical Care Insurance Commission (MCIC) at the accepted fee schedule – a measure that not only inconvenienced patients and would allow extra-billing but was contrary to the principle that services should be free at the point of service.[9] Not wanting to undercut Lloyd, Douglas was silent on the issue. However, many CCF supporters saw this as a unilateral surrender by the Lloyd government, with nothing obtained from the CPS in return. Some began to take matters into their own hands. They established pro-medicare citizen groups, which issued newsletters to members setting out the benefits of a universal medical care program and the unreasonableness of the college's intransigence.

As 1 July crept closer, the college ensured that its members would provide emergency services, although these were limited to some hospitals in a few of the province's cities. The government and the MCIC feared the worst and began to recruit doctors from outside Saskatchewan to fill in for the strikers. The single most important source was Britain, because these doctors (unlike those from the United States) were automatically eligible to practise in the province, based on the college's historic rules. The lead recruiter was Graham Spry, T.C's longtime friend and agent general for Saskatchewan in Britain.

Saskatchewan House in London had long been in the business of recruiting doctors for the province, but it would now do so on a scale never contemplated or planned. Spry had already picked up the pace for permanent recruitment when he was joined by MCIC board member Dr. Sam Wolfe in early June. Wolfe was one of the most outspoken pro-medicare doctors in the province and would eventually co-author a book that chronicled the strike. A left-wing activist in the CCF who was knowledgeable about health policy, Wolfe was on friendly terms with Douglas.[10]

Sam Wolfe was born in Toronto in 1923, just two years after his Jewish parents had emigrated from an area bordering Poland and the Soviet Union. After serving as an X-ray technician in the Canadian military during Second World War, he received free tuition and a stipend to attend medical school at the University of Toronto. The Douglas government and its socialist agenda attracted Wolfe to Saskatchewan while a medical student, and he worked for a summer at the mental hospital in Weyburn and later returned to work as an intern. When he graduated in 1950, he moved to Saskatchewan and went into rural practice as a salaried municipal doctor. He then did a one-year specialization in psychiatry at the University of Saskatchewan in the program established by Griff McKerracher. Afterwards, he joined the faculty of medicine at the University of Saskatchewan but soon took a leave to complete his PhD in public health at Columbia University in New York.[11]

Having convinced the rest of the MCIC board and its chair, Don Tansley, that a major recruiting effort in Britain was justified "because there was reciprocity" between the two countries for physician licensing – allowing British physicians to practise in Canada merely by becoming a member of the elevant provincial college of physicians and surgeons – Wolfe flew to London in June to assist Spry in recruiting physicians prepared to practise in Saskatchewan. On the way, he stopped in Toronto to recruit Canadian doctors, including a young and idealistic physician, Dr. Theodore Tulchinsky, who would not only leave Toronto to practise in Saskatoon but would become Douglas's son-in-law when he married Douglas's younger daughter, Joan, who had been adopted in 1945.[12] Adding to the permanent doctors being recruited by Spry, Wolfe focused on hiring temporary doctors in anticipation of the strike. A week before the strike, after Wolfe returned to Canada, Spry pulled out all the stops to encourage doctors to move to Saskatchewan, including placing ads in newspapers and medical journals as well as hosting workshops and interviews for interested doctors.[13]

In response to the negative publicity being seeded in Britain by the CMA about the nature of the Saskatchewan health insurance plan, Spry contacted newspapers and provided news releases attempting to set the record straight. Beyond explaining the type and amount of remuneration doctors could expect in Saskatchewan under the new medical care plan, Spry enumerated the ways in which it differed from the National Health Service (NHS), challenging CMA propaganda, which described the two as almost identical. It was a delicate line. Of course, Spry was trying to attract doctors who believed in the merits of universal coverage; therefore some identification with the NHS was useful. However – and this seemed to be the more critical factor – Spry needed to convey to those less idealistic doctors who perhaps felt constrained by the NHS that, unlike the NHS, the Saskatchewan program was a simple health insurance plan in which both general practitioners (GPs) and consultants (specialists) could set up private practices and earn considerably more than under the NHS.[14]

The strike was the result of major miscalculations by both sides. Douglas always thought there were enough doctors in the province who would accept, however grudgingly, the inevitability of universal medical care. These doctors, many of them rural GPs, were pragmatic individuals who were genuinely concerned about their patients and could see at least some merit in making sure patients were not financially prevented from accessing care. These doctors, he felt, would push the leadership of the CPS to negotiate the best arrangement possible within the new scheme on their behalf. While recognizing that the "rich" specialists who dominated the college were adamantly against the government, T.C. continued to believe that rank-and-file GPs would attenuate the CPS's decisions.[15] However, to his government's great detriment, he seriously "underestimated the solidarity of the medical profession."[16]

If T.C. miscalculated, so too did the college, underestimating the provincial government's determination to implement medicare both during and after Douglas's tenure as premier. The CPS continued to believe that the government was bluffing and would collapse as soon as the strike began. The Lloyd cabinet would withdraw the legislation, the CPS assumed, rather than subject the province's population to a withdrawal of medical services beyond emergency services provided by doctors in a few select hospitals.

The day the strike started, Spry sent a message summarizing the situation to two influential British friends, Labour peer Lord Stephen Taylor, one of the originators of the NHS, and Richard Titmuss, "the high priest of the welfare state" at the London School of Economics and someone T.C. had already consulted with in London in 1960 to review his medical care plan.[17] The strike, Spry explained, was the fault of the doctors. Members of cabinet had met "representatives of the profession several times in the previous week," but the "compromises proposed by the Government were rejected or found insufficient." The real objective of the CPS, the government believed, was "to crack the medical care scheme and crack the Government." Although the government was "determined to stand firm on the basic principle of a universal, prepaid scheme," it nonetheless would remain "open to proposals which will re-assure the profession, particularly with respect to the point that private practice may continue."[18]

On day three of the strike, Spry sent a note to newspaper editors throughout the United Kingdom, inviting them to a news conference to explain the crisis from the Saskatchewan government's perspective. He also made a plug for more doctors, being careful to add that, while "a number" of UK doctors had been working on a permanent basis in Saskatchewan for years, the MCIC was "now offering to general practitioners and specialists in the United Kingdom (as well as elsewhere) short-term appointments of one to three months to fill vacancies created by the withdrawal of services."[19]

Journalists from the rest of Canada, the United States, and the United Kingdom flooded into Saskatchewan to report on the conflict. This was the first such strike in Canada and, because such occurrences were extremely rare in the rest of the world, it naturally drew considerable attention.[20] Until then, a withdrawal of services by doctors was almost unthinkable. Indeed, the college was emphatic that, because it had put together a volunteer roster of doctors to provide emergency services in selected hospitals in the larger centres, this action was not a strike. However, the CPS's emergency coverage was so spotty that most residents felt they had to go without medical services during the walkout.

Even media sympathetic to the doctors did not hesitate to characterize the event as a strike.[21]

The death of a child – along with allegations and counter-allegations about whether the strike was to blame – made headlines everywhere and was the top news story of the year in Canada.[22] The head of the Legal Medicine Department at Harvard Law School phoned Premier Lloyd and offered his services at no charge to investigate the child's death and any others that "might be related to professional negligence by delinquent physicians." Although he personally felt that "socialized medicine" was "stultifying," he also believed that "no doctor" had "the right to strike."[23]

Spry held a second press conference in London on 5 July to set out the nature of the plan being implemented by the Saskatchewan government, emphasizing that it was not "a State or complete Health Scheme on the British model, but a fee payment plan."[24] Again, Spry used the media to fan publicity for his campaign to convince yet more UK doctors to go to Saskatchewan to replace those on strike.[25] Most of these temporary doctors engaged in short-term practices in rural Saskatchewan, while others joined the rapidly forming community clinics.[26] These clinics were consumer cooperatives set up by avid supporters of the government's plan. Many of these advocates were in the left wing of the CCF and felt such the development of such clinics was overdue: they had long advocated for major reform of the way health services were delivered to the public, not merely in the way they were financed. Convinced that the government was too timid in its dealings with the college, and far too compromising in its willingness to accept the fee-for-service business model of practice, some community clinic activists wanted to forge a new model of primary care group practice based on salary, with the integration of other health professionals, including nurses and social workers, into cooperative clinics.[27] If the provincial government was not prepared to establish government-owned clinics with salaried doctors and other health professionals, as had originally been promoted by the Health Services Planning Commission in the mid-1940s, advocates would use the model of consumer cooperatives, long established in Saskatchewan through its extensive system of credit unions and co-op retailers, to pursue what they saw as a superior approach to health care.[28]

One individual who played a leading role in the establishment of community clinics was Stan Rands. Rands had joined the Psychiatric Services Branch (PSB) of the Department of Public Health in 1950. He was hired despite Stanley Knowles warning T.C. that Rands was a doctrinaire socialist and a "very apt pupil" of Watson Thompson.[29] As described earlier, T.C. and his education minister at the time, Woodrow Lloyd, had fired Thompson in 1946 for using the Saskatchewan government's Adult Education Division to disseminate what they perceived as Marxist propaganda. During the 1950s, Rands worked to improve the plight of the mentally ill and change the custodial model of mental hospitals to sites where treatment was provided and promoted. Along with his other PSB colleagues, he advocated in favour of a wholesale shift from large mental hospitals to community-based psychiatric treatment.[30]

By the early 1960s, Rands had become increasingly disillusioned with the Douglas government. As far as he was concerned, the original medicare bill did not go far enough. Although it improved access by ensuring that everyone's medical expenses were pre-paid, the bill reinforced the business model of medical practice based on fee-for-service payment to physicians. In his view, Douglas-style medicare kept the "authoritarian" doctor-patient relationship intact, "thus reinforcing capitalist class relations." For Rand, decisions concerning "the kind of care and quality of service" should be in the hands of patients and the community, not the "monopoly of doctors."[31]

Rands wanted socialized medicine in the way it had been originally conceived by Henry Sigerist, Mindel Sheps, and the State Hospital and Medical League, in which private physician offices would be replaced by public primary care clinics integrated with publicly administered polyclinics and hospitals. One development since the mid-1940s was of great interest to Rands: the rise of non-profit group medical practices in the United States, which combined primary care clinics with the specialist and diagnostic services offered in polyclinics. Group practices offered GP services in concert with those of other health professionals, especially nurses and social workers, as well as a few medical specialists, all under one roof. Whether owned and managed by a labour union or charitable foundation, these group practices employed physicians and other clinicians on a salaried basis, on the theory that doctors' own monetary gain should not influence how they deal with their patients. Rands would leave the government in 1962 to become the inaugural head of the Community Health Services Association, the umbrella organization for the community clinics in the province.[32] In his new position, he was able to work with community clinics throughout Saskatchewan to put into practice his ideal of a better health care system, going beyond the mere insurance coverage provided by medicare.[33]

Another individual who played an important role in the establishment of community clinics was Sam Wolfe. Impatient with what he described as "the timidity" of the Lloyd government in dealing with

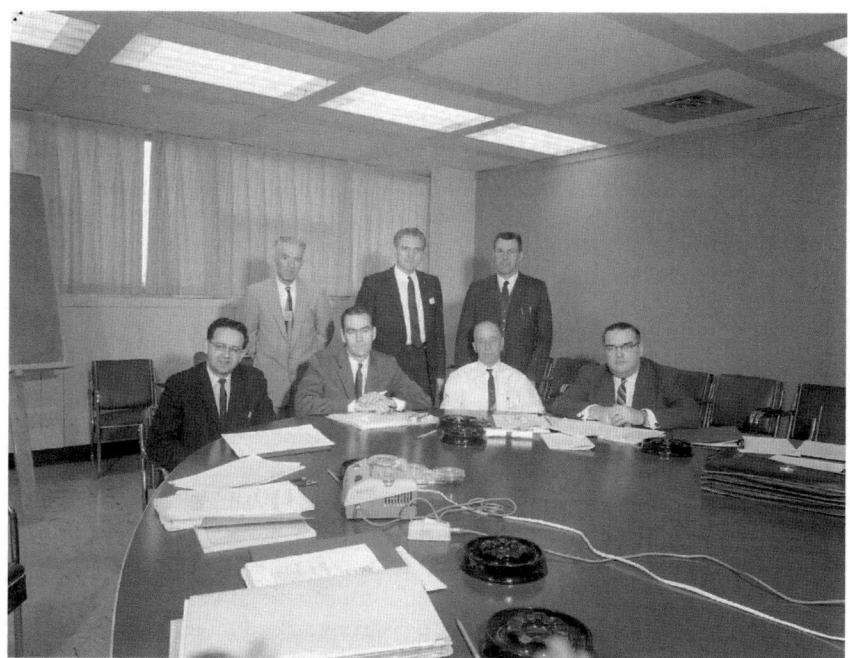

Members of the Medical Care Insurance Commission, 1962. Sitting (left to right): Dr. Sam Wolfe, Donald Tansley (chair), Stuart Robertson, Burns Roth. Standing (left to right): A.V. Kipling, George Taylor, Dr. Orville Hjertaas (founder of the community clinic in Prince Albert (PAS 61-817-01)

the CPS, Wolfe took direct action. He assumed the medical directorship of the nascent community clinic in Saskatoon, developing it into what would become the most successful clinic of its type in the province.[34] Like Rands, Wolfe wanted more than just health insurance, and was keen to set up a model group practice in the province. Another physician, Dr. Orville Hjertaas, who had worked for the Health Services and Planning Commission before returning to the full-time practice of medicine in 1946, was the catalyst in setting up a community clinic in Prince Albert. Like Wolfe, he attracted much opprobrium from organized medicine for his promotion of community clinics and his willingness to accept appointment to the government's Medical Care Insurance Commission. Rands, Wolfe, Hjertaas, and many other activists rapidly established twenty-five community clinics throughout the province during the doctors' strike.[35]

## The KOD Rally and the Arrival of Lord Taylor

Fascinated by this new and unexpected development, Spry carefully monitored the growth in community clinics from the United Kingdom.[36] The day before a London news conference he had organized in response to British interest in the developing doctors' strike, Spry had sent a note to the House of Lords to tell his old friend Lord Stephen Taylor that Premier Lloyd wanted Taylor to fly to Saskatchewan as soon as possible.[37] For many weeks, Spry had been pushing the idea of injecting an outside mediator to secure an agreement between the government and the CPS. Spry recommended Lord Taylor to the premier as the man for the job. Although a Labour peer who had been intimately involved with the establishment of the NHS, Taylor was moderate in his politics and highly sympathetic to the interests of the medical profession. Seizing on the idea, Premier Lloyd reached out – twice – to the CPS in the first five days of the strike to suggest a mediator. Although he didn't raise Lord Taylor's name, he had decided, based on Spry's description, that Taylor was best suited for the job.[38]

On 8 July, Spry updated Taylor on the medicare conflict. A supremely confident man, Taylor told Spry he would need only a week to mediate a settlement. Spry was struck by his friend's self-assured cheekiness but must have wondered if it were misplaced. Not only was the CPS refusing mediation, but even if the doctors ultimately agreed to a conciliator, would they agree to Lord Taylor? After all, not only was he associated with helping establish the NHS, but he was travelling to the province at the premier's request.

For his part, Taylor well understood medical politics, and he spoke to the secretary of the British Medical Association and the editors of *The Lancet*, asking both if they might produce an editorial that would make Taylor more "acceptable to the Canadian doctors." This, along with Lord Taylor's telegram requesting a meeting with Dr. Arthur D. Kelly, the CMA's experienced and highly influential general secretary, produced the desired effect on the leading voices with organized medicine in Canada.[39] A few days later, Spry drove Taylor to the airport and gave him all the money he had left in petty cash – $55 in Canadian currency.[40]

Graham Spry asked George Cadbury to pick up Taylor at the Toronto airport and brief him on the local situation for a few hours before his connecting flight to Regina. After retiring from the Douglas government in 1951, Cadbury had gone to work for the United Nations but then chose to move to Toronto when he retired in the early 1960s. Volunteering his time to work on national policy for the NDP, Cadbury resumed his friendship with T.C. when his former boss ran for the

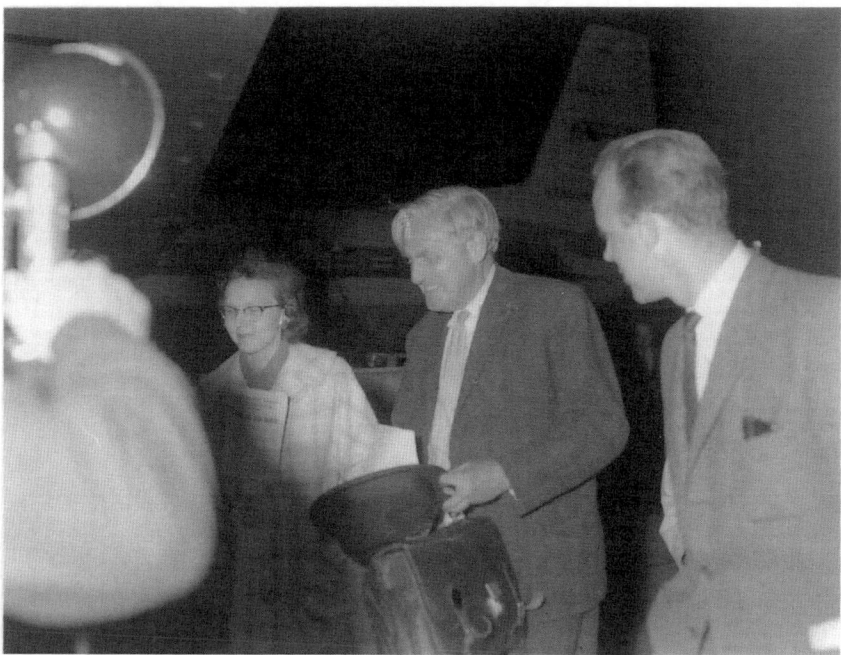

Lord Taylor arriving at night at the Regina airport, 16 July 1962 (PAS R-LP1841)

national leadership in 1961. The doctors' strike mobilized Cadbury, who acted as a listening post in central Canada, sending Douglas and his assistant, Tommy Shoyama, in Regina daily reports on how the central Canadian media were responding to the strike.[41]

Cadbury and Taylor took an immediate dislike to each other. Taylor found Cadbury too similar to the "intellectual Labour theorists in Britain," but he used the conversation with Cadbury to begin to understand what he described as "the true nature of the doctors' fears and the government's misapprehensions" about the doctors.[42] Cadbury confided in Shoyama that he was worried about Taylor's evident sympathy for the doctors and his egotistical desire to be the hero of the day by forging a deal between the two warring sides. The problem, Cadbury felt, was that Taylor might "force the government to make new concessions."[43]

By the time Taylor arrived in Regina, the city had calmed down just days after the most public event during the doctors' strike. On Wednesday, 11 July, KOD held a rally in front of the Legislative Assembly just a couple of blocks from T.C.'s home on Angus Crescent. To whip up

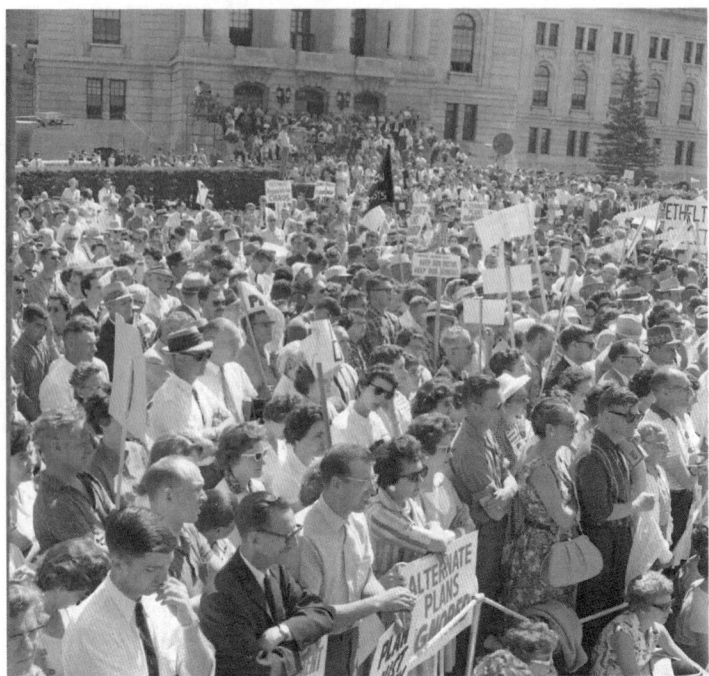

Keep Our Doctors rally in front of the Saskatchewan Legislative Assembly, 11 July 1962 (PAS R-PS62-229-25)

enthusiasm for the big event, the KOD had held public rallies and organized television panels throughout the province days before.[44] The rally produced great theatre. The crowd with their anti-medicare signs became iconic images of the strike. There were also anti-foreign and anti-Semitic effigies of doctors, a reference to the non-Canadian physicians who were being flown in by the MCIC to provide services during the strike. Effigies of both Douglas and Lloyd, with the caption "Down with Dictators," were carried by two women after being removed from a makeshift gallows.[45]

Those assembled in front of the legislature listened to speech after speech denouncing medicare, calling the newly arriving doctors from Britain the "garbage of Europe."[46] Douglas was very much on the minds of the protestors. In their petition to the provincial government that day, his election defeat was presented as evidence of the extent of opposition to the medical care plan, with the petition stating that "the former premier of this province expressly made" the medicare bill "the primary issue" in his federal election campaign.[47] Ross

The Doctors' Strike and the Cost of Peace 387

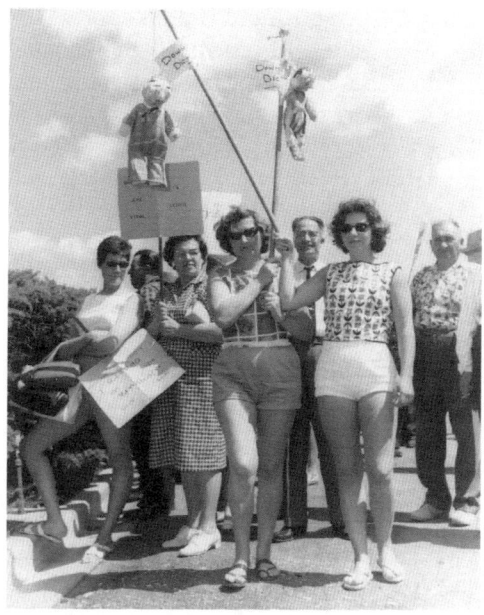

KOD protesters with effigies of T.C. and Woodrow Lloyd (PAS R-B3980)

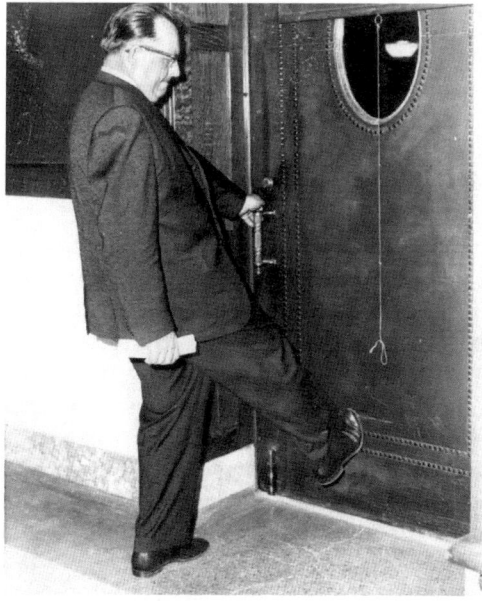

Ross Thatcher pretending to kick in the door to the chamber of the Saskatchewan Legislative Assembly, the day of the KOD rally (CP 2701055)

Thatcher demanded the government hold a special session of the legislature that afternoon. When Lloyd refused, Thatcher walked up to the assembly door and posed for a photograph, pretending to kick in the doors.[48]

## The Momentum Shifts

A few days after the rally, T.C. took the offensive, describing the withdrawal of services to the *Regina Leader-Post* as "illegal and immoral." Commenting on that newspaper's heavily biased support of the doctors, Douglas pointed out that the media in central and eastern Canada looked upon the strike with "repugnance and distaste" and hoped that the "good sense of the doctors and the public would bring an end to it."[49] As T.C. himself must have realized after his outburst, the momentum was finally shifting from the doctors to the government, and he no longer felt the need to restrain himself, becoming even more scathing in his attacks on organized medicine in the weeks and months ahead.

The KOD rally marked the beginning of the end for the anti-medicare forces. Expecting well over 10,000 people to join the demonstration on the legislature grounds, organizers were disappointed that only 4,000 people actually attended.[50] More importantly, doctors, particularly those who worked in smaller communities, were beginning to feel the disapprobation, if not the wrath, of their friends and neighbours for not providing services. To their patients' relief but the doctors' great discomfort, medical services were increasingly being provided by the 110 doctors who came, mainly from Britain, to work in the smaller hospitals not served on an emergency basis by the CPS as well as in the community clinics.[51]

The city specialists who dominated the college knew they would not be able to keep their members, especially the rural GPs and hospital doctors, on strike for much longer. For guidance, they consulted senior officials in the CMA, who, in turn, pointed to Lord Taylor and a compromise that would protect the sanctity of independent practice for doctors and keep alive the physician-based insurance companies. From the perspective of those leading the CPS as well as the CMA, the objective was to get the best deal possible in a way that would make it easier for a future government to undo the CCF's plan and replace it with a multi-payer form of medicare, which had always been organized medicine's preference.

The next opportunity for mediation between the government and the doctors was in Saskatoon, where the CCF-NDP provincial convention was being held, just a week after the KOD rally. Douglas had originally been scheduled to speak the same day as Woodrow Lloyd and Bert Herridge, the latter the NDP's new house leader in Ottawa. At the last minute, the president of the CPS, Harold Dalgleish, asked to have an opportunity to address the delegates, a request accepted by Lloyd and the provincial party, partly to reciprocate for the college's agreement to let Lloyd speak to its members back in April.[52]

The day before Douglas, Lloyd, and Dalgleish were to address the delegates, the forces in contention had assembled in Saskatoon. The doctors were assisted by a delegation of senior officials from the CMA, including Dr. William Wigle, the president-elect, and Dr. Arthur D. Kelly. Watching the doctors' strike unfold from his position as executive director of the Community Health Association in Detroit, Fred Mott had sent a telegram to Kelly the week before, urging "that responsible leaders of Canadian medicine exert influence to end [the] tragic strike in Saskatchewan" and that "unless service to people remains the guiding ethical commandment, professional freedom will indeed by [sic] endangered in both our nations."[53]

On next day, eight hundred members of the CCF-NDP's provincial council assembled in the Bessborough Hotel's main convention hall. Lloyd, who was the first to address the delegates, devoted his entire speech to medicare, making it clear that the government had no intention of backing down.[54] Lloyd reminded those present of all that had been achieved in Saskatchewan by the CCF under Douglas, including the free cancer care program, the air ambulance services, major advances in mental health services, hospital coverage, and the trial medical care program in the Swift Current Health Region. These programs, he argued, delivered "service and satisfaction" without discouraging "individual initiative" or creating stifling bureaucracies:

> On the contrary they have encouraged and supported research, they have made possible specialized training and special facilities. Money barriers – standing between problem and solution, between people and needed services – have been removed. They have received better financial support than would otherwise have been the case. The talents of the profession have been freed rather than hindered: they have been used in the interests of any person who can benefit from such skills. As a result lives have been saved, pain relieved and suffering alleviated. We have seen in these programs a more complete application of what has been called the "ancient wisdom" of the profession of medicine. It is this kind of freedom and this result that the people of Saskatchewan wish to extend by way of the Medical Care Insurance Plan.[55]

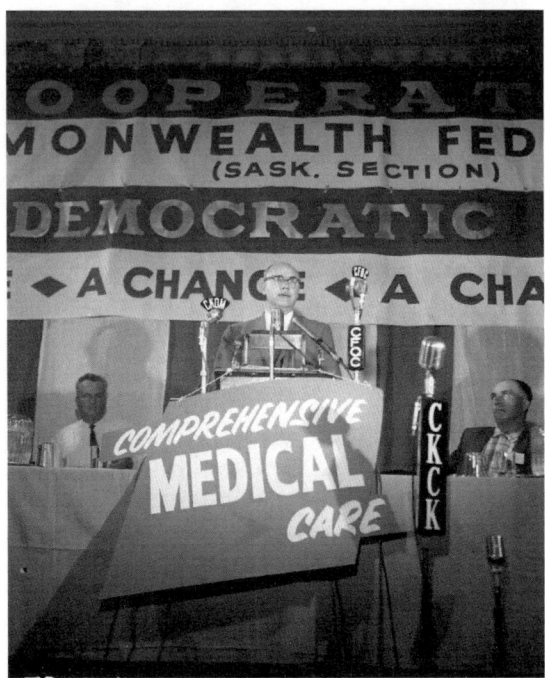

Woodrow Lloyd speaking (PAS S-SP-B52528(2))

Then, referring directly to the college and its efforts to have the government withdraw the legislation, Lloyd stated:

> There are those who are concerned not that the medical care insurance plan will not work but that it will work too well. They are concerned that if it does work it will become part of the warp and woof of Saskatchewan society. They are concerned they realize that satisfaction is contagious, that Canadian public opinion is on the move in this direction, that other provinces of Canada and areas beyond are watching carefully the Saskatchewan scene. Our answer to them is – give the Plan a fair trial. Then let the people judge in the light of actual experience rather than on the basis of suspicion without foundation in fact, or hysteria arising from fear. That's the way democracy works. That process should be observed and its results accepted.[56]

When Lloyd was done, he turned the stage over to Harold Dalgleish. His speech elaborated on written proposals the college had made to the government days before, proposals firmly rejected by Lloyd. These included the right of doctors to opt out of medicare and "assign to any agency" their "right to payment from" the Medical Care Insurance Commission, and permission for the two doctor-led insurance companies in the province to collect government-set premiums on behalf of their members. Then Dalgleish said something new: the CPS was prepared to negotiate, even if the government did not suspend the bill. It was clear that events had forced the college to alter its approach to the government, as some of its members, particularly family doctors serving smaller communities, unable to deny friends and neighbours or continue to live without any income, had quietly gone back to their offices.

Dalgleish well knew that the college's united front was beginning to collapse and that the doctors needed the most face-saving way to call an end to the strike. There were other factors that contributed to the CPS's new line as well. The government had called into question how the college, with the tacit support of hospital administrators and the Saskatchewan Hospital Association (SHA), was using its regulatory powers to delay the registration of newly arrived British doctors and blocking their ability to get hospital privileges. The week before his speech, Lloyd had sent a telegram to the college and the SHA, letting them know that he was ready to appoint a royal commission to examine their actions.[57] Underneath this lay the threat that, if the college were found to have flagrantly abused its power, it could have its powers of self-regulation stripped, giving the government the authority to step in as the profession's sole regulator.[58]

For T.C., Dalgleish's new offer meant little, since, based on what he had just heard, the CPS's position on the substance of the bill had not changed. No longer willing to contain himself, that afternoon he delivered before the convention the most stinging indictment of organized medicine and its allies yet heard.[59] To a chorus of cheering supporters, he "accused the doctors of undermining parliamentary democracy, of using propaganda, intimidation and blackmail and of punishing the sick, needy and helpless through their campaign against the government's Medicare Act."[60] He reproached Dalgleish and the CPS for not respecting the outcome of the 1960 election, an outcome that could not be used, as the college had, to support the proposition that a majority of Saskatchewanians were "behind the doctors," and he "condemned the doctors for pouring $90,000 into advertising during the 1960 campaign" against medicare "to help defeat the CCF."

Douglas accused the doctors of being the "cat's paws of the [provincial] Liberal party," with both groups using what he called "McCarthy tactics." Their campaign was abetted by the Sifton press in Regina and Saskatoon, which, before and during the doctors' strike, produced articles and editorials that were "dangerously close to causing insurrection." In his opinion, "the Sifton news media" had "reached an all-time low in a record that was never very high."[61] Both the Liberals and the doctors were fully supported by the KOD, the membership of which, he bluntly stated, read "like a roster of the Liberal party."[62] Their tactics were nothing less than an attempt to subvert democracy. "Fascism," he argued, "will come to this country not in brown shirts, or black shirts, but in dress shirts."[63]

Douglas then said he would have handled the doctors in the same way as Premier Lloyd, but "I don't think I could have kept my temper this long." He then suggested that Dalgleish had received a more attentive and polite hearing from the CCF-NDP than the one Lloyd received from the college at its general assembly months before.[64] Anger and extreme frustration were evident in his speech. These emotions matched those felt by many of the delegates who had fought for Douglas's medical care plan since 1959 and who had also endured much in the process, and they too had come to despise organized medicine.

While these emotions were understandable, given everything that Douglas had suffered at the hands of the college and its allies for over two years, this venting was hardly helpful to the Lloyd government, which had to find a way to end the strike and make the medical care plan actually work. There is nothing about T.C.'s speech or Lloyd's reaction to it in the biography *Woodrow*, written by Lloyd's daughter Dianne Lloyd, but the premier, who scrupulously refrained from using such inflammatory language himself and had done everything possible to discourage verbal or other retaliation by pro-medicare supporters in his own ranks, must have been left with some concerns about both the tone and substance of T.C.'s remarks.[65] After all, it was Lloyd, much more than Douglas, who had to live with the consequences.

## Lord Taylor and the Saskatoon Agreement

After his speech, Dalgleish returned to the Medical Arts Building about three blocks from the CCF-NDP convention. There, he and the rest of the college executive along with some CMA brass met with Lord Taylor. Pointing out that he was not being paid for his services by the government, Taylor emphasized his own medical credentials and his position as a person who understood the average physician's concerns, hopes, and aspirations.

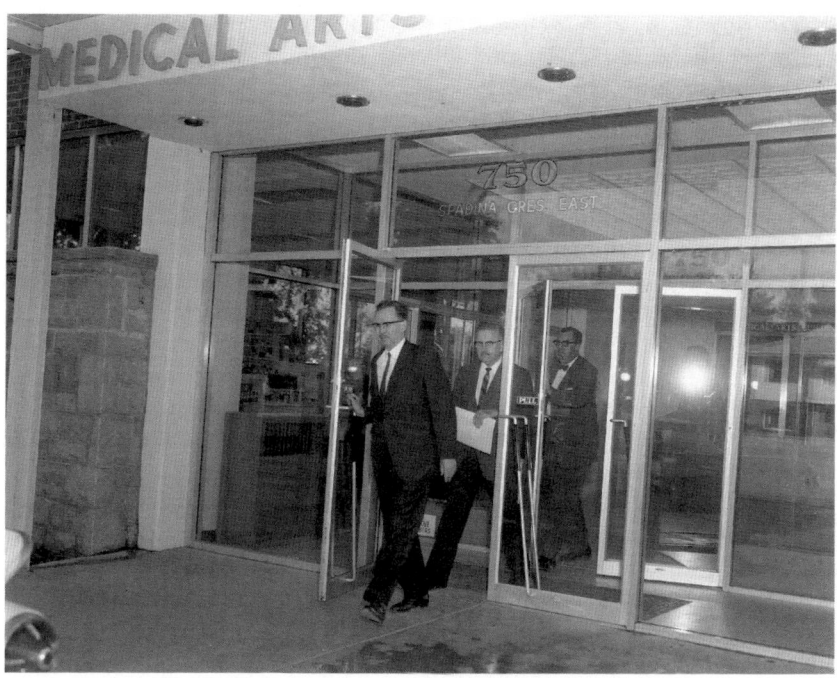

Dr. Harold Dalgleish, leaving the Medical Arts Building in Saskatoon just before finalizing the Saskatoon Agreement (PAS S-SP-BB134-4)

Dalgleish and the college had already been briefed on Taylor by Dr. A.D. Kelly, the CMA's general secretary, who told them that the British peer, as a doctor himself, could at least understand their perspective. Within minutes after the preliminary introductions, Taylor began to ingratiate himself with the assembled doctors.[66] Repeating what he had already told the media, which had thronged around him when he first landed in Saskatchewan, he admitted he had come at the invitation of the government but was receiving no money for his work other than a one-week fishing trip after he was done. He was aided in his efforts by both his appearance and his manner. Tall and patrician with his white hair and shaggy eyebrows, Taylor had the peculiar habit of stuffing his handkerchief in his mouth when he got excited.[67]

Kelly described Taylor's meeting with the doctors in a summary written shortly after the event:

> Although the guest could not be classified as a mediator, he immediately began to act as one. He told the Council what he had learned in his

brief stay in Saskatchewan and very skillfully dissected the essentials of Dr. Dalgleish's speech. He said that as a doctor he was in favour of the new proposals which established a useful function of the prepaid [Medical Services Incorporated and Group Medical Services] plans and that he would endeavour to convince the Premier and the Cabinet of their merits. As a politician he doubted that government would agree to the plans acting as tax collectors and advised the Council not to press the point. By sheer force of an attractive and aggressive personality he rapidly reached the stage where Council was agreeing to his transmission of the doctors' case to Government and after two hours of discussion he departed to do just that.[68]

After his first session with the college, Lord Taylor returned to the Bessborough Hotel, where he proceeded to convince the provincial government to allow Medical Services Incorporated (MSI) and Group Medical Services (GMS) to be used to reimburse doctors. The government agreed, as long as it remained the sole source of financing and the sole determiner of the terms of medical care coverage. As language was found acceptable to both sides, Taylor began to move more quickly between the cabinet and its chief officials hunkered down in the stately Bessborough and the college mere blocks away at the newly constructed modernist Medicare Arts Building. During it all, Taylor used histrionics to get each side to give up something here and something there. To some extent, his behaviour broke the tension and relieved at least some of the anxiety that had descended on both sides during the many months of epic struggle. In a four-part series for the *Canadian Medical Association Journal* in 1974, Lord Taylor clearly revelled in his own antics: "Every now and then I exploded with violent wrath and the strongest possible language. I think there were a number among the doctors and among the cabinet who enjoyed these episodes far more than I did. Both sides thought I was hamming it up, and in the end I got a pseudo-Oscar ... for my acting ability from 'my chums and mates of the Saskatchewan Government.' This was quite undeserved! I was just being my natural self."[69]

As Lord Taylor was going back and forth between the government team and the doctors, T.C. boarded an airplane to attend a meeting of the NDP executive being held in Kingston, Ontario.[70] While Douglas, of course, had no direct role in these negotiations, he remained in close touch with Lloyd and his old team, especially Tommy Shoyama. Although Shoyama had left the NDP to return to the Lloyd government a few weeks after the June federal election, he continued to work during his free time on a voluntary basis for Douglas for many months,

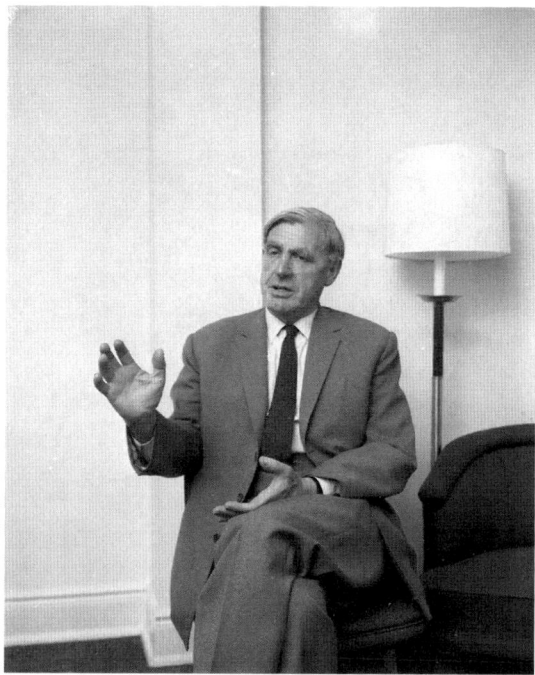

Lord Taylor in Saskatoon (PAS S-SP-B5315(2))

presumably with Lloyd's blessing. Barely taking a break after Douglas's shattering federal election bid, Shoyama carefully assessed the strengths and weaknesses of the Saskatchewan government's proposal and the CPS's counterproposal in that frantic week leading up to the 1 July deadline.[71]

Once the strike began, Shoyama was part of an elite team assembled by Lloyd to strategize his cabinet's strike management. This tiny group was then assigned to work with Taylor on the many draft proposals of what would soon become known as the Saskatoon Agreement. During the strike, Shoyama received daily reports on the situation, especially the extent to which the airlift of British doctors was filling the gaps left by the strikers, information that he shared regularly with both Douglas and George Cadbury.[72] The other three key members of Lloyd's strike strategy committee were Al Johnson, Don Tansley, and Dr. Graham Clarkson. Johnson had just returned to his position as deputy provincial treasurer after an extended leave to do his PhD at Harvard.[73] Tansley had worked for years as second-in-command to Johnson in the

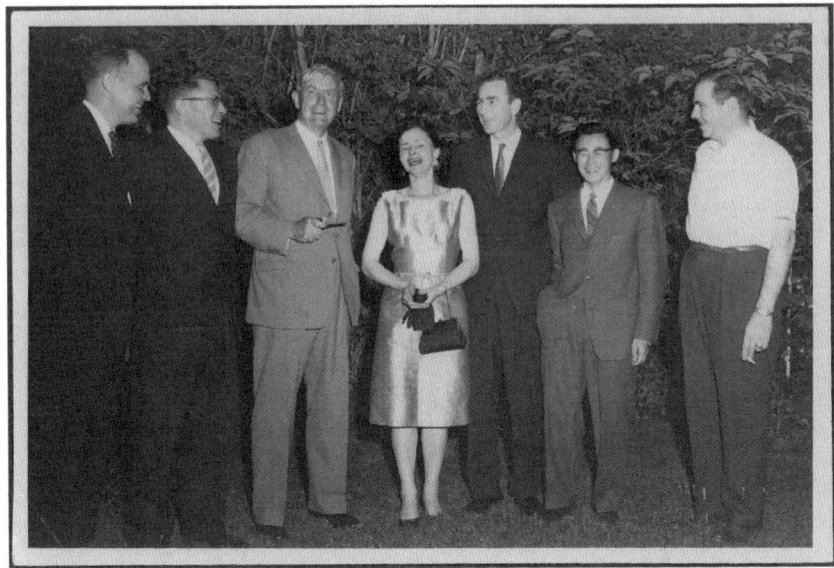

Lord Taylor with government strategists Al Johnson (second from left), Don Tansley (fifth from left), Tommy Shoyama (sixth from left), and Tim Lee (far right) (LAC, A.W. Johnson fonds, R12503, vol. 38, photo no. 31)

treasury department, but now, as MCIC chair, he was responsible for getting the plan implemented. Tansley, in turn, depended on Clarkson, who had been seconded from the Department of Public Health to serve as the MCIC's medical director.

Shoyama, Johnson, Tansley, and Clarkson were chiefly responsible for the drafting of the Saskatoon Agreement.[74] For days following the CCF-NDP convention, Shoyama and his colleagues were ensconced in the Bessborough Hotel editing a provisional agreement that Lord Taylor was conveying back and forth with the doctors at the Medical Arts Building.

### The Legacy of the Saskatoon Agreement

In the end, the doctors obtained important concessions. They were able to be paid in four different ways. The first option involved them being reimbursed directly by the government through the MCIC, the approach intended by Douglas in the original medicare bill. The second

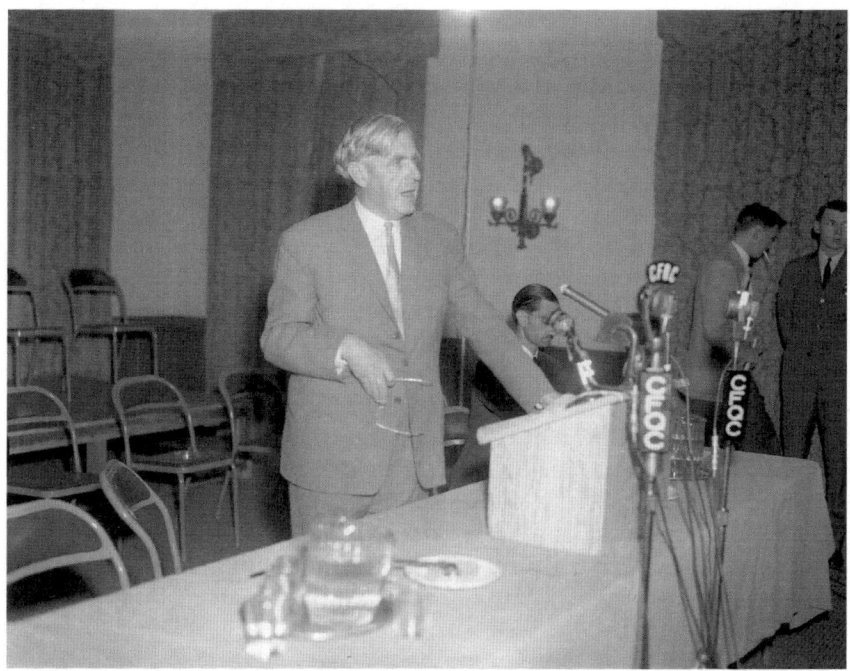

Lord Taylor, with Graham Clarkson in the background, at a Saskatoon Agreement news conference (PAS S-SP-B5134-7)

option involved the right by doctors to be reimbursed by one (or more) of the three private insurance carriers, the two largest of which were the physician-based MSI and GMS companies. Two other options were available to physicians who wanted to opt out of both the government plan and the voluntary plans. In both cases, the patient would pay the physician directly, but, in the third option, the doctor would provide the necessary information so that the patient could be reimbursed by the MCIC. In the fourth option, both physician and patient would agree to direct payment without reimbursement.[75]

This choice-of-payment concession gave doctors two things: the right to opt out of the plan and, not as obviously, the right to extra-bill patients. Douglas had few problems with opting out, believing doctors should have such a right if they practised entirely outside the medicare system and were in no way subsidized by public taxation. However, he felt that extra-billing was inimical to universal access and that it should never have been allowed.

To explain how extra-billing was implied in the Saskatoon Agreement requires further analysis of the options. In the first payment option, doctors could participate directly in the plan by seeking reimbursement for patient fees, which were set at 85 per cent of the CPS fee schedule, since doctors no longer had to pursue patients for payment. In the second and third options, doctors could opt out of dealing with the government or the MCIC in any way, leaving this task to the patient. Both of these options offered doctors the possibility of extra-billing their patients by charging the full amount of the fee in the fee-for-service (FFS) schedule, a practice that was neither prohibited nor set out as an explicit right.[76] The implicit right to charge above the agreed tariff turned out to be the more permanent concession, one that would be taken full advantage of by the Thatcher administration after the defeat of the Lloyd government in May 1964. Permanently opposed to user fees, Douglas was irked by this provision because it posed a potential financial barrier to access. As will be seen, Douglas would fight extra-billing for the next two decades and would support the provisions in the Canada Health Act of 1984 that finally penalized provincial governments that continued to permit physician extra-billing and hospital user charges.[77]

In the second payment option, there was no getting around the fact that doctors were de facto accepting payment from the government. Although they received cheques from the insurance carriers, MSI and GMS were not in fact writing or controlling independent health insurance policies. They simply acted as a pass-through or a post office, and, within a few years, due to the low profit margins they generated from acting in this capacity, they decided to focus exclusively on supplementary insurance.

While the fourth payment option gave physicians an unqualified right to opt out of public payment – direct or indirect – there was never much chance of this approach becoming the entry point for a two-tier system in Saskatchewan. The economic elite was simply too small and preferred to work with existing MSI and GMS carriers. However, to the extent that the Saskatoon Agreement became the template for medicare in other provinces, including those with more sizeable wealthy populations clustered in large cities, the possibility of a two-tier system remained ever-present.

The right of doctors to continue practising medicine as physician businesses paid on a FFS basis was not a concession, since it had always been accepted, albeit grudgingly, by the Douglas government. However, in the Saskatchewan Agreement, this entrepreneurial right went well beyond what T.C. thought it encompassed – that is, the freedom of doctors to choose their patients and "their place and nature of practise."[78] It was now used by the CPS to choke off alternative models of practice, especially the community clinics, which had sprung up during the doctors' strike and posed some threat to the dominant mode of private business FFS practice.

Clause 14 of the Saskatoon Agreement bluntly stated that it was "not for the Commission [MCIC] to appoint doctors" in underserviced areas of the province or areas where "few or no doctors have enrolled for direct payment by the Medical Care Insurance Commission." It would be up to "citizens" alone – without the direct assistance of the MCIC – to establish community clinics. However, the wording made it clear that "the interests" of clinic doctors had to "be safeguarded from" any "improper citizen pressure" from these consumer cooperatives, and that "the role" of the cooperative "in the provision of insured services must be limited to that of landlord."[79] This clause put the governance of the community clinics into a straightjacket, preventing the boards from being more innovative in their organization of health services for fear of putting "improper citizen pressure" on the clinic doctors.[80]

How this clause ended up in the Saskatoon Agreement is not difficult to uncover. Lord Taylor had little sympathy for the community clinics that had sprung up, and he derided what he called the left-wing theorists in the CCF-NDP who were in favour of "cooperative consumer controlled medical clinics." The problem with the clinics, according to Taylor, was that they were opposed by the "majority of doctors" and therefore stood in the way of an agreement with the CPS. In addition, he felt the clinics "were not generally compatible with the highest standards of medical care" but never explained how he had come to this conclusion.[81]

On the question of community clinics, Lord Taylor differed sharply from Douglas, Cadbury, Shoyama, and, from afar, his old friend Spry – none of whom could be called "theoretical" socialists but who were nonetheless supporters of the community clinic movement.[82] On the sixth day of the strike, for example, Shoyama and his wife joined the community clinic in Regina. They were among its founding members, and Shoyama continued to support the clinic movement long after his move to Ottawa in 1964.[83]

If clause 14 was not enough to choke the clinics, they faced ongoing discrimination by the college. Using its power over regulation as a weapon (and with the active collusion of some hospitals), the CPS prevented clinic doctors from obtaining hospital privileges. This had already become an issue by the time the Saskatoon Agreement was being drafted, so the government insisted on, and the CPS conceded to, a clause that stated that there "must be no discrimination against any doctor" for choosing one or another mode of practice. "In particular," the agreement went on, "there must be no discrimination against any doctor in the matter of hospital privileges."[84]

Knowing the hostility being directed towards both the community clinics and the doctors who were staffing the new clinics, T.C. was keen to see the community clinics protected to the greatest extent possible, a concern he communicated directly to the Lloyd cabinet.[85] Upset by what the government saw as a clear breach of the Saskatoon Agreement by the CPS, the Lloyd government ordered a royal commission to review the charges of discrimination, and what it viewed as the abuse of the powers of self-regulation, by the college against clinic doctors.[86]

Preoccupied with getting the new payment system working, the government – through the MCIC – required all doctors, including clinic doctors, be paid by FFS. This meant that, if clinics wanted to adopt a salary mode, the only way to do so was to have the clinic doctors collect their FFS billings from the MCIC and then pool the proceeds, to be redistributed according to a salary scale. This left almost no money for the hiring of non-medical personnel within such clinics without getting loans and indebting the clinics over the long haul. It would take another decade and a different NDP government for the community clinics to replace this unworkable FFS system with a global funding arrangement more suited to their aspirations.[87]

The end result was that, contrary to what T.C. desired, the community clinics were hampered from their inception.[88] Isolated by the college, improperly funded by the MCIC, these clinics never had the opportunity to pose a challenge to FFS practice in Saskatchewan and, through the use of the Saskatoon Agreement as a template for medicare in other provinces, the rest of Canada. Although Douglas would regularly extol the benefits of multidisciplinary group practice from the 1960s until the 1980s, its discouragement lay at the heart of the compromise with organized medicine in 1962.[89]

# 14 The Hall Commission and the Leftward Tilt of Canadian Politics

*Without your program as a successful one in being, I couldn't have produced the unanimous report for the Canada-wide universal health recommendations in 1964. If the scheme had not been successful in Saskatchewan, it wouldn't have become nation-wide.*
Justice Emmett M. Hall writing to T.C. Douglas, April 1971[1]

*I more than anyone could show that the NDP was irrelevant because the kind of economic and social improvements looked for by people who might be marginal NDP voters could in truth be ensured by voting for a Liberal government.*
Tom Kent reflecting on his 1963 electoral bid against Tommy Douglas[2]

Tommy Douglas was head of the federal New Democratic Party from 1961 until 1971. Compared to his two decades leading the CCF in Saskatchewan, where he distinguished himself as Canada's most activist premier and was supported by an effective cabinet and outstanding civil service, this decade of leadership would prove far less fruitful and far more frustrating. In contrast to the Saskatchewan years, this part of T.C.'s life was marked by constant stress and strain, with, at times, little to show for his effort. While, as premier, he had led a well-oiled and powerful political and bureaucratic machine able to accomplish most of the goals he had set out for his party and his government, the NDP lacked cohesion, and the national office had considerably less talent than his government had assembled in Regina.

In addition, perpetual elections had exhausted both T.C. and the NDP's meagre financial and human resources. From the time he assumed leadership until 1968, a period of less than seven years, four federal elections were called. These repeated campaigns overwhelmed the NDP's paltry financing and its tiny core of professional staff. In between the elections, Douglas, long accustomed to delegating the daily business of politics and government to trusted associates while acting as the chief conductor and communicator of change, now led an undisciplined caucus facing parties with little respect for, much less fear of, the NDP. In sum, he had gone from being the unquestioned leader of North America's most progressive government to the leader of a marginal party that never seriously threatened to form the official opposition, let alone the government, in Ottawa.

Fully aware that he faced an uphill struggle against almost overwhelming odds, Douglas nonetheless was assiduous in trying to put political pressure on the main parties, when they formed governments, to adopt his own party's programs and policies. In this, he was assisted by a left-leaning contingent within the Liberal cabinet and a federal bureaucracy enriched by the influx of public servants who had served his government for many years in Saskatchewan. In this way, he ultimately succeeded in seeing through the adoption and implementation of national medicare. Even if Douglas and the NDP never came close to governing nationally, his version of medicare, with its strong form of universality, gave the country a social democratic hue.[3]

## Contending with the Sixties

The world Douglas inherited as national leader of the NDP was changing rapidly. Without doubt, in the late 1950s he was seen as the ideal leader of the New Party as the demand for a makeover of the CCF intensified. A proven leader, his mixture of idealism and pragmatism had produced an enviable record of achievements. Within a few years, however, he would increasingly be seen as yesterday's man, part of a generation shaped by the Great Depression, unlike the baby boomers beginning to emerge with perspectives shaped by post-war prosperity.[4]

But well before the Vietnam War protests and the emergence of the New Left, there was a major shift in the nature of the policy environment in Canada and in the partisan debates concerning the welfare state. Before Diefenbaker and his new brand of populist conservatism had shattered both the CCF and the Liberal Party in 1958, Douglas knew exactly where he and the CCF stood in relation to the two main parties. The CCF was in favour of building an all-encompassing welfare state that would include comprehensive coverage of all needed health services, while the federal Liberals and Progressive Conservatives (PCs) had to be forced, kicking and screaming, to make even the most incremental of reforms.

This all began to change, first with Diefenbaker pushing the PCs towards a more populist centre of gravity and a more progressive position on social policy that challenged traditional Bay Street orthodoxy. Then came the more significant change: the leftward shift of the Liberal Party of Canada under Pearson. From the Kingston Conference in September 1960 to the National Liberal Rally of January 1961, the Liberal Party adopted a detailed program on the welfare state, including health policies that met the social democrats partway.[5] Pearson attracted a new group of social policy reformers, such as Tom Kent, Pearson's chief policy advisor, as well as ministers such as Walter Gordon, Allan MacEachen, and Judy LaMarsh.

These social reform Liberals held some appeal among a number of older CCFers, including Frank Underhill, who had been one of the key figures (along with Frank Scott and Graham Spry) in the League for Social Reconstruction in the 1930s.[6] Underhill's philosophical shift from the CCF to the Liberal Party was underscored when his book of essays *In Search of Canadian Liberalism*, published in 1960, was dedicated to Mike Pearson.[7] In the elections of 1962 and 1963, Underhill proclaimed his support for Pearson and the Liberals rather than Douglas and the NDP.[8] Once elected, the Pearson government hired some of the closest former advisors in the Saskatchewan government, the most prominent being Tommy Shoyama and Al Johnson.

These changes meant that, from the time Douglas took over as NDP leader, he had to work much harder to demonstrate how his party differed from the Liberals in its policy program. Both Douglas and those in the Liberal Party whose perspective was closest to his own party understood the stakes of the competition. Early on, this was illustrated in Gordon's reaction to Kent's detailed social policy paper, which, according to Pearson, was "the most intellectually brilliant" contribution to the Kingston Conference: "I must shake the hand that has strangled the New Party before it's born," Gordon told Kent.[9]

In addition, Douglas's prairie populist appeal and his famed ability to reach out to the common person would, at critical times, be overshadowed by Diefenbaker's similar attraction and talent. But soon, both would see their populist brand of politics become a relic of the past. Their downhome bonhomie would be supplanted by the youthful, cosmopolitan, and "cool" image projected by the newly elected Kennedy administration in the United States. Without a populist bone in his body and as someone who could never compete with Diefenbaker or Douglas on the hustings, Pearson benefited as the first national leader whose image was remade based on extensive and expensive public opinion surveys.

Impressed by Theodore White's book *The Making of the President: 1960*, the Liberal strategists hired a Kennedy pollster to conduct opinion surveys on how voters perceived leaders, the first time such a technique was applied to politics in Canada. Based on the results, Pearson traded in his bow tie for a straight tie.[10] And rather than focus the campaign on Pearson – the polling showed that he "lacked a clear image," and was seen as a "diplomat" seemingly "unfitted for domestic politics – the Liberals emphasized the team surrounding their leader in the 1962 election.[11] Their polling also told them some disconcerting news – that many Canadians continued to have an image of Diefenbaker as an "honest, sincere, straightforward man," despite his many gaffes and disabilities in managing a government.[12] Liberal strategists told candidates how they could best deal with both the Diefenbaker government and the NDP:

> The enemy is the government. If we pay much attention to the New Party, we foster the idea that we are not the only alternative. We must be on guard against both Tories and Socialists trying to represent the election as a fight between them. For that reason, a close-up attack by us on Douglas, or on the New Party generally, would hurt us more than it would help.
>
> In the attack we do make, we should talk always about the Socialists, never the New Party. We should stick to three main points: (1) They are doctrinaire. (2) We speak for all groups, not one. (3) We are for individual freedom and they don't care enough about it; the best example is provided not by any elaborate argument about their policies, or about what has happened in Saskatchewan, but the very basis of their party. It is organized and financed by trying to tell the individual union member what party to support.[13]

Something more fundamental was also changing in Canadian society with the advent of the 1960s. The emerging zeitgeist favoured building a welfare state – to the point that not one of the parties could afford to oppose the extension of publicly financed health coverage for fear of losing public support. A focus on social welfare should have helped the NDP, but both establishment parties quickly pivoted to portray themselves as offering newfound support for such policies. For Douglas, this realignment challenged his earlier view that the country's electorate was about to consign the Liberal Party to the dustbin of history, with left-wing Liberals joining the NDP, and right-wing or "business Liberals," as they were called, migrating to the Tories.[14]

On a socio-cultural level, Canada was rapidly becoming a secular society. The 1960s would constitute an inflection point between Canada as a predominantly Christian society and as a more secular and religiously pluralistic society.[15] Douglas's basis for his political ideology, built as it was on the social gospel, was rarely understood, much less shared, by the sixties generation, thus separating him from most younger members of the NDP and the left more broadly defined. Despite sharing similar causes, especially opposition to the Vietnam War and support for the liberation movements in the Third World, younger progressives began to perceive Douglas's Christian convictions as old-fashioned or even peculiar.

**The First Months of the Hall Commission**

The origins of the Royal Commission on Health Services (the Hall Commission) predate Douglas's assumption of the leadership of the federal NDP and his departure as premier of Saskatchewan. Some backtracking in the narrative is required to explain why the Hall Commission was established and examine Douglas's evolving relationship with the commission and its chair, Justice Emmett Hall.

Unlike many of the interest groups traditionally supporting the Progressive Conservative Party, Prime Minister John G. Diefenbaker was not against medicare as a matter of principle. In fact, his experience with hospital insurance had been very positive. However, after witnessing the controversy in Saskatchewan over medicare in the 1960 election, he wanted to avoid making a decision on the issue and so established a commission to study it.

Just before the Christmas parliamentary break in 1960, Diefenbaker announced his intention to appoint a royal commission to examine the whole question of health services. In the House of Commons, he read a letter he had received from the Canadian Medical Association (CMA) on 12 December, using it, as well as requests from other groups and individuals, as his justification for a study. The CMA letter pronounced on the effectiveness of doctor-sponsored insurance plans, in opposition to the single-payer approach embraced by Douglas's government in Saskatchewan.[16] The Liberals and the CCF (soon to become the NDP) responded by criticizing Diefenbaker's avoidance of the issue and the delays a commission would cause.[17]

Diefenbaker's ministers were divided on the type of person who should be appointed chair of the commission. The more progressive ministers, including the PM, felt that the person should be "favourably disposed toward welfare legislation," while the true-blue Conservatives argued that the chair should not be "a person predisposed to recommend vast and expensive public plans." All could agree, however, that "a judge would be particularly appropriate as chairman of the Royal Commission because of the wide differences of opinion in the general field of health services." Diefenbaker had already put forward the name of an old friend of his from Saskatchewan, Emmett Hall, whom he had arranged to be appointed chief justice of the Saskatchewan Court of Appeal.[18] Diefenbaker phoned Hall, who agreed to consider the offer, but before the PM received a final answer, the appointment was announced publicly. Despite being put into an awkward position, Hall agreed to the appointment.[19]

The two men had been close political allies for years, and few were surprised at the decision. Diefenbaker's classmate at the University of Saskatchewan's law school, Hall had switched allegiance from the Liberal Party to the PCs in the early 1940s, and, as the *Saskatoon Star-Phoenix* unambiguously proclaimed upon his appointment, "the commission chairman is a Progressive Conservative."[20] While the reasons for Hall's conversion are contested – was it his dissatisfaction with federal Liberal policies, as he himself suggested, or was it the refusal of Jimmy Gardiner (the federal Liberal government's regional minister) to appoint him to the bench – he was without any doubt a personal supporter of Diefenbaker and his brand of populist and, at times, progressive conservatism.[21]

Initially, Douglas had reservations about Hall, concerned he "was by no means a convinced proponent of medicare or any form of government sponsored pre-paid medical insurance plan."[22] Hall had strong anti-socialist leanings. Born into an Irish Roman Catholic family in Quebec, Emmett was only nine when the family moved to Saskatchewan. As a strong Catholic, he shared that church's concerns about socialism in general and the CCF in particular when it emerged as a political party in the 1930s.

From the beginning, however, Hall's personal antipathy to the CCF was balanced by his belief in collective rights and in fundamental justice, beliefs that sometimes put him at odds with his well-heeled and complacent friends and colleagues who formed part of the Canadian elite – hence the subtitle *Establishment Radical* used by Dennis Gruending for his biography of Hall. Although, in the 1930s, Hall had not hesitated to accuse those who supported the Republican cause in Spain of being communists, he was nonetheless sympathetic to the unemployed and felt that the trekkers involved in the Regina Riot of 1935 had been treated unfairly. He disturbed many in his circle when he accepted an invitation by Peter Makaroff, a well-known CCF lawyer and pacifist, to help him defend the men accused of causing the riot.[23] While T.C. respected Hall's courage in the mid-1930s, he also remembered when

The Hall Commission and the Leftward Tilt of Canadian Politics  407

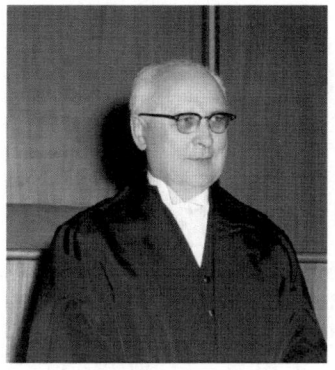

Emmett M. Hall, chief justice of the Saskatchewan Court of Appeal, 31 July 1962. While chairing the Hall Commission, he was appointed by the Diefenbaker government to the Supreme Court of Canada in January 1963 (SPL B-11153-1)

Hall, as a PC candidate in the 1948 provincial election, called Douglas a Nazi for suggesting bias among the judges who found a section of the Saskatchewan Trade Union Act unconstitutional.[24]

Whatever his views on Hall in 1960, T.C. nonetheless saw an opportunity for the Saskatchewan government to influence the royal commission's thinking, and his cabinet agreed, months before the commission began meeting, to start work on a major submission.[25] This optimism stood in contrast to the more negative views of Douglas held by both Diefenbaker and Hall, who felt that the Saskatchewan premier was shamelessly using medicare to support his campaign to become the leader of the New Party and then challenge both the PCs and the Liberals at the federal level. In late May 1961, Diefenbaker wrote Hall, confirming that "he had reports that Premier Douglas intends to announce the introduction of a Health Insurance Plan in the Province," and the "fact that he is not going to give up the Premiership until November would give support to the idea that he will have a Fall session and bring in legislation to act as a boost in his federal ambitions."[26]

T.C. might have had more qualms about Hall if he had known the extent to which Diefenbaker had influenced Hall to select the members of the commission from a list of twenty individuals the PM had provided.[27] Among those finally selected by Hall were individuals who, at first glance, would hardly be sympathetic to Douglas-style medicare, including Wallace McCutcheon, the vice-president and general manager of Argus Corporation and board chair of one of the largest insurance companies in the country; Arthur Van Wart, past president of the CMA; Dr. Leslie Strachan, from London, Ontario, dentist and past president of the Ontario Dental Association; and Dr. David Baltzan, a Saskatoon surgeon and professor of clinical medicine and the PM's close friend.[28] All four could be expected to share the CMA's opposition to single-payer medicare and, instead, support the extension of private health insurance. In contrast, the two other members approved by Hall, Alice Girard, past president of the Canadian Nurses Association, and Professor O.J. Firestone, a professor from the University of Ottawa who had served as an economist in the government of Canada for almost two decades, were more open to argument on the merits of a publicly financed and administered system.[29]

As the editors of the *Ottawa Citizen* put it, the "commission's effectiveness" could be damaged "by the fact that a majority of its members" were "associated with the medical and related professions" and therefore overly swayed by the CMA's adamant opposition to a universal scheme.[30] One wag suggested that "putting the prospects of a national medical care scheme in the hands of that commission – composed as it is of the past president of the C.M.A. and the head of Argus Corporation – is like asking Colonel Sanders to protect your chicken farm."[31]

Despite these signs, during the spring and early summer of 1961 (just before the New Party convention), Douglas and Hall exchanged letters in which T.C. promised that the Saskatchewan government would do everything possible to support the commission. "All of us recognize," wrote Douglas, "the important part which the provincial administrations must play in any health plan for the future." He assured Hall that his government would "co-operate in the fullest possible extent, recognizing as we do the important task at hand."[32] Part of the reason for Douglas's attitude was the fact that this was a commission with a strong Saskatchewan flavour, appointed by a Saskatchewan-based PM, with a Saskatchewan-based chair and a Saskatoon-based surgeon. (Baltzan had treated and cared for Diefenbaker's own ailing mother in Saskatchewan. Diefenbaker also thanked Douglas for the high quality of her care under the provincial hospitalization plan, donating $5,000 towards a medical research fellowship in the name of his parents as a token of appreciation.[33])

The commission was scheduled to hold public hearings throughout Canada but, given the growing intensity of the struggle between the Saskatchewan government and doctors over medicare, the five days of hearing set for Regina in January 1962 had the potential to be particularly explosive.[34] With the national media in attendance, T.C. believed that the Regina hearings would provide an opportunity to argue in favour of a universal single-payer plan and rebut organized medicine's arguments for a targeted, multi-payer, means-tested plan, although Hall was committed to preventing his commission from being

## The Hall Commission and the Leftward Tilt of Canadian Politics 409

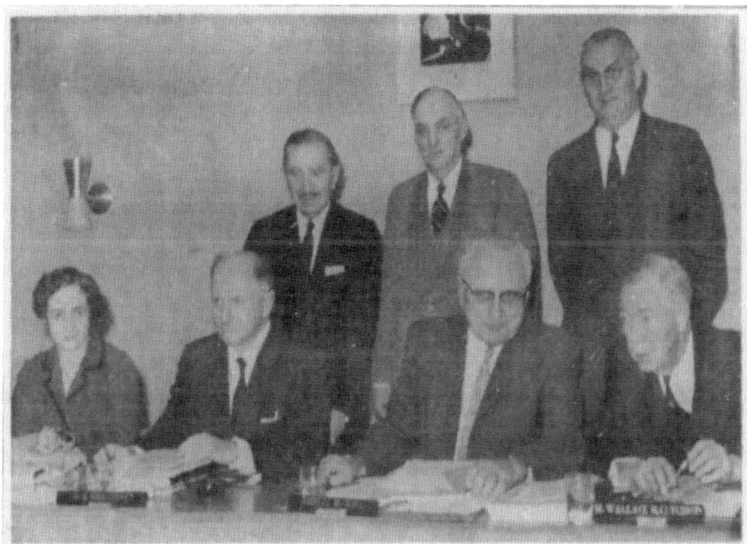

HEARING STARTS: The Hall royal commission on health services began its hearings in Regina Monday and is expected to sit for a full week. Commission members shown here are: seated, Miss Alice Girard, Montreal; Prof. O. J. Firestone, Ottawa; Chief Justice Emmett Hall, Regina, chairman; M. Wallace McCutcheon, Toronto. Standing: Dr. David Baltzan, Saskatoon; Dr. Arthur Van Wart, Fredericton; and Dr. C. L. Strachan, London.

Newspaper photograph of Hall Commission members at the start of the Regina hearings on 22 January 1962 (*Regina Leader-Post*, 22 January 1962, 1)

weaponized by either side in the ongoing dispute between the doctors and the government in Saskatchewan.

By 22 January 1962, when Hall opened the first day of his Saskatchewan hearings, Douglas, by then the national leader of the NDP, was still ensconced in his Regina office, having not yet moved to Ottawa. The extensive document outlining the Saskatchewan government's arguments on the merits of medicare and federal participation in a comprehensive scheme of universal health coverage, which had been prepared over months under his watchful eye, had been formally submitted to the Hall Commission well in advance of the hearing.[35] Hall tried to set the tone with an opening statement that made it clear the commission members were fully cognizant of the "disagreement [that] exists between the government and the College of Physicians and Surgeons. But we have ... no intention of taking sides one way or the other." Knowing what was likely to come, he also warned against observers and the media inferring the position of the commission from the questions its members would be asking of presenters.[36]

The oral argument for the provincial government was presented by Bill Davies, the minister of health, who had replaced Walter Erb two months earlier. After presenting the highlights of the written submission, Davies was subjected to a severe cross-examination by Hall and the other commissioners, especially McCutcheon and doctors Van Wart and Baltzan. The commissioners probed Davies on why Saskatchewan had rejected the CMA's recommended approach of subsidizing private medical care insurance in favour of a universal, compulsory plan. Davies response, that the government plan would finance "better medical care" than could be obtained by subsidizing private insurance, triggered an aggressive, at times rude, cross-examination by McCutcheon.[37]

NDP MP Frank Howard would subsequently raise the question in Parliament of the Hall Commission's partiality. A colourful trade unionist from British Columbia who was referred to by one Conservative MP as "the anarchy wing of the N.D.P," Howard had just hosted a "stunned and leaderless" NDP caucus in his office to deal with the defection of Hazen Argue.[38] Howard criticized Diefenbaker for punting the matter of national medicare to the commission, which was made up "to a large extent of people who are hatchet men for the government in office." He then complained of the attack by commission members on "Saskatchewan's health minister, Mr. W.G. Davies, in which there were accusations by the royal commission about political control, about the inefficacy of the plan in Saskatchewan," and about the Saskatchewan government's desire to be "bailed out" of its expensive medical care plan by getting transfer money from Ottawa.[39] In Howard's view, these comments demonstrated the hostility of the commissioners to a Saskatchewan-style plan before they had had time to complete their fact finding.

**The 1963 Federal Election and a New Direction**

With a seat in the House of Commons secured after a by-election in Burnaby, British Columbia, in October 1962, T.C. left Saskatchewan and entered Parliament after an absence of almost two decades. His first order of business was to grapple with a disintegrating Diefenbaker cabinet. By the end of that year, the infighting within the PC government had become endemic, and a faction attempted to jettison Diefenbaker and move the government back to its more traditionally conservative position. Douglas was approached by Wallace McCutcheon to support the government in a confidence vote. By this time, McCutcheon had

# The Hall Commission and the Leftward Tilt of Canadian Politics 411

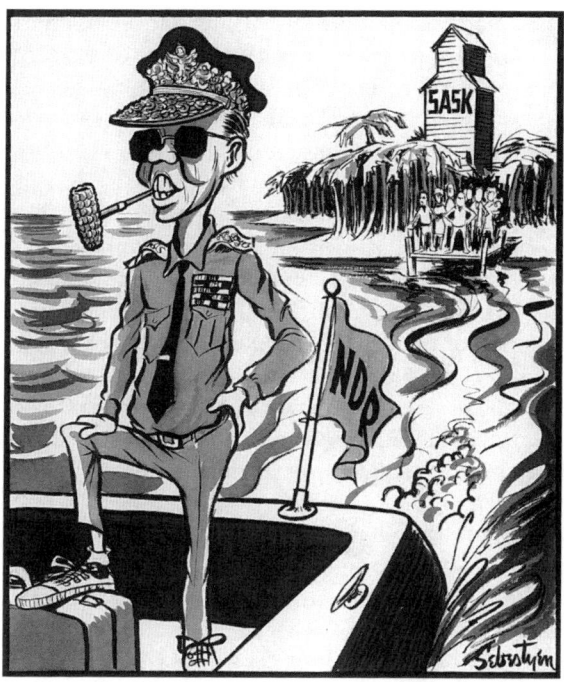

Political cartoon in the *Saskatoon Star Phoenix*, 16 October 1962, six days before the Burnaby-Coquitlam by-election, contrasting T.C.'s departure from Saskatchewan (with the caption "I will not return") with General Douglas MacArthur's evacuation from the Philippines during the Second World War, when MacArthur was reported to have said, "I will return" (PAS S (A918), file 496)

left the Hall Commission for the Senate and a cabinet appointment to help Diefenbaker shore up support for himself among the PCs on Bay Street.[40]

McCutcheon tried to convince Douglas and his NDP caucus to support the PCs in a critical parliamentary vote of confidence in return for a promise that Diefenbaker would be deposed by his caucus within forty-eight hours. T.C. could not agree, as he believed that the NDP needed to register its non-confidence because the PC government was no longer "able to govern." No fan of the senator's attacks on creeping socialism and big government, Douglas made it clear that the NDP was hardly keen to see Diefenbaker quit, only to be replaced by McCutcheon and his friends on Bay Street.[41] As one of the founders of Argus

Corporation, a wealthy financier, and right hand of Canadian business tycoon E.P. Taylor, McCutcheon was a caricature of a cigar-smoking Toronto financier who represented everything Douglas deplored about the Canadian establishment.[42] In an interview a few years after the election, Douglas stated his reasons for ultimately pulling his party's support for the Diefenbaker government:

> We had every reason politically to support the government. We had gone through an election in June 1962. I had been defeated; I had gone through a byelection in October in Burnaby-Coquitlam and I had just entered the House. The funds of our party were completely depleted, people were tired after the election. Nobody wanted an election ... From the standpoint of political strategy, it would have been wise for us to have kept the government in office at least for a year or so. But you couldn't do it; it was so apparent that the government was disintegrating before one's eyes.[43]

The result was another federal election on 8 April 1963, a little less than nine months after Douglas's 1962 election defeat and just over five months after his by-election victory.[44] T.C. faced a new challenge in this campaign: his opponent was Tom Kent, a candidate whom Liberal strategist Keith Davey called "the most left-wing liberal I have ever known."[45] Kent, a Rhodes scholar, was an editorial writer for the *Manchester Guardian* and the *Economist* before he moved from Britain to Canada to become editor of the *Winnipeg Free Press* in 1954. He was a self-described progressive Liberal, who was perceived by many of the old guard in his party as a social democrat little different than Douglas.[46] One press wag referred to the contest as the "battle of the Toms."[47]

Kent was parachuted into the Burnaby-Coquitlam riding as the Liberal's best hope of challenging Douglas.[48] To emphasize the Liberals' relationship with organized labour, Kent chose the former president of the International Woodworkers of America as his campaign manager and received the support of a few other prominent unionists in the constituency.[49] Keith Davey's political logic was that Douglas could be defeated only by someone who represented similar values. Even if Kent did not win, his more progressive campaign style and the publicity focused on constituencies in which party leaders were running could help the Liberals win other marginal seats against the NDP. Kent also hoped that his candidature would "compel" T.C. "to spend more time in his riding and be less effective in the national campaign."[50]

The Liberal medical care plan first devised by Kent was buffed up for the 1963 campaign.[51] To separate the "fiscally responsible" Liberals from the NDP, Kent emphasized that the Liberal plan would cover the

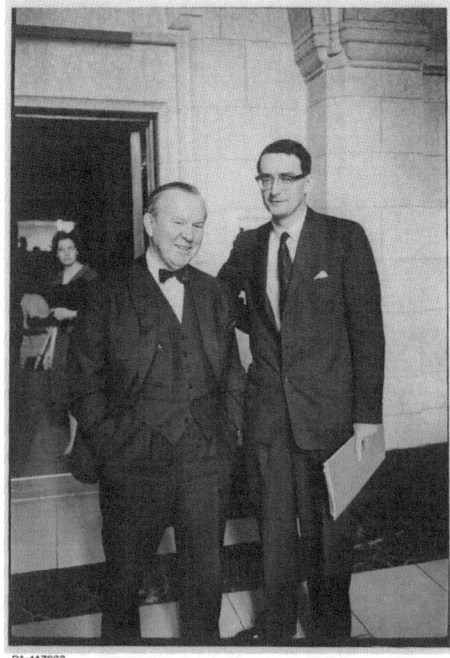

Lester B. (Mike) Pearson with Tom Kent (LAC PA-117098)

population in stages: the first stage would include schoolchildren and seniors.[52] And once medical care for the whole the population was covered, the Liberal platform stated that a future government would then "broaden its health plan to cover other burdensome costs, with priority for prescribed drugs and children's dental services."[53] For many voters, this seemed little different from the NDP platform promise of "fully comprehensive health care including dentists, drugs and appliances," so Douglas did his best to convey what he felt were critical differences.[54]

First and foremost, the NDP plan was universal, unlike the Liberal proposal involving deductibles as well as taxable benefits that would be clawed back at tax time. In response to Kent's billing as the architect of the Liberal medical care plan, Tom Berger, an NDP MP for Vancouver-Burrard running for re-election, simply responded, "What medical care plan?"[55] For Douglas, especially in Socred British Columbia, it made more sense to attack the plan proposed by Alberta premier Ernest Manning, which he found far more objectionable. Douglas characterized Manning's scheme – which would soon become known as

"Manningcare" when implemented in Alberta later in the year – as a form of "tin cup medicare." The plan was fatally flawed, as it segregated the population "into the haves and the have nots" and then required the have-nots "to undergo the humiliation of a means test."[56] But, in the end, medicare and social policy in general were not key issues in the 1963 campaign. Instead, it focused on questions of defence, foreign affairs, and the personalities of Diefenbaker and Pearson. While T.C. and his NDP candidates placed considerable emphasis on domestic issues and kept "hammering away at such matters as medicare, family allowances, education, pensions, and economic growth," they could not make these the salient issues.[57]

As the campaign wore on, the Liberals found that they were losing their lead in public opinion. In a desperate effort to shore up support, they promised "sixty days of decision," an action plan that left health care out of the mix.[58] This lack of emphasis on medicare was reflected in the all-party candidates' debate in Port Coquitlam on 22 March 1963, where the media did not even mention medical care in its extensive reporting on the event. The *Vancouver Sun* described the boisterous crowd cheering and applauding Douglas while booing and insulting Tom Kent in response to Pearson's apparent willingness to accept nuclear weapons on Canadian soil.[59] Kent blamed trade union organizers for what he felt was harassment, and while he "could not believe that Tommy Douglas relished these proceedings on his behalf," Douglas nonetheless did nothing to restrain the crowd.[60] Smarting from his treatment at the debate, Kent soon struck back, describing Douglas as "a voice out of the past," out of touch with the realities of 1960s Canada.[61]

The defence and foreign policy concerns of the campaign did not play to the NDP's strengths on domestic policy and likely contributed (along with a strapped campaign budget) to a slightly worse result for the party than ten months earlier. Nationally, the party was left with seventeen seats, compared to the nineteen it had held, and it remained the fourth party behind Social Credit, which its kept twenty-four seats.[62] Nine of the NDP seats were won in British Columbia, the new citadel of NDP strength, with another six in Ontario and two in Manitoba. In Saskatchewan, where loyalty to Diefenbaker was most pronounced, the NDP could not win a single seat. The one piece of good news for the NDP was that, despite the challenge from Kent, Douglas won the battle of the two Toms. If he had not done so, he no doubt would have had to resign, and the party would have been forced into a potentially divisive leadership campaign.

For the Liberals, the election proved to be a victory "of a sort," as Kent put it.[63] With 128 seats to the PCs' 96, the Liberals had missed obtaining a majority by only two seats. Diefenbaker prevented a Liberal majority by again sweeping the Prairies and scoring well in the Maritime provinces, where his personal magnetism continued to pull in the votes. Douglas was not surprised by this trend, as he understood Diefenbaker's close connection with farmers and the inhabitants of small towns and how the election had made him a "giant revived by his contact with the people."[64] For T.C., the silver lining of this otherwise very disappointing result was that a minority government offered his party greater influence in Parliament. As for Kent, he would go on to serve as Pearson's chief policy advisor, a role, paradoxically, in which he would end up exerting far more influence on the direction of the government than any ministerial position he might have attained had he been elected.

**Rumours of Merger**

Since the Liberals depended on the NDP to get their legislative agenda through Parliament and to prevent it from being defeated on a confidence question like the budget, it was hardly surprising that a few members in each party wanted to come up with more formalized agreement, perhaps even a coalition government. Because of the dominance of the two-party model at the federal level, the nuances of the different options short of full fusion between parties were not well understood by the media.[65] As a consequence, when word of tentative discussions reached the press, the word "merger" was immediately applied, upsetting Douglas, who viewed the Liberals as the NDP's permanent rival. As he saw things, there was room for only one of these two parties in the long run, and, as in the United Kingdom, it was the Liberal Party, a relic of the past, that should give way to the NDP, which would become home for former centre-left Liberals.

The rumours of a merger started shortly after the 1963 election and carried into the following year. When the media reported that Douglas himself had attended a high-level meeting with key Liberals in the spring of 1964, all hell broke loose. Based on Douglas's own recollection of the meeting, he along with David Lewis and MP Doug Fisher had gone to see the PM, Keith Davey, and Walter Gordon at Gordon's Ottawa apartment. Pearson was to have been at the meeting but, being ill (and insisting to Douglas that it was not a diplomatic flu), he phoned Douglas at Gordon's apartment. T.C. claimed the discussion initially focused solely on the possibility of an agreement to support the Liberals' legislative agenda, and he set out the NDP's expectations in terms of medicare, the Canada Pension Plan, and improvements to Old Age Security.

When Davey and Fisher eventually swung "the conversation" to the idea of a merger, T.C.'s recollection was that he stopped the discussion dead, stating that "any type of merger or even any type of continuing organizational structure" was "completely out of the question." Instead, he wanted to discuss how both parties could cooperate on individual votes and policies, thereby getting "the most" out of the current session. Gordon agreed with Douglas, and the discussion of the merger ended.[66]

However, a Canadian Press article that appeared weeks later called into question Douglas's version of events. "Well-informed political sources" said that the Liberals had "made changes in their party structure" to meet the requirements laid down by Douglas, Lewis, and Fisher at the meeting with Gordon and Davey. The article also alleged that Pearson had "agreed to the talks to explore a basis for co-operation between the minority Liberal government and the New Democrats for this Parliament" and the "eventual union of the two parties after the next federal election."[67] The article harmed T.C.'s reputation and raised suspicions among veteran members of the party, that the NDP – under the influence of big labour – was gradually moving towards absorption by the Liberal Party of Canada.

T.C. received a distraught letter from Grace MacInnis. The daughter of J.S. Woodsworth, the wife of a former CCF MP, and a respected socialist politician in her own right, MacInnis demanded that Douglas give her a straight answer.[68] He admitted that he and other MPs and officials of the NDP had met with "some of the Liberals from time to time" on issues of common interest to get certain legislation "through Parliament," but he denied any "discussions aimed at bring about a merger with the Liberals."[69] Former Quebec CCF activist Thérèse Casgrain also asked T.C. if there was any truth to his making a deal with the Pearson Liberals. Denying any discussion of a merger, Douglas said that he "would resign as federal leader if the party decided on such a course."[70]

## Walter Gordon's Budget and the Canada Pension Plan

The two big-ticket social policy items in the Liberal's 1963 platform were pensions and medicare. What would become known as the Canada Pension Plan was slated to begin first, as it was considered the easier and faster of the two to accomplish – this, despite the fact that the newly appointed minister of national health and welfare, Judy LaMarsh, was more invested in medicare than pensions.

Other factors were also at play in determining the Pearson government's policy priorities. However much reform-minded Liberals viewed medicare with favour, the virulence of the doctors' strike in Saskatchewan, to say nothing of the opposition of the Liberal Party in Saskatchewan, had cooled the ardor of many in the party. As historian Penny Bryden so aptly put it, the population in Saskatchewan "was only beginning to recover from the doctors' strike: history had not yet cast the government as the dragon-slayer in this epic battle, and it was far from clear that the public was fully behind health insurance in Saskatchewan, let alone across the rest of the country."[71] Add to that the opposition of provincial governments, especially those in Alberta and Ontario, which had joined forces with organized medicine and the insurance companies to oppose a universal plan, and it is little wonder that the Pearson government decided to proceed with pensions rather than medicare.[72] Further, there was the question of money. As LaMarsh herself recalled, the pension plan "was the first thing to start with ... because it would be self-funding and we didn't know how much money there would be to start with Medicare."[73]

So, the social reformers within the cabinet, including Judy LaMarsh, finance minister Walter Gordon, and labour minister Allan J. MacEachen, along with Tom Kent, expected to get the Canada Pension Plan up and running as quickly as possible, to be immediately followed by the Liberal medicare plan. However, they were stopped in their tracks by the hostile reception to Gordon's first budget. As a charter member of the progressive wing of the Liberals, Gordon was highly supportive of the Canada Pension Plan. However, to the horror of the business community and its friends in the Liberal Party, Gordon's tax measures included a 30 per cent withholding tax on the sale of Canadian-owned corporations to non-residents, which reflected his desire to reduce the level of foreign ownership.[74]

When Pearson failed to come to the assistance of Gordon, the ensuing controversy over the budget forced a policy reversal on the measure, which permanently damaged Gordon's reputation and status within cabinet. Before the budget, he was the most powerful member of cabinet, to some extent because of his very close relationship with Pearson. After the budget, he lost his lustre, and the progressive ministers were forced to retreat, in part because the botched budget raised questions among the more conservative members of cabinet about the ability of the government to finance expensive social measures such as medicare.[75]

Sympathetic to Gordon's views on foreign ownership, Douglas also agreed with his takeover tax but felt that Gordon had destroyed himself by bringing in advisors from Bay Street, who, knowing his revenue measures in advance, had helped launch a lobby against the tax.[76] As for the old guard in the Liberal cabinet, T.C. believed they had always wanted one of their own to be finance minister and were just waiting for any opportunity to throw Gordon "to the wolves."[77]

As much as the question of using external advisors had hurt Gordon's reputation, his real problem was with his own Department of Finance bureaucrats, some of whom were incompetent and others (such as Simon Reisman) entirely unsympathetic to his objectives.[78] Desiring greater competence and an individual who shared his progressive vision, Gordon tried to recruit Al Johnson, Douglas's long-time deputy provincial treasurer, a position Johnson still held under Premier Woodrow Lloyd. In her history of the Pearson Liberals, Penny Bryden posits that Gordon, because he "realized the ramifications" of the budget debate for his ability to fund and "implement progressive social policies," wanted to "shore up defences by bringing in one of the masterminds behind Saskatchewan's medical programs."[79] Johnson accepted the offer but on condition that he be given a few months to complete his work with the Lloyd government, and he did not move to Ottawa until the spring of 1964.[80]

In the aftermath of the budget debate, the federal-provincial negotiations on the Canada Pension Plan began in earnest. For the next eighteen months, Judy LaMarsh, Tom Kent, and the rest of the social policy team would be completely absorbed in negotiating a pension plan acceptable to the provinces. Putting aside medicare for the time being, Douglas and his caucus colleagues pushed for a more comprehensive pension plan than the Liberals – and most provincial governments at the time – were willing to countenance.[81] As LaMarsh made clear in a public statement in July 1963, "the Canada Pension Plan is *not* intended to be comprehensive" or "to provide all the retirement income which many Canadians wish to have. This is a matter of individual choice and, in the Government's view, should properly be left to personal savings and to private pensions plans."[82]

Whatever deficiencies the Liberal plan had, Douglas felt he had to support the Canada Pension Plan as a major improvement from the status quo. After all, it has been a major part of the NDP's platform in both the 1962 and 1963 elections. His hope was that, once implemented, the plan would be shored up and made more comprehensive with time, and that eventually private plans would not be required.[83]

**The Hall Commission Report**

In the end, the Canada Pension Plan would prove devilishly difficult to negotiate with the provinces, involving machinations that further fractured the Pearson cabinet. Action on medicare would have to wait considerably longer than the Liberal progressives or Douglas and the NDP desired. However, when the much-anticipated Hall Commission report was finally delivered in June 1964, the Pearson government would be forced to begin planning for medicare, even while still finalizing the Canada Pension Plan. As for Douglas and the NDP, the Hall Commission report provided much-needed leverage in its ongoing efforts to push the federal government into action, efforts resisted by a powerful coalition of forces, including organized medicine, the business lobby, and almost every provincial government in the country.

On 16 June 1964, the Pearson government received a 914-page document from commission chair Justice Emmett Hall.[84] The commission ultimately rejected organized medicine's view that, since the current system of private health insurance covered most Canadians, the only government intervention required was to subsidize the payment of premiums for the means-tested poor. As it discovered in its research, less than half of the population had private medical insurance coverage and even this was often inadequate. It was in the "public interest," then, that general taxation be used to provide universal health coverage.[85] The Hall Commission had rejected the Manningcare model in favour of the single-payer universal model of hospital and medical care coverage in Saskatchewan.

The recommendations proved to be a shock to the CMA, which had lobbied the Diefenbaker government to set up the royal commission four years prior to counter the Douglas government's drive towards universal medicare in Saskatchewan. In a press conference called shortly after the report's release, the CMA could only splutter that any effort to impose such a plan against the doctors' wishes could lead to a "withdrawal of services," as had happened in Saskatchewan two years earlier.[86] As the *Ottawa Citizen* described in its front-page coverage, the Hall Report went much "further toward socialized medicine than most people expected" – further than anticipated not only by organized medicine but by the Pearson cabinet itself.[87]

As was the case for hospital insurance, the Hall Commission recommended cost-shared financing of provincial programs by the federal government. Eligibility for cost sharing would depend on provincial governments having medical care insurance programs that met federal requirements. In addition to physician services, the Hall Commission urged that universal coverage be extended, as finances permitted over time, to prescription drugs, prosthetics, and home-care services, while targeted coverage for children and social assistance recipients be provided for dental services and optical services. Added to this already ambitious menu was "a complete reorganization and reorientation" of "mental health services and important changes in the Hospital Insurance Program."[88]

Beyond medical care, which was defined as the "next essential service," the commission was careful to say that the provinces should retain "the right to determine the order of priority" in introducing coverage for other services.[89] However, Hall and his commissioners were clear that the goal was a comprehensive health program, exactly what T.C. had been pushing the federal government towards for twenty years.[90]

Readily acknowledging the cost implications of its recommendations, the Hall Commission devoted three chapters – an entire section of the report – to financing.[91] To implement comprehensive health coverage by 1971 would cost both orders of government $466 million.[92] Although the commission argued that this was more than affordable, the figure was seized on by the anti-medicare lobby to argue that universal coverage was simply too expensive.

Emmett Hall had insisted on the inclusion in the commission's report of a "Health Charter for Canadians," declaring what he personally felt should be the basic principles, values, and objectives of Canada's reconfigured health system. Comprehensive universality was the goal, but it was to be based on a respect for the constitutional division of power, "freedom of choice," and "free and self-governing professions and institutions."[93]

The day after the report was tabled in Parliament, Don McGillivray, the parliamentary correspondent for Southam News, reported breathlessly on the significance of its recommendations:

> The Hall Commission has startled Ottawa by calling for a complete and compulsory national health program – a giant $4,000,000,000 addition to the already expansive structure of the Canadian welfare state.
>
> Coupled with the Canada Pension Plan already in the works, it could give Canada a unique combination of British-type health insurance and American-style social security, which might add up to the most generous and expensive welfare system in the world.[94]

Based on the experience of the Swift Current Health Region since 1946, the Hall Commission used detailed information on the cost of medical care in the country's only pilot medicare project.[95] Drawing more broadly on the Saskatchewan experience with hospital insurance, the commission well understood that the extension of universal health coverage beyond acute care and diagnostics would put enormous demands on existing facilities and health human resources. To face this challenge, it recommended new health funds and grants to finance the expansion and improvement of existing health facilities and health professions, including university education and professional training. And to improve the state of health services research, the commission urged the broadening of the mandate of the Medical Research Council and to ramp up Canada's statistical capacity and infrastructure in the field. Drawing on the experience of the National Health Grants, the idea was for the federal government to leverage its spending power and act as the spark for pan-Canadian improvements in establishing a high-quality health system.[96]

For T.C., the most appealing feature of the report was the fact that it endorsed his vision of single-payer and single-tier coverage as the template for the national scheme. In a private letter with a union official, he admitted that the "report went further than we dared hoped" and that he would "be supporting it all along the way."[97] He told the press that he was "particularly pleased" with its acceptance of universality rather than the targeted subsidy schemes being pushed by organized medicine, the insurance lobby, local and national chambers of commerce, and some provincial governments. If implemented, Douglas went on, it would mean that Canada would have the type of health plan he had long advocated.[98]

The three most significant factors that had swayed the Hall Commission were the proven effectiveness of the Saskatchewan hospital plan in terms of its low administrative cost and its coverage of all Saskatchewan residents on the same terms and conditions; the experience of the Swift Current Health Region's medical care plan as the only pilot of medicare of its type in the country; and the effectiveness of federal government cost sharing and standard setting through the Hospital Insurance and Diagnostic Services Act of 1957. Although not stated in the report explicitly – this would have been politically unwise – the Hall Commission essentially recommended the adoption of the Saskatchewan approach to universality on a national basis.[99] Each of these initiatives had T.C.'s fingerprints all over them.

## Antipathy to Saskatchewan-Style Medicare

At the same time, Douglas was far from confident that the Pearson government would accept the Hall Commission's recommendations regarding the single-payer and single-tier design of national medicare. The forces of opposition had been strengthened immensely by the actions of provincial governments in Alberta, British Columbia, and Ontario. The year before, Ernest Manning had worked directly with the

Alberta Medical Association and private insurance companies to set up a voluntary, multi-payer medical care plan in Alberta. The basic design features were almost identical to the multi-payer, voluntary hospital insurance plan that his government had operated from 1950 until it was reconfigured into a compulsory and universal hospital plan to meet the eligibility requirements for federal cost sharing in 1958.[100]

In contrast to Douglas, who was trying to replace the market for health insurance, Manning was committed to both the market and the "insurance principle," and wanted to minimize redistribution through the tax system. Manning's voluntary insurance-based approach was intended to "maintain the responsibility of the individual in providing for his medical requirements, with the state assuming its responsibility to assist [only] to the extent necessary to bring medical services within the financial reach of all the people."[101] Manningcare was championed by organized medicine and insurance companies throughout Canada as the template for other provinces and the model that should be promoted by the Pearson government.[102]

In Ontario, in April 1963, the PC government under Premier John Robarts introduced a medical care bill based on a targeted subsidy approach similar to the one that Manning had implemented.[103] And, like Manning, Robarts's government had worked with organized medicine and private insurance carriers to create the plan. However, in the face of vehement attacks by the NDP and the Liberals in the Legislative Assembly of Ontario that the proposal was "a 100 percent capitulation to the insurance companies and the medical profession," the bill was not passed.[104] Instead, Robarts decided to set up a committee under University of Waterloo president Gerald Hagey to study the plan and make suggestions for improvement.[105] As Robarts had explained to the media after his government's brief had been submitted to the Hall Commission, he did "not believe that a compulsory scheme" was "necessary," given the number of Ontario residents already in private insurance plans. However, he was not as dogmatic as Manning on the issue and added that "if the result of the many studies going on indicate the need for compulsion," then his government was willing to reconsider.[106] However, the makeup of the Hagey Committee almost guaranteed that it would, in the end, endorse the basic approach reflected in the government's bill, one that the media referred to as "Robartscare" to distinguish it from both Saskatchewan-style medicare and Alberta-style Manningcare.

Then there was W.A.C. Bennett's Social Credit government in British Columbia. From the time the medicare plan had been proposed in Saskatchewan, the NDP opposition in British Columbia under leader

Robert Strachan had been pushing for a similar plan.[107] In his brief to the Hall Commission in February 1962, months before the doctors' strike in Saskatchewan, Strachan stressed that access "to the finest medical care available is a basic human right which must be made available to every person in Canada regardless of his means." This could be achieved, Strachan argued, only through a compulsory and publicly administered plan, as private insurance should never "be allowed to profit from a health scheme." He went further than his CCF confreres in Saskatchewan, stating that medicare "legislation must spell out clearly the fact that the patient's right to health services is an enforceable legal right and must ensure that no person eligible for medical care can be refused such care by the medical profession." Having observed the College of Physician and Surgeons of Saskatchewan stymie Douglas's efforts to introduce medicare since 1960, Strachan told the Hall Commission that the "medical profession should not have either the moral or legal right to obstruct or defeat a national or provincial health plan."[108]

Premier Bennett could not have disagreed more. His minister of health spoke for the Socred government when he attacked the way in which Douglas and then Lloyd had implemented medicare as "the most shameful and fearsome anti-democratic behaviour that we have ever witnessed in this country."[109] Still, the NDP posed a major threat to Bennett. In the province's 1963 provincial election, the "New Democrats led with their *pièce de resistance*, a comprehensive medicare scheme."[110] The idea was popular enough among voters that the Socreds felt they had to respond with an alternative scheme, one that would provide the benefits of medicare without the compulsion or the higher taxes associated with the Saskatchewan model, in an election that Bennet described as a choice between a "construction crew" of Social Credit and a "wrecking crew" of socialists. The promise proved enough to dampen support for the NDP. Bennett won the election handily, even in working-class areas that had been previously held by the NDP.[111]

After the election, Bennett put together a working group with members from the ministry of health and the British Columbia Medical Association. Together, they worked out a plan in which the government would take care of bad risks through a public plan while the not-for-profit private insurance carriers would take care of everyone else. By excluding the for-profit carriers, Bennett hoped that his plan would better fit what he thought might be the shared-cost eligibility requirements in any future federal scheme. By the time the Hall Commission had delivered its recommendations, Bennett had just introduced the legislative framework for his multi-payer "Bennettcare" plan.[112]

Meanwhile, in Saskatchewan, after twenty years in government, the CCF under Woodrow Lloyd were struggling in the provincial election campaign of 1964. While many factors contributed to the government's vulnerability, there was little question that the civil society opposition to medicare that had sprung up in the weeks and months leading up to the doctors' strike had solidified into a force fiercely opposed to the CCF government. Despite growing acceptance of the Saskatoon Agreement, most doctors distrusted, even hated, the CCF-NDP.[113] As could be expected, the Sifton press, in an editorial that would be similar in tone to many others during the campaign, blamed Douglas for the doctors' aversion to the provincial government:

> The then Premier of Saskatchewan, Mr. T.C. Douglas, who departed from a seriously split province to become national leader of the New Democratic Party, had publicly promised that the medicare legislation would never be implemented before agreement had been reached that the doctors were satisfied with its terms.
>
> That promise was never kept. The resultant controversy precipitated a provincial crisis, involving all Saskatchewan residents. It threatened to erupt in violence.[114]

The Liberals under provincial leader Ross Thatcher were the natural beneficiaries of this antipathy and, by the time of the provincial election on 22 April 1964, the Liberals had managed to attract enough PC and Socred support to win a majority – thirty-two seats compared to the CCF-NDP's twenty-six – even though their popular vote percentage was only a sliver above that of Woodrow Lloyd's party. The only consolation for Douglas and his federal party was the provincial Liberals' abrupt change of tactics by pledging "not to change the existing Medicare legislation by as much as a comma."[115] Although the NDP-CCF's relationship with a majority of doctors remained strained, the polarization in the general public had eased, and many members of the public who had previously exhibited anxiety about the coming of medicare now wanted to keep the program. In the end, medicare did not feature as a major election issue, despite the CCF-NDP's best efforts to make it so. The Lloyd government lost in large part because the party had been in office for two decades and a slim majority decided it was time for a change.[116]

In T.C.'s view, while the Hall Report may have tipped the scale towards his model of medicare, he knew that forces within the federal Liberal government preferred a targeted, means-tested approach, if only because it would cost less and might not require a tax increase. He

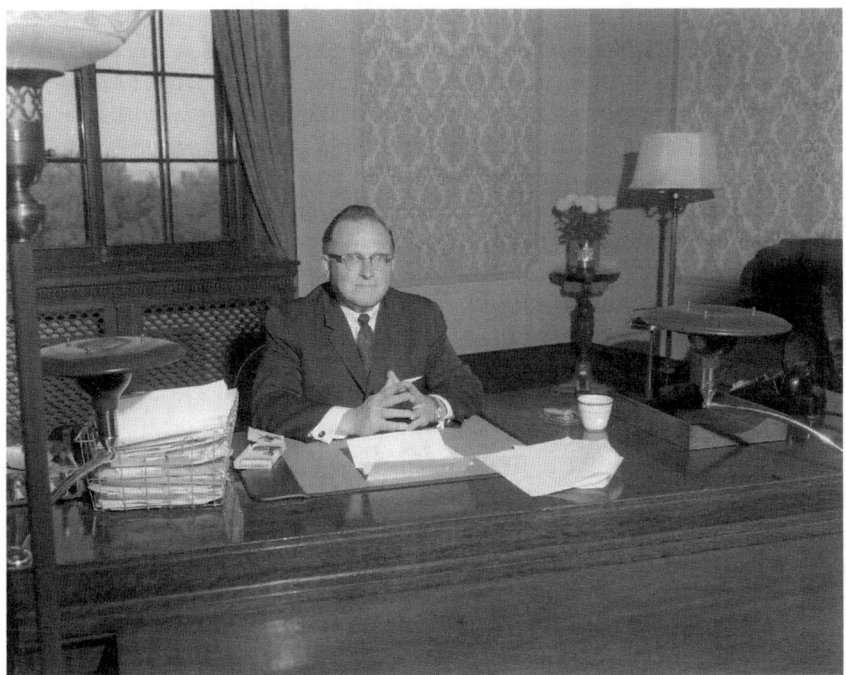

Ross Thatcher in the premier's office c. 1964 (PAS, *Regina Leader-Post*, Thatcher negative no. 1)

feared that the Liberals might play their old game of promising medicare in the next election but letting it drop if they won a majority. When interviewed by the press on his reaction to the report, he reminded everyone of the fact that the recommendations were similar to those in the federal government's Green Book proposals of 1945, and, as he had with the King and St-Laurent administrations, he stewed over the possibility the Pearson government might not follow through.[117]

**The 1965 Federal-Provincial Conference**

Fortunately for Douglas, the Hall Commission had recommended that the first ministers meet within six months to finalize the fiscal and administrative arrangements for a comprehensive, pan-Canadian medicare program.[118] Using this in the House of Commons, T.C. demanded to know when the prime minister would convene the premiers. Pearson's initial answer – that his government would first have to study the report and come to its own conclusions before it contacted the premiers to find a date convenient to all parties – was too vague for Douglas's liking. He followed up with a supplementary query: would the prime minister commit to calling a meeting within the six months recommended by the Hall Commission? Pearson's final response was that he did "hope" that a federal-provincial conference could be held within six months, "subject to the wishes of the provinces."[119] It would, in fact, take over a year before a first ministers' conference was convened to deal with the Hall Commission's recommendations.

The delay was due not only to the unfinished business of the Canada Pension Plan. From the time the Hall Report was submitted until well into 1965, the Pearson government was wracked with the decision of whether to call an election to try to win a majority. Although he prevaricated on the timing of an election, Pearson desperately wanted a majority. In his view, the minority position of his government never allowed him to stand "at ease," in part because Douglas and his NDP caucus had made "instability" inescapable.[120]

Walter Gordon was an early proponent of calling a summer election, in the hope that it would stack both the backbench and the cabinet with more progressives. Gordon convinced Pearson that medicare could be used as part of the election platform. But, since the Liberals had already promised medicare in the 1963 election, the government would have to show some progress, by calling a federal-provincial conference as recommended by the Hall Commission.[121]

Towards the end of January 1965, Justice Emmett Hall submitted his commission's considerably shorter second (and final) volume, along with his proposed news releases.[122] While this volume summarized detailed studies on health professions and sectors and added no new recommendations, Hall used the opportunity to "provide the definitive rebuttal of the CMA" and other anti-medicare groups that the commission provoked with the first volume.[123] Hall had already spent months on a national speaking tour defending his recommendations and explaining why a targeted, subsidy-based approach could never deliver as good access and quality as a universal, publicly administered plan. He also used the opportunity to attack the arguments made by organized medicine. In the public hearings, he had had a bellyful of "those damn doctors" and their "propaganda." In his view, they presented "not a shred of evidence to support their opposition to a government sponsored plan."[124]

In speech after speech, Hall sharpened his message, and by the time he spoke to the Winnipeg Community Welfare Planning Council in January 1965, he had already inserted the text of his speech into the second volume of the report.[125] In the speech, he openly described the arguments of organized medicine as "just plain nonsense." Moreover, although his commission had recommended in favour of fee-for-service payment, he argued that no method of payment was "sacrosanct" and that the belief by doctors in their "absolute right" to set fees was a "19th century concept that" had "no validity in the 20th century."[126]

In the months between the first and second volumes of the commission's reports, Hall's own views had hardened. Although he had not addressed the subject in volume 1, Hall decided to reject physician extra-billing in volume 2. He also proposed that governments should not cover the fees of those patients seeing physicians who chose to opt out of a provincial medicare scheme. Both these "suggestions" – there were no formal recommendations in volume 2 – so upset one member of the commission, Dr. David Baltzan, that he insisted on adding his own dissenting view.[127] Hall eventually and reluctantly agreed, "but rather than putting it into the introduction as Baltzan had asked, Hall instructed that it be placed on … the last page in the body of the second volume," together with a few errata to volume 1, to minimize the impact of Baltzan's dissent.[128] Not surprisingly, the public release of volume 2 in February 1965 triggered the CMA to renew its attack on the Hall Commission.[129]

Hall's actions also disturbed Judy LaMarsh, who felt it was improper for any royal commissioner, much less a sitting member of the Supreme Court of Canada (Diefenbaker had appointed Hall to the top court in January 1963), to play an advocacy role after the delivery of a report. She was especially annoyed that Hall had put pressure on the government to hold federal-provincial meeting on the commission's recommendations.[130] Whatever the internal views of Pearson's cabinet, the delivery of the commission's final volume increased pressure on the Liberals to set out their own position.

Back in Saskatchewan, over the space of four years, medicare had gained broader acceptance as the benefits of the program became more obvious. In response to its growing popularity, even Ross Thatcher, in the election campaign of April 1964, had to promise not to get rid of the plan. When Thatcher defeated Woodrow Lloyd and the CCF-NDP, he stayed true to his word and kept medicare in place. Although there remained a hardcore of doctors who (unlike their patients) continued to harbour animosities towards the program, they saw how government funding resulted in an appreciable gain in their personal incomes. With the growing popularity of the program came increased demands for medicare across Canada. As Malcolm Taylor expressed it, by the mid-1960s, the Saskatchewan scheme was a constant spectre at every [federal] Liberal Cabinet meeting when medicare was discussed." In Parliament, Douglas, Stanley Knowles, and the other NDP MPs "never let" the Pearson government forget that Saskatchewan-style medicare was working.[131]

In the federal throne speech, delivered a little less than two months after volume 2 of the Hall Report was tabled, the Pearson government stated its intention to "improve the quality of Health services" and ensure "that all Canadians can obtain needed health care, irrespective of the ability to pay." Consistent with this, the federal government committed to meet with the provincial governments "at an early date" so it could "discuss with them the way in which federal and provincial action can most effectively contribute to programs that will provide health services to Canadians on a comprehensive basis."[132] Not enough for Douglas, he lambasted the government the next day in the House for delaying action on the Hall Commission now that it had "the most extensive and exhaustive report on this subject that has been printed in the English language."

The report's main conclusions were not hard to understand, T.C. argued: "first, that Canada needs medicare; second, it says that Canada can afford medicare; and third, it says the government should take action immediately within six months of receiving the report to call a federal-provincial conference in order to begin laying plans for its implementation." He told the House he was worried about any meeting between the PM and the premiers, because "several of the provinces [sic] phony medicare plans" had been proposed simply to forestall federal cost sharing of universal programs throughout Canada. "If the federal government fails to act, and to act promptly, these plans will become established," and we will be set "back 25 years in our march toward national, comprehensive medicare."[133]

These concerns, shared by organized labour and other pro-medicare interests in the country, were reiterated by other NDP MPs.[134] Referring to a resolution passed by Winnipeg City Council, "urging the establishment of a Federal-Provincial health plan along the lines recommended by the Hall Commission," Stanley Knowles asked the PM whether he would reply in the affirmative. Although Pearson brushed off the question at first, when asked a second time, he responded by saying he would reply in a "friendly way," purposely avoiding the term "favourable."[135] Regardless, behind the scenes, there was considerable activity as the federal government prepared its position for the first ministers' conference. Moreover, T.C. was likely aware of this, as one of his former chief officials, Al Johnson, was in the middle of this new burst of activity.

## Al Johnson and the Federal Offer

Johnson along with a bevy of Saskatchewan civil servants had moved from Regina to Ottawa in the immediate aftermath of the change in the federal government in April 1963.[136] He arrived at an opportune time. Still smarting from the interminable federal-provincial meetings over the Canada Pension Plan, Pearson wanted to be sure that some kind of deal on medicare could be made before he called a first ministers' conference. Thus, he and Judy LaMarsh dispatched some of their chief officials to gather information from the ten provincial capitals.[137]

Now responsible for federal-provincial fiscal relations, Johnson took the lead in the discussions with provincial governments on a national health program.[138] Most of the premiers seemed to be quite receptive to the idea, except for Ernest Manning, who wanted nothing whatsoever to do with universal medicare.[139] Ontario was less than enthusiastic, but John Robarts had, unlike Manning, at least shown some flexibility. The hardest nut to crack was Quebec premier Jean Lesage. He had made it clear after national hospital insurance program that Quebec would never again accept a cost-shared program. Alberta could be ignored but, given their demographic and political weight, the two central Canadian provinces were key to any agreement on national medicare, as they had been on pensions.

Johnson had an idea. Rather than subjecting any province to a set of conditions enforced by bilateral federal-provincial agreements and regular federal monitoring, as was the case for the hospital insurance program, he suggested something much simpler. If the provincial government could establish a program conforming to four simple principles – public administration, universality, comprehensiveness, and portability – then the federal government would simply transfer to the province its per capita share of the cash (and part tax transfer in the case of Quebec). After clearing the idea with his bureaucratic and political masters, Johnson and Claude Morin, Lesage's deputy minister of intergovernmental affairs, discussed the idea for two hours in the bar of Ottawa's Chateau Laurier. Morin took the idea to Lesage, who agreed to it. Pearson now had a workable proposal he could present to the premiers. According to Tom Kent, Johnson had "originated the kind of solution that, once you have heard it, you kick yourself for having failed to think of it," and Kent gave him full credit for providing a way forward.[140]

What Pearson, Kent, and LaMarsh may not have been aware of is that Johnson got the idea for the principles from his old boss, Tommy Douglas, in particular Douglas's speech setting out his government's intention to implement universal medical care in December 1959.[141] While flexible on the administrative details for medicare in Saskatchewan – eventually worked out in detail by the Thompson Committee – he expected the final plan to conform to five basic principles, including universal coverage and public administration, two of the four federal criteria in Johnson's proposal.[142] The four eligibility criteria for provincial participation in medicare "were immediately submitted" to and approved by cabinet "as the definitive national approach" to be presented at the four-day first ministers' conference slated to begin on 19 July 1965.[143]

When the premiers assembled in Ottawa, they were in a more conciliatory and constructive mood than usual, which boded well for Pearson.[144] The first ministers faced an enormous agenda, ranging from economic development and fiscal relations to transportation and social security, so each had brought sizeable delegations. Among the participants were some top officials from Douglas's time as premier, now spread out as key advisors in three governmental delegations.[145]

These former Douglas advisors included Johnson, who, with Kent, was a critical federal official – the two men were seated just behind Pearson and next to Claude Morin, Premier Lesage's top official. The Saskatchewan delegation included Graham Clarkson, the former executive director of the Medical Care Insurance Commission and now the deputy minister of health, and Art Wakabayashi, who had been one of Johnson's senior officials and whom Johnson had recommended to Thatcher to take over his position as deputy provincial treasurer.[146] In New Brunswick, the former Douglas regime was represented by Donald Tansley, Johnson's former second-in-command at treasury, who, at Douglas's request, was seconded to the MCIC to become its first permanent head. Tansley was joined by Robert McLarty, who had left the treasury department in Saskatchewan to join Tansley's new team under New Brunswick Liberal premier Louis Robichaud. No longer premier, Douglas had no standing at the first minister's conference, but he nonetheless exercised influence through this powerful group of his former officials.

In his opening statement, Pearson made it clear that medicare would be the "most important" item among the many in the disparate agenda "because it can most closely affect the daily lives of all Canadians." According to the PM, the release of the first volume of the Hall Report increased public interest in medicare and triggered considerable discussion concerning the ways in which it might be implement. While the pre-conference discussion by federal and provincial officials led him to conclude "that all provincial governments rank high among their objectives the establishment of a health services plan which will enable their residents to have access to comprehensive physicians' services on a prepaid basis," there were nonetheless "considerable differences" among the provincial governments as to "the type of plan" they favoured. Such "circumstances" Pearson argued, "create the necessity for a federal role."[147]

However, instead of insisting on a one-size-fits-all program, Pearson explained that the federal government would be willing to contribute to any provincial design that met the four "criteria" of comprehensiveness, universality, public administration, and portability:

> First, the scope of benefits should be, broadly speaking all the services provided by physicians, both general practitioners and specialists. A complete health plan would include dental treatment, prescribed drugs, and other important services, and there is nothing in the approach we propose to prevent these being included, from the start or later, if this were the general wish. We regard comprehensive physicians' services as the initial minimum.
>
> Secondly, we would propose that the plan should be universal. That is to say, it should cover all residents of a Province on uniform terms and conditions ...
>
> Thirdly, I think it will readily be agreed that a federal contribution can properly be made available only to a plan which is publicly administered, either directly by the provincial government or by a provincial non-profit agency.
>
> Fourthly, and finally, I think it is important to recognize the mobility of Canadians; each provincial plan should therefore provide full transferability of benefits when people are absent from the Provinces or when they move their homes to another Province.[148]

Pearson explained why the federal proposal was not a shared-cost program similar to the arrangement on hospital coverage under the Hospital Insurance and Diagnostic Services Act of 1957. For one, the new proposal did not "require detailed [bilateral] agreements" with the provinces. If a provincial government's plan met the four criteria, that government would be free to run the program the way it saw fit.[149] As for federal funding, this too would change. Instead of sharing the cost of medical care with the provinces after those costs had been incurred provincially (carefully monitored by federal inspectors to ensure eligibility under the terms of a bilateral agreement), Pearson offered a "fiscal contribution of pre-determined size" – an amount subsequently set at 50 per cent of the province's per capita share of the total national cost – subject only to the provincial government continuing to adhere to the four criteria.[150] Consistent with another Hall Commission recommendation, the federal government offered a generous $500 million Health Resources Fund for infrastructure and the training and education of new health professionals to grease the wheels.

While Manning remained opposed to the plan on ideological grounds and the premiers of Nova Scotia and Prince Edward Island fretted about the cost of the programs, the Quebec premier had agreed in advance of the conference, thanks to the solution proposed by Johnson. Four Liberal premiers – Joey Smallwood, Louis Robichaud, Jean Lesage, and Ross Thatcher – agreed, with few reservations. Although they too had some reservations, the PC premiers of Ontario and Manitoba, along with the sole Social Credit premier, Bennett of British Columbia, agreed to cooperate with Ottawa. The media speculated that Robarts, given his past opposition to universal medicare, was now driven mainly by partisan politics, especially the desire to take away a potential election issue from Pearson, speculating that the Liberals would have been in an even more advantageous position if the majority of premiers had opposed the plan.[151]

With most of the premiers agreeing to work within the federal framework, the Liberals could finally tell Canadians that they were on the verge of implementing a national program.[152] Pearson had been looking for a way to say that his government had made progress on medicare since the 1963 election and the Hall Commission Report. Now, with the most bullish member of the cabinet in favour of an early election, Walter Gordon enthused to the press that medicare was "right near the top" of the list of past campaign promises the Liberals wanted to complete before going to the electorate for a new mandate. From his perspective, enough provinces were supportive of the plan to "get it off the ground." As the finance minister, he also affirmed, based on the Saskatchewan medicare program cost of roughly $25 per person, that the cost would be sustainable for the federal government, although he would not speculate as to whether medicare would necessitate an increase in federal taxes.[153]

Pearson tried to downplay medicare as a "springboard to an election."[154] However, his statement that national medicare could be operational by 1 July 1967 seemed ready made for the coming election campaign.[155] Little surprise was evinced when, on 8 September, Pearson announced an election for 8 November 1965.

# 15 National Medicare

The prime minister's announcement of an impending federal election turned out to be a happy coincidence for Ernest Manning: the same day as Pearson's announcement, the premier of Alberta had already reserved time on television stations across the country for a thirty-minute lecture on what he saw as the many dangers of the federal medicare plan.[1] In the broadcast, Manning took direct aim at Douglas-style medicare, as reflected in Pearson's four eligibility principles. If these were accepted, Manning argued, then Canada "will have embarked on the road to a complete welfare state" that "will affect every family and every taxpayer and the individual rights of every citizen." While Manning did not "question for one moment the sincerity of the Prime Minister and his government in advocating this program," they nonetheless had been hoodwinked by their "socialist advisers," no doubt a reference to Tom Kent and Al Johnson.[2]

Of most concern to Manning was the insistence on universality, "in which participation is compelled by the state and not left to the voluntary choice of the citizen himself." For the Alberta premier, this violated the "fundamental principle of free society, namely the right of each citizen to exercise freedom of choice in matters relating to his own and his family's welfare." He particularly objected to the plan "being advocated as a program to provide free medical services." He believed that if taxpayers were not misled by socialists like Douglas, they would never favour "governments spending" taxpayer "money to pay for medical services for those who can well afford to buy their own medical insurance."[3]

In contrast, his Manningcare scheme, if adopted nationally, would be only "a fraction of the cost to Canadian taxpayers." It would also protect against a government bureaucracy becoming a monopoly insurer, "a flagrant violation of the basic principles of a free enterprise society."

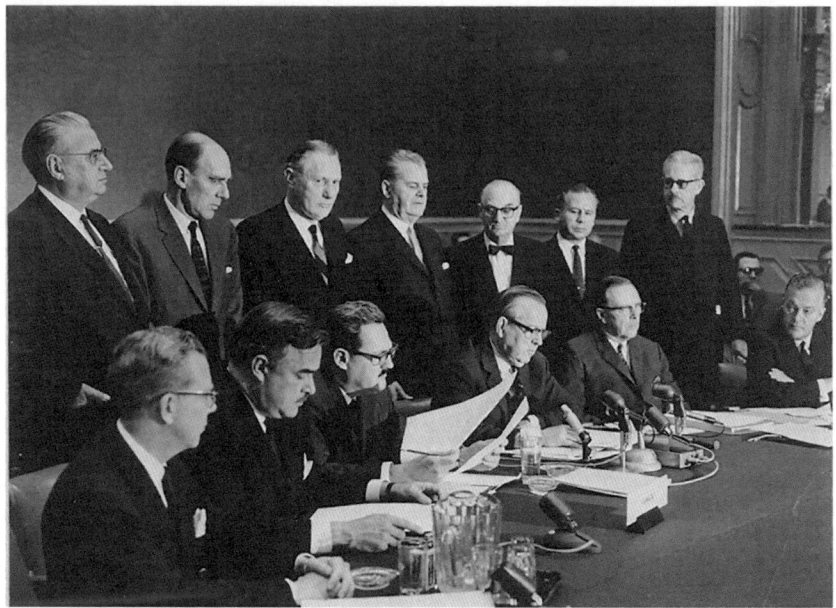

First Ministers' scrum with Ernest Manning (sitting far left) watching the prime minister answer questions, October 1964 (LAC C-094169)

The "false philosophy that medicare services are a right," rather than a personal responsibility for which you pay at least part of the cost, "leads men to demand all they can get of the so-called 'right' at the state's expense."[4] As in the battle for national hospitalization in the mid-1950s, Manning was once again squaring off against Douglas, but this time he would take his message beyond Alberta and beyond the federal-provincial conference table in Ottawa. He would take his message to the people of Canada through the medium of television.

Manning's television time was paid for by an anti-medicare coalition made up of life insurance companies, chambers of commerce, and organized medicine. All had an interest in making sure the public and their political representatives throughout the country knew there was an alternative to universal medicare. From Douglas's perspective, this coalition – for which Manning was the public advocate – was the most formidable opponent of medicare. Of course, the coalition had some strong allies in Parliament beyond the two dozen Socred MPs, including the business Liberals in the Pearson cabinet and the Bay Street Conservatives in the Diefenbaker opposition.

## The Federal Election of 1965

By promising to implement the recommendations of the Hall Commission, the Liberals had made it difficult for the NDP to distinguish the Liberal program from the NDP platform promise of comprehensive health insurance. Not even the PCs, given Diefenbaker's warm support for the Hall Report, seemed to be against medicare.[5] In public, Douglas said he welcomed "the opportunity of going to the Canadian people and offering them a real alternative" to what he described as the Pearson government's "ineptitude and indecision," but in private he could see little upside for his party in the election.[6]

The NDP had not yet financially recovered from the 1963 election, and much of its meagre resources had to be invested in Quebec, where it was fielding seventy-one candidates in a bid to become a truly national party. While a Gallup poll showed a slight improvement in popular support for the NDP early in 1965, the numbers rolling in months later told Douglas that Pearson could score a majority government, eliminating his party's limited leverage.[7]

And then, very early in the campaign, came disastrous news from Quebec. Three prominent leftists, Pierre Trudeau, Jean Marchand, and Gérard Pelletier, joined the Liberal Party as candidates. Trudeau had been a member of the CCF in Quebec until the mid-1950s. Marchand was a prominent labour leader who had led striking workers in the famous Asbestos Strike of 1949. An intellectual and editor-in-chief of *La Presse*, Pelletier was a long-time progressive voice in the province. The New Party movement had been created, in part, to attract unionists and leftist Quebeckers, yet the three chose to join the Liberals, albeit only after much wooing by the Pearson Liberals. The underlying message of this Liberal coup in obtaining the "three wise men" of Quebec was that the NDP was not a contender for power. As Jean Marchand explained at the time, "if we believe in this country and we want to do something for the country, we have to do it in Ottawa – and we have to do it in the party which has a chance to be in power."[8]

Given voter fatigue, the 1965 election campaign generated little interest. The Liberals felt that it was enough to say that they were keeping their long-held promise to deliver national health insurance. As for the NDP, its campaign platform on the theme of building a just society emphasized the pioneering role of the Saskatchewan CCF in establishing a beachhead for medicare in Canada and promised that, if elected, the party "would act immediately to implement the full recommendations of the Hall Commission report," which went well beyond covering physician services.[9] An NDP campaign leaflet criticized the Pearson government for doing "nothing to implement the Hall Royal Commission report which recommended the kind of Medicare enacted by a New Democratic government in Saskatchewan" and claimed that only the NDP could "be relied upon to enact a national plan."[10] As the election wore one, Douglas released a statement in which he contested the sincerity of the Liberals and the Progressive Conservative. "Everyone" was "now jumping on the medicare bandwagon," but only the NDP could be trusted to implement it:

> There is only one Party in Canada with a proven record in medicare. When I was Premier of Saskatchewan in 1960 we had an election in which the main issue was medicare. We were re-elected at that time, and before the next election medicare in Saskatchewan was a reality.
>
> In 1963 the Liberals promised medicare in their campaign ... Where is medicare? From which party are Canadians likely to get real medicare? From those who make a promise and carry it out? Or those who ignore their promises?
>
> The Hall Commission gave Canadians a blueprint for Medicare. But only the New Democrats will put their carefully drawn plan into action.[11]

T.C. carried the same message as he spoke across Canada, afflicted as always by knee pains. He exhausted himself and Cliff Scotton, his only election staffer. A young Desmond Morton was seconded from the Ontario NDP office partway through the campaign to help out. Morton carried T.C.'s bags and wrote his media releases, taking on a similar role to Tommy Shoyama's in the 1962 election. By 1965, Shoyama was a senior research economist for the federal government's relatively new Economic Council of Canada and therefore could not assume such a visible partisan role.[12] In a revealing essay written over a decade later when he was a history professor at the University of Toronto, Morton described the grueling campaign:

> Travelling with Tommy in the 1965 followed a pattern. He spent his weekends with Irma in their Burnaby apartment, secluded from all but the most urgent of all-candidate meetings. It was the price of his osteomyelitis. At dawn each Monday, we would join him for the first flight from Vancouver, heading east as far as we could go, then coming westward through the week. The final flight on Friday night would drop us back over the mountains. An exhausted Tommy Douglas would then have two days to recuperate while his raw speech-writer [Morton] would take refuge in a dreary motel to draft the forthcoming week's press releases and speech fragments on a slim, portable Olivetti [typewriter].

At each airport, an invariable ritual was played out. A modest gaggle of party supporters, all who could be mustered from their daily work, would be treated to Tommy's most blinding smile and a handshake. Next, flanked by [Cliff] Scotten and the local organizer, Douglas would march purposely down the airport corridor to the washroom. The purpose, with characteristic practicality, served both the calls of nature and the need, free from prying media, to sort out local issues. Next came a press conference timed, if possible, to catch afternoon newspapers and evening television. Ideally, rest would follow. It rarely did.[13]

In Morton's account, the final week proved to be the best for Douglas and the NDP, with huge rallies from Montreal to Vancouver. In Maple Leaf Gardens in Toronto, for example, it was clear that the 12,000 people inside and "the thousands more who milled outside" had come to see Douglas. Although "weary by now" and "visibly in pain," he was energized by the enthusiasm and gave the fiery – and funny – speech everyone had hoped for. By election night, the momentum turned into a 5 per cent increase for the party in the popular vote, but this produced only four more seats than in 1963. Nonetheless, Morton saw the result as a "personal triumph" for T.C.[14] The party had moved from the fourth to the third position in Parliament, enough to publicly declare victory. Although he felt disappointed that the party had again not come close to becoming the official opposition, T.C. smilingly told the press that the election had turned the NDP from "a splinter party" to "a major party."[15]

As for the Liberals, the election produced only two more seats, well short of a majority. They simply could not convince the electorate that their obtaining a majority government was a good enough reason to hold an election. In the end, the campaign had not be fought on any "clearly defined major issue."[16] For Douglas, another factor in the Liberal's poor showing was Diefenbaker, who, in his view, "had tremendous recuperative powers" and, despite his loosening grip on his own party, continued to be popular in the more rural areas of the country.[17] After months of debilitating infighting, Diefenbaker was rejuvenated by the campaign and the opportunity to barnstorm outside Ottawa. The result was that the PCs, despite all their internal conflict, went down only two seats in the election, with heavy losses in Ontario compensated for by gains in the Prairies and the Maritimes.

T.C. must have felt just a little personal vindication after the disappointing election results of 1962 and 1963 along with his personal defeat in 1962. While obtaining twenty-one seats was only an incremental improvement over the nineteen seats it had won in 1962 and the seventeen in 1963, the NDP's share of the popular vote, almost 18 per cent, was higher than that ever before achieved by the CCF or the NDP at the federal level. More importantly, Douglas's party was now in a powerful position to dictate at least some of the policy agenda to the minority Liberal government. In a cover piece in the *Star Weekly*, T.C. was characterized as the "Strong Man in the Middle." The election was enough for Douglas to return to the notion that he might live to see the day that Canada would "return to a two-party system, with one party left of centre and one right," and that left-of-centre party might be his own alone or some combination of his party joined by progressive Liberals.[18]

Immediately following the election, Douglas was quick to rule out a coalition with a minority Liberal government.[19] While the NDP would support individual pieces of legislation, it would remain in opposition. Douglas criticized the uselessness of the election. Pearson's "only justification" for calling it "was to obtain a majority which the Canadian people have refused to give him." It was now time to "get back to the work which the last parliament was forced to abandon." In particular, the time had come to give "Canada a comprehensive, universal Medicare plan."[20]

**Preparing the Medical Care Act, January–June 1966**

Following the election, Pearson replaced Judy LaMarsh with Allan J. MacEachen as minister of national health and welfare, in part because of MacEachen's proven ability to get legislation through the House of Commons.[21] While Pearson had originally appointed LaMarsh as minister of national health and welfare because he thought this was an appropriate portfolio for a woman, the ensuing (and, for Pearson, unexpected) protracted federal-provincial struggle over the Canada Pension Plan, particularly with Jean Lesage's Quebec, had tested his patience and put in question the competence of his minister. MacEachen, he thought, would be able to shepherd national medicare without the fuss and federal-provincial conflict that accompanied the pension plan. Unfortunately for Pearson and his government, this was not to be.[22] Indeed, compared to the pension plan experience, national medicare would be subject to more extreme objections and foot dragging by several provincial governments. Worse, cabinet itself was divided on both the substance and the timing of medicare, revealing Pearson's fragile position in his own government and contributing to his eventual decision to resign as leader and prime minister.

While MacEachen, like LaMarsh, very much wanted medicare to be implemented, the progressives in the Pearson cabinet had lost the support of a key ally. Assuming the blame for the timing and the poor outcome of the election, Walter Gordon resigned as finance minister and moved to the backbench. He was replaced by Mitchell Sharp, a fiscal conservative, under whom the department reverted to its traditional position of opposing expensive new programs, a crucial change in how the file would be managed over the next two and a half years.[23] Without question, the election outcome meant a more "uncertain future for medicare."[24]

From January 1966 until the beginning of medicare's implementation thirty months later, Douglas used his party's position in the minority government to keep the pressure on a government that often seemed on the verge of delaying, if not retreating from, medicare. In January 1966, Douglas made a major speech on medicare in Parliament. The basic message was to get on with the job without any further delay. Reminding the government of the "excellent blueprint" it had received from the Hall Commission eighteen months earlier, he could only hope that Pearson and his ministers would "have the courage to follow the report" and "to believe that the great bulk of the Canadian people will support" them "if courageous steps are taken."

Douglas then paid credit to the leader of the opposition and reminded the members that it was the Diefenbaker government, not the Liberals, that had made the plan possible by removing the double majority provision in the Hospital Insurance and Diagnostic Services Act. This had allowed for provinces to come into the scheme at different times, but the provinces that were first ready and willing to come in, Douglas believed, encouraged the others to follow suit, despite the pressure they were under from the many interest groups lobbying against a universal scheme. He then changed tack to "plead with the Prime Minister not to allow this befogging of an important issue by some people, who seem to be more interested in keeping the private insurance companies in the medicare field than in getting progressive legislation on the statute books, to keep him from doing the things he started out to do."[25]

Ten days later, MacEachen and the country's provincial ministers of health met in Ottawa to begin a two-day meeting. Noting that the federal government had expected, but not received, all the provincial positions on the question of medicare by the end of 1965, MacEachen asked each health minister to set out their respective positions by the second day of the conference. To this, four health ministers simply refused, in large part because their premiers were not yet prepared to give a final answer. A fifth, the minister from Alberta, Dr. Donovan Ross, made it clear that his province was sticking with its multi-payer subsidy approach.[26] Since only Saskatchewan had a plan that met the criteria set out by Pearson the summer before, while other provinces such as

Alberta, Ontario, and British Columbia were on a different track, Ross hoped the federal government would "rethink" its original position favouring a Saskatchewan-style "compulsory" program.[27] Only the ministers from Newfoundland, New Brunswick, and Saskatchewan gave a clear affirmative answer. Quebec's response was more complicated, but the upshot was that if the provincial government's conditions on tax abatement and lack of conditionality were met, it too would sign up.[28]

Beyond describing the original double-majority rule under the 1957 hospital insurance law as "unfortunate," MacEachen felt it was too early to state how many provinces would be required, and with what percent of the population, before Ottawa was prepared to proceed. Among the provincial ministers of health, Davey Steuart from Saskatchewan expressed the view that those provinces that had eligible programs should be able to get federal funding as soon as possible. Unless Ottawa proceeded immediately with legislation, T.C. posited, many provinces would continue to "just sit on the fence." Since Steuart felt that some provincial governments had exaggerated the cost of medicare in Saskatchewan to justify blocking the national plan, he reminded everyone that the Saskatchewan plan, which then cost $25 per capita, would not likely cost more than $28 per capita by 1967.[29] Given what unfolded in the months to come, Steuart's intervention had little impact, not only on the positions of other provinces but on Steuart's own premier, Ross Thatcher.[30]

A health ministers' communique following the meeting stated that, while "several provinces accepted the federal proposals and indicated their readiness to commence programs" by 1 July 1967, some provinces still "were unprepared to make definite commitments at this time." However, at the end of the communique, MacEachen reiterated Ottawa's "adherence" to the four criteria first announced by the PM the summer before and "its objective to commence federal contributions to provincial medical care plans on a nation-wide basis by July 1st, 1967."[31] Since no province had rejected the federal proposal outright, MacEachen told the press that he remained optimistic about the 1 July 1967 start date.[32] At least one journalist speculated that the minister was willing to proceed with a small coalition of willing provinces in an effort to put fiscal pressure on the more reluctant ones, as their taxpayers would be paying for something they were not yet receiving.[33]

A month after the meetings, no federal draft legislation had yet been placed before cabinet, which continued to debate approaches. Based on his reading of the provincial governments, MacEachen requested a decision from cabinet so that he or the PM could announce "that the federal government would commence payments" on 1 July 1967 "to any provinces having established plans which met federal requirements." In his view, this public notice would give provincial governments both the incentive and time to prepare eligible plans so they could receive federal contributions by 1 July the following year. While at least one minister supported MacEachen, many others did not, and a few began to make noises about the advantages (at least from a public finance standpoint) of the multi-payer subsidy approaches implemented in Alberta and British Columbia and being seriously considered in Ontario. Pearson came down on the side of the majority supporting a delay in the announcement.[34]

As the drafting of Bill C-227 – the Medical Care Act, as it would become known – continued, the CMA was furiously lobbying MacEachen on two key criteria: public administration and universality. Given past Liberal electoral promises that the federal version of medicare, unlike the Saskatchewan plan, would get the support of the medical profession, MacEachen tried to compromise without losing the essence, if not the details, of the plan recommended by the Hall Commission. In a meeting with the CMA leadership, he promised that extra-billing would not be banned in the legislation as long as the "profession accepts" its "responsibility" to avoid "abuses and excesses which would impair universality or access to patient services."[35] As for public administration, MacEachen discovered what he felt was a modest compromise with the CMA as well as the dissident provincial governments.

## Debating and Passing the Medical Care Act, July–December 1966

On 12 July, six months after Douglas's speech in Parliament pushing the government to get on with medicare, MacEachen presented Bill C-227 in the House. After he paid due credit to Paul Martin Sr. for establishing the foundation upon which medicare would be built – the National Health Grants program followed by national hospital insurance – he remarked that the time had finally come to accept that access to medical care "should be available to every citizen of our country," irrespective of ability to pay. "This effort," MacEachen suggested, "springs not only from a deepening of our humanitarian concern for our fellow citizens, but from a realization that we cannot afford the social and economic consequences of our failure to do so."[36]

MacEachen was then interrupted by oppositions MPs, including Diefenbaker and Douglas. All were incensed at the fact that, while the press gallery had received advance copies of his lengthy speech, they had not. Apologizing for the oversight and promising to make copies available, MacEachen carried on. He made it clear that Pearson's

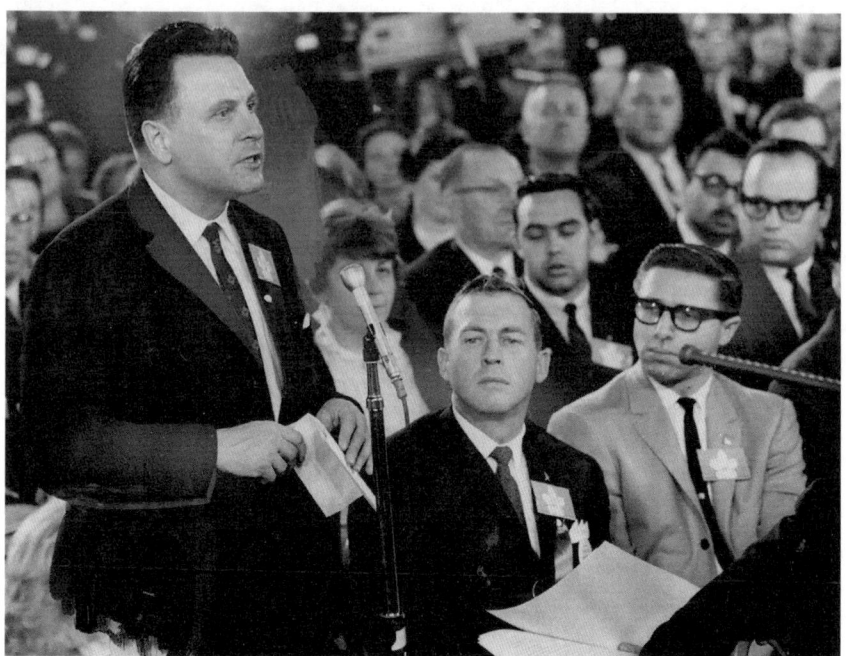

Allan J. MacEachen in 1966 in the midst of the debate over the federal government's Medical Care Act (MacEachen Institute for Public Policy and Governance, Dalhousie University)

four principles remained his government's firm position. Universality, as defined by Pearson based on the Hall Commission's report, was non-negotiable:

> Hon. members may ask why the federal government considers the principle of universal coverage to be so important. I believe that if the considerable expenditures which will have to be made to provincial programs are to be justified, then the federal government must have the assurance that as many people as possible will benefit. That is the case for the federal government. From the national point of view it is also essential to ensure that there is no differentiation in coverage between the residents of one province and another if federal funds are to be provided.[37]

While the bill limited coverage to physician services, MacEachen emphasized that the Medical Care Act should be seen as a floor rather than a ceiling for universal coverage and that there was "nothing to deter" provincial governments from "including additional benefits." Moreover, MacEachen said he had already "assured the provincial governments that as soon as there is a consensus on the timing of further benefits to be provided over and above physicians' services, the federal government would consider enlarging appropriately and in due course the scope of benefits to which it would be prepared to contribute."[38]

When T.C. responded as leader of the NDP, he commended MacEachen and Martin for the work they had done. As for the criticism MacEachen received "from many quarters about the drain on the federal treasury and about the increased costs which can be anticipated," he reminded everyone that Canadians were already paying for medical care. "It is already costing" Canadians in excess of $600 million a year for physician care. National medicare would redistribute that cost "so that instead of the burden being placed on the sick, it is distributed over the entire population on a basis that has some relation to ability to pay."[39] Heckled by Conservative and Social Credit MPs at this point about the burden on taxpapers, he quickly responded: "People who pay taxes also pay doctors' bills" but "most of us would rather pay taxes when we are well than pay doctors' bills when we are sick."[40]

Addressing the scepticism concerning MacEachen's estimated cost for a national medical care plan, T.C. pointed to the Saskatchewan experience. While it was accurate that hospital costs went up 26 per cent three years after hospital coverage was introduced, this dramatic growth in costs "levelled out" once the backlog of pent-up demand was cleared. Moreover, this experience was not repeated in the years after medicare was introduced, due to the fact that pent-up demand for physician care was not nearly as significant as had been the case for hospital coverage.[41]

On other points, T.C. was more critical. Why was federal cost sharing limited to physician care? Could the floor "not be sufficiently flexible" to encourage individual provinces, once they covered medical services, to expand beyond them, with the encouragement of the federal treasury? In moving towards comprehensive health coverage, the provinces could progress at their own pace, selecting, for example, "optometric care" or "mov[ing] into the field of prescribed drugs."[42]

Douglas then took aim at the federal government's evolving definition of "public administration." Pearson had been clear in the federal-provincial conference the year before that, to be eligible, a public body, not a consortium of private insurers, needed to manage the provincial medical care program. But, as Pearson put it, there would still "be scope for the continuation of private insurance" for non-medicare services. However, during the election campaign, as reported in the press, Pearson had told an Alberta audience that provincial governments would be "free to delegate" the "administration of federally-supported medicare to private agencies."[43]

In T.C.'s view, this completely contradicted "the principle" that Pearson had presented to the premiers in July 1965. In fact, the definition of "public administration" had been altered from that used in the Hospital Insurance and Diagnostic Services Act to permit non-profit insurance companies from participating. According to Malcolm Taylor, this was "an obvious shift in strategy" to enable W.A.C. Bennett's multi-payer plan based on non-profit carriers to qualify and to appease the premiers of Alberta and Ontario.[44] Taylor argued that this new definition would allow provincial medical plans "to be turned over to private insurers, with resulting higher costs associated with marketing, advertising and duplicate administrations." He pointed to the Saskatchewan plan, where less "than 6 cents out of every dollar paid by the public for medicare goes to administration whereas ... in private plans this cost can range anywhere from 16 cents to as high as 30 cents and in many cases works out at an average of 23 cents to 27 cents on the dollar."[45]

As for the Progressive Conservative health critic's suggestion that the government consider delaying implementation to allow the provinces more time to prepare, T.C again drew on his own experience. There was "something about human nature whereby we never do things until we have to do them." Unless the pressure of a deadline was present, governments would never be 100 per cent ready, so it was best for the federal government to "cling to its target date of July 1, 1967." Besides, Canadians had "waited far too long for a step which has already been taken by most of the countries of western Europe."[46] For these and other reasons, T.C. had been fretting about the timing of the bill for many weeks.

**A Question of Timing**

T.C. was anxious to see the bill passed before the summer recess of Parliament. If it was not, he feared that some provincial governments would delay their own preparatory work on provincial bills while others, especially those in Ontario and Alberta, and in Quebec, where the Union Nationale had just defeated the Liberal Lesage government, would have time to mount a major offensive against medicare.[47]

Privately, MacEachen had come to the same conclusion. Months before, he told his cabinet colleagues that delaying action on the bill would remove the pressure on provincial governments to join the national scheme. In fact, both MacEachen and Pearson had initially planned the medical care bill to go from first to third reading before the summer recess and had made announcements both inside and outside the House of Commons to that effect. However, to MacEachen's great irritation, he discovered just before first reading that the Liberal house leader had made a deal with the PC opposition to delay second reading until the fall session.[48]

T.C. felt Pearson should overturn that deal. Pointing out that the NDP was not party to the agreement with the Liberal house leader, Douglas was upset that the Liberals had already delayed the bill far too long. Now that the bill had finally arrived in the house, he argued that all MPs had "a duty to the people of Canada" and a "debt to posterity to see that this legislation is put on the statute books of Canada before we leave here for a summer holiday."[49]

Stanley Knowles piled on. As he pointed out, it had been forty-seven years since the Liberals first proposed health insurance, and the "chances were 'slim'" that the Liberals would meet their own deadline of implementation of 1 July 1967 if second reading were delayed until autumn.[50] Knowles's reference to the original Liberal promise of 1919 got under the skin of Liberal MP John Munroe, who said he was fatigued with Knowles and the NDP constantly making the same argument and reminded the house that it took Douglas, when he was premier of Saskatchewan, almost two decades to implement medical care coverage.[51] The next day, MacEachen announced that, contrary to his personal wishes, the bill would not proceed to second reading until the fall. T.C. continued to argue vehemently against delay, but the government's decision was supported by the official opposition.[52]

That summer, the forces of opposition to the medical care bill grew. Sensing an opportunity to delay the bill and renegotiate the four criteria, provincial premiers and finance ministers lobbied key members of the Pearson cabinet. By early August, the federal cabinet was solidly divided into two warring factions: the fiscal conservatives who felt that "the strong negative reaction from many provinces provided" the Pearson government with a golden opportunity "to re-open the whole question" of the Medical Care Act "and possibly defer its implementation," and the progressives who insisted that the government "stand by" its "pledge" to make medicare "available on July 1, 1967."[53] Although Pearson was initially noncommital, it would soon become clear which faction held the upper hand.

In early September, all hell broke loose. Finance Minister Mitchell Sharp announced in a CBC television interview that, due to the government's budgetary deficit and inflationary pressures, the implementation date of medicare would likely have to be delayed for one year.[54] Sharp then confirmed the decision a day later in his budget speech in the House of Commons.[55] As both Douglas and MacEachen had predicted, the delay signalled to anti-medicare interests in the country "a weakening" of federal resolve.[56] Premier Robarts applauded the decision, stating that this would allow the time for the Pearson government to "hammer out some of the difficulties" he and other premiers had with the existing legislation. The CMA viewed the postponement as a "reasonable, useful and progressive step."[57]

At the time of the announcement, Douglas was on the campaign trail assisting the provincial NDP in an election in British Columbia. He lashed out at Sharp, stating that inflation could never be cured by cancelling medicare and that Sharp's reasoning amounted to "sheer economic illiteracy." Speaking at an NDP reception in Vancouver, he told party faithful that medicare would not "infuse new money into the economy"; it would simply shift payment for individuals from an out-of-pocket or insurance payment when they received the service to payment through taxation.[58]

The press was divided on the issue, the majority supporting Sharp and the provinces, the minority against the delay. The *Ottawa Citizen* aptly set out the contending positions:

> From the viewpoint of social justice, there was never a time when medicare was more badly needed. The cost of medical treatment is soaring and those on fixed or low incomes, many of whom are elderly and therefore prone to illness, feel the pinch most severely.
>
> From the viewpoint of the conservative mind, however, there is never a good time for major social change. Only unremitting popular clamor and the clear threat of political disaster can justify so big a step. Thus any convenient excuse will do as an argument for postponing change. Inflation is the latest excuse for postponing medicare, as so many other excuses have been found over many years of tedious argument.[59]

As the same editorial pointed out, "every delay" gave additional "hope and comfort to those" hoping "to block a national health plan," including the "medical associations, the insurance companies, [and] the drug manufacturers," who now "have been granted an extra year in which to lobby and campaign against medicare." Tying this into the speculation concerning Pearson's weakness as a PM and his imminent resignation, the *Citizen* predicted that Sharp would "now become the leadership candidate of all those Liberals – and there are many – who want to slow down the pace of change," while prominent progressive such as Allan MacEachen or Jean Marchand would become the leadership candidate for centre-left Liberals.[60]

Fuelling this speculation was a series of cabinet leaks.[61] Soon, journalists on the hill were openly writing about the split in the Pearson cabinet. One of these was Peter C. Newman, who would, in 1968, reveal the full extent of these divisions in his personality-driven account of the Pearson years. With Sharp's announcement, MacEachen almost resigned, and Marchand made it clear that if the health minister quit, Marchand would join him. However, both were convinced to stay on board when a compromise was reached in cabinet on the amendment changing the date of implementation, which would allow medicare "to be implemented earlier than July 1968, provided economic conditions changed."[62] However, immediately following the cabinet meeting, Sharp convinced Pearson that this change of wording would look like a retreat on the budget measures. Pearson not only accepted Sharp's argument but backed his position at a Liberal caucus meeting in early October, when the PM told the caucus that, if they disagreed with the decision to defer medicare, he would resign immediately.[63] With the prime minister in Sharp's corner, MacEachen told Pearson he would stay but would not tolerate any implementation delay beyond July 1968.

## Passage of the Medical Care Act and a Shift in Federal-Provincial Fiscal Relations

In mid-October 1966, in the midst of the Liberal government's turmoil, the medicare bill moved to second reading, kicking off eight days of debate. In Parliament, MacEachen expressed his regret at the postponed implementation date but reiterated that the bill would constitute a major milestone in the Canadian welfare state.[64] On the seventh day of the debate, T.C. delivered a lengthy speech in the House.[65] He applauded the fact that the Liberals did not this time insert "a joker" into the legislation, as they had in 1957, by requiring a double majority before it could be implemented. He also complimented the Liberals on rejecting "tin cup" medicare in favour of full universality, as implemented in Saskatchewan and recommended by the Hall Commission.

Douglas restricted his criticisms to three issues.[66] The first was the definition of medical care, which was limited to physicians. He suggested the definition should be revised to include optometrists and be flexible enough for those provincial governments that so desired to include osteopaths and chiropractors. The second issue was the threshold for universality, which MacEachen had relaxed largely to meet the criticisms of the Ontario and BC governments. If provincial governments attained 90 per cent population coverage in the first two years of the operation of their medical plans, they were eligible, as long as they reached 95 per cent coverage afterwards.[67] The third issue was the delay in the implementation date, which he pledged that the NDP would oppose "with all the powers at our command" so that "medicare comes into effect, as the government promised, on Canada's 100th birthday."[68]

T.C. could certainly have raised other issues about the limitations of the bill. Perhaps the most significant was the lack of clarity on user fees. The failure to prohibit such fees was a sop to premiers such as Manning who insisted on their right to impose deterrent fees to control utilization. Although MacEachen felt he had come to an understanding with the CMA on the issue, the verbal agreement that physicians would strictly limit extra-billing was unenforceable, and it would become a major flashpoint by the late 1970s and eventually lead to the Canada Health Act in 1984.[69] At this point, however, the only assurance MacEachen was prepared to offer Douglas and the NDP was that Ottawa would subtract the amount of extra-billing permitted by a provincial government from its per capita share of the federal cash transfer.[70]

Still, a flawed medicare act was better than none. Fully aware of the divisions within the federal cabinet as well as MacEachen's precarious position, T.C. ended his speech fulsomely supporting the legislation, because "it will give to our people freedom from fear and freedom from want" and "will enhance human dignity and extend social security in this country."[71] After a final statement by David Lewis, all NDP MPs voted in favour of the law on second reading on 25 October. Six weeks later, on 8 December, every member of the house except for two Social Credit MPs voted to pass the bill.[72] The Senate approved the bill just before Christmas, and the Medical Care Act came into force by year's end, with the amended start date of 1 July 1968.

Similar to the brief, ten-section-long, Hospital Insurance and Diagnostics Services Act (HIDSA) of 1957, the Medical Care Act had only nine sections.[73] Unlike HIDSA, however, it was not accompanied by bilateral agreements involving federal audits of provincial spending, administration, or performance. Instead, provincial governments simply had to pass their own medical care insurance laws implementing the federal act's criteria to be eligible for federal transfers, the formulation designed by Al Johnson to meet the Quebec government's demand for a less conditional approach.[74] These criteria were set out in section 3 of the Medical Care Act. They included public administration, defined as "a public authority appointed or designated" by the provincial government, as well as universal access to medical services on "uniform terms and conditions."

Sections 4 and 5 defined the amount of the contribution. While the purpose was to cost share eligible provincial spending on medical care, the 50 per cent was calculated on the basis of a province's per capita share of all spending on physician care by participating provinces. This differed from HIDSA, where only 25 per cent of the federal contribution was calculated in this way and the other 25 per cent was based on the actual spending of a province. This formula was designed to discourage provincial governments from spending more than they needed in the expectation of direct federal cost sharing.

The real sleeper in the act was section 8, a single but overly long sentence marking a major sea change from HIDSA, yet hardly commented upon at the time by Douglas or anyone else. Admittedly, the change was hard to spot in its Byzantine legalize:

> At least six months before the 31st day of March, 1973, the Government of Canada shall review the provisions of this Act respecting the amount and manner of payment of contributions payable by Canada pursuant to section 3 with a view to formulating proposals for any changes therein that appear then to be necessary or desirable with respect to the amount and manner of payment, whether by the transfer or allocation of specified tax revenues by Canada and the making of equalization payments and other fiscal adjustments by Canada in lieu of the contributions that would otherwise be payable pursuant to section 3 or in any other manner, of the contributions to be paid by Canada pursuant to this Act for years commencing after that day.[75]

What lay behind this section was a major rethinking of shared-cost social policy programs in Ottawa, led by Al Johnson. Almost immediately after his move to Ottawa in 1964, Johnson had started work on a restructuring of federal fiscal relations with the provinces.[76] At the request of Premier Lesage, no less, he was put in charge of the federal-provincial working committee for the ministerial Tax Structure Committee.[77] This work was spurred in large part by the Pearson government's desire to answer Quebec's charge that federal conditions on provincial social programs were an "intolerable invasion of provincial jurisdiction."[78] Johnson was also motivated by earlier provincial experiences in Saskatchewan with shared-cost conditional programs, which had generated an arsenal of ideas on how to improve fiscal federalism, including a major revamping of the equalization program.[79]

Johnson's proposal was radical and involved nothing less than the phasing out of shared-cost programs. The first stage was a transitional period – the five years identified in section 8 – needed to establish the program. In this phase, a cash transfer, calculated as a per capita provincial share of aggregate provincial spending on medical care, would be provided. The second, permanent, stage would see Ottawa replace the cash transfer with a permanent reduction of a selected federal tax (Johnson assumed personal income tax) to allow "an equivalent province tax increase." Since such a "tax transfer" would yield less in those provinces with a shallower tax base, such provinces would "receive an equalization payment bringing their tax yield to the national average."[80]

After the transitional period, there would be no federal enforcement under what Johnson called a block transfer regime for programs labelled "established." Instead, provinces would be held accountable to the agreed-upon criteria through their own provincial legislation. The advantage of the proposal, from Johnson's perspective, was that it cut the ground from underneath Quebec's demands for greater provincial autonomy and tax-abatement compensation for contracting out of shared-cost programs, and would allow Ottawa to treat all provinces the same.

Pearson, along with Johnson's ministers, first Walter Gordon and then Mitchell Sharp following the election of 1965, saw great merit in his proposal. As Sharp put it to his provincial counterparts when he presented the proposal as the new federal position in September 1966, a "block grant–established program" regime would mean that all provinces would receive more taxation authority for their expanding social policy responsibilities and would produce a more "uniform application of federal laws in all provinces."[81]

Regardless of the merits of this program, a worsening economic situation was creating concerns about the implementation of medicare in 1968, dividing the federal cabinet on whether it could proceed, despite the implementation date set out in legislation.

**The Continuing Campaign to Delay Implementation**

The decision to amend the Medical Care Act to change the implementation date from 1967 to 1968 should have ended the debate on timing, but it did not. Instead, the question continue to be a flash point both inside and outside government as opposition to medicare grew. Even some medicare-friendly provinces began to change their positions. The Liberal government in New Brunswick, for example, became so concerned about the cost of the program and the opposition of the provincial medical association that Premier Robichaud joined with other premiers to ask for further postponement.[82]

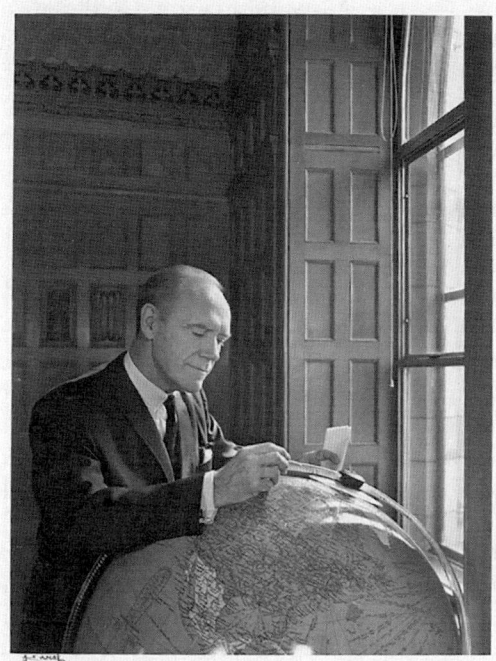

Karsh portrait of Mitchell Sharp (LAC, Yousef Karsh, R4515-38, e006608789)

In November 1967, Mitchell Sharp announced that medicare would cost $1 billion in its first year, contradicting the $885 million that MacEachen and his department had estimated.[83] Douglas angrily attacked Sharp's "fantastic estimate" in the House of Commons. Using figures drawn from the Saskatchewan experience with medicare, he accused Sharp of using the inflated figure as a "dishonest attempt to frighten" the Canadian public and "stampede" the provinces into postponement.[84]

As 1967 came to a close, the anti-medicare lobby by provincial governments, insurance companies, and organized medicine reached a crescendo. On 14 December, Pearson announced his decision to retire, and the previous differences on medicare became chasms as leadership aspirants, including Sharp and MacEachen, began to size up their chances at succeeding the PM.

In January 1968, a full-fledged cabinet crisis erupted. On one side was Sharp, supported by more conservative Liberals; the CMA; the business establishment, including Bay Street financiers and the

Canadian Manufacturers' Association; and almost all provincial governments, some of whom wanted the legislation cancelled entirely but were willing to settle for either a major revision or, at a minimum, a major deferral of implementation.[85] On the other side was MacEachen and the dwindling centre-left reformers in cabinet, supported by the NDP, labour unions, church groups, and a majority of the Canadian public, who wanted the federal government to enact medicare as it had promised to do.

From his side, Douglas encouraged a campaign by labour unions and sympathetic farm organizations to prevent medicare from being "either watered down or postponed once again."[86] The many letters sent to the prime minister were part of a national campaign to countervail the letters Pearson was receiving from anti-medicare proponents such as the CMA.[87] They were followed up by telegrams, petitions, resolutions, and cards sent to all federal politicians, with the key message that the government of Canada needed to keep its promise and that "no further delays" would "be tolerated" by Canadians.[88]

Inside cabinet, the two sides feuded through the month of January 1968. In a meeting on 10 January, Sharp used the opposition of premiers and what he perceived as a deterioration in federal revenues to argue in favour of a much more gradual phasing in of medicare, in which coverage would be limited to a subset of physician services in the first stage. MacEachen argued vehemently against this option. He also reminded his colleagues that the continuing opposition within cabinet had weakened his negotiating position with the provinces. Paul Martin Sr., as the acting PM in Pearson's absence that day, intervened on MacEachen's behalf, arguing it was "politically impossible to make any change in the legislation" now that it had passed. Further, he urged cabinet members to make a more concerted effort to explain the fiscal as well as the social benefits of medicare to the media and the public.[89] When Pearson got news about the tenor of the meeting, all he could do was fret over the rifts developing in his cabinet and make sure he was present at the next meeting.[90]

The ongoing warfare in the Pearson cabinet, accompanied by regular leaks to the media, encouraged the anti-medicare forces. In response, T.C. told the press that his party would "fight tooth and nail" against any further delay or any further amendment to the legislation. And if it were "postponed again," his party would bring down the government on a confidence vote and make medicare's delay "a key election issue."[91]

On 18 January, cabinet met again, this time with Pearson in the room. The PM summarized his discussions with provincial premiers. All except two, he explained, were emphatic in their demands for a postponement. Moreover, even Ross Thatcher, a premier of a province that would be eligible for federal cost sharing immediately on the 1st of July, said he was willing to see a postponement if the federal government would provide a financial contribution to some other social program in Saskatchewan. Given this information, Pearson felt the cabinet needed to postpone implementation, or possibly amend the Medical Care Act to provide more limited coverage at the front end. Sharp then added that the provincial finance ministers he had met with were "simply not prepared to face additional costs relating to Medicare." These statements precipitated another fight in cabinet, as ministers presented their positions on one side or other of the debate. MacEachen, now joined by more than just Marchand, threatened to resign if cabinet did not keep the act as it was and proceed with implementation in July.[92]

In the face of such deep divisions and threats of resignation, Pearson delayed any decision until his colleagues had some time to cool down. However, a major leak to the media from one member of cabinet created an even hotter and more distrustful environment for the next cabinet meeting, once again held in Pearson's absence. The government looked to the world like it was falling apart, and the few ministers who had not taken strong sides on the issue of timing tried to use the media's perception of a cabinet crisis to work out a compromise. They emphasized the vulnerability of the government on the issue of medicare, "not only because of divisions within the party but also because of the leadership convention in the offing." The leaking had to stop, and the time had come to show outward unity, whatever the private opinions of ministers. MacEachen demanded an immediate decision but, given Pearson's absence, the majority felt it best to wait for the next meeting.[93]

On 30 January, the cabinet again met, with Pearson in the chair. The PM repeated his position on the need for a gradual phasing in of medicare "over a period possibly of three years, with emphasis on early coverage of the more needy categories." Urging his centre-left ministers to reconsider their positions, he assured them that the amendment to the Medical Care Act "would not be complex." Yet MacEachen and the pro-medicare ministers held their ground, some arguing that provincial support for "phasing-in was just a screen for their basic philosophical opposition" to universal medicare. Moreover, the purpose of letting some provinces come in immediately was that it placed public pressure on the others to follow suit. "The federal plan was to put a gun to" the "heads of the provincial governments," without which "it would never get done." On the other side, Sharp was equally immovable, telling his colleagues that if medicare "were considered purely in terms of the effect on the economy and the stability of the Canadian dollar the right thing was not to proceed."[94]

Pearson was forced into a corner. Hanging in the balance was the potential resignation of MacEachen and possibly other key ministers such as Marchand. Despite his own favourable view of the phasing-in approach, Pearson reluctantly came down on the side of proceeding on time with the legislation as it stood. However, the cabinet conclusions clearly reflected Pearson's anger with MacEachen and the minority who had held firm with him. The PM expressed "regret at the failure of some Ministers to be more flexible with regard to a formula for phasing-in the Medicare program, or for otherwise obtaining more provincial participation."[95] Implementation would begin that year on 1 July after all, by which time the Liberals would have a new leader.

# 16 Defender of Medicare

*I'm telling you that, unless those of us who believe in Medicare raise our voices in no uncertain terms, unless we arouse our neighbours and our friends and our communities, we are sounding the death knell of Medicare in this country, and I for one will not sit idly by and see that happen.*

T.C. Douglas in 1982[1]

The last three years of T.C.'s leadership of the NDP were mired in internal dissent and ideological warfare. Things outside the party were little better for Douglas. Facing off against the fluently bilingual and charismatic Pierre Trudeau, he sometimes looked and sounded like a man from another generation. And so, when T.C. lost his seat in Burnaby in the Trudeaumania election of 1968, journalists began writing his political obituary.[2]

Even after he re-entered the House of Commons following a by-election in February 1969, Douglas had limited influence on the majority Liberal government. After he retired as leader in 1971, he would remain an MP for another eight years, but his interventions in the Commons gradually diminished. He used his dwindling influence in the 1970s to push for an expansion of Medicare (the capitalized version of the word denoting both hospital and medical care coverage). He also defended Medicare's underlying principles when he felt these were under attack. He was especially opposed to the replacement of shared-cost federal financing of Medicare with a new block grant, which he said accelerated the prevalence of user fees in some provinces, eroding equitable access to health services.

Working assiduously with civil society actors, Douglas consistently pressured the federal government to pass remedial Medicare legislation, which eventually came in the form of the Canada Health Act in 1984. A few months after the passage of the act, T.C. was seriously injured in an accident. Already suffering from terminal cancer, he began to decline rapidly. When he died on 24 February 1986, his influence as Canada's chief advocate for comprehensive health coverage should have disappeared. However, the opposite happened, as his memory and legacy have ever since been used to defend Medicare or urge its expansion.

**The Trudeaumania Election of 1968**

From the moment he announced his resignation in December 1967, Pearson became a lame duck prime minister. Once the leadership candidates were announced, T.C. told the press that Paul Martin Sr. would be hard to beat.[3] Such an observation may have been wishful thinking. After all, he had known Martin since they were rookie MPs in the mid-1930s. They had had their clashes, but Douglas knew Martin to be a progressive who had fought hard to get national hospital coverage accepted by the cautious St-Laurent government and as one of the few ministers to support Allan MacEachen (another leadership hopeful) in his struggle to implement the Medical Care Act by 1967.

On 6 April 1968, the Liberals chose their new leader from a crowded field of nine candidates. It took four rounds of voting for a victor to finally emerge. Contrary to Douglas's prediction, Martin received less than 12 per cent of the vote in the first round and withdrew.[4] MacEachen, who had received an even smaller percentage than Martin on the first ballot, stubbornly held out until the third, when he was eliminated. In the final ballot, Pierre Trudeau came out with a bare majority, successfully defeating the right wing's preferred candidate, Robert Winters, with John Turner coming in a distant third.

Trudeau accentuated a perception of T.C. that Tom Kent had first given expression to in the 1963 federal election. To both, Douglas seemed a throwback to an earlier era, a politician who had come of age in the 1930s and 1940s. His social gospel–rooted socialism seemed old fashioned amid the growing secularism of the 1960s. And then there was the cool factor. As one of the Liberal leadership candidates put it during his convention speech before the vote, the NDP might "pose as swingers, but can you see Tommy Douglas doing the frug?" To great laughter and applause, he described the Douglas "socialists" as "a party with their heads in the clouds and their feet in another century."[5]

Some factions within the NDP, the Ontario group in particular, also saw T.C. as an outdated leader poorly suited to contest Trudeau. The first challenge to his leadership came during the federal NDP convention in 1967 from an Ontario-based group of delegates led by Stephen Lewis and Terry Grier. The son of David Lewis and not yet thirty, Stephen Lewis had become a prominent member of the Ontario legislature. Another Young Turk, Grier was the former assistant secretary of the federal party and a major organizer for the Ontario NDP. They brought together other young, urban NDP delegates to oust John Brockelbank, T.C.'s old colleague from Saskatchewan and a Douglas loyalist, from the position of party president. In the weeks following, Grier canvassed members of the federal council about holding an early leadership convention to choose a new leader to "bring new life and momentum to the party."[6]

Some two months before the federal Liberal leadership convention, the Ontario caucus dispatched Stephen Lewis to see Douglas in Vancouver and try to convince him to relinquish the leadership. As Lewis subsequently recalled, "We had moved into a new age, a new era, and Tommy's magnificent appeal from the previous era was just a little out of synch." Although he continued to be "admired" and even "loved," these feelings no longer translated into new votes for the NDP.[7] Lewis's visit came as a surprise to T.C., who had earlier convinced him to enter the Ontario legislature and had read with pride his maiden speech in 1964, which called upon the Ontario government to implement Saskatchewan-style medicare. Moreover, the young politician was the son of the man he felt, more than himself, should have been the first leader of the NDP. Now, here he was in a Vancouver hotel room, telling him his time had passed. As Lewis remembered the scene, "Tommy sitting in a corner chair, myself perched on the edge of the bed, putting to him a view that was shared by a majority of [Ontario] caucus members, and Tommy, as I recall, saying he'd think about it but that it was not his instinct [to quit]."[8]

Although the younger Lewis vehemently denied that his father had had anything to do with the request, the fact remained that many in the party saw David Lewis as Douglas's natural successor, and T.C. must have struggled with the suspicion that his old ally felt it was time for him to move on. David too denied that he was behind the effort but, as he explained to Doris French Shackleton in an interview just a few years later, defended his son by saying that "at least he had the guts to say it to his face."[9]

Stephen Lewis's intervention misfired, actually fortifying T.C.'s instinct to remain as leader for the 1968 election. If Stephen had been acting on behalf of his father, then the argument based on the need for a generational shift in the party was hardly satisfied by having David Lewis – who was only five years younger than Douglas and whose politics had also been shaped by the Great Depression – assume the leadership.[10] From this point forward, the tension between the two

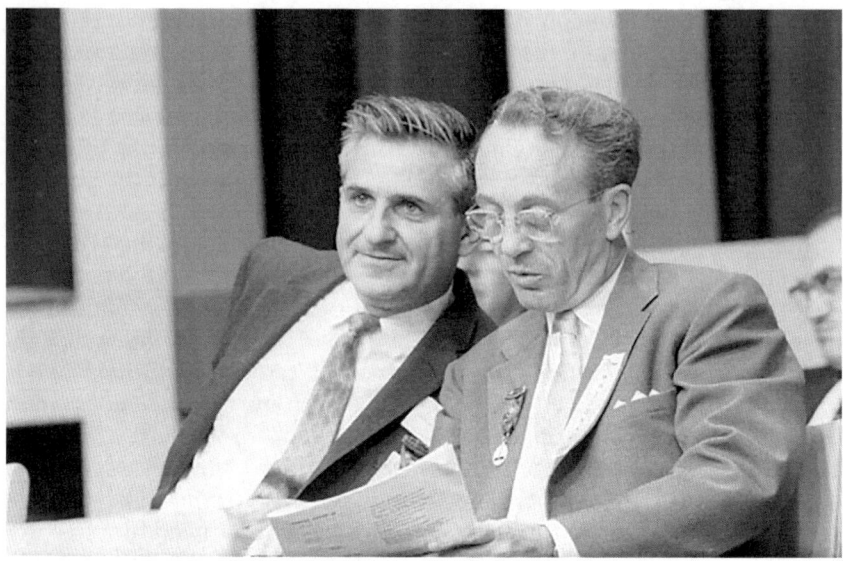

David Lewis and Tommy Douglas in 1961, when they were still close allies (LAC, Horst Ehricht, PA-180405)

most senior leaders within the NDP was palpable. Only loyalty to the party, which they both had been so instrumental in shaping and then reshaping, mitigated what threatened to become a highly publicized and damaging rupture.

For these two NDP stalwarts, it was a sad end to what had been a very long and productive relationship. Each man had qualities the other did not, and when they worked together, they were a very effective team. As recounted to Douglas's biographer Walter Stewart in a private exchange with an NDP insider who knew and admired both, "each man would have preferred more of what the other had."[11]

By 1968, young left-wing activists were beginning to alter the course of the NDP in a movement that would soon become known as "the Waffle."[12] Although older than this emerging generation, the new Liberal leader seemed more in tune with the youth culture that had emerged in the 1960s than Douglas, as was later captured by John Lennon's positive perception of the PM during Lennon's famous Montreal "bed-in" with Yoko Ono in 1970.

On 23 April 1968, just three days after assuming the mantle of PM, Trudeau called for a federal election, to be held on 25 June.[13] More than ever, this was a television election targeting a national audience, and the Liberal campaign team used "engaging visuals" designed to emphasize the impression of a "swelling wave of popular support" for their new leader. This was to be a campaign in which image would occupy central stage and issues of public policy would be "soft-pedalled."[14]

For T.C., policies such as medicare were what an election should be all about. For Trudeau and the Liberals, however, medicare was done and the issue dead, the word not even appearing in the party's policy statement.[15] Of course, the reality was that medicare was in the process of being implemented, although only the governments of Saskatchewan and British Columbia had said that they were ready to begin their plans on 1 July, and each were making problematic demands, which Douglas wanted to highlight during the election campaign.

In the case of Saskatchewan, Ross Thatcher's Liberal government had just introduced what it called "deterrent fees" on both hospital and physician care. Thatcher insisted these fees were modest enough that they did not contravene the federal criteria of universal access under the federal act, an argument that Allan MacEachen did not contest.[16] Douglas strongly disagreed, and criticized Thatcher's "tax on the sick."[17] The Saskatchewan NDP, then in opposition, condemned the deterrent fees, while the community clinics launched a public movement, Citizens for the Defence of Medicare, "which held protest marches" and sponsored a petition that would be signed by 35,000 residents.[18] Even Canadian author and television celebrity Pierre Berton flew to Saskatchewan from Toronto, sponsored by the Regina community clinic, to give a speech against the deterrent fees.[19] Months later (well after the federal election), Les Benjamin, the NDP MP representing Regina–Lake Centre, presented a private member's bill in Parliament requiring the federal government to withdraw its medicare transfers from those provinces permitting user fees, on the basis that such fees were contrary to the criteria of the Medical Care Act. After a debate that lasted an hour, the bill was consigned to the bottom of the long list of private member's bills, with almost no chance of being raised again during the session.[20]

Meanwhile, in British Columbia, Premier W.A.C. Bennett insisted that his multi-payer design based on physician, cooperative, and labour-based insurance carriers met the criteria of public administration.[21] With Bennett and Thatcher claiming compliance, the other eight provincial governments were left either to complain about what they viewed as the overly rigid requirements of the Medical Care Act and to continue to call for changes before they would join, or to express their concern about the impact of the program on their budgets and the need for more time.[22]

The opposition parties had to respond to these provincial positions as they prepared to fight the Trudeau Liberals. While the PCs claimed to be "fully committed" to medicare, they also criticized the Liberal "government's 'take it or leave it' attitude toward the provinces" and said it had "resulted in a situation where citizens of eight of the ten provinces will be contributing tax monies to a program from which they receive no benefits." If elected, the PCs promised to call a first ministers' conference, "not to lay down ultimatums, but to ask provincial authorities to agree on a concensus [sic] program that would bring Medicare to those who need it throughout the country on a basis that the provinces could afford."[23] It was not hard to see that the federal conservatives, led by Robert Stanfield, were open to a targeted subsidy approach, as had long been promoted by organized medicine and some provincial governments and had been operating, in the case of Manningcare in Alberta, since 1963.[24]

The NDP's voluminous speakers' notes for federal candidates set out the many missteps of the Liberals, especially the delayed response to the Hall Commission Report and the deferred implementation of the Medical Care Act. The notes also highlighted the shortcomings of the legislation and the Liberals' approach to implementation, including the relatively permissive 90 per cent coverage standard for universality and the "loop-hole" in its redefinition of public administration, potentially allowing private carriers to be part of provincial Medicare plans, both of which paved the way for British Columbia's plan to be eligible by 1 July 1968.

The NDP then laid out the planks of its platform, the most important of which was the promise to extend universal health coverage to the services provided by "dentists, nurses, therapists, medical-social workers and other medical and paramedical personnel as well as the provision of drugs and prosthetic appliances." Using "existing federal medicare legislation" as a starting point, "the NDP would encourage the provinces to expand their medicare programs as rapidly as possible in order to make them truly comprehensive" and would also "provide the necessary funds and other incentives to help meet shortages in personnel and facilities."[25] It was the same position the NDP had been advocating since Douglas became leader in 1961.

Irrespective of the position on medicare laid out by the NDP, Douglas was unable to make it a factor in the election. More than problems or policies, it was image, particularly the image of the respective party leaders, that seemed to be the critical factor in the minds of Canadians tuning into their televisions each night during the campaign.[26] As journalist and Douglas biographer Walter Stewart put it, the NDP leader seemed "petulant" beside Trudeau and, although T.C. always delivered "lively, provocative speeches" in front of the crowds, he "might as well have shouted into the closet back in his Burnaby apartment."[27]

A growing number within the party worried that their aging leader's image contrasted poorly with Trudeau's magnetism. He "seemed old and passé like Pearson and Diefenbaker," while Trudeau, even when arguing with the New Left, seemed tuned into the present.[28] They saw how, by the second week of May, Trudeau campaign stops were drawing mobs of adoring fans, resembling a pop star's tour. As Peter Newman described the scene at the time, there were "hordes of teeny-boppers, running with long manes blowing like banners in the wind, full of vitality, excitement, laughter, shrieking in a kind of wild ecstasy that rises to a squawk when one of their number is kissed."[29]

In contrast to Trudeau's "mod" campaign, Douglas insisted the election be fought on issues. In early May, he told a group of reporters in Montreal that an election "was too important to be just a beauty contest," and he challenged Trudeau "to step out of the screen of platitudes" he had offered in place of real policies.[30] NDP events across the country, organized by local party associations, had Douglas speaking to the party faithful about what the NDP could accomplish if given more seats. But, despite its personal importance to Douglas, medicare took a backseat to issues such as inflation, the economy, and foreign ownership of Canadian resources and companies.[31] Although the sixties movement had a strong left-progressive character, and Trudeau was openly criticized by vocal New Left activists at some campaign stops, Douglas seemed unable "to capitalize on the progressive bent of the sixties," despite the NDP's left-wing identity and policy platform.[32]

The one bright spot was the first-ever televised leaders' debate, held by the CBC just over two weeks before election day.[33] The initial CBC–Radio Canada–CTV proposal was limited to the Liberal and Tory leaders, a format that Douglas called discriminatory and against which the NDP threatened to mount a national protest. The threat worked, and the program was expanded to include Douglas for the full debate, with Créditiste leader Réal Caouette joining for the last forty minutes.[34] As the candidates entered the debate, polls were showing that the election would be a cakewalk for Trudeau.[35] With the confidence such a lead provided and the comfort Pierre Trudeau had with the medium of television, the media predicted that Trudeau would easily dispatch Douglas and Tory leader Robert Stanfield.[36]

However, it was T.C. (sitting on a raised platform to add some height) who ended up coming across as more dynamic than the distant and seemingly disengaged Trudeau. The *Montreal Gazette*, for example,

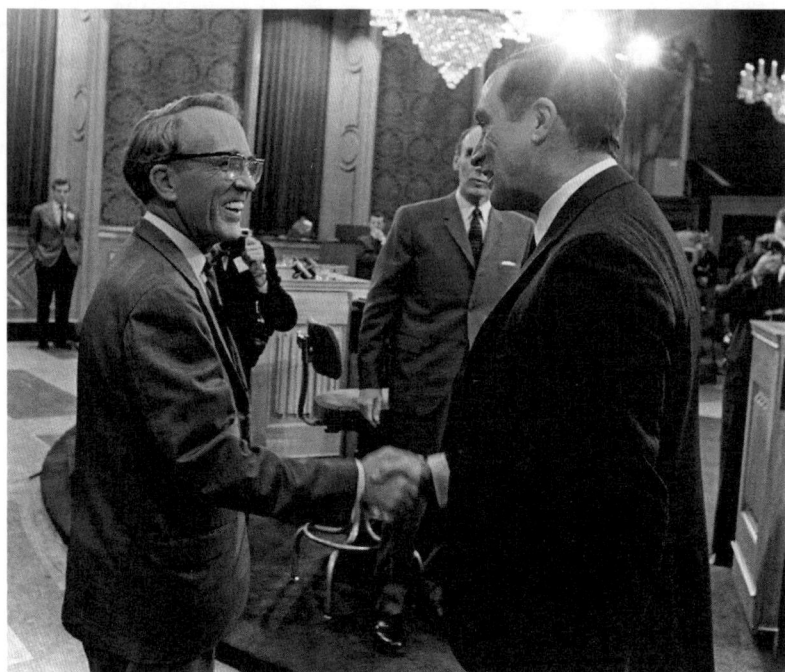

T.C. and Pierre Trudeau shaking hands just before the first televised election debate in the 1968 election, with Robert Stanfield looking on, 9 June 1968 (CP 2872975)

reported that "Mr. Douglas – that old platform speaker par excellence that he is – used contrast in approach to good effect" and provided "the only semblance of rousing political oratory" that evening.[37] Party staff in Ottawa were jubilant. According to one of Douglas's aides, the "debate did one thing which we weren't able to do up to that point in the election campaign, and that was excite our own workers," who were almost "ready to throw in the towel" because of Trudeau's momentum and appeal.[38]

T.C. had been highly motivated to best Trudeau in the debate. As a former member of the CCF, Trudeau had been approached by Douglas to run as a candidate in Quebec over a decade earlier. Trudeau's refusal plus his subsequent decision to join the Liberals had deeply upset T.C. He was also irked by Trudeau's ripping off the NDP's "just society" theme from the 1965 election and using it as his own at the Liberal leadership convention: T.C. loved telling election crowds that Trudeau's version of the term was "a just society with a means test."³⁹ In the weeks leading up to the debate, Trudeau kept repeating the phrase "just society," even while declaring that he was "a pragmatist" rather than an idealist.⁴⁰ As a former four-term premier, Douglas demonstrated that the two concepts were not only compatible but could be a potent combination when balanced properly. T.C. could only have been rankled to hear this false dichotomy spoken by someone whose own experience in government was so limited.

The question of health policy was never raised in the televised debate, although Douglas did make a point of saying that mental health was a problem in Canada in part because psychiatric hospitals had not been included under national hospital coverage.⁴¹ Indeed, medicare was not an election issue except in Saskatchewan, where NDP candidates pointed out that the Thatcher government's deterrent fees were contrary to the criteria of universality in the federal Medical Care Act. In sharp contrast to 1962, Douglas now "attracted large and noisy crowds" when he spoke in the province. As recounted by twenty-two-year-old NDP candidate Lorne Nystrom, Dalton Camp, the Tory most responsible for Diefenbaker's fall from leadership (and therefore highly unpopular in Saskatchewan), had said that medicare would fail at the implementation stage. That very night, after talking to Douglas, Nystrom's team created a one-page handbill, headlined "Medicare Dead Duck: Dalton Camp," highlighting "Douglas' role as the father" of medicare and the Tories as its potential destroyers.⁴²

The NDP scored a major comeback in Saskatchewan, electing six MPs, bettering the Tories' five and Liberals' two. Overall, however, that province was the exception. Trudeaumania won the day and gave the Liberals a majority government, the first for the party since the St-Laurent era. Trudeau's candidates came out on top in the most urban and populous provinces – Ontario, British Columbia, and especially Quebec. The Liberals reaped 45.2 per cent of the popular vote, leaving 31.4 per cent for the Tories and 17.4 per cent for the NDP. Trudeau's victory came largely at the expense of the PCs, while the NDP managed, barely, to hold its own with twenty-two seats, the same number it had held when Parliament was dissolved.⁴³ While the NDP clung to its working-class base, Trudeaumania had whittled away at the NDP's middle-class supporters in central Canada and British Columbia.⁴⁴ The most prominent casualty of Trudeaumania was Douglas, who lost his seat in Burnaby.

The overall result triggered considerable disappointment within NDP ranks. The party had once again failed to make a breakthrough in Quebec, despite its dynamic provincial leader, Robert Cliche, and its policy of *deux nations*. Federally, its share of the popular vote dropped slightly from the 1965 election. Not only had the party lost its federal leader, but some of the NDP's brightest lights – potential future leaders of the party, including Cliche, Charles Taylor, and Laurier LaPierre – lost their electoral bids.[45]

In a bittersweet twist, the NDP regained the Regina constituency where T.C. had been humiliated in 1962.[46] But, by losing his seat in Burnaby, Douglas's already shaky hold on the leadership was brought into further question in the media and by members of his own party. Within days after the election, Douglas met with the NDP's national executive and "announced his intention to step down at the 1969 convention."[47] His statement triggered a flurry of speculation in the press.[48] In keeping with a headline in the *Globe and Mail* that proclaimed "Douglas Likely to Quit as NDP Leader," his political obituary appeared in numerous newspaper columns.[49] One editorial by Charles Lynch was particularly dismissive:

> Tommy Douglas' best work is done, and he recedes into the minor-league hall of fame occupied by his predecessors, J.S. Woodsworth and M.J. Coldwell. Like theirs, his career has been one of extreme usefulness to his party and to his country. The only thing that ever eluded him was success. In Canada, it seems, old socialists just fade away ...
>
> Tommy Douglas will be remembered not as the leader of the New Democratic Party, which was launched with such high hopes in 1961 (it was supposed to supplant the Liberals as the party of the left, you may remember). Rather, his place in history will rest on his record as premier of Saskatchewan, when he led the only socialist government ever to be elected in North America, and preached the message of the New Jerusalem on the western plains ...
>
> Insofar as national politics is concerned, the name of Tommy Douglas will occupy a small place in history, for his national leadership of the NDP produced little that was memorable.[50]

## Double, Double, Toil and Trouble

As in 1962, T.C. was knocked to the ground bleeding, but now, at the age of sixty-three, he seemed intent on passing the torch of leadership. He might continue as an MP, but he would not allow any NDP MP to step aside for him, as had happened in 1962.[51] Then, one month after the election, the unexpected occurred.

In late July 1968, Colin Cameron, the NDP MP for a constituency with the unwieldy name of Nanaimo–Cowichan–The Islands, died at the age of seventy-one.[52] The riding executive immediately asked

Douglas to step in. Still debating his own retirement, Douglas delayed his decision until early September. When the answer came back, it was yes. Despite everything, he wanted to get back into the ring one more time, his sixth election battle in less than seven years. He now had to wait for the PM to call a by-election the following February, a long time for a party leader to remain outside Parliament.[53]

For the fall session of the House of Commons, David Lewis assumed the role of parliamentary leader, and the speculation grew that Douglas would, whatever the outcome of the by-election, exit as leader. Typical of the commentary at the time, a *Financial Post* column suggested that, although "New Democrats naturally grieve at the absence of Douglas," it nonetheless "appears that the team functions quite as effectively under its new parliamentary leader, David Lewis." According to the *Post* editorialist, "Lewis at his best displays greater capacity to command the House and sharper incisiveness in criticism than Tommy Douglas."[54] And behind Lewis were several talented newcomers to Parliament, including York University political scientist Ed Broadbent and thirty-two-year-old Manitoba MP Ed Schreyer.[55]

The by-election date was eventually set for 10 February.[56] The long wait favoured T.C., as it allowed time for Trudeaumania to sag, especially in the West. The NDP's main campaign brochure emphasized Douglas's past achievements, especially his hospital and medical care insurance programs in Saskatchewan. As he had done when he was the MP for Weyburn, T.C. promised to provide voters in the constituency with regular reports from Ottawa as well as a local office where anyone could drop in to voice their concerns.[57] On election night, Douglas would win a convincing 57 per cent of the vote, his final political comeback.[58]

Before the by-election, many in the NDP assumed there would be a leadership race at the national convention slated for October 1969. However, the Ontario provincial council, the very organization that had tried to get Douglas to step aside the year before, now begged him not to retire. Although the Ontario group still felt the NDP desperately needed a younger leader, they could not agree on that candidate, and many of the Ontario Young Turks (with the obvious exception of Stephen Lewis) did not want David Lewis to become leader.

By the spring of 1969, a consensus had emerged within the national NDP: Douglas should continue as leader until an obvious contender for the job appeared. On 5 May, Douglas issued a press release stating that he would stay on until either a special leadership convention in 1970 or the next biennial NDP conference in 1971 but would "under no circumstances" stay beyond that time.[59] In the press conference that followed, T.C. got a cheap laugh out of the assembled journalists by telling them he had slipped a little mentally in recent years "but on Parliament Hill that's not noticed at all."[60] Douglas claimed that his announcement reflected the unanimous decision of the MPs in the federal caucus, implying the agreement of deputy leader David Lewis.[61] Despite the fact that he would have preferred T.C. to have stepped down at that year's NDP convention, and swallowing his anger that many of his colleagues had put him into the same category of "aged leader" as Douglas, Lewis reluctantly went along with the consensus, to preserve party unity.[62]

To the press, T.C. defended the long wait as an opportunity to encourage the "broadest possible choices for future leadership," preferably someone under the age of fifty. He then reeled off the names of several potential leaders, including Broadbent, Schreyer, LaPierre, and Taylor, adding the name of David Lewis only when it was raised by the press.[63] Perhaps the most perceptive editorial appeared in the *Montreal Star*. Commending Douglas for stating his intention to retire in or before 1971, and therefore not making the same mistake as St-Laurent and Diefenbaker by staying on too long, the author then commented on the two senior figures in the party:

> Under the circumstances this is probably their best bet but the price to be paid for it is Mr. Douglas' less effective leadership for the next year or two – normally it would be two years but the way is open to the party to call a leadership convention earlier if it chooses.
>
> There is an element of sadness and frustration in this for both men. Mr. Douglas has been over-taken by time and, once one of the sharp goads of the House of Commons, he is now among its most predictable seeming members. It is a long time since the leader of the NDP has made his listeners sit up with a start, realizing that he had said something fresh and particularly pertinent to the moment.
>
> It is a feat which Mr. Lewis still accomplishes with reasonable regularity and it must be a frustrating experience for him to realize that he is capable of making his party's performance considerably more impressive than the man actually at the helm. There must also be for him the added sting of feeling himself in his prime, reasonably capable of many years more effectiveness and yet too old to be the man the party wants – 20 years too old if Mr. Douglas is right in his belief that the party should choose a man in his late thirties or early forties.[64]

It was indeed ironic that, despite T.C.'s clear preference for a younger leader to take the helm, he nonetheless delegated much of the running of the national party and its parliamentary business to David Lewis. While this may have suited Douglas as he prepared his exit, it nonetheless worked against his desire to facilitate a shift in leadership to a newer generation. The very opposite occurred: Lewis used his delegated power and resulting influence to consolidate his control over the party and its members. And when the time came for the leadership, Lewis would draw extensively on accumulated favours and connections to give himself the best possible crack at securing the position of leader.

**Shirley Douglas and the Black Panthers**

To add to his leadership troubles, Douglas also faced a family crisis in 1969. Just weeks before the NDP's October convention, he discovered that his daughter Shirley had been arrested by the Federal Bureau of Investigation (FBI) in Los Angeles for allegedly purchasing hand grenades for the Black Panthers, although no explosives were found in a search of her home.[65] After studying at the Royal Academy of Dramatic Art in London, England, Shirley became a theatre and film actor, including a role in Stanley Kubrick's *Lolita*. Tommy and Irma had always been extremely supportive of her life in the arts when she was a teenager in Regina, where she had started with a role in Regina's Little Theatre in 1950 followed by two summer stints at the Banff School of Fine Arts.[66]

After marrying her second husband, Donald Sutherland, Shirley moved to California, where her twins, Kiefer and Rachel Sutherland, were born. She was shocked by the social and racial inequalities she witnessed in the United States. As she recalled five years later, "there is no way of understanding the poverty in Los Angeles until you've seen it." She was especially struck by the fact that "so many children" had to go "to school without breakfast" and decided to do something about it.[67]

Joining with like-minded celebrities such as Marlon Brando, Vanessa Redgrave, Jean Seberg, Jane Fonda, Richard Burton, Elizabeth Taylor, and Paul Newman, Shirley became part of "the Friends of the Black Panthers" and helped fund a breakfast-for-children program sponsored by the Panthers.[68] This immediately attracted the attention of a secret FBI unit attempting to disrupt and discredit any potential Black Power coalition with the New Left.[69] At the time of her arrest, Donald Sutherland was on set in Yugoslavia for the filming of *Kelly's Heroes*. The news of the arrest first reached his right-wing co-star Clint Eastwood, who, with a "big shit-eating grin," gave Sutherland the news: "Shirley's been arrested in LA for trying to buy hand grenades for the Panthers from

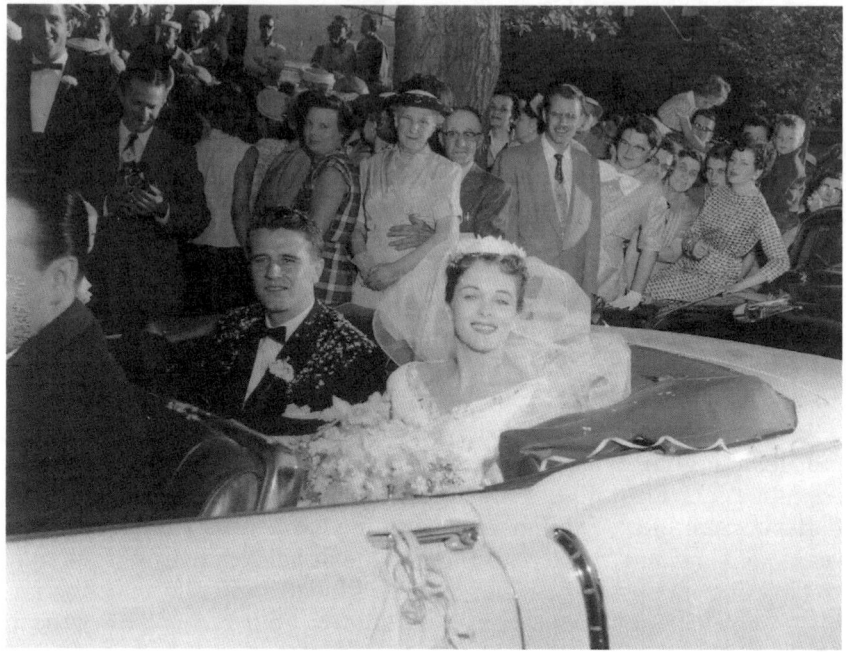

Wedding picture of Shirley Douglas and Western brewery heir Timothy E. Sicks in 1957. Her second marriage was to Donald Sutherland (1966–70) (PAS R-LP1022)

an undercover FBI agent – and she tried to pay him with a personal cheque!" At this point, Eastwood "fell on the ground laughing."[70]

As the news of the arrest travelled from California to Canada, Douglas called a press conference to get ahead of the story.[71] He made two things clear to the attending journalists. First, he did not believe there were any grounds for the arrest. Second, he was "proud of the fact that" his daughter believed, as he did, "that hungry children should be fed whether they are Black Panthers or White Republicans."[72] After pointing out that the FBI had laid two hundred charges against individuals connected with the Black Panthers but only one had gone to trial – evidence of harassment, in his view – he announced he would fly down to LA to be with his daughter.[73] Upon landing, Douglas was mobbed by journalists curious about the leader of the "Canadian Communist Party." When they asked him whether he was disappointed that his daughter wasn't present to greet him, Douglas defiantly asked, "Who says she's not?" At that moment Shirley appeared, walking up to her father through the pack of journalists.[74]

When Shirley finally came to trial in February 1970, the charges were dismissed by the judge for lack of evidence. Although there was "a strong case" that Shirley had been framed as part of the FBI's counterintelligence targeting of the Black Panther Party, she still faced a campaign by US immigration officials to deport her. After many legal battles, she returned to Canada in 1978 and was thereafter barred from working in the United States.[75] As for her father, the Security Service of the Royal Canadian Mounted Police (RCMP) followed his every move. T.C. had been under surveillance by the RCMP for decades, but his daughter's alleged affiliation with the Black Panthers, combined with his own anti–Vietnam War activities and the growing influence of the New Left within the NDP, made him more than ever a person of interest to the domestic intelligence service.[76]

## Douglas and the Waffle

Meanwhile, in Canada, a domestic version of the New Left was turning the NDP inside out. It came in the form of what became the Waffle caucus, which some critics would soon label a party within a party. Just weeks before Douglas was in LA, the members of this caucus had released its manifesto, "For an Independent Socialist Canada." The Waffle members vowed to turn the NDP, which they felt had consistently moved to the centre of the ideological spectrum in search of votes, into a "truly socialist party" – although the manifesto provided little detail on what it meant by "socialism" – or it would "become irrelevant." The first concern of the party, the Waffle proclaimed, should be "the development of socialist consciousness" rather than electoral politics – the party needed to be "radicalized from within" and "without."

More than its call for "a true socialist party," it was the Waffle's zealous nationalism and anti-Americanism that proved particularly controversial both inside and outside the party.[77] The manifesto called for struggle for "national survival" against an imperialist United States, "an empire characterized by militarism abroad and racism at home." This "American empire is held together," the manifesto declared, by global "military alliances" and "giant monopoly corporations" that treat subservient countries like Canada solely as "a resource base and consumer market."[78]

Much of the drafting and redrafting of the manifesto had been done by James Laxer, a history graduate student at Queen's University, and Mel Watkins, an associate professor of economics at the

University of Toronto.[79] Watkins had received considerable public attention as the chair of the federal Task Force on the Structure of Canadian Industry and its nationalistic report on foreign ownership and Canadian industry – almost immediately known as the Watkins Report – released the year before.[80]

The Waffle manifesto's vociferous anti-Americanism turned off many NDP moderates, including David Lewis, who hit back immediately. While he accepted the Waffle's view of the corporate domination of Canada (and other countries) by the United States, he rejected the "excessively strident way" in which the manifesto attacked the United States, and he said that he would never sign the document. In response to the manifesto's statement that capitalism in Canada "must be replaced with socialism, by national planning of investment and by the public ownership of the means of production," Lewis reminded the Waffle that its declaration was almost identical to the final statement in the Regina Manifesto of 1933 and that the majority of NDP members had long "rejected the idea of complete public ownership."[81] And Douglas, of course, had been a major supporter of the Winnipeg Declaration of 1956, which had tried to make it clear that the party wanted a balance of "public ownership, private ownership and co-operative ownership in a planned economy" rather than the elimination of private property.[82]

While the deputy leader had his say, the leader remained strangely quiet. Although the wording of the manifesto was very much a product of the 1960s, the notion that "the main business of socialist parties is not to form governments but to change minds" went back much further.[83] T.C. had always opposed the notion, not because he did not believe in changing minds, but because he felt that only real change, as demonstrated by something tangible, could shift the views of the public beyond the party activists. We can only speculate at Douglas's silence. Perhaps he felt he would exacerbate the damage to the party if he were provoked into debating its political and policy differences in public. Or he may have been concerned that any statement he would make could potentially provoke a premature leadership challenge at the NDP convention.

At the press conference where he had fired back at the Waffle, Lewis was asked whether he might consider challenging Douglas for the leadership. Despite his earlier commitment, and upset at what he saw as T.C.'s lack of fortitude in dealing with the Waffle, Lewis now left the door open to a contest with Douglas.[84] Lewis was in a strong position, with growing support in Ontario as well as Quebec.[85]

The NDP convention began on Monday, 27 October, in Winnipeg. Just three months earlier, the NDP had, in a major upset, been elected

Defender of Medicare 471

as the government of Manitoba.[86] The provincial leader, now premier, was Ed Schreyer, who had given up his seat in Parliament the day after he was elected leader of the Manitoba NDP.[87] Enough Liberal and Conservative voters were attracted to Schreyer's very moderate brand of social democracy that he was able to pull off this unexpected victory. It had taken a quarter-century since Douglas had first won office in Saskatchewan, but the NDP finally formed the government in another province.[88]

At thirty-three years of age, Schreyer may have been as young as many members of the Waffle who gathered in Winnipeg for the convention, but he had little in common with the New Left and its program: he was a moderate New Democrat who would have been comfortable as a left-leaning Liberal. As the headline speakers on the convention's first evening, Schreyer and Douglas spoke to the delegates. Schreyer emphasized political pragmatism and the need for the NDP to tailor its program to be more attractive to middle-of-the-road voters. "It is simply wrong," he said, "to promise the electorate the moon when you know that all you can reasonably expect to deliver are some sizeable rock samples."[89] He warned against party policies that "are so far out in front the public can't even see us."[90]

In contrast to Schreyer's emphasis on incrementalism, Douglas made an impassioned appeal to the delegates' idealism, but that idealism had been battle tested during his seventeen years as federal leader. To the New Left Wafflers in the crowd, Douglas represented the Old Left, while Schreyer represented the centre-left liberalism of the New Right in the party, the direction the NDP would likely go under Lewis's leadership.

T.C. was acclaimed leader at the convention, with both David Lewis and Mel Watkins among the names sponsoring his nomination. However, he was seen by both factions as a caretaker and therefore irrelevant. As noted in the *Montreal Gazette*, Douglas "was no longer a force in the minds of delegates."[91] Weeks before the convention, political columnist Charles Lynch had predicted that, with "Douglas' lame-duck leadership" secure for the next year or two, the Waffle would end up providing some much-needed dramatic tension for the convention.[92] Debate centred on the Waffle manifesto, which had been submitted as a resolution. In response, Lewis and the federal NDP council led the charge with a counter-resolution that avoided its anti-American rhetoric even while criticizing American ownership in the Canadian economy.[93]

Although T.C. endorsed the alternate statement – and made it clear he would have to resign if the anti-American Waffle manifesto was adopted – he urged delegates not to get mired in rhetoric and to remember that the NDP was a political party, not a debating society. The representative of the United Steelworkers Union at the convention was even blunter: "Our objective is to gain power. We must persuade the Canadian people we have the answer to problems, and not scare the hell out of them."[94] A lengthy debate ensued, and the Waffle lost the vote on its resolution, but Douglas (perhaps unlike Lewis) felt the debate had been a healthy one, as the influx of new ideas prevented the NDP from degenerating "into a mutual admiration society." Afterwards, he told the press that if the NDP "get to the place where there is complete agreement, then no social action is possible."[95]

**The Quebec Doctors' Strike and the October Crisis of 1970**

A caretaker he may have been, but T.C. had one more major leadership moment before he relinquished his position at the 1971 NDP convention. This was the October Crisis of 1970, a time of great upheaval in Quebec. Adopting the tactics of liberation movements in some areas in the Third World, the Front de Libération du Québec (FLQ) used violence, including bombing the Montreal Stock Exchange in 1969, in its effort to free Quebec from the rest of Canada.

An often overlooked fact is that the October Crisis coincided with significant unrest associated with the implementation of medicare in Quebec. The latter eventually culminated in a strike by specialists, which had important parallels with the 1962 strike in Saskatchewan. "While there was no direct connection between the specialists' strike and the October crisis," according William Tetley, a minister in the Quebec government at the time, "the turmoil that prevailed in the health-care system in October 1970 added to the climate of tension in which the crisis unfolded" and "added to the pressures bearing down on the newly elected Bourassa government."[96]

Quebec was in social and political ferment, and the polarization within the province concerning the implementation of national medicare was intense. On one side, organizations representing wage labourers, teachers, and farmers demanded "the introduction of state medicine along the lines of the British National Health Service, salaried service rather than fee-for-service" payment for doctors, and financing through general tax revenues only.[97] The opposition was led by physicians, particularly the Federation of Medical Specialists, who insisted on the right to opt out but still allow their patients, after having paid the specialists directly, to be reimbursed by the public plan. The specialists were heavily supported by the insurance industry, the Quebec Manufacturers Association, and the Quebec Chamber of Commerce, all of whom rejected a universal plan in favour of targeted public subsidies for the purchase of private health insurance. The newly elected Liberal government under Premier Robert Bourassa was caught in a vice between the two blocs and tried to appease the specialists by allowing up to 3 per cent of physicians in any of Quebec's administrative regions to opt out and have their patients reimbursed up to a maximum of 75 per cent of the fee schedule.[98] The Bourassa bill was not nearly enough for the doctors and the business lobby, and it was far too much for the powerful provincial unions.

In September 1970, the Quebec specialists served the government with an ultimatum accompanied by a strike threat, and frantic negotiations ensued. The government came back with a new compromise on opting out, with doctors split into three categories: 1) doctors who opt in and collect their entire fees from the Quebec Health Insurance Board; 2) doctors who opt out but agree to charge patients no more than the physician fee schedule which their patients then collect back; and 3) non-participants who determine their own fees and whose patients pay them without any government reimbursement. The Quebec government also made it clear it was prepared to deploy back-to-work legislation in the event of a strike.[99]

On 5 October, the day the FLQ kidnapped a British diplomat and Quebec's minister of labour, Bourassa offered to increase the medical services fund by $20 million, for an average increase of $3,000 per physician. It was still not enough, and on 8 October the specialists began a province-wide strike, which would soon end in the midst of the larger events of the October Crisis.[100]

In response to the FLQ kidnappings, and at the invitation of the Quebec government, Ottawa proposed to use the War Measures Act to suspend civil liberties and give the police greater powers to arrest suspects. The FLQ responded by killing the kidnapped labour minister and deputy premier, Pierre Laporte.[101] The NDP caucus meeting to prepare for the session in Parliament that day crackled with tension. Contrary to his usual demand for consensus, T.C. simply said that he would oppose the War Measures Act, leaving the impression that those MPs who disagreed could vote otherwise, as they had their "own political careers to think about." He then went into the House to condemn the killing but also to oppose the bill. "Right now," he said, "there is no constitution," and the "government now has the power by Order in Council to do anything it wants – to intern any citizen, to deport any citizen, to arrest any person or to declare any organization subversive or illegal."[102]

During T.C.'s speech, MPs "rocked with howls of anger and cries of 'shame.'" He suggested that the government already had enough resources and power to deal with the situation: the ability to use troops to supplement the police and to use the Criminal Code, which could perhaps be amended, with his party's support, to "make it easier for police to search for weapons." But the War Measures Act, with its power to search without warrant and to detain people without laying charges, was like "using a sledgehammer to crack a peanut."[103] In the end, fifteen members of his party voted with their leader while four joined the Liberals and Tories in support of the measure.[104]

T.C.'s position drew a storm of popular protest. His office overflowed with hate mail. One former supporter told Douglas that his speech in Parliament "was a disgrace," both for T.C. and his party.[105] It was only years later, with hindsight and a reappraisal of the use of the act, that Douglas's controversial position would be validated on both human-rights and political grounds. In 2001, one of Trudeau's cabinet members during the crisis, Eric Kierans, recalled that it was "Douglas who stood in the House, day after day, and hammered the government for suspending civil liberties" and "showed political courage of the highest order."[106]

Months later, on 21 April 1971, Douglas gave his last report as leader at the biennial federal NDP convention. In it, he talked about his party's achievements in the ten years since the New Party convention of 1961. Although his speech focused on present issues such as foreign ownership, he began with a reflection on the achievements of the past, including medicare.[107]

The leaders' election that followed came down to a contest between David Lewis and Waffle representative James Laxer. On the final ballot, Lewis won, but Laxer managed to garner nearly 40 per cent of the vote. Once he took control, Lewis used his position to keep Laxer off the national council and Watkins out of the executive, a move that very much disappointed Douglas, who felt that the Waffle had earned the right to have its views represented, even if he did not endorse some of them or its efforts to create a party within a party.[108]

## Implementing and Altering "National" Medicare in the 1970s

Douglas would remain an MP within the NDP parliamentary caucus until his retirement in 1979. During these years, he kept a close watch on the implementation and direction of medicare. But he moved on to other issues, especially energy, leaving the health critic role to others, most notably Stanley Knowles and later Ed Broadbent, Lewis's successor as NDP leader.

By 1971, all provincial governments had met the federal criteria under the Medical Care Act and had implemented medicare.[109] Not all had gone the way Douglas hoped, although he would not have been surprised at the tactics used by the specialists in Quebec.

In the case of Saskatchewan, the federal government, while not keen on the deterrent fees imposed by the Thatcher government, did not deem them a significant enough barrier to access that they contravened the universality criteria under the act. In any case, the issue was soon dealt with when the provincial NDP, which promised to reverse this policy, defeated the Liberal government in June 1971 and promptly eliminated deterrent fees.[110] While the new government saw user fees as a direct "attack on accessibility," it did not perceive premiums in the same way, provided they "were reasonable and so long as access to care did not depend on paying the tax."[111] But as the provincial tax base expanded with the resource boom of the late 1960s and early 1970s, premiums – which Douglas, during his time in government, had seen as regressive and undesirable but still essential to avoid raising general taxes "too high, too quickly" – were no longer needed, and the Blakeney government repealed them.[112]

In British Columbia, the original multi-payer Bennettcare was adjusted slightly to meet the more relaxed federal eligibility introduced by Allan MacEachen in 1966. In its original form, coverage under Bennettcare had reached 89.2 per cent of BC residents by the end of 1965. By increasing subsidies, the provincial government was able to clear the 90 per cent population coverage threshold set by MacEachen. With the establishment of the Medical Services Corporation, a statutory body responsible for overseeing the non-profit insurance carriers plus managing a public option, the administration of British Columbia's medical care plan was accountable to the minister of health and the Legislative Assembly of British Columbia. Over the next few years, due to the thin profit margins, the private health insurers incrementally dropped out of the BC medicare plan to focus on the more profitable business of supplementary health insurance.[113]

In Nova Scotia, the provincial government worked with the main private health insurance provider in a structure unique to that province. Before Robert Stanfield became leader of the federal Progressive Conservative Party in September 1967, he had been premier of Nova Scotia for over a decade. During that time, his government had a close relationship with the Nova Scotia Medical Society and its non-profit medical care insurance company, Maritime Medical Care Incorporated. Similar to other provincial medical associations, the NS medical society initially decried the concept of universality in favour of a targeted, subsidy-based approach. However, Stanfield and the society came to a compromise, which was then reviewed by Ottawa. After extensive discussions with the province, MacEachen approved the unique arrangement.[114] In the result, Maritime Medical Care Incorporated acted as the government's financial and administrative agent, with the government remaining the bargaining agent with provincial physicians in determining the fee schedule.[115]

In Alberta and Ontario, the multi-payer Manningcare and Robartscare plans were converted into single, publicly administered plans to meet federal eligibility under the Medical Care Act. However, physician extra-billing was tolerated – to some extent, even encouraged – by both provincial governments, a challenge to the concept of universality that would soon become a major flashpoint in the country and ultimately lead to the passage of the Canada Health Act in 1984. In the eyes of many observers at the time, physician extra-billing as well as hospital user charges would be exacerbated by a major change in the federal financing of health care, a change presaged in section 8 of the Medical Care Act.[116]

As discussed in the preceding chapter, the federal government had been trying to replace shared-cost financing of social programs with a block grant involving the transfer of tax room rather than cash. Although unable to convince the provinces to agree to the change in the early 1970s, the Trudeau government used the stagflation crisis of the mid-1970s to once again propose a mechanism involving a permanent tax transfer with an escalator tied to national economic growth rather than provincial health spending.

**Established Programs Financing**

In 1975, the federal government notified the provinces that Ottawa "wanted out of its commitments under the hospital insurance program by 1980 and for medical care by 1982."[117] To add further pressure on the provinces, the federal government introduced a bill to put a ceiling on its contribution to medical care coverage. Both moves were intended to force the provincial governments to the bargaining table and to accept a new transfer mechanism.

The Trudeau government proposed a block transfer to replace shared-cost financing for both Medicare and postsecondary education.[118] This new transfer would be made up of two roughly equal parts. The first involved a permanent tax transfer in which Ottawa would cede tax room (known as tax points) to the provinces so that they would be responsible for raising revenue through their own taxes for future Medicare spending. The second part was an annual cash transfer with an escalator tied to the rate of growth of the gross national product (GNP). For years, health costs had been growing faster than government revenues, and the federal government wanted to free itself from what it viewed as a perpetually inflationary cost. Provincial governments would be able to use the federal money not just for hospital and medical care coverage but for other areas of health. Provincial spending would no longer be monitored by federal officials to determine if it was eligible for cost sharing by Ottawa.

The proposal was presented to the premiers by Prime Minister Trudeau at a federal-provincial conference that began on 14 June 1976. Trudeau promised that, in return, the provincial governments would have greater flexibility in the use of federal funds from the proposed block transfer.[119] Although this first meeting did not immediately result in an agreement, Douglas was left very troubled about the Trudeau government's intentions. Unlike Al Johnson, who had originally devised the new approach shortly after he left Regina in 1964 for a senior post in Ottawa, T.C. feared that the more permissive mechanism laid the groundwork for a Balkanization of Medicare. He also felt that the current system of federal cost sharing of Medicare through annual cash transfers, with an escalator tied to aggregate provincial spending on Medicare, required Ottawa to work with the provinces to improve the functioning of the system, if only to save money.

An irony for Douglas was that his former close advisor Tommy Shoyama was now the federal deputy minister of finance and, as such, the official primarily responsible for the latest version of the federal block transfer proposal. After the federal election of 1962, Shoyama had returned to his old job heading up the Economic Advisory and Planning Board in Saskatchewan rather than moving to Ottawa with Douglas, even though Douglas and also David Lewis and the other top NDP brass in Ottawa had encouraged Shoyama to make the jump to the federal civil service.[120] In 1964, after the defeat of the Lloyd government, Shoyama did move to Ottawa, but not to become an NDP advisor, despite a continuing close affiliation with the party.[121] Instead, he began his meteoric rise as a civil servant in the federal Liberal government. After a stint in the Economic Council of Canada, he succeeded Al Johnson as an assistant deputy minister of finance responsible for federal-provincial programs. Then, in 1975, after a brief term as deputy minister of energy, mines, and resources, he was appointed finance deputy.[122]

As the chief official responsible for Established Programs Financing (EPF) – the name for the block funding mechanism – Shoyama may have tried explaining the logic behind the plan to T.C. If so, it had no appreciable impact, and Douglas would become one of its fiercest critics. On 17 June 1976, T.C. blasted the Trudeau government for what he viewed as a dangerous change to the financing of medicare. In his lengthy speech to Parliament, one of only a few permitted an ordinary MP, T.C. noted how the Trudeau government had set the table for this momentous shift in federal financing.

First, there was the Lalonde Report, released in 1974. Named after Minister of National Health and Welfare Marc Lalonde, this report focused on the factors beyond health services that determine health outcomes, such as lifestyle, the environment, and human biology.[123] The report dovetailed with Douglas's arguments in favour of expanding universal coverage to include more prevention-based primary care, home-care services, long-term care, and population-based prevention programs. However, instead of using the report as the basis to encourage such services through universal coverage, the federal government was refusing to work with the provinces to transform the health system. Douglas congratulated Lalonde for writing the report but then, just as quickly, condemned him "for having done nothing about the policy he enunciated" in it.[124] Beyond this, the Lalonde Report also provided a justification for the federal government to allow the provinces the flexibility to reallocate spending from hospitals and doctors to other areas of health, and even non-health, spending that would have as much – perhaps more – impact on improving the health of their respective populations.[125]

For some in the Trudeau cabinet, the Lalonde Report provided an argument to reduce the level of federal Medicare funding. In fact, the federal government had introduced a bill the year after the report, in 1975, that had capped transfers to the provinces under the Medical Care Act. Despite their strenuous efforts, Douglas and his NDP colleagues were unsuccessful in killing that bill.[126] At the same time, T.C. feared that the Trudeau government was trying to upset what he had always seen as a shared commitment for Medicare between Ottawa and the provinces. He was aghast when, that same year, the federal government notified the provinces that it would not be renewing its shared-cost commitments under the Hospital Insurance and Diagnostic Services Act and the Medical Care Act. This was done to force the provinces to the negotiating table to replace shared-cost financing with a block transfer formula based in part on a permanent federal tax transfer. Since the escalator for the cash portion of the transfer would be based on economic growth rather than provincial spending, the provinces would alone take the risk of health spending continuing to outpace both inflation and the growth in provincial revenues.[127]

T.C. believed that the Trudeau government had no intention of continuing to support, much less expand, the system of universal health coverage that the Diefenbaker and Pearson administrations had committed to. For Douglas, it felt like a stunning reversal of a policy and was actually intended to dismantle health insurance in Canada, all under the guise of cost control. While agreeing that health care costs had "risen rapidly," he pointed out that health costs in other countries without universal health coverage had grown "to a far greater extent than they have risen in Canada." Specious arguments on cost, in his view, only served those who wanted to see Medicare rolled back:

> Those who oppose health insurance – usually those who are comfortably well off and who do not worry about meeting their health care costs – point to the United States where health care costs are met on an individual basis. In that country ... our American neighbours spend a higher percentage of their gross national product on health care – they have no [universal] health insurance program – than we do in Canada, where we have a health insurance program. We have the best health insurance program in the western hemisphere: not the best in the world, but certainly the best in the western hemisphere. This does not mean, of course, that we should be satisfied to let the cost of health care continue to escalate without our doing anything to limit that escalation. All of us want to eradicate any abuse of or wastage in health insurance programs. But we ought not to fall into the trap, as some members have in the course of this debate, of laying the blame at the feet of the public for over-utilization.[128]

Douglas's fear was that a tax transfer would benefit the wealthy provinces to the detriment of the less wealthy ones and, over time, would force the smaller and poorer provinces to reduce the quality of services, leading to different standards of care across the country. "Are we to return to the situation we once had," he asked the House, "when the standard of services enjoyed by Canadians was determined by the financial affluence of the province in which they resided? If we take this retrograde step, we will remove the cornerstone of confederation and weaken the bonds which hold this nation together." But what disturbed him even more was that "the less affluent" provinces would be driven to use "deterrent fees and user service charges" to "meet their health care costs in a period of declining tax revenue." This would destroy "the concept of uniform health insurance benefits" and result in "a patchwork of health programs across the country." For Douglas, this was a "negation of the kind of" country that Canadians had "been striving to create over the last quarter of a century." He ended with a ringing declaration that "a nation which is not prepared to make adequate health services available to all its citizens, regardless of income or residence, is a nation which is in danger of losing its vision, and when a nation loses its vision, the people perish."[129]

Beneath these concerns laid Douglas's distrust and dislike of the prime minister. Douglas had revealed his true feelings towards Trudeau years earlier, in a wide-ranging interview with the press as he was leaving the NDP leadership. First acknowledging the PM's intellectual competence, his mastery of constitutional law, and his proven ability to run a tighter ship than Pearson, he then became very personal:

> I think he thinks in theoretical terms that, you know, we should do something for the poor and the needy. But, in terms of understanding a young person out of work, or a student who can't get money to go back to university, or the problems of an unemployed man with five kids ... well, he doesn't understand because he's never come up against it.
>
> I don't know whether he's ever worked with, or lived with, day in and day out, people who are really up against the crunch. And he reacts like this when he's crossed in the House of Commons. You get all the marks of the arrogance of the spoiled little rich boy who always had what he wants, and who bites the carpet and kicks his feet when he's thwarted.[130]

However accurate the substance of his assessment, Douglas's bitter tone was accentuated when, immediately following this assessment, he was asked to give his opinion of Stanfield. The contrast could not have been starker: Stanfield, Douglas opined, was "a man of undoubted integrity and genuine interest and concern for people."[131] T.C. never forgave Trudeau for abandoning the CCF and joining the Liberals. And he must also have been frustrated that Al Johnson and Tommy Shoyama, his talented former policy advisors, had worked assiduously to replace the shared-cost financing of Medicare with a mechanism that Douglas thought inimical to a national system.[132] To add insult to injury, in addition to Johnson and Shoyama, T.C. and his NDP colleagues also had to contend with Don Tansley, the former head of Saskatchewan's Medical Care Insurance Commission, being in the employ of the federal government in what they perceived as a highly objectionable role. Trudeau had appointed Tansley as the administrator of the Anti-Inflation Board, a measure roundly criticized by Douglas and the NDP as favouring business to the detriment of labour and ordinary Canadians.[133]

## Retirement and SOS Medicare

Despite Douglas's grave concerns about the Trudeau government's intentions in terms of the future of Medicare, he and the tiny coterie of NDP MPs did not have the parliamentary clout to alter the federal government's trajectory. Moreover, the NDP government in Saskatchewan, although very much opposed to the change in funding – and supported in this by the governments in the four Atlantic provinces – eventually capitulated to the federal proposal to end shared-cost financing of Medicare.

As described by Malcolm Taylor, the federal-provincial negotiations were "lengthy, often bitter, and always complex."[134] By December 1976, all ten provinces had accepted EPF, the Saskatchewan NDP government very grudgingly so, in exchange for greater flexibility in spending federal transfer money and no longer having reporting requirements, especially those required under the old hospital insurance legislation and bilateral agreements. The new block transfer regime came into effect in April 1977.

That year, Douglas had told his constituency association in Nanaimo that he would not be seeking the nomination for the next federal election. The Trudeau years had been frustrating ones for him, as he felt that much of what he had helped build from the mid-1940s until the late 1960s was being torn down. After a lifetime of public service and a crushing work schedule, Douglas began to look forward to spending more time with Irma, his children, and his grandchildren. Still, he fully intended to continue agitating for the policies he felt were needed – especially health policies – as he explained in a letter to Iain Gow, a public administration professor at the Université de Montréal.

> In the forty-three years since I was first elected to Parliament, I have been privileged to see vast changes in the social and economic structure in Canada – much of it for the better. I derive some satisfaction from the fact that I had some part in promoting progress such as Hospital Insurance and Medicare, which are now part of our national life. If I have been privileged to make some small contribution to making life a little more secure for the average citizen, then I feel my years in public life have not been in vain.
>
> Although I am leaving Parliament, I have no intention of curtailing my political activities and I hope I will have the necessary health and strength to continue to raise my voice and exercise any influence I can on the important issues facing our country.[135]

As Douglas predicted, the amount of physician extra-billing and hospital user charges increased under the new EPF regime. By the federal election of 1979, an election in which he was not a candidate, user fees had become a hot-button issue.[136] In response, the PCs promised to examine the issue, if elected. And, following their defeat of the

Trudeau Liberals, the new (and short-lived) Clark government, through Health Minister David Crombie, appointed Emmett Hall to review the situation.[137]

In the weeks preceding the federal election of 22 May, the NDP, under the leadership of a Ed Broadbent, made the erosion of Medicare under the federal and provincial governments a major political issue. The NDP had already joined in the fight alongside the Canadian Labour Congress (CLC), which unveiled its own plan to "save and improve Medicare."[138] Of course, this was not enough for T.C., who wanted to see as much public pressure as possible brought to bear on the federal government. Now a private citizen, he used his extensive influence with trade unions and church groups and drew on the resources provided by the Douglas-Coldwell Foundation, which had been established in 1971 to honour T.C. when he retired as leader of the NDP, to forge a broader Medicare coalition. To preserve what had been achieved in terms of universal health coverage as well as carry on the project of expanding Medicare over time, T.C. had concluded that a larger and more permanent civil society organization was required.

Months after the election, in early November, the Douglas-Coldwell Foundation joined with the CLC and the Canadian Federation of Nurses Unions, to host an "SOS Medicare" conference in Ottawa. This meeting of pro-Medicare civil society groups and individuals was intended to examine the emerging threats to Medicare, including the EPF and the growth in physician extra-billing and hospital user charges in the 1970s. T.C. felt his main objective had been achieved when the Canadian Health Coalition, a partnership of labour unions, health provider organizations, faith-based groups, and women's organizations, was formed at the conference. Joining Douglas in the SOS Medicare sessions was the PC federal minister of health, David Crombie, as well as Monique Bégin, the former Liberal minister of health, who would soon resume the post after the fall of the Joe Clark government in early 1980. Also present was Hall, then preparing his report on the impact of the block transfer and provincial health spending and the growth in physician extra-billing and user fees. In his own speech, Douglas lauded Hall:

> It is time that we took a look at the present system to see whether or not we are carrying out the vision that was contained in the report of Mr. Justice Emmett Hall. I am delighted that Mr. Crombie, the minister of national health and welfare, appointed Mr. Justice Hall to conduct this inquiry into public health care. I have complete confidence in his competence and integrity. I am sure that his report will provide a blueprint on how we can

work together, irrespective of political party or region or profession or interest, to make Medicare what it was intended to be: a program that would provide in Canada a society which had freedom from fear and freedom from want.[139]

Leaning into a theme he had been developing since the early 1970s, Douglas also stressed that it was not enough to simply protect the Medicare status quo. He reminded everyone that his original intention, going back to the Saskatchewan government in the 1940s – a vision now shared across the partisan spectrum – involved two phases for Medicare:

> The first was to remove the financial barrier between those who provide health services and those who need them. We pointed out repeatedly that the first phase was the easiest of the problems we faced. In governmental terms, of course, it means finding the revenue, it means exercising controls over cost, but in the long term it was the easiest problem to surmount.
> 
> Phase 2, however, would be a much more difficult one: altering our delivery system so as to reduce costs by putting the emphasis on preventive medicine rather than treatment and drugs. I think we have to realize now that we have not yet grappled seriously with the second phase. We must now move increasingly toward group practice, whether it be community clinics, cooperative clinics, [or] clinics set up by the doctors themselves. Only through group practice of this kind will it be possible to focus mainly on the prevention of illness instead of the treatment of illness. Only in that way are we going to be able to keep the costs from becoming so excessive that people will be easily convinced that Medicare is too expensive to maintain.[140]

In other words, Medicare was a journey, not a destination, and for Douglas, the perpetual reformer, the hardest part of the journey had not yet begun. He expressed the hope to his audience "that from time to time we will gather" as interested citizens so "that we may be able to build in Canada a program that will provide the maximum amount of health" and that will enable all Canadians to "enjoy good health and provide them with remedial services when that good health is no longer present ... without fear of the financial burdens which have crippled so many people in other places and other times."[141] This hope dovetailed with the establishment that day of the Canadian Health Coalition. This group along with its provincial chapters would become a permanent advocate for the protection of single-payer and single-tier Medicare in Canada.

Despite their partisan differences, Douglas, Crombie, and Bégin all agreed that Medicare was in trouble.[142] The real question was what to do about it. The answer would soon become clear after the defeat of Joe Clark's government by the Trudeau Liberals in February 1980, the reappointment of Bégin as minister of health, and the release of Emmett Hall's report that September.[143] The review by Hall was hampered by a lack of staff and money as well as the demand that the study be finalized within twelve months. Although less than enthusiastic, given these constraints, the veteran health policy expert Malcolm Taylor agreed to lead the research for the study.[144]

On the first question of whether provincial governments had used EPF to divert health transfers to non-health spending, the Hall Report's answer was a definitive "no": the "proportions of provincial budgets allocated to health, before and after EPF, were identical." However, on the second question of user fees, there was little question that they had increased over time. To the suggestion by some provincial governments that these fees did not impede the universality of access, Hall shot back: "If extra-billing is permitted as a right and practised by physicians in their sole discretion, it will, over the years, destroy the program, creating in that downward path a two-tier system incompatible with the societal level which Canadians have attained."[145] On this question, Hall provided Bégin with the rationale for what would ultimately become the Canada Health Act, passed in Parliament in 1984.

**The Sun Sets**

While Douglas continued to agitate for change outside of the parliamentary system, he became ill and, in the summer of 1981, was diagnosed with cancer that was too far advanced to be treated. Already thin, he began to shed more weight, and any public interventions became ever more painful and difficult. In November 1982, he spoke at a conference on medicare organized by the Canadian Centre for Policy Alternatives, a left-leaning think tank close to organized labour and the NDP. A somewhat sarcastic editorial on the conference in the *Canadian Medical Association Journal* described Tommy Douglas, "medicare's political Messiah," as joined by other "pioneers of medicare," including its "codifier and scribe," Emmett Hall; "its most successful tactician," Claude Castonguay of Quebec; and Sam Wolfe, the doctor "who broke" the "1962 doctor strike and wrote to tell about it."[146]

At the conference, Douglas explained the danger posed by user fees, and how they would soon produce two classes of people in the country, "those who come under the general program and are paid for out of government funds and those who pay a little extra to doctors who want a little extra." As the proportion of extra-billing increases, "people will get to the place where they're saying – I'm paying almost as much in extra billing as I pay through taxes." They will inevitably say, "Let's scrap the plan. Who needs it?," and the country will get two classes of physicians: those who extra bill and those who don't. Douglas warned that many of the doctors who engaged in extra-billing "would be the most competent doctors and the most proficient surgeons," leaving people who would not, or could not, "accept extra billing ... to go to less competent doctors and less competent surgeons," as had been the case before Medicare.[147]

In 1983, Douglas gave his last great speech, to the NDP's national convention in Regina, where hundreds of delegates had come to celebrate the fiftieth anniversary of the Regina Manifesto. Once again, he reiterated the centrality of universal health coverage to the fabric of a civilized country. After being introduced by Allan Blakeney, the seventy-eight-year-old appeared gaunt and drawn, but he came alive with a couple of introductory jokes. What followed was well described by Walter Stewart:

> It was The Speech. He had given it many times before, but like every great speech, it improved with age. He had the timing just right, the pauses in just the right places, the lifted hand, the pointed finger, the long sentences broken by abrupt ones, the jokes interspersed with sombre warnings. It was a sermon, really – not surprising in a man who had trained as a preacher – a political sermon that drew on his experience, and his humanity, and his faith, to lift that crowd for forty-five minutes, and make it believe.[148]

After the speech, everyone rose out of their seats, cheering, waving their arms, weeping, and clapping non-stop for almost twenty-five minutes, a thunderous outpouring of love and admiration. They knew it was their last chance to say goodbye to the man and to everything he represented.

In the debates over Medicare in Parliament, Douglas had a worthy successor in Bill Blaikie, an ordained minister in the United Church of Canada. From a working-class family in Winnipeg, Blaikie was himself highly influenced by the social gospel traditions of Woodsworth, Knowles, and Douglas, which made him a unique figure at this point in the House of Commons. First elected to Parliament in 1979 and serving as NDP health critic, Blaikie, in speech after speech, demanded to know why it was taking Bégin and her fellow Liberals so long to follow up on Hall's second report. He was so dogged that she accused him of waging "guerilla warfare" on the issue.[149] Between January and August 1982 alone, Blaikie intervened on at least fifteen separate days.[150] Outside the House of Commons, relations were less strained, and Bégin worked with the NDP caucus to gather evidence from constituents on extra-billing and user charges.[151]

While the drama over the Canada Health Act unfolded in the country, T.C. faced challenges of another sort. In June 1984, while taking his daily three-kilometre walk in his Ottawa neighbourhood, he was struck by a city bus. At seventy-nine years of age, Douglas had hearing aids but, according to Irma, rarely wore them. While trying to cross the Ottawa River Parkway, he forgot that one of the bus lanes changed direction during rush hour. He did not see or hear the bus coming straight at him. Unable to stop, the bus driver swerved, but the corner of the bus hit Douglas straight on, causing rib fractures, chest injuries, and a concussion. Landing in the intensive care unit of the Ottawa Civic Hospital, his condition was deemed serious but stable.[152] His scheduled trip to Regina to be the keynote speaker at the fortieth anniversary celebration of the election of North America's first socialist government had to be cancelled.[153]

After his release from hospital, Douglas's condition worsened as his cancer spread. He died surrounded by his family in his Ottawa home on the morning of Monday, 24 February 1986. He was eighty-one.[154] The next day, party leaders and members across the political spectrum sang the praises of the principled but "tough and steely little Scotsman," emphasizing his achievement in leading the first socialist government in North America and in pioneering Medicare.[155] Prime Minister Brian Mulroney described him as "one of our great humanitarians." Liberal leader John Turner called Douglas "a living legend to the people of Saskatchewan." NDP leader Ed Broadbent called Douglas "a great man" who had "changed the course of history" and whose life embodied "the truth that reason and passion" go "hand in hand" in any "political life seriously undertaken."[156]

Of all of his achievements, the most important "in terms of its impact on our nation," according to Broadbent, was the Douglas government of Saskatchewan's introduction of universal health coverage, "an act that was soon picked up by other governments and became part of our national legislative heritage."[157] John Paul (Jean-Paul) Harney, a former NDP MP who was then relaunching the NDP's provincial party in Quebec, described how he had been transformed by one of Douglas's speeches on medicare in the weeks just before the doctor's strike in Saskatchewan in the summer of 1962:

Defender of Medicare 487

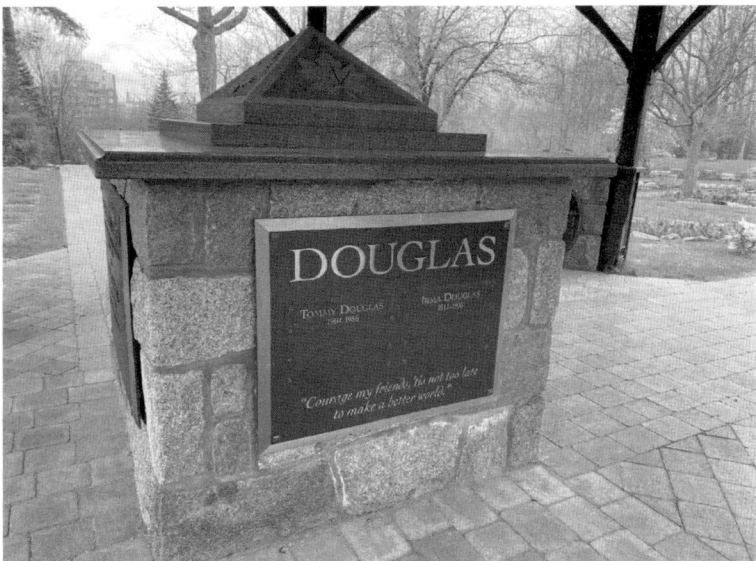

Marker for T.C. Douglas at Beechwood Cemetery, Ottawa (Gregory P. Marchildon, 2023)

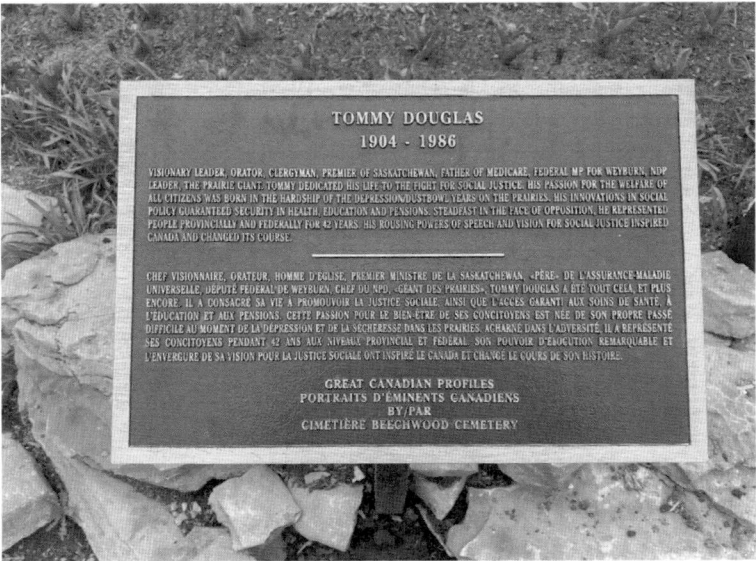

Historical plaque at Beechwood Cemetery (Gregory P. Marchildon, 2023)

> I had just recently come from Quebec where eloquence was not a scarce commodity, but Tommy applied eloquence to something beyond partisan or sectoral purposes; his speech was reason and passion bent to eminently practical proposals which when they were brought to pass would change men's lives.
>
> I had already accepted medicare as a good idea. The fact that it made sense was one of the reasons why I had joined the NDP and become one of its candidates.
>
> But as I listened to Tommy Douglas speak, the idea of medicare took on flesh, it began to be peopled by the ordinary men and women of this country whose lives would be immeasurably bettered by a publicly-run, tax-supported universal medical insurance plan.[158]

As a politician both in government and in opposition, he married his idealism to his political pragmatism to achieve as much as he could. As an editorial-cum-obituary in the *Ottawa Citizen* put it, he "gave voice to the better part in all of us." Although he spent a half century "fighting the battles of democratic socialism," he tried to avoid "the politics of sanctimony." He "won genuine victories – though not as many as he wanted." He did it all "in the hard and unforgiving business of politics, a business he practised with skill and relentless energy."[159]

Frank Scott, the McGill intellectual, put it best years earlier when comparing the first leaders of the CCF:

> There was J.S. Woodsworth – philosophical, spiritual. M.J. Coldwell – the supreme parliamentarian, superbly good. But Tommy was it. Tommy related the whole thing to people, to every type of person. He was never, very terrifying in his ideas even when putting forth bold CCF policy. And he was able to put it into words that made it seem perfectly sensible and reasonable to ordinary people. And he was therefore the best.[160]

In death, Douglas continued to be relevant to Medicare as it once again became a contested policy in the 1990s and the early twenty-first century. He had been so instrumental in the establishment of Canada's most iconic policy, and through it a constituent part of the identity of Canadians. His name would be regularly invoked to not only defend Medicare but to improve, expand, and build within the principles he had long ago articulated while premier of Saskatchewan.

# Conclusion

*I don't mind being a symbol, but I don't want to become a monument. There are monuments all over the Parliament Buildings, and I've seen what the pigeons do to them.*[1]

Tommy Douglas

The prominence of most public figures declines sharply after they leave public life. Within a generation or two, they are largely forgotten, except by the occasional student of history: only a few manage to exert any influence after they leave office, and even fewer continue to do so generations after their death. Tommy Douglas falls into the last category, almost exclusively due to his formative role in establishing a beachhead for universal health coverage (UHC) in North America. In Canada, he remains an icon of Medicare, the signature social policy for generations of Canadians.[2] Outside Canada, his name has drawn the attention of those pursuing universal health coverage in their own countries.[3]

For the very same reasons, Tommy Douglas also attracts the ire of those opposed to the principles of Medicare in Canada. For them, he represents what they see as Canadian Medicare's faulty foundation. In their view, Douglas's model of single-payer and single-tier UHC, as enshrined in the Canada Health Act, is the reason for the poor performance of Canada's health system relative to other comparable countries.[4] In contrast, supporters of this model see the shortcomings as resulting from governance, regulation, and delivery that have nothing to do with the criteria of the Canada Health Act and that in no way diminish the values of universality and single-tier delivery that Douglas fiercely advocated in his lifetime.[5]

In recent years, this debate has become shriller. It has also been the subject of extensive scrutiny in the courts. The most exhaustive review was in the *Cambie Surgeries* trial in British Columbia, led by orthopaedic surgeon Dr. Brian Day, a long-time critic of Canadian Medicare and a former president of the Canadian Medical Association. In a trial that ran from 2016 until 2019, dozens of experts from Canada, the United States, the United Kingdom, and other countries submitted reports to the court that focused on Medicare's design, probing the implications of the strong form of universality in British Columbia, and in Canada more generally. Some of these experts, perhaps fewer than half, were then examined and cross-examined on their respective reports.[6]

In 2020, in a momentous 880-page ruling, the Supreme Court of British Columbia decided that these values and principles as operationalized in BC law, did not infringe sections 7 (individual right to life, liberty, and security) or 15 (individual right to equal protection and equal benefit) of the Canadian Charter of Rights and Freedoms.[7] In 2021, the BC Court of Appeal heard arguments as to why the trial court decision should be overturned, and when that court dismissed the application a year later, Day appealed the decision to the highest court in the country.[8] On 6 April 2023, the Supreme Court of Canada dismissed Day's leave to appeal, leaving in place the BC provisions protecting the single-tier nature of Medicare. Reacting to the decision, Day said it was "a very sad day for Canadians," arguing that, because of it, people would continue "to suffer and die on wait lists." In contrast, the NDP government of BC proclaimed that "our nation's highest court supports the principles of universal health care, where access to medical care is determined by a patient's needs, not their ability to pay their way to the front of the line."[9] Of course, the *Cambie* decisions hardly ended the debate on the single-tier and single-payer nature of Canadian Medicare, and there are likely to be more political and legal challenges in the future.

In one respect, the critics of Medicare are correct when they point the finger at Douglas and his central responsibility for the design of UHC in Canada. Four of the five criteria in the Canada Health Act were drawn from the Medical Care Act of 1966, whose criteria, in turn, were drawn directly from T.C.'s articulation of the operating principles of the medical care plan he proposed in a radio speech in 1959. However much the critics object, these principles remained important to Canadians as values worth defending. Moreover, how this "pan-Canadian" system works on a daily basis owes much to what Douglas developed in Saskatchewan. While some form of UHC may have emerged in Canada without Douglas, it is highly doubtful it would have exhibited the strong universality of his design.

If Douglas had never existed and if the CCF had never gained office in Saskatchewan 1944 and stayed in government for five successive terms, the result for medical insurance would more likely have been targeted, rather than universal, coverage. Consistent with the demands of organized medicine and business interests, private health insurance would have remained (and perhaps would continue to remain) the predominant form of coverage for most Canadians. While various provincial governments – perhaps with fiscal assistance from Ottawa – would strive to fill the gaps in coverage so that poorer and more marginalized Canadians would have access to some form of needed health care, the result would still reflect a two-tier system, one for those with the capacity to pay and another for those without the means to access high-quality private care.

Canada's single-payer and single-tier design can be traced directly to T.C.'s first term in office in 1944–8. As both minister of health and premier, Douglas had more direct control over the health policy agenda than he would ever enjoy again in his life. Able to attract a highly talented group of advisors and public servants, he achieved an astonishing transformation during his government's first term in office. Douglas operated on two tracks simultaneously. The first was his work with local governments to change the organization of the health system through health regions and to increase the supply of doctors and other health professionals, hospitals, medical care, and public health infrastructure in rural areas. This track also required new approaches, infrastructure, and health human resources for the care and treatment of mental illness as well as pathbreaking research and innovation in the field.

The second track was to increase availability by making health services free at the point of access. Within months of taking office, the Douglas government provided free hospital and medical care coverage for public assistance recipients, mental hospital residents, and all cancer patients in the province. T.C. then spurred his government to provide universal coverage for hospital care and diagnostic services for all residents. Rolled out in 1947, the plan became the template for national hospital insurance in the rest of Canada by the end of the 1950s, with the help of the federal spending power and the support of both Liberal and Progressive Conservative administrations in Ottawa.

Both tracks were extremely expensive for a government still dealing with the devastation of the Great Depression. Both were difficult to achieve, the first track because it required the commitment and initiative of numerous local governments acting in tandem, the second because it required the design and implementation of the first government-run single-payer and single-tier hospital coverage program in the world. However, the second track was more quickly pursued, as it relied less on the cooperation of local governments (except, of course, for the collection of premiums). The second track also had the tantalizing allure of potential federal cost-shared dollars if the federal government fulfilled its post-war reconstruction promises to partner with the provinces to introduce national health insurance.

Given the challenge of creating a novel program of government coverage within an almost impossible timeline, the implementation of a successful universal hospital coverage program was nothing short of miraculous, particularly when compared to the troubled implementation of the almost identical program in British Columbia two years later. Experts from near and far came to Regina to study the program and went away with a positive impression, irrespective of the ideological orientation of the governments they served. Moreover, the design features decided at that time – access based on the simple fact of citizenship rather than contribution, the government as single payer, and the insistence on a single tier of services – would become the template for both universal hospital and universal medical care coverage throughout Canada in the 1950s and 1960s.[10] Hospital insurance also proved politically successful for the government, keeping it in office in the election of 1948 and, in Douglas's view, being the most important ingredient in the government's recipe for victory in 1952.

What was even more remarkable was the fact that T.C. and his government continued with track one after his first term in office. Building its public health, medical, and hospital infrastructure in rural and remote areas, creating an air ambulance service that saved countless lives, and improving the plight of the mentally ill and their treatment may have pleased leading health experts and advocates throughout Canada, but these initiatives were hardly vote-getters. Still, T.C. persisted, understanding that health insurance was insufficient on its own to achieve the revolution he sought in health. The innovations of the Douglas government in these less-prominent health fields influenced other provincial governments.

But it was hospital coverage in Saskatchewan that had the most direct impact. While, for years, T.C. was, despite his best efforts, ineffectual in convincing the King and St-Laurent governments to re-engage the provinces on the Green Book proposals of 1945–6, he did play an important role in getting hospital insurance on the federal-provincial agenda a decade later. Because of its administrative success, his single-payer hospitalization program – not the multi-payer program in

Alberta – provided the operating principles for federal cost sharing. In turn, the federal fiscal contribution allowed the Douglas government to extend universal coverage to physician services.

Unlike hospital insurance, implementing universal medical care coverage quickly became a political nightmare. Although there had always been some opposition to the idea of a government-managed system of universal coverage, organized medicine had hardened against the idea in the 1950s and saw Saskatchewan as the battlefront where the idea had to be stopped before it spread to the rest of Canada or even the United States. Supported by a powerful coalition of provincial governments, the insurance industry, and almost every chamber of commerce in the country, the doctors fought both Douglas and the program. As we have seen, Douglas was also distracted with his federal NDP leadership and was trying to work through a minister of health who wanted peace with organized medicine at almost any price.

Universal medical care coverage would be implemented in the province, but only after T.C.'s defeat as a federal candidate. More importantly, it could be implemented only through a compromise that allowed some of the less desirable features of private medical practice to continue and even thrive. This book began with a glimpse at this pivot point in Douglas's life and career in 1961. Before this date, he was on the ascent, establishing and then consolidating an ambitious health reform program that has never been equalled in Canada. After 1961, though, T.C. experienced a descent, in part self-inflicted through mistakes he made in the introduction of medicare. These mistakes were exacerbated by his decision to take on the federal leadership of the NDP. Admittedly, he did this in part because he could not convince the person he felt most suited for leadership to take on that role, but he also became federal leader because he felt he had the ability to eventually lead the NDP to government in Ottawa. His political life as a federal opposition politician from 1961 until 1979 was a disappointment compared to what he had managed to achieve in government in the 1940s and 1950s. Although he refused to show it publicly, Douglas likely felt the disappointment more than anyone else in his party.

In retrospect, T.C.'s herculean efforts to pass his medicare bill in 1961 constitute the inflection point of his political life. Before, he was innovating and creating, while after, he was largely criticizing and defending and could only cajole, heckle, embarrass, and preach as the leader of a third (or fourth) party. Even from this limited station in life, however, he was persevering and, at times, successful. The transition from the Liberal plan for medicare in the early 1960s to the plan actually adopted in the mid-1960s reflects Douglas's value and preferences.

In the last years of his life, T.C. was limited to advocacy outside the chambers of government, and his influence waned accordingly. Since his death, however, his influence as a symbol of the ethos of Medicare has actually grown with time, his name evoked to defend the principles of universality and public administration, as well as to pursue the enlargement of universal coverage. His continuing posthumous reputation as the originator of Canadian Medicare is deserved, given the ferocity of his effort, his consistent focus, and his gritty tenacity. We should all be so lucky to have one good idea to commit to until the end.

His doggedness reflected a rare constitution, one that had no qualm about sacrificing his personal popularity in the cause of ensuring access to the benefits of modern medicine for all, including those who might not have felt they needed it or wanted it, let alone those who complained about those who didn't deserve it. At the same time, he inspired members of his government, ministers and civil servants, to persevere and overcome the formidable challenges to implementing UHC in Saskatchewan twice. In the first instance, he led the establishment of UHC for hospital and diagnostic services, a program that was implemented nineteen months before the National Health Service began operating in the United Kingdom. In the second, he proceeded with covering medical care despite the resolute opposition of organized medicine and a potent anti-medicare coalition of business and a print media long associated with Liberal interests.

T.C. may not have wanted to become a monument, but he has become one, and the engraving on the monument is invariably "Tommy Douglas: The Father of Medicare." In almost every contemporary reference to him, popular or scholarly, Douglas and Medicare are fused in any opening statement. This label may not be fair to the other major policy breakthroughs achieved by his provincial government between 1944 and 1961, or the other social policies he pursued as a MP and federal party leader, but it is the one that will nevertheless be remembered for generations to come.

Perhaps this is as it should be. However, for Douglas, Medicare was only a way station towards a much more comprehensive form of UHC. From the early 1960s until his death in 1984, T.C. was unwavering in his pursuit of broadening Medicare. More importantly, he recognized that health insurance alone would never be enough to create a healthier society. This required a major reorganization of services in which the prevention of illness and the promotion of healthier lifestyles were integrated. Long before "population health" became a common term, he understand the importance of income, education, and food security as the key determinants of health. For T.C., the purpose of government policy was to create an environment that allowed all citizens to live up to their fullest potential.

In a sense, T.C. achieved sainthood after his death. And in death he became acceptable to the Canadian establishment in a way he never was in life, in part because the movement and ideas he represented has become such an accepted feature of the Canadian social landscape. As Jonathan Eig points out in his biography of Martin Luther King Jr., the process of "canonizing" such historical figures also can defang them.[11] Their "complicated politics and philosophy" become so simple as to be acceptable to almost everyone.

We should remember how polarizing and how divisive Douglas was in his lifetime. Motivated by principle, he had the courage and tenacity to try to change the way things were. But T.C. also possessed an innate pragmatism. He knew what he needed to do within a democracy to convince the public of the need to change. He knew how to find and work with talented individuals to figure out the concrete steps required to transform a set of laudable policy objectives into an effective and sustainable program.

# Notes

**Preface**

1 *Building on Values: The Future of Health Care in Canada* (Ottawa: Commission on the Future of Health Care in Canada, Commissioner Roy J. Romanow, 2002), 271–2.
2 A.B. McKillop, "Engaging History: Historians, Storytelling, and Self," in *Thinkers and Dreamers: Historical Essays in Honour of Carl Berger*, ed. Gerald Friesen and Douglas Owram (Toronto: University of Toronto Press, 2011), 34.
3 Jill Lepore, "Historians Who Love Too Much: Reflections on Microhistory and Biography" *Journal of American History* 88, no. 1 (2001): 129.
4 McKillop, "Engaging History," 47.

**Introduction**

1 Bernard Crick, as quoted by Ben Kisby, "'Politics Is Ethics Done in Public': Exploring Linkages and Disjunctions between Citizen Education and Character Education in England," *Journal of Social Science Education* 16, no. 3 (2017): 8.
2 These exceptions include historian Michael Bliss (see, for example, "Michael Bliss: Tommy Douglas Era Has Passed," *National Post*, 26 Jan. 2012, http://nationalpost.com/opinion/michael-bliss-tommy-douglas-era-has-passed) and physician and anti-medicare activist during the 1962 doctors' strike, Noel Doig, *Setting the Record Straight: A Doctor's Memoir of the 1962 Medicare Crisis* (Saskatoon: Indie Ink Publishing, 2012).
3 Gregory P. Marchildon, "The Single-Tier Universality of Canadian Medicare," in *Universality and Social Policy in Canada*, ed. Daniel Béland, Gregory P. Marchildon, and Michael J. Prince (Toronto: University of Toronto Press, 2019), 49–62.

4 Roderick J. Barman, "Biography as History," *Journal of the Canadian Historical Association* 21, no. 2 (2010): 62.
5 Louis W. Banner, "Biography as History," *American Historical Review* 114, no. 3 (2009): 589; Lucy Riall, "The Shallow End of History? The Substance and Future of Political Biography," *Journal of Interdisciplinary History* 40, no. 3 (2010). The latter phrase was first coined by Michael Holroyd in his essay "The Case against Biography," in *Works on Paper: The Craft of Biography and Autobiography*, ed. Holroyd (London: Counterpoint, 2002), 3–9.
6 This was a common refrain in the oral interviews provided by those who knew T.C. best. Allan Blakeney, for example, said that none of even his closest political colleagues felt they knew Douglas: Provincial Archives of Saskatchewan (PAS), Dennis Gruending fonds, R-1379, box 14, file II.54.3, interview with A.E. Blakeney for Gruending's biography of Blakeney, 16 June 1989.
7 Lawrence Goldman, "History and Biography," *Historical Research* 89, no. 245 (2016): 405.
8 Robert I. Rotberg, "Biography and Historiography: Mutual Evidentiary and Interdisciplinary Considerations," *Journal of Interdisciplinary History* 40, no. 3 (2010): 320.
9 Jonathan Eig, *King: A Life* (New York: Farrar, Strauss and Giroux, 2023), 7.
10 For a concise summary of these biographies, see Gregory P. Marchildon, "Thomas Clement Douglas," *Dictionary of Canadian Biography*, vol. 21 (2021), http://www.biographi.ca/en/bio/douglas_thomas_clement_21E .html.
11 Gregory P. Marchildon, "The Douglas Legacy and the Future of Medicare," in *Medicare: Facts, Myths, Problems, and Promise*, ed. Bruce Campbell and Greg Marchildon (Toronto: Lorimer, 2007), 36–41.
12 Nelson Wiseman and Benjamin Isitt, "Social Democracy in Twentieth Century Canada: An Interpretive Framework," *Canadian Journal of Political Science* 40, no. 3 (2007): 567–89; Patrik Marier, "A Swedish Welfare State in North America? The Creation and Expansion of the Saskatchewan Welfare State, 1944–1982," *Journal of Policy History* 25, no. 4 (2013): 614–37; Gregory P. Marchildon, "Social Democratic Solidarity and the Welfare State: Health Care and Single-Tier Universality in Sweden and Canada," *Canadian Bulletin of Medical History / Bulletin canadien d'histoire de la médecine* 38, no. 1 (2021): 177–96.

## 1. Medicare: The Agony and the Ecstasy

1 *Journals of the Legislative Assembly of Saskatchewan*, Second Session, 1963, 18: Bill No. 1, The Saskatchewan Medicare Care Insurance Act; "Care Bill Provides Payment by Premiums, Public Funds," *Regina Leader-Post* (*LP*),

13 Oct. 1961, 1; "Compulsory Health Plan Legislation Introduced by Erb," *Saskatoon Star Phoenix*, 13 Oct. 1961, 3. The word "medicare" was not used in Canada until this bill made its appearance. However, after "medicare" was implemented throughout Canada, the term gradually came to be used for all universal coverage services, including hospital and diagnostic care. In this book, "medicare" (lowercased) is used only for universal medical care coverage while "Medicare" (uppercased) is used for universal hospital, diagnostic, and medical care coverage.
2 As the historical benchmark for the postwar welfare state, Sweden is the obvious comparator to Saskatchewan. See Patrik Marier, "A Swedish Welfare State in North America? The Creation and Expansion of the Saskatchewan Welfare State, 1944–1982," *Journal of Policy History* 25, no. 4 (2013): 614–31. For a direct comparison concerning the policy of universal health coverage, see Gregory P. Marchildon, "Social Democratic Solidarity and the Welfare State: Health Care and Single-Tier Universality in Sweden and Canada," *Canadian Bulletin of Medical History / Bulletin canadien d'histoire de la médecine* 38, no. 1 (2021): 177–91.
3 On the Liberal newspapers owned by Clifford Sifton and his sons, see Mitch Diamantopoulos, "The Foundations of Agrarian Socialism: Co-operative Economic Action in Saskatchewan, 1905–1960" *Prairie Forum* 37, no. 2 (2012): 124–5, and Dennis Gruending, "Paternalism on the Prairies," in *Canadian Newspapers: The Inside Story*, ed. Walter Stewart (Edmonton: Hurtig Publishers, 1980), 144–5.
4 C. Marie Fenwick, "'Building the Future in a Steady but Measured Pace': The Respectable Feminism of Marjorie Cooper," *Saskatchewan History* 54, no. 1 (2002): 25–8.
5 *Debates*, Legislative Assembly of Saskatchewan (DLAS), 11 Oct. 1961, 3–13.
6 DLAS, 11 Oct. 1961, 7–10.
7 DLAS, 12 Oct. 1961, 34–5.
8 DLAS, 11 Oct. 1961, 3–14.
9 The provincial medical association (the Saskatchewan Division of the Canadian Medical Association, later known as the Saskatchewan Medical Association) had been subsumed into the regulatory college, the College of Physicians and Surgeons of Saskatchewan, in 1936 as a cost-saving measure during the Great Depression (a parallel development occurred Alberta and British Columbia). The two bodies were not separated again until the latter half of the 1960s. See Malcolm G. Taylor, *Health Insurance and Canadian Public Policy: The Seven Decisions That Created the Canadian Health Insurance System and Its Outcomes*, 2nd ed. (Montreal and Kingston: McGill-Queen's University Press, 2009), 241, and C. David Naylor, *Private Practice, Public Payment: Canadian Medicare and the Politics of Health*

*Insurance, 1911–1966* (Montreal and Kingston: McGill-Queen's University Press, 1986), 95–6.
10 "Doctors Ponder Course of Action on Care Plan," *LP*, 11 Oct. 1961, 1.
11 A.W. Johnson with Rosemary Proctor, *Dream No Little Dreams: A Biography of the Douglas Government of Saskatchewan* (Toronto: University of Toronto Press, 2004), 270.
12 The classic piece was by Escott Reid, "The Saskatchewan Liberal Machine before 1929," *Canadian Journal of Economics and Political Science* 2, no. 1 (1936): 27–40 (reprinted in *Politics in Saskatchewan*, ed. Norman Ward and Duff Spafford (Toronto: Longmans Canada, 1968), 93–104). Also see David E. Smith, *Prairie Liberalism: The Liberal Party in Saskatchewan, 1905–71* (Toronto: University of Toronto Press, 1975).
13 Dale Eisler, *Rumours of Glory: Saskatchewan and the Thatcher Years* (Edmonton: Hurtig Publishers, 1987), 20.
14 The reasons for this are more fully explained in chapter 10.
15 Eisler, *Rumours of Glory*, 11–59.
16 DLAS, 11 Oct. 1961, 28.
17 DLAS, 13 Oct. 1961, 4–5.
18 DLAS, 13 Oct. 1961, 9.
19 DLAS, 13 Oct. 1961, 9.
20 Douglas, quoting Ross Thatcher in DLAS, 13 Oct. 1961, 9.
21 DLAS, 13 Oct. 1961, 10.
22 DLAS, 13 Oct. 1961, 10–11.
23 DLAS, 13 Oct. 1961, 11.
24 DLAS, 13 Oct. 1961, 12.
25 DLAS, 13 Oct. 1961, 12.
26 DLAS, 13 Oct. 1961, 19.
27 DLAS, 13 Oct. 1961, 25–6.

## 2. The Making of a Preacher-Politician

1 See R.H. Campbell's *Carron Company* (Edinburgh: Oliver and Boyd, 1961) and "The Industrial Revolution: A Revision Article," *Scottish Historical Review* 46, no. 141 (1967): 37–55; T.M. Devine, *The Scottish Nation, 1700–2000* (London: Penguin, 2000), 106–16; Christopher A. Whatley, *The Industrial Revolution in Scotland* (Cambridge: Cambridge University Press, 1997); and Chris Evans, "The Industrial Revolution in Iron in the British Isles," in *The Industrial Revolution in Iron: An Introduction*, ed. Chris Evans and Göran Rydén (London: Routledge, 2004), 15–27.
2 Library and Archives Canada (LAC), Peter Stursberg fonds, MG 31 D78, vol. 33, file 19, transcript of T.C. Douglas memoirs interview with Peter Stursberg, Ottawa (hereafter T.C. Douglas memoirs interview with Stursberg), 29 April 1980, 4.

3 LAC, RG 150, Canadian Expeditionary Force, accession 1992-93/166, box 2626-45, item 3622277, Thomas Douglas personnel record (hereafter referred to as Thomas Douglas war record), https://www.bac-lac.gc.ca/eng/discover/military-heritage/first-world-war/personnel-records/Pages/item.aspx?IdNumber=362277.
4 T.C. Douglas memoirs interview with Stursberg, 5–9.
5 LAC, Passenger Lists, 1865–1935, RG 76-C, microfilm roll T-4824, T.C. Douglas, age seven, arrived in Saint John, New Brunswick, on 18 April 1912.
6 T.C. Douglas memoirs interview with Stursberg, 10–11.
7 Daniel Hiebert, "Class, Ethnicity and Residential Structure: The Social Geography of Winnipeg, 1901–1921," *Journal of Historical Geography* 17, no. 1 (1991): 68. On the North End specifically, see Russ Gourluck, *The Mosaic Village: A History of Winnipeg's North End* (Winnipeg: Great Plains Publications, 2010).
8 T.C. Douglas, *The Making of a Socialist: The Recollections of T.C. Douglas*, ed. Lewis H. Thomas (Edmonton: University of Alberta Press, 1982), 13. On the North End's political influence, see Nelson Wiseman, *Social Democracy in Manitoba: A History of the CCF/NDP* (Winnipeg: University of Manitoba Press, 1983), 5, 10.
9 Jan Oussoren, *From Baptist Preacher to Social Gospel Politician: T.C. Douglas's Transition* (Vancouver: Vancouver School of Theology, Chalmers Institute, 1998), 7; Thomas H. McLeod and Ian McLeod, *Tommy Douglas: The Road to Jerusalem* (Edmonton: Hurtig Publishers, 1987), 11.
10 McLeod and McLeod, *Tommy Douglas*, 11.
11 James S. Woodsworth, *Strangers within Our Gates: Or, Coming Canadians* (Winnipeg: Missionary Society of the Methodist Church, Canada), 3; McLeod and McLeod, *T.C. Douglas*, 11.
12 Dave Margoshes, *T.C. Douglas: Building the New Society* (Toronto: XYZ Publishing, 1999), 2.
13 Stuart Houston and Bill Waiser, *Tommy's Team: The People behind the Douglas Years* (Calgary: Fifth House, 2010), 191.
14 Margoshes, *T.C. Douglas*, 5.
15 Douglas, *Making of a Socialist*, 14–15.
16 Vincent Lam, *Tommy Douglas* (Toronto: Penguin Canada, 2011), 16; Douglas, *Making of a Socialist*, 13.
17 Douglas remembered this surgery taking place "about 1913 or 1914": see Douglas, *Making of a Socialist*, 7. According to Houston and Waiser (*Tommy's Team*, 194), Dr. Stanley Smith "performed, without charge, at least three operations on young T.C. under anaesthetic" over "the course of slightly less than three years" (*Tommy's Team*, 194).
18 Houston and Waiser, *Tommy's Team*, 192.
19 This account draws on my entry on Douglas in the *Dictionary of Canadian Biography*, vol. 21 (hereafter *DCB* Douglas entry), http://www.biographi.ca/en/bio/douglas_thomas_clement_21E.html.

20 In his recollections of 1958 (Douglas, *Making of a Socialist*, 7), Douglas erroneously refers to Dr. Stanley Smith as Dr. R.J. Smith. See the biography of Dr. Stanley Smith in Houston and Waiser, *Tommy's Team*, 191–6.
21 Douglas, *Making of a Socialist*, 7.
22 Thomas Douglas war record.
23 T.C. Douglas memoirs interview with Stursberg, 12.
24 Thomas Douglas war record.
25 Oussoren, *Baptist Preacher*, 9. According to Douglas (*Making of a Socialist*, 2), Andrew Clement was originally a member of the Plymouth Brethren but "he later became a Baptist and lay preacher."
26 Douglas, *Making of a Socialist*, 26.
27 T.C. Douglas memoirs interview with Stursberg, 20; Douglas, *Making of a Socialist*, 28.
28 Thomas Douglas war record. T.C.'s father was hospitalized with a condition then known as disordered action of the heart (DAH), commonly referred to as soldier's heart, in France for a month (12 Jan.–13 Feb. 1917), a cardiac condition common in soldiers with nervous conditions, sometimes made worse by being poisoned in gas attacks. See Tim Cook, *Lifesavers and Body Snatchers: Medical Care and the Struggle for Survival in the Great War* (Toronto: Allen Lane, 2022), 173–93; Mark Osborne Humphries, *A Weary Road: Shell Shock in the Canadian Expeditionary Force, 1914–1918* (Toronto: University of Toronto Press, 2018), 10–13, 184–8; and Edgar Jones, "Terror Weapons: The British Experience of Gas and its Treatments in the First World War" *War in History* 2, no. 3 (2014): 355–75. Although there is no indication in Thomas Douglas's service file that he was gassed, beyond a diagnosis of DAH, Thomas and Ian McLeod (*Tommy Douglas*, 16) suggest that he suffered from both poison gas and "bouts of despair" following the war. T.C. Douglas himself stated that his father suffered from "serious complications from having been gassed overseas" (Douglas, *Making of a Socialist*, 40).
29 T.C. Douglas memoirs interview with Stursberg, 20.
30 According to Thomas Douglas's war record, T.C.'s father was finally demobilized on 20 May 1919, the day after he was released from No. 12 Canadian General Hospital. His file notes that he arrived in Winnipeg on 2 June 1919.
31 Uduak Idiong, "Third Force: Returned Soldiers in the Winnipeg General Strike of 1919," *Manitoba History*, no. 34 (Fall 1997): 15–22.
32 Reinhold Kramer and Tom Mitchell, *When the State Trembled: How A.J. Andrews and the Citizen's Committee Broke the Winnipeg General Strike* (Toronto: University of Toronto Press, 2010), 184–99.

33 Reinhold Kramer and Tom Mitchell, "'Daniel deLeon Drew up the Diagram': Winnipeg's Seditious-Conspiracy Trials of 1919–20," in *Canadian State Trials*, vol. 4: *Security, Dissent, and the Limits of Toleration in War and Peace, 1914–1939*, ed. Barry Wright, Eric Tucker, and Susan Binns (Toronto: University of Toronto Press for the Osgood Society for Canadian Legal History, 2015), 233–5; Douglas, *Making of a Socialist*, 30.
34 *DCB* Douglas entry.
35 Douglas, *Making of a Socialist*, 20.
36 McLeod and McLeod, *Tommy Douglas*, 6–10. On the Labour Party, see Andrew Thorpe, *A History of the British Labour Party* (Basingstoke, UK: Palgrave Macmillan, 2008).
37 Kenneth O. Morgan, *Keir Hardie: Radical and Socialist* (London: Weidenfeld & Nicolson, 1975).
38 Kenneth O. Morgan, *Kenneth O. Morgan: My Histories* (Cardiff: University of Wales Press, 2015), 89–90.
39 McLeod and McLeod, *Tommy Douglas*, 16, 14.
40 McLeod and McLeod, *Tommy Douglas*, 16.
41 Douglas, *Making of a Socialist*, 33–4.
42 *DCB* Douglas entry.
43 Sandra Beardsall, "'One Here Will Constant Be': The Christian Witness of T.C. 'Tommy' Douglas," in *Baptists and Public Life in Canada*, ed. Gordon L. Heath and Paul R. Wilson (Hamilton: McMaster Divinity College Press, 2012), 147.
44 Beardsall, "'One Here Will Constant Be,'" 146–7.
45 Beardsall, "'One Here Will Constant Be,'" 148.
46 Douglas, *Making of a Socialist*, 39; Beardsall, "'One Here Will Constant Be,'" 149.
47 T.C. Douglas memoirs interview with Stursberg, 23–4. For T.C., DoMolay was a lifelong association. In 1970, T.C. was the keynote speaker at the all-Canada conclave of DeMolay Association in Winnipeg. LAC, Thomas Clement Douglas fonds, MG 32 C 28, vol. 91, file 8, letter, Bill Agerbak and Ron Collett (Manitoba DeMolay Association) to T.C. Douglas, 1 June 1970.
48 On Mark Talnicoff (later Talney) and his relationship with Douglas, see Houston and Waiser, *Tommy's Team*, 97–103.
49 T.C. Douglas memoirs interview with Stursberg, 27.
50 T.C. Douglas memoirs interview with Stursberg, 23.
51 Oussoren, *Baptist Preacher*, 16.
52 Douglas, *Making of a Socialist*, 51.
53 Oussoren, *Baptist Preacher*, 15.
54 Houston and Waiser, *Tommy's Team*, 84.

55 Susan Mann Trofimenkoff, *Stanley Knowles: The Man from Winnipeg North Centre* (Saskatoon: Western Producer Prairie Books, 1982), 11–20, 185.
56 Houston and Waiser, *Tommy's Team*, 82.
57 Doris French Shackleton, *Tommy Douglas: A Biography* (Toronto: McClelland & Steward, 1975), 31–2.
58 Lam, *Tommy Douglas*, 14. In his biography, which is part of John Raulston Saul's series "Extraordinary Canadians," Lam uses the phrase "practical Christian" as the theme animating Douglas's life from 1904 until 1924.
59 Douglas, quoted in Shackleton, *Tommy Douglas*, 32.
60 Houston and Waiser, *Tommy's Team*, 37.
61 Douglas, *Making of a Socialist*, 50.
62 Houston and Waiser, *Tommy's Team*, 37; Douglas, *Making of a Socialist*, 46.
63 Houston and Waiser, *Tommy's Team*, 37.
64 Mark Talnicoff came from a Jewish-Russian family that had left Odessa to escape the 1905 pogrom – the most extreme of its type in the Russian Empire. How he became a Baptist is not explained by Houston and Waiver (*Tommy's Team*, 197–203). In 1940, Mark and Nan left for the United States, where he anglicized his name from Talnicoff to Talney; he died in Portland, Oregon, in 1992. Robert Weinberg, "The Pogrom of 1905 in Odessa: A Case Study," in *Pogroms: Anti-Jewish Violence in Modern Russian History*, ed. John D. Klier and Shlomo Lambroza (Cambridge: Cambridge University Press, 1992), 248–89.
65 Eleanor J. Stebner, "The Education of Stanley Howard Knowles," *Manitoba History*, no. 36 (1998): 48.
66 LAC, Stanley H. Knowles fonds, MG 32 C59, vol. 525, file 505, letter, Stanley Knowles to Ronald J. Wormsbecker (chair, T.C. Douglas Calvary Centre, Weyburn), 1 February 1988.
67 Douglas, quoted in Margoshes, *Tommy Douglas*, 37.
68 Irma Douglas, quoted in Shackleton, *Tommy Douglas*, 49.
69 Douglas, *Making of a Socialist*, 54.
70 Oussoren, *Baptist Preacher*, 22–3.
71 Gregory P. Marchildon, "The Great Divide," in *The Heavy Hand of History: Interpreting Saskatchewan's Past*, ed. Marchildon (Regina: Canadian Plains Research Center, University of Regina, 2005), 56.
72 Gregory P. Marchildon, "War, Revolution and the Great Depression in the Global Wheat Trade, 1917–39," in *A Global History of Trade and Conflict since 1500*, ed. Lucia Coppolaro and Francine McKenzie (London: Palgrave Macmillan, 2013), 148–53.
73 Bill Waiser, *Saskatchewan: A New History* (Calgary: Fifth House, 2005), 282.
74 Waiser, *Saskatchewan*, 122–31.
75 Census population, 1931, for the three largest cities in Saskatchewan: Regina (53,209), Saskatoon (43,291), and Moose Jaw (21,209), Statistics

Canada table, https://www65.statcan.gc.ca/acyb02/1937/acyb02_19370191033-eng.htm; Waiser, *Saskatchewan*, 285.
76 Robert Bothwell, John English, and Ian M. Drummond, *Canada, 1900–1945* (Toronto: University of Toronto Press, 1987), 253–5.
77 Robert A. McLeman et al., "What We Learned from the Dust Bowl: Lessons in Science, Policy, and Adaptation," *Population and Environment* 35, no. 4 (2014): 417–40.
78 Gregory P. Marchildon, Jeremy Pittman, and David J. Sauchyn, "The Dry Belt and Changing Aridity in the Palliser Triangle, 1895–2000," in *Drought and Depression: History of the Prairie West*, vol. 6, ed. Gregory P. Marchildon (Regina: University of Regina Press, 2018), 15–23; Gregory P. Marchildon, Suren Kulshreshtha, Elaine Wheaton, and David J. Sauchyn, "Drought and Institutional Adaptation in Alberta and Saskatchewan, 1914–1939," *Natural Hazards* 45, no. 3 (2008): 391–411.
79 John G. Diefenbaker, *One Canada: Memoirs of the Right Honourable John G. Diefenbaker*, vol. 1: *The Crusading Years, 1895–1956* (Toronto: Macmillan of Canada, 1975), 170.
80 "Monday's Dust Storm Causes Havoc in City," 28 May 1931, 1; "Weyburn Again in Grip of Dust Storm," 18 June 1931, 1; and "Heat Wave Aftermath Further Menace to Parched Crops in Southern Part of Province," 18 June 1931, 1, all in the *Weyburn Review*.
81 "Weyburn Farmers Petition Government for Relief," *Weyburn Review*, 30 July 1931, 1; "Weyburn Rural Council Copes with Relief Problem Facing the Farmers," *Weyburn Review*, 6 Aug. 1931, 1.
82 See Gregory P. Marchildon and Don Black, "Henry Black, the Conservative Party and the Politics of Relief," *Saskatchewan History* 58, no. 1 (2006): 4–17, and Blair Neatby, "The Saskatchewan Relief Commission, 1931–34," in *Historical Essays on the Prairie Provinces*, ed. Donald Swainson (Montreal and Kingston: McGill-Queen's University Press, 1978), 54. On 27 August 1931, almost the entire front page of the *Weyburn Review* was devoted to relief efforts, including a headline about the Saskatchewan government's imminent announcement of a provincial relief policy.
83 Waiser, *Saskatchewan*, 297.
84 Douglas, *Making of a Socialist*, 56–9; McLeod and McLeod, *Tommy Douglas*, 42. According to T.H. McLeod, out of that small group of boys "came three United Church ministers, two university teachers, one university registrar and business manager, which, out of a small group in a small town, wasn't a bade take" and a "great deal of it was due to Tommy" – Provincial Archives of Saskatchewan (PAS), Jean Larmour oral history of CCF government, R8444 to R8448, transcript of interview with T.H. McLeod, 25 Nov. 1981 (hereafter Larmour interview with T.H. McLeod), 1–2.
85 Larmour interview with T.H. McLeod, 1–5.

86 T.C. Douglas, "The Highlights of the Dirty Thirties," in *The Dirty Thirties in Prairie Canada: 11th Western Canada Studies Conference*, ed. R.D. Francis and H. Ganzevoort (Vancouver: Tantalus Research, 1980), 163.
87 "Churches – Calvary Baptist Church," *Weyburn Review*, 27 Nov. 1930, 4.
88 "Churches – Calvary Baptist Church," *Weyburn Review*, 14 May 1931, 4.
89 Oussoren, *Baptist Preacher*, 30–5. The author of numerous books and articles on social justice, Arthur E. Holt wrote in 1920 that social justice was the essential foundation for both Christian faith and a trusting community here on Earth: "Social Justice and the Present Duty of the Church," *Biblical World* 54, no. 2 (1920): 136–9.
90 Oussoren, *Baptist Preacher*, 38–41.
91 Douglas, *Making of a Socialist*, 65.
92 Stephen Endicott, *Bienfait: The Saskatchewan's Miners' Struggle of 1931* (Toronto: University of Toronto Press, 2002), 103.
93 University of Saskatchewan Archives and Special Collections (USAS), Charles and Sophia Dixon fonds, MG 224, report entitled "What about the Estevan Coal Strike?" by a Baptist minister to A.J. Macauley, president of the United Farmers of Canada (Sask. Section), 25 September 1931. Although Douglas is not named as the Baptist minister in the report, it was almost certainly Douglas who wrote the report, as there is no evidence of any other Baptist minister who visited the strikers.
94 "Churches – Calvary Baptist Church," *Weyburn Review*, 24 Sept. 1931, 4.
95 Endicott, *Bienfait*, 74–5.
96 *Weyburn Review*, 22 Oct. 1931, 8; Oussoren, *Baptist Preacher*, 57.
97 Douglas, *Making of a Socialist*, 69.
98 Steve Hewitt, "September 1931: A Re-interpretation of the Royal Canadian Mounted Police's Handling of the 1931 Estevan Strike and Riot," *Labour/Le Travail* 39 (1997): 159–78.
99 McLeod and McLeod, *Tommy Douglas*, 36.
100 Douglas, "Highlights of the Dirty Thirties," 167.
101 *Weyburn Review*, 24 Sept. 1931, as quoted in McLeod and McLeod, *Tommy Douglas*, 36.
102 McLeod and McLeod, *Tommy Douglas*, 36. On Macphail, see Terry Crowley, *Agnes Macphail and the Politics of Equality* (Toronto: Lorimer, 1990); on Williams, see J.F. Conway, *The Prairie Populist: George Hara Williams and the Untold Story of the CCF* (Regina: University of Regina Press, 2018).
103 Douglas, *Making of a Socialist*, 70.
104 Douglas, *Making of a Socialist*, 70.
105 Walter Stewart, *M.J.: The Life and Times of M.J. Coldwell* (Toronto: Stoddard, 2000), 95; McLeod and McLeod, *Tommy Douglas*, 35–7.
106 Walter D. Young, *The Anatomy of a Party: The National CCF, 1932–61* (Toronto: University of Toronto Press, 1969), 21.

107 Kenneth McNaught, *A Prophet in Politics: A Biography of J.S. Woodsworth* (Toronto: University of Toronto Press, 2001), 259–60.
108 George Hoffman has covered the early history of the Farmer-Labor Group in a trilogy of articles: "The Saskatchewan Farmer-Labour Party, 1932–1932: How Radical Was Its Origin?" *Saskatchewan History* 28, no. 2 (1975): 52–64; "The Entry of the United Farmers of Canada Saskatchewan Section into Politics: A Reassessment," *Saskatchewan History* 30, no. 3 (1977): 99–109; and "Frank Eliason: A Forgotten Founder of the CCF," *Saskatchewan History* 58, no. 1 (2006): 18–31.
109 Young, *Anatomy of a Party*, 41 and 303–4.
110 Douglas, quoted in McLeod and McLeod, *Tommy Douglas*, 47. Other names were suggested by attendees at the one-day Calgary meeting, including by M.J. Coldwell (the organizer of the Saskatchewan delegation), who put forward "The Social Democratic Party" as his preferred name: see Stewart, *M.J. Coldwell*, 99.
111 PAS, CCF fonds, II, file 235, item 23182, letter, Frank Eliason to members of the Political Directive Board of the Saskatchewan Farmer-Labor Group, 12 July 1933.
112 "Coldwell Will Address Labor Rally on Monday," *Weyburn Review*, 1 Sept. 1932, 1; "Coldwell and Douglas Speak at Labor Meet: Provincial Farmer-Labor Leader Says No Hope for Farmer or Laboring Man under Present Economic System," *Weyburn Review*, 8 Sept. 1932, 1. Since the event took place during the harvest, only 200 people attended. "Throughout the Province," *Regina Leader-Post* (*LP*), 3 Sept. 1932, 3.
113 C.M. Fines, "The Impossible Dream: An Account of People and Events Leading to the First CCF Government, Saskatchewan, 1944" (unpublished manuscript, Trinity College, Toronto, 1982), 1: 114.
114 Established by the Baptist Union of Western College, Brandon College (chartered as a university in 1967) was affiliated with McMaster University (itself founded as Toronto Baptist College in 1881) between 1911 and 1938. See Charles M. Johnston, *McMaster University: The Toronto Years*, vol. 1 (Toronto: University of Toronto Press, 1976), and Charles G. Stone and F. Joan Garnett, *Brandon College: A History, 1899–1967* (Brandon: Brandon University, 1969).
115 See Erika Dyck and Alexander Deighton, *Managing Madness: Weyburn Mental Hospital and the Transformation of Psychiatric Care in Canada* (Winnipeg: University of Manitoba Press, 2017), 98–103, and Gregory P. Marchildon, "A House Divided: Deinstitutionalization, Medicare and the Canadian Mental Health Association in Saskatchewan, 1944–1964," *Histoire sociale / Social History* 44, no. 88 (2011): 305–29.
116 T.C. Douglas, "The Problems of the Subnormal Family" (MA thesis, McMaster University, 1933).

117 David Chariandy, "Canadians of Tomorrow: J.S. Woodsworth and the New Ethnicities," in *Human Welfare, Rights, and Social Activism: Rethinking the Legacy of J.S. Woodsworth*, ed. Jane Pulkingham (Toronto: University of Toronto Press, 2016), 266–86. In her book *Facing Eugenics: Reproduction, Sterilization, and the Politics of Choice* (Toronto: University of Toronto Press, 2013), Erika Dyck reviews Douglas's thesis in the context of the dominant views of the day and concludes that, while it reflected the "reformist view on the issue as it was understood in Canada at the time," his thesis nonetheless "favoured a more empowering outcome" than the general left-wing reformist views of the day (39), through his emphasis on the "integration and acceptance" (38) of "subnormal" families within society. On the broader context of such views during the interwar years, also see Alex Deighton, "The Nature of Eugenic Thought and Limits of Eugenic Practice in Interwar Saskatchewan," in *Eugenics at the Edges of Empire: New Zealand, Australia, Canada, and South Africa*, ed. Diane B. Paul, John Stenhouse, and Hamish G. Spencer (Cham, CH: Palgrave Macmillan, 2018), 63–84.
118 See Angus McLaren, *Our Own Master Race: Eugenics in Canada, 1885–1945* (Toronto: McClelland & Stewart, 1990), 9; Jana Grekul, Arvey Krahn and Dave Odynak, "Sterilizing the 'Feeble-Minded': Eugenics in Alberta, Canada, 1929–1972," *Journal of Historical Sociology* 17, no. 4 (2004): 358–84.
119 This evidence is repeated by Michael Shevall in "A Canadian Paradox: T.C. Douglas and Eugenics," *Canadian Journal of Neurological Sciences* 39, no. 1 (2012): 38, but Shevall's argument, popularized in the *National Post*, that his earlier advocacy of eugenics has been airbrushed out by his biographers was not accurate (see, for example, McLeod and McLeod, *Tommy Douglas*, 39–41). See Michael Shevell "Tommy Douglas, the Young Eugenicist," *National Post*, 24 March 2012, https://nationalpost.com/opinion/michael-shevell-tommy-douglas-the-young-eugenicist
120 Douglas, "Problems of the Subnormal Family," 28–9.
121 Douglas, "Problems of the Subnormal Family," 30.
122 Douglas, "Problems of the Subnormal Family," 34.
123 Douglas, quoted in the *Weyburn Review*, 27 July 1932; see McLeod and McLeod, *Tommy Douglas*, 48.
124 Michiel Horn, "Frank Underhill's Early Drafts of the Regina Manifesto 1933," *Canadian Historical Review* 54, no. 4 (1973): 398. Also see Michiel Horn, "The LSR, the CCF, and the Regina Manifesto," in *Building the Co-operative Commonwealth: Essays on the Democratic Socialist Tradition in Canada*, ed. J. William Brennan (Regina: Canadian Plains Research Center, University of Regina, 1985), 25–41.
125 T.C. Douglas memoirs interview with Stursberg, 50–1.
126 Young, *Anatomy of a Party*, 313.

127 Young, *Anatomy of a Party*, appendix A, Regina Manifesto, 304–13.
128 Fines, "The Impossible Dream," 1: 133.
129 Young, *Anatomy of a Party*, 309–10.
130 McLeod and McLeod, *Tommy Douglas*, 48.
131 The official designation on the party's letterhead was "Saskatchewan Farmer-Labor Group (C.C.F.)." There was a movement to shorten up the name to simply the CCF before the 1934 election: "Farmer-Labor Party Changed," *LP*, 26 June 1933, 5.
132 McLeod and McLeod, *Tommy Douglas*, 49.
133 "Douglas Named for Weyburn," *LP*, 6 Nov. 1933, 8.
134 Stewart, *M.J. Coldwell*, 88, 94–5.
135 McLeod and McLeod, *LP*, *Douglas*, 50; Fines, "The Impossible Dream," 1: 149–50.
136 "Douglas Is Choice of Weyburn Farmer-Labor Party," *Weyburn Review*, 9 Nov. 1933, 1, 4; Oussoren, *Baptist Preacher*, 74.
137 Fines, "The Impossible Dream," 1: 149–50.
138 "Farmer-Labor Man Speaker Tuesday Night," *LP*, 25 Nov. 1933, 3; "Farmer-Labor Man Speaker," *LP*, 5 March 1934, 2; "Douglas Stuart Speakers," *LP*, 9 March 1934, 33; "Douglas Speaker," *LP*, 16 April 1934, 3. In the 1931 census, Regina had a population of 53,209 people compared to Saskatoon's population of 43,291: *Canada Year Book, 1937*, https://www65.statcan.gc.ca/acyb02/1937/acyb02_19370191033-eng.htm.
139 "Farmer-Labor Land Policy Address Theme," *LP*, 20 March 1934, 9.
140 T.C. Douglas memoirs interview with Stursberg, 53–5.
141 John Manley, "'Communists Love Canada!' The Communist Party of Canada, the 'People' and the Popular Front, 1933–1939," *Journal of Canadian Studies* 36, no. 4 (2002): 59–86.
142 Nelson Wiseman, "Ethnicity, Religion, and Socialism in Canada: The Twenties through the War," *Canadian Ethnic Studies* 47, no. 2 (2015): 2.
143 "Pastor Invites Kerr to Debate," *LP*, 24 April 1934, 3.
144 As quoted in George Hoffman, "The 1934 Saskatchewan Provincial Election Campaign," *Saskatchewan History* 36, no. 2 (1983): 49. On the influence of the Ku Klux Klan in Saskatchewan, see Patrick Kyba, "Ballots and Burning Crosses," in *Politics in Saskatchewan*, ed. Norman Ward and Duff Spafford (Toronto: Longmans Canada, 1968), 105–23, and James M. Pitsula, *Keeping Canada British: The Ku Klux Klan in 1920s Saskatchewan* (Vancouver: UBC Press, 2013).
145 See the letters to the editor section in *LP*: 3 May 1934, 4; 7 May 1934, 4; and 15 May 1934.
146 Saskatchewan Farmer-Labor Group, *Handbook for Speakers: Compiled from Reports of Conferences held in Saskatoon and Regina, January 7 and February 11 Respectively, 1933* (Saskatoon: Farmer-Labor Group, 1933), 15.

147 On Gardiner's political acumen, see Norman Ward and David E. Smith, *Jimmy Gardiner: Relentless Liberal* (Toronto: University of Toronto Press, 1990), and David E. Smith, "James G. Gardiner," in *Saskatchewan Premiers of the Twentieth Century*, ed. Gordon L. Barnhart (Regina: Canadian Plains Research Center, 2004), 93–103. In his own account (*Making of a Socialist*, 76), Douglas veers between saying he had a good chance to win the seat as part of a general Farmer-Labour victory over the two establishment parties and admitting he had no chance at all against Dr. Eaglesham, given the fact that he "was a very fine old family doctor who had brought half the people in our community into the world" (79).
148 McLeod and McLeod, *Tommy Douglas*, 55.
149 Patrick Kyba, "J.T.M. Anderson," in *Saskatchewan Premiers of the Twentieth Century*, ed. Gordon L. Barnhart (Regina: Canadian Plains Research Center, 2004), 129–34.
150 Neatby, "The Saskatchewan Relief Commission," 4–17.
151 T.C. quoted in T.C. Douglas memoirs interview with Stursberg, 58.
152 Kyba, "J.T.M. Anderson." On the history of the Conservative Party in Saskatchewan (rebranded as "Progressive Conservative" in 1942), see Dick Spencer, *Singing the Blues: The Conservatives in Saskatchewan* (Regina: Canadian Plains Research Center, 2007).
153 Conway, *Prairie Populist*, 101–19.
154 PAS, CCF fonds, II, file 235, letter, W.D. Summers to members of the Political Directive Board of the Saskatchewan Farmer Labor Group (CCF), 25 April 1934 (item 27813), and 29 June 1934 (item 23184-5).
155 Hoffman, "The 1934 Saskatchewan Provincial Election Campaign," 51–2. Peter R. Sinclair, "The Saskatchewan CCF: Ascent to Power and the Decline of Socialism," *Canadian Historical Review* 54, no. 4 (1973): 419–33.
156 PAS, T.C. Douglas fonds, R-33.2, III, 37(1-5-3), letter, J.G. Gardiner to Rev. Peter Strang, 11 April 1934.
157 James Naylor, "Socialism for a New Generation: CCF Youth in the Popular Front Era," *Canadian Historical Review* 94, no. 1 (2013): 56–67.
158 I have relied on the account provided by McLeod and McLeod, *Tommy Douglas*, 57. Doris French Shackleton also provides an unreferenced one-paragraph account in *Tommy Douglas*, 78. McNaught, *A Prophet in Politics*, 282n1.
159 Douglas, quoted in McLeod and McLeod, *Tommy Douglas*, 57.
160 Naylor, "CCF Youth," 65. For the United States, see Paul C. Mishler, *Raising Reds: The Young Pioneers, Radical Summer Camps, and Communist Political Culture in the United States* (New York: Columbia University Press, 1999).
161 PAS, CCF (Sask. Section) fonds, B7, II-195 – National Office, 1935–1936, Minutes of National Council Meeting of the CCF, Winnipeg, 30 Nov.–1

Dec. 1935, 6, where Jack King, national secretary of the CCYM, defended the support of the organization on the grounds that the Saskatchewan branch members all belonged to the League Against War and Fascism.

162 Naylor, "CCF Youth," 68; PAS, CCF (Sask. Section) fonds, B7, II-195 – National Office, 1935–1936, Minutes of National Council Meeting of the CCF, Winnipeg, 30 Nov.–1 Dec. 1935.

163 PAS, John (Jack) Gregory King fonds, F44, file 23 – CCYM – Sask. Section, A.A. MacLeod's letter to the membership of the Canadian League Against War and Fascism (on league letterhead highlighting T.C.'s position in the organization), 8 March 1938.

164 T.C. Douglas memoirs interview with Stursberg, 53–4.

## 3. Federal Member of Parliament, 1935–1944

1 T.C. Douglas, *The Making of a Socialist: The Recollections of T.C. Douglas*, ed. Lewis H. Thomas (Edmonton: University of Alberta Press, 1982), 79; Library and Archives Canada (LAC), Peter Stursberg fonds, MG 31 D78, vol. 33, file 19, transcript of T.C. Douglas memoirs interview with Peter Stursberg, Ottawa (hereafter T.C. Douglas memoirs interview with Stursberg), 29 April 1980, 60.
2 Douglas, *Making of a Socialist*, 80.
3 Douglas, *Making of a Socialist*, 80–1.
4 Roy J. Romanow interview with author, 19 March 2003.
5 Douglas, *Making of a Socialist*, 60–1.
6 Douglas, *Making of a Socialist*, 81.
7 I would date his first major entrée into politics as his organizing of a Labour Day rally in Weyburn, in which he, along with M.J. Coldwell, spoke on behalf of the Independent Labor Party, including Douglas's Weyburn chapter of the ILP – the Weyburn Independent Labor Party. "Throughout the Province," *Regina Leader-Post* (*LP*), 5 Sept. 1932, 3.
8 Desmond Morton's filmed interview with T.C. Douglas, 26 Feb. 1975, University of Toronto Archives, Desmond Morton fonds, B1999-0023.
9 Provincial Archives of Saskatchewan (PAS), Jean Larmour oral history of the CCF government, interview with T.C. Douglas, R-8353.1-2, 15 June 1981, transcript, 10.
10 James Struthers, *No Fault of Their Own: Unemployment and the Canadian Welfare State, 1914–1941* (Toronto: University of Toronto Press, 1983), ch. 3; Lorne Brown, "Unemployed Struggles in Saskatchewan and Canada, 1930–1935," in *Drought and Depression: History of the Prairie West Series*, vol. 6, ed. Gregory P. Marchildon (Regina: University of Regina Press, 2018), 123–6.
11 "Meetings, Radio to Gain Regina Sympathy Planned by Strikers," *LP*, 13 June 1935, 2.

12 Bill Waiser, *All Hell Can't Stop Us: The On-to-Ottawa Trek and Regina Riot* (Calgary: Fifth House, 2003).
13 Douglas, quoted in Bill Waiser, "Wiping Out the Stain: The On-to-Ottawa Trek, the Regina Riot, and the Search for Answers," in *Canadian State Trials*, vol. 4: *Security, Dissent, and the Limits of Toleration in War and Peace, 1914–1939*, ed. Barry Wright, Eric Tucker, and Susan Binnie (Toronto: University of Toronto Press for the Osgood Society for Canadian Legal History, 2015), 429.
14 Tommy Douglas, "The Highlights of the Dirty Thirties," in *The Dirty Thirties in Prairie Canada: 11th Western Canada Studies Conference*, ed. R.D. Francis and H. Ganzevoort (Vancouver: Tantalus Research, 1980), 169.
15 "Meetings, Radio to Gain Regina Sympathy Planned by Strikers," *LP*, 13 June 1935, 2. The number of organizations within the Citizens' Emergency Committee would eventually reach thirty-one. See J. William Brennan, "From 'Honest Connie' to 'Rockpile Rink': The Political Rise and Fall of Cornelius Rink in 1930s Regina," *Urban History Review / Revue d'histoire urbaine* 40, no. 2 (2012): 43n70.
16 See Brennan, "From 'Honest Connie' to 'Rockpile Rink,'" 36–8; C.M. Fines, "The Impossible Dream: An Account of People and Events Leading to the First CCF Government, Saskatchewan, 1944" (unpublished manuscript, Trinity College, Toronto, 1982), 1: 173–91.
17 Waiser, *All Hell Can't Stop Us*, 125.
18 University of Saskatchewan Archives and Special Collections (USAS), Sophia Dixon fonds, MG 224, series 1, box 4, file – Citizen's Defence Movement, letter, Jack C. King (National Office of Citizen's Defence Movement) to all supporters, 21 Feb. 1936.
19 "Meetings, Radio to Gain Regina Sympathy Planned by Strikers," *LP*, 13 June 1935, 2.
20 Waiser, *All Hell Can't Stop Us*, 105.
21 This number was based on the number of registered trekkers who left Regina four days after the riot: "Relief Camp Strikers Come from Every Point," *LP*, 5 July 1935, 3.
22 Fines, "The Impossible Dream," 189. Fines describes the Regina Riot in telling detail. Although he does not say explicitly that he witnessed the Regina Riot, as one of the chief city officials supporting the trekkers, he may have seen at least some of the riot.
23 "C.C.F. Names MacLean for Regina Fight," *LP*, 26 June 1935, 1.
24 T.C. Douglas memoirs interview with Stursberg, 72; Waiser, "Wiping out the Stain," 429; Robert A. Wardhaugh, *Mackenzie King and the Prairie West* (Toronto: University of Toronto Press, 2000), 186.
25 McLeod and McLeod, *Tommy Douglas*, 146–7.
26 "Meetings, Radio to Gain Regina Sympathy Planned by Strikers," *LP*, 13 June 1935, 2.

27 "Officer Hurt in Riot Makes Good Progress," *LP*, 23 July 1935, 3.
28 *LP*, 10 June 1935, 3 (notice of Dr. MacLean speaking at Scott Collegiate on "State Health Services").
29 Douglas, *Making of a Socialist*, 326.
30 Waiser, *All Hell Can't Stop Us*, 243.
31 PAS, John (Jack) Gregory King fonds, F44, file 13 – Citizen's Legal Defence Committee, Aug. 1935–June 1936. Waiser, *All Hell Can't Stop Us*, 262.
32 PAS, John (Jack) Gregory King fonds, F44, file 20 – Parliamentary contacts: letter, M.J. Coldwell to Arthur Evans (Citizens Defence Committee), 20 Feb. 1936; M.J. Coldwell to J.G. King, 8 May 1936; T.C. Douglas to J.G. King, 11 and 18 May 1936; 2 and 9 June 1936. Jack King (1909–44) moved in 1947 from Regina to Toronto, where he worked with the Canadian League Against War and Fascism and served as secretary of the Canadian Committee to Aid Spanish Democracy (and may have been a member of the Mackenzie-Papineau Battalion in the Spanish Civil War). From 1939 until 1941, he was the business manager of the leftist labour newspaper the *Canadian Tribune*, which was edited by A.A. MacLeod, a prominent member of the CPC. He joined the Royal Canadian Air Force in 1942 and was posted overseas in 1943. On 13 August 1944, he was killed at the Kolar Airfield near Mysor, India. This information was obtained in the biographical sketch in the PAS finding aid for the John (Jack) Gregory Kind fonds, SAFA 68.
33 "Eight Hundred at C.C.F. Gathering," *LP*, 10 July 1935, 13.
34 McLeod and McLeod, *Tommy Douglas*, 36–7.
35 T.C. Douglas memoirs interview with Stursberg, 60–2.
36 "Candidate to Be Chosen by Weyburn C.C.F.," *LP*, 15 June 1935, 15.
37 McLeod and McLeod, *Tommy Douglas*, 59.
38 Robert Bothwell, John English, and Ian M. Drummond, *Canada, 1900–1945* (Toronto: University of Toronto Press, 1987), 256.
39 John Ibbitson, *The Duel: Diefenbaker, Pearson, and the Making of Modern Canada* (Toronto: Signal, 2023), 71. In Saskatchewan, when a four-wheeled Bennett buggy was converted into a more compact two-wheel vehicle, it was sometimes referred to as an Anderson cart, named after Premier J.T.M. Anderson, the leader of the Co-operative government, a one-term coalition administration (1929–34) that united Conservatives with Progressives. Dale Johnson, "Bennett Buggies a Prairie Hallmark in the '30s," *LP*, 23 May 2014, AA2.
40 Larry A. Glassford, *Reaction and Reform: The Politics of the Conservative Party under R.B. Bennett, 1927–1938* (Toronto: University of Toronto Press, 1992), 142–66. On the dramatic change in Bennett's agricultural policies, see Gregory P. Marchildon, "The Prairie Farm Rehabilitation Administration: Climate Crisis and Federal-Provincial Relations during the Great Depression," *Canadian Historical Review* 90, no. 2 (2009): 283–91,

and Gregory P. Marchildon and Carl Anderson, "Robert Weir: Forgotten Farmer-Minister in R.B. Bennett's Depression-Era Cabinet," in *Drought and Depression: History of the Prairie West*, vol. 6, ed. Gregory P. Marchildon (Regina: University of Regina Press, 2018), 277–83.
41 Glassford, *Reaction and Reform*, 170–96.
42 Bill Waiser, *Saskatchewan: A New History* (Calgary: Fifth House, 2005), 315.
43 Wardhaugh, *Mackenzie King*, 176.
44 Marchildon, "The Prairie Farm Rehabilitation Administration," 277–82; Gregory P. Marchildon, "War, Revolution and the Great Depression in the Global Wheat Trade, 1917–39," in *A Global History of Trade and Conflict Since 1500*, ed. Lucia Coppolaro and Francine McKenzie (London: Palgrave Macmillan, 2013), 147–58.
45 Douglas, *Making of a Socialist*, 78,
46 "Dr. MacLean's Nomination," *LP*, 27 June 1935, 4.
47 Michiel Horn, *The League for Social Reconstruction: Intellectual Origins of the Democratic Left in Canada, 1930–1942* (Toronto: University of Toronto Press, 1980), 73.
48 T.C. Douglas memoirs interview with Stursberg, 51.
49 League for Social Reconstruction, *Social Planning for Canada*, ed. Michael Bliss (1935; Toronto: University of Toronto Press, 1975), 394.
50 League for Social Reconstruction, *Social Planning for Canada*, 396.
51 League for Social Reconstruction, *Social Planning for Canada*, 395–8.
52 McLeod and McLeod, *Tommy Douglas*, 63.
53 Alan Whitehorn, *Canadian Socialism: Essays on the CCF-NDP* (Toronto: Oxford University Press, 1991), 72.
54 USAS, Sophia Dixon fonds, MG 224, series 1, box 6, file – CCF Pamphlets, *Canada through C.C.F. Glasses* (Vancouver: Commonwealth Press, 1934), by Grace MacInnis and Charles J. Woodsworth (the daughter and son of J.S. Woodsworth).
55 *LP*, advertisement for Douglas and MacLean speaking together in Regina, 11 Oct. 1935, 2; "Political Items," *LP*, 9 Sept. 1935, 15.
56 McLeod and McLeod, *Tommy Douglas*, 63–4.
57 Douglas, quoted in McLeod and McLeod, *Tommy Douglas*, 64.
58 Douglas, quoted in McLeod and McLeod, *Tommy Douglas*, 64, based on a taped interview with A.M. (Sandy) Nicholson, 11 Feb. 1975.
59 Alvin Finkel, "Obscure Origins: The Confused Early History of the CCF in Alberta," in *Building the Co-operative Commonwealth: Essays on the Democratic Socialist Tradition in Canada*, ed. J. William Brennan (Regina: Canadian Plains Research Center, University of Regina, 1985), 102–9; Alvin Finkel, *The Social Credit Phenomenon in Alberta* (Toronto: University of Toronto Press, 1989), 22–6.
60 On the Social Credits entry into Saskatchewan in the 1935 election and the party's strategic arrangements with six CCF candidates, see Ken

Andrews, "'Progressive' Counterparts of the CCF: Social Credit and the Conservative Party in Saskatchewan, 1935–193," *Journal of Canadian Studies* 17, no. 3 (1982): 59–62.
61 The literature on the origins of Social Credit in Alberta and Canada is rich, but the main works include C.B. Macpherson, *Democracy in Alberta: Social Credit and the Party System* (1953; Toronto: University of Toronto Press, 2013); Finkel, *The Social Credit Phenomenon*; and Edward Bell, *Social Classes and Social Credit in Alberta* (Montreal and Kingston: McGill-Queen's University Press, 1993).
62 Andrews, "'Progressive' Counterparts of the CCF," 59–61.
63 As quoted in McLeod and McLeod, *Tommy Douglas*, 61; "Nomination," *LP*, 1 Oct. 1935, 2.
64 Douglas, *Making of a Socialist*, 87–9; "Two Remain with Double Nomination," *LP*, 1 Oct. 1935, 1–2; "C.C.F. in Two Ridings Stick to Nominees," *LP*, 2 Oct. 1935, 1; "Executives Stick by Own Candidates," *LP*, 3 Oct. 1935, 7;"Executives Stick by Own Candidates," *Saskatoon Star Phoenix*, 3 Oct. 1935, 7.
65 "Douglas Case to Be Studied by Executive," *LP*, 9 Oct. 1935; "Party's Action on T. Douglas Still Pending," *LP*, 10 Oct. 1935, 1, 4; Douglas, *Making of a Socialist*, 89; John C. Conway, *The Prairie Populist: George Hara Williams and the Untold Story of the CCF* (Regina: University of Regina Press, 2018), 136–7.
66 Just before he died in 1921, the three newspapers constituted Sir Clifford Sifton's principal business interests. After his death, Sir Clifford's youngest son, Victor Sifton, took ownership control of the Sifton newspapers. D.J. Hall, *Clifford Sifton*, vol. 2: *The Lonely Eminence, 1901–1929* (Vancouver: UBC Press, 1985), 320–6.
67 Resolution quoted in "Douglas Says Not Running on 2 Tickets," *LP*, 10 Oct. 1935, 8.
68 Andrews, "'Progressive' Counterparts of the CCF," 61. Andrews names the other candidate (72n18). They included Douglas's friend Dr. Hugh MacLean as well as Jake Benson, the other CCF candidate accused of going further than accepting the endorsement of Social Credit.
69 "King's Party Wins 166 Seats – Young, Weyburn Liberal, Loses," *LP*, 15 Oct. 1935, 1.
70 "Weyburn Swings C.C.F.; Coldwell Also Wins Seat," *LP*, 15 Oct. 1936, 3.
71 Andrews, "'Progressive' Counterparts of the CCF," 60.
72 "King's Party Wins 166 Seats – Young, Weyburn Liberal, Loses," *LP*, 15 Oct. 1935, 1.
73 McLeod and McLeod, *Tommy Douglas*, 66.
74 PAS, CCF fonds, II, file 128, letters: George Williams to M.J. Coldwell, 4 Oct. 1935, and Jack G. King to G.H. Williams, 4 Nov. 1935. Andrews, "'Progressive' Counterparts of the CCF," 72n17.

75 PAS, CCF fonds, B7, file II-235, minutes of meeting of Political Directive Board of the CCF (Sask. Section), Regina, 14 Dec. 1935, items 23261–3.
76 PAS, CCF fonds, B7, file II-235, minutes of meeting of Political Directive Board of the CCF (Sask. Section), Regina, 14 Dec. 1935, item 23263.
77 Douglas, *Making of a Socialist*, 92.
78 Tom Douglas's date of death is recorded in his service record: LAC, RG 150, Canadian Expeditionary Force, accession 1992-93/166, box 2626-45, item 3622277, Thomas Douglas personnel record accessed online: https://www.bac-lac.gc.ca/eng/discover/military-heritage/first-world-war/personnel-records/Pages/item.aspx?IdNumber=362277.
79 According to his service record, Tom Douglas was born on 21 November 1878.
80 Douglas, *Making of a Socialist*, 348.
81 Making matters worse was the prevailing attitude of the time that "that shell shock was synonymous with cowardice." See Mark Osborne Humphries, *A Weary Road: Shell Shock in the Canadian Expeditionary Force, 1914–1918* (Toronto: University of Toronto Press, 2018), 185.
82 Douglas, *Making of a Socialist*, 93.
83 T.C. Douglas memoirs interview with Stursberg, 61–71.
84 T.C. Douglas memoirs interview with Stursberg, 77.
85 T.C. Douglas memoirs interview with Stursberg, 73.
86 T.C. Douglas memoirs interview with Stursberg, 74–5.
87 *House of Commons Debates*, Government of Canada (*HCD*), 11 Feb. 1936, 127–8. Douglas, quoted in L.D. Lovick, *Tommy Douglas Speaks: Till Power Is Brought to Pooling* (Lantzville, BC: Oolichan Books, 1979), 53–4.
88 McLeod and McLeod, *Tommy Douglas*, 243, where Franklin Roosevelt is described as one of his "political role models."
89 PAS, John (Jack) Gregory King fonds, F44, file 23, letter, A.A. MacLeod (national chairman, Canadian League Against War and Fascism) to members, 8 March 1937. In addition to Douglas being listed as vice chairman, members included Frank Underhill and Graham Spry. The league was one of many organizations that fit within the Popular Front strategy of the Communist International (Comintern) against fascism. A.A. (Alexander Albert) MacLeod was a prominent member of the CPC (and the Labor-Progressive Party when the CPC was outlawed) who eventually became a member of the Provincial Parliament in Ontario (1943–51) representing the Labor-Progressive Party. According to one scholar of the Popular Front in Canada, CCF members of such anti-fascist groups used CPC members as much as they used CCF members: John Manley, "'Communists Love Canada!' The Communist Party of Canada, the 'People' and the Popular Front, 1933–1939," *Journal of Canadian Studies* 36, no. 4 (2002): 72.

90 James Naylor, "'Pacifism or Anti-Imperialism?' The CCF Response to the Outbreak of World War II," *Journal of the Canadian Historical Association / Revue de la société historique du Canada* 8, no. 1 (1997): 222.
91 On 3 January 1940, the *Saskatchewan Commonwealth* published Douglas's attack on the USSR under the title "I Am Disgusted." PAS, CCF fonds, B7, file II-305, "Douglas Is Disgusted," by W.W. Turple, n.d., items 36036–41.
92 Thomas R. Davies, "Internationalism in a Divided World: The Experience of the International Federation of League of Nations Societies, 1919–1939," *Peace & Change* 37, no. 2 (2012): 231–2; William A. Angel, *The International Law of Youth Rights* (Leiden, NL: Brill Nijhoff, 2015), 114–17.
93 James Naylor, "Socialism for a New Generation: CCF Youth in the Popular Front Era," *Canadian Historical Review* 94, no. 1 (2013): 68.
94 Greg Donaghy, *Grit: The Life and Politics of Paul Martin Sr.* (Vancouver: UBC Press, 2015), 47; McLeod and McLeod, *Tommy Douglas*, 72.
95 Douglas, *Making of a Socialist*, 106.
96 This was Nicholson's recollection: Archives of Ontario, A.M. Nicholson fonds, F80.1, sound recording of A.M. Nicholson interview with T.C. Douglas, 15 June 1980.
97 Kevin P. Lavery, "'Youth of the World, Unite So That You May Live': Youth, Internationalism, and the Popular Front in the World Youth Congress Movement, 1936–1939," *Peace & Change* 46, no. 3 (2021): 269–85.
98 Paul Martin, *A Very Public Life*, vol. 2: *So Many Worlds* (Toronto: Deneau, 1985), 186–7.
99 Douglas, *Making of a Socialist*, 106–9.
100 See Michael Petrou, *Renegades: Canadians in the Spanish Civil War* (Vancouver: UBC Press, 2008).
101 Douglas, *Making of a Socialist*, 106–8.
102 Douglas, *Making of a Socialist*, 108. The Nuremberg gathering was the Eighth Congress of the Nazi Party and took place on 8 September 1936. According to the *LP*, more than 500,000 Nazi stormtroopers were scheduled to be present when Hitler opened the congress ("Million Attend Eighth Congress of Nazi Party," 8 Sept. 1936, 1). Given the political makeup of the World Youth Congress, it is interesting that, as the *LP* reported, Hitler's main theme for this gathering was the official launching of the Nazi's "crusade 'to save the world from Bolshevism.'"
103 "Peace Rally to Hear Douglas," *LP*, 31 Oct. 1936, 3; "Douglas Says Canada World Policy Wrong," *LP*, 31 Oct. 1938, 10.
104 Douglas, *Making of a Socialist*, 109. On the Deutscher Bund Canada's activities in Saskatchewan in the 1930s, see Jonathan F. Wagner, "Heim Ins Reich: The Story of Loon River's Nazis," *Saskatchewan History* 24, no. 2 (1976): 45–9.
105 Donaghy, *Life and Politics of Paul Martin Sr.*, 48. Martin too spent a few months travelling in Europe and gave speeches upon his return.

"Moncton Girl to Be Regional Secretary of League Society," *Ottawa Citizen*, 19 Oct. 1936, 3; "Paul Martin Returns Home," *Ottawa Citizen*, 23 Oct. 1936, 2. The "limited" nature of their friendship did not extent to parliamentary debate, of course. One particularly personal exchange occurred in April 1938, when Douglas, upon being interrupted by Martin, suggested that if Martin had been in the chamber instead "of having a nap outside," he would not have asked his question. When Martin objected that he was regularly in the House, Douglas apologized for suggesting that Martin "was asleep but he looked like he were" sleeping in the House of Commons, to which Martin replied, "You are putting me to sleep." This exchange was report in "Fussy about Interpretations," *LP*, 29 April 1938, 3.

106 Naylor, "'Pacifism or Anti-Imperialism?'" 214–16. The pacifist camp included Stanley Knowles and Carlyle King, while the isolationists included Frank Scott and Frank Underhill. As Naylor points out (225), this conflict within the party was largely kept behind closed doors except in Saskatchewan, where King and George Williams (the party's most vocal interventionist) carried on a very public spat.
107 Douglas, *Making of a Socialist*, 122.
108 T.C. Douglas memoirs interview with Stursberg, 82–4.
109 Douglas, *Making of a Socialist*, 122.
110 CBC Radio Archives, "Canadian Prime Minister Addresses War in Europe in 1939," 3 Sept. 1939, https://www.cbc.ca/player/play/1402779919
111 This conference was held on 6–7 September 1939. Naylor, "'Pacifism or Anti-Imperialism?'" 213.
112 McLeod and McLeod, *Tommy Douglas*, 83.
113 *HCD*, 9 Sept. 1939, 53–8.
114 *HCD*, 8 Sept. 1939, 41–7.
115 Woodsworth, quoted in McLeod and McLeod, *Tommy Douglas*, 82.
116 McLeod and McLeod, *Tommy Douglas*, 84.
117 Douglas, *Making of a Socialist*, 124.
118 Carlyle King, quoted in McLeod and McLeod, *Tommy Douglas*, 103. Although there was considerable tension and mistrust between King and Douglas initially, they worked constructive together when King was president of the Saskatchewan CCF between 1945 and 1960. Brett Quiring, "Carlyle King," in *Saskatchewan Politicians: Lives Past and Present*, ed. Quiring (Regina: Canadian Plains Research Center, University of Regina, 2004), 119–20.
119 Douglas, quoted in McLeod and McLeod, *Tommy Douglas*, 85.
120 Douglas, *Making of a Socialist*, 130.
121 Douglas, *Making of a Socialist*, 131.
122 Douglas, quoted in *T.C. Douglas: A Biographical Essay* (Ottawa: New Democratic Party, 1971), 7.

123 Daniel Béland, Gregory P. Marchildon, Michele Mioni, and Klaus Petersen, "Translating Social Policy Ideas: The Beveridge Report, Transnational Diffusion, and Post-War Welfare State Development in Canada, Denmark, and France." *Social Policy & Administration* 56, no. 2 (2012): 319.

124 Leonard Marsh, *Report on Social Security for Canada*, ed. Allan Moscovitch (1943; Montreal and Kingston: McGill-Queen's University Press, 2017), x–xiii; Horn, *League for Social Reconstruction*, 68; Antonia Maioni, *Parting at the Crossroads: The Emergence of Health Insurance in the United States and Canada* (Princeton, NJ: Princeton University Press, 1999), 69.

125 Heather MacDougall, "Into Thin Air: Making National Health Policy, 1939–45," *Canadian Bulleting of Medical History / Bulletin canadien d'histoire de la médecine* 26, no. 2 (2009); 284–303; Maioni, *Parting at the Crossroads*, 66–8.

126 Advisory Committee on Health Insurance, *Health Insurance: Report of the Advisory Committee on Health Insurance* (Ottawa: House of Commons Special Committee on Social Security, presented by the Hon. Ian Mackenzie, 16 March 1943); A.E. Grauer, "Canada's Program of Social Security: The Marsh Report and the Report of the Advisory Committee on Health Insurance," *Public Affairs* 6, no. 4 (1943): 181–7; J.J. Heagerty, "The Proposed Canadian National Health Bill," *American Journal of Public Health* 34, no. 2 (1943): 117–22.

127 AO, A.M. Nicholson fonds, taped recorded interview, A.M. (Sandy) Nicholson and T.C. Douglas, 15 June 1980.

128 Heagerty, "Proposed Canadian National Health Bill," 117–22.

129 Maioni, *Parting at the Crossroads*, 69; PAS, Jean Larmour oral history of the CCF government, R-8398 to R-8402, interview with T.C. Douglas, 14 Nov. 1982, transcript 1, 135–8.

130 "Canada Able to Make Own Plans Says Beveridge," *Ottawa Citizen*, 24 May 1943, 1; London School of Economics and Political Science (LSE), Sir William Beveridge papers, Beveridge/11/35/speeches, radio address by Sir William Beveridge entitled "The Beveridge Report on Social Security," Ottawa, 23 May 1943.

131 LSE, Sir William Beveridge papers, Beveridge/11/31/1, Committee on Reconstruction; "Hoping Canada to Adopt Marsh Security Plans," *Ottawa Citizen*, 25 May 1943, 1; "After-War Employment Big Issue – Beveridge," *Ottawa Citizen*, 25 May 1943, 7.

132 "Marsh Report 'Remarkable' Says Beveridge," *Ottawa Journal*, 25 May 1943, 12.

133 "Social Architects Meet," *Montreal Daily Star*, 26 May 1943, 8.

134 LSE, Sir William Beveridge papers, Beveridge/11/38/2, press clippings, and Beveridge/11/36, itineraries for the United States and Canada, 1943; "Peace Jobs Can Be Made for All, but Plan Now, Urges Beveridge," *Montreal Gazette*, 26 May 1943, 7; "Beveridge Lists Security Needs: Canadian Club Hears British Economist," *Montreal Daily Star*, 27 May 1943, 3.

135 LSE, Sir William Beveridge papers, Beveridge/11/38/2, press clippings.
136 Coldwell letter (apparently to Dr. Hugh MacLean), quoted in Conway, *The Prairie Populist*, 189.
137 Thomas, *Making of a Socialist*, 139–46; McLeod and McLeod, *Tommy Douglas*, 96–106; Shackleton, *Tommy Douglas*, 117–20.
138 McLeod and McLeod, *Tommy Douglas*, 111.
139 A.W. Johnson with Rosemary Proctor, *Dream No Little Dreams: A Biography of the Douglas Government of Saskatchewan, 1944–1961* (Toronto: University of Toronto Press, 2004), 39–40.
140 T.C. Douglas radio broadcast, 9 Feb. 1943, referenced in Johnson with Proctor, *Dream No Little Dreams*, 50–1.
141 *The CCF Program for Saskatchewan* (Regina: CCF Sask. Section, Nov. 1943; reprinted April 1944), 7–8.
142 Douglas, *Making of a Socialist*, 225.
143 "Political Parties Outline Election Stands," *LP*, 20 May 1944, 4. The wording in the article was identical to the *Election Manifesto by the Government of Saskatchewan: May 16th, 1944* (a wording that would be prohibited under the election laws of any province today), found in USAS, Sophia Dixon fonds, MG 224, series 1, box 6, file – CCF Election Materials.
144 "Political Parties Outline Election Stands," *LP*, 20 May 1944, 4.
145 Shackleton, *Tommy Douglas*, 124.
146 PAS, T.C. Douglas fonds, R-33.1, X, 395a (10-1-1), Executive Council, Saskatchewan provincial election 1944 results. Strum would then be elected president of the Saskatchewan CCF, the first woman to head a political party in Canada. She lobbied Douglas, unsuccessfully, to appoint a female cabinet minister: entry for Gladys Strum in Canadian Plains Research Center, *Encyclopedia of Saskatchewan* (Regina: Canadian Plains Research Center, 2005), 913. Her campaign brochure's motto was "Woman's Influence Begins at Home – Who Can Say Where It Ends." USAS, Sophia Dixon fonds, MG 224, series 1, box 6, file – CCF Election Materials.
147 Fines, quoted in Shackleton, *Tommy Douglas*, 125.
148 This optimism was expressed by the leader of the national CCF, M.J. Coldwell, in his book *Left Turn, Canada* (Toronto: Duell, Sloan and Pearce, 1945).

## 4. Sigerist, Sheps, and Socialism

1 Henry E. Sigerist, *Henry E. Sigerist: Autobiographical Writings*, ed. Nora Beeson (Montreal and Kingston: McGill-Queen's University Press, 1966), 188.
2 Sigerist, *Henry E. Sigerist*, 188.

3 In the twelve-page condensed version of the CCF program issued before the election of 1944, there was a ten-point program covering three and a half pages, but nothing on the CCF's proposed health program: CCF (Sask. Section), *CCF Program for Saskatchewan: Condensed Summary* (Regina: Canadian Co-operative Federation, Saskatchewan Section, 1944). Also see Michael Owen, "Toward a New Day: The Larger School Unit in Saskatchewan, 1935–1950," in *A History of Education in Saskatchewan: Selected Readings*, ed. Brian Noonan, Dianne Hallman, and Murray Scharf (Regina: Canadian Plains Research Center, University of Regina, 2006), 33–49.
4 *The CCF Program for Saskatchewan* (Reprint, Regina: CCF Sask., 1944), 7.
5 *The CCF Program for Saskatchewan*, 7.
6 Dr. Hugh MacLean was so fascinated by what was going on in New Zealand that he and Dean McHenry, an associate professor of political science at the University of California in Los Angeles, toured that country (McHenry received a Carnegie fellowship to do so) and then produced a piece summarizing the development of universal health coverage there: Hugh MacLean and Dean E. McHenry, "Medical Services in New Zealand," *Milbank Memorial Fund Quarterly* 26, no. 2 (1948): 148–81. What their piece makes clear is that, while hospital care was universally free to all New Zealanders as a right beginning in 1939, this free access applied only to public hospitals. As for care by general practitioners, this was provided by private doctors on a fee-for-service basis, with patients paying their doctors and then seeking reimbursement from the social security scheme. Doctors retained the right to extra-bill, so patients were in effect subsidized rather than fully covered by the New Zealand scheme for physician services. Philippa Mein Smith, *A Concise History of New Zealand* (Cambridge: Cambridge University Press, 2012), 161–5.
7 Provincial Archives of Saskatchewan (PAS), Jean Larmour oral history of CCF Government (hereafter Larmour history), R-8358 to R-8362, T.C. Douglas interview transcript 4, 4 Sept. 1981, 17–18, and R-8393 to R-8397, T.C. Douglas interview transcript, 1 Oct. 1982, 89–94.
8 *The Trade Union Act*, SS 1944(2), c. 69. Judy Fudge and Eric Tucker, *Labour before the Law: The Regulation of Workers' Collective Action in Canada, 1900–1948* (Toronto: University of Toronto Press, 2004), 272–3.
9 Carmella Patrias, "Socialists, Jews and the 1947 Saskatchewan Bill of Rights," *Canadian Historical Review* 87, no. 2 (2006): 266–92. In T.C. words, "the strength of this act is not in the fact that it will force equality but rather, that it puts into words the belief of the people of Saskatchewan in the inherent right of all Canadians to equality in education, employment, the right to own and occupy property, the right to access to public places" (284).

10 A.W. Johnson with Rosemary Proctor, *Dream No Little Dreams: A Biography of the Douglas Government of Saskatchewan, 1944–1961* (Toronto: University of Toronto Press, 2004), 37–41, 60–3.
11 Thomas H. McLeod, and Ian McLeod, *Tommy Douglas: The Road to Jerusalem* (Edmonton: Hurtig Publishers, 1987), 120; C.M. Fines, "The Impossible Dream: An Account of People and Events Leading to the First CCF Government, Saskatchewan, 1944" (unpublished manuscript, Trinity College, Toronto, 1982), 2: 374–5.
12 PAS, Larmour history, R-8393 to R-8397, T.C. Douglas interview transcript, 1 Oct. 1982, 88–9.
13 Corman, quoted in McLeod and McLeod, *Tommy Douglas*, 123. J.W. (Jack) Corman (1884–1969) was attorney-general from 1944 until he retired in 1956. Although originally a Liberal, and then a Social Credit candidate in the 1938 provincial election, he agreed to run for the CCF in 1944, in part because he was promised a cabinet post. This was not a difficult promise for Douglas to keep, as Corman's legal skills were conspicuously absent among a caucus made up of farmers, teachers, and preachers. Ed Whelan and Pemrose Whelan, *Run It by Jack: Tommy Douglas' First Attorney General, J.W. Corman* (Regina: Whelan Publications, 2002).
14 PAS, Larmour history, R-8387 to R-8392, interview with T.C. Douglas, 24 June 1982, transcript 1, 87.
15 Kathleen Carlisle, *Fiery Joe: The Maverick Who Lit Up the West* (Regina: University of Regina Press, 2017), 59–188; John Richards and Larry Pratt, *Prairie Capitalism: Power and Influence in the New West* (Toronto: McClelland & Stewart, 1979), 109–17; Johnson with Proctor, *Dream No Little Dreams*, 66–77.
16 John F. Conway, *The Prairie Populist: George Hara Williams and the Untold Story of the CCF* (Regina: University of Regina Press, 2018), 210.
17 PAS, Larmour history, R-8393 to R-8397, T.C. Douglas interview transcript, 1 Oct. 1982, 92–3. On the relationship between the CCF and the Roman Catholic Church, see Gregory Baum, *Catholics and Canadian Socialism: Political Thought in the Thirties and Forties* (Toronto: Lorimer, 1980), and Robert H. Dennis's two articles: "Beginning to Restructure the Institutional Church: Canadian Social Catholics and the CCF, 1931–1944," CCHA *Historical Studies* 74 (2008): 51–74, and "Faith on the Prairies: Social Catholics and the CCF in the Generation before Vatican II," CCHA *Historical Studies* 85 (2019): 7–32.
18 Lisa Dale-Burnett, "Beatrice Janet Trew," in *Saskatchewan Politicians: Lives Past and Present*, ed. Brett Quiring (Regina: Canadian Plains Research Center, University of Regina, 2004), 230–1. Trew was defeated in the 1948 election but went on to play major roles in the CCF's national council and the leftist Saskatchewan Farmers Union. She was also a member of

the Advisory Planning Committee on Medicare (Thompson Committee), which is discussed at length in chapter 10.
19 Cristine DeClercy, "Women and the Public Sphere in Saskatchewan, 1905–2005," *Prairie Forum* 32, no. 2 (2007): 357–82. No women were elected in the 1948 election, but Douglas could have appointed Marjorie Cooper, first elected in 1952 and re-elected in the 1956 and 1960 elections. On the more general subject of the relationship between leftist parties (the CCF and the CPC) and women, see Joan Sangster, *Dreams of Equality: Women on the Canadian Left, 1920–1950* (Toronto: McClelland & Stewart, 1989), and "The Role of Women in the Early CCF, 1933–1940," in *Beyond the Vote: Canadian Women and Politics*, ed. Linda Kealey and Joan Sangster (Toronto: University of Toronto Press, 1989), 118–38.
20 PAS, Larmour history, R-8436, David Levin interview transcript, 26 Nov. 1981. A civil servant, Levin pointed to the example of Marie Parr, a leading innovator in social welfare policy and program formulation and implementation who received little credit or promotion within the bureaucracy.
21 Johnson with Proctor, *Dream No Little Dreams*, 61.
22 PAS, T.C. Douglas fonds, R-33.1, box X.395, file X (10-1-1), Memorandum on Provincial Reorganization by T.H. McLeod, 28 June 1944.
23 There is an extensive literature on the Douglas government's contributions to the modernization of public administration in Canada, best summarized by Johnson with Proctor, *Dream No Little Dreams*, 117–49. On the development of central agencies, see Ken Rasmussen and Gregory P. Marchildon, "Saskatchewan's Executive Decision-Making Style: The Centrality of Planning," in *Executive Styles in Canada: Cabinet Structures and Leadership Practices in Canadian Government*, ed. Luc Bernier, Keith Brownsey, and Michael Howlett (Toronto: University of Toronto Press, 2005), 184–207; Christopher Dunn, *The Institutionalized Cabinet: Governing the Western Provinces* (Montreal and Kingston: McGill-Queen's University Press, 1995), 3–40; and Robert I. McLaren, "George Woodall Cadbury: The Fabian Catalyst in Saskatchewan's 'Good Public Administration,'" *Canadian Public Administration* 38, no. 3 (1995): 471–80.
24 PAS, Larmour history, R-8358 to R-8362, interview with T.C. Douglas, 4 September 1981, transcript 4, 17.
25 "C.C.F. Cabinet Takes Office," *Regina Leader-Post* (*LP*), 11 July 1944, 1. Lieutenant governors were appointed by the federal cabinet on the advice of Jimmy Gardiner, and were invariably Liberal partisans during the King–St-Laurent administrations. They included John M. Uhrich (1948–51), who had been minister of public health in successive provincial Liberal administrations in the province from 1923 until 1944, and William J. Patterson (1951–58), the former Liberal premier from 1935 until his

defeat by the CCF in 1944. The Progressive Conservative government under John G. Diefenbaker appointed Frank Bastedo (1958–63), a former president of the federal PC Association in Regina, to the office. Norman Ward, "The Politics of Patronage: James Gardiner and Federal Appointments in the West, 1935–57," *Canadian Historical Review* 58, no. 3 (1977): 195; *Saskatchewan Executive and Legislative Directory, 1905–1970* (Regina and Saskatoon: Saskatchewan Archives Board, 1971).

26 McLeod and McLeod, *Tommy Douglas*, 118. In 1948, Hugh MacLean told Henry Sigerist that he had convinced Douglas to "take the health portfolio instead of the one he had in mind" and that Douglas agreed but "insisted" that MacLean give the CCF convention "an outline of the tentative health program" Douglas had in mind. Letter, MacLean to Sigerist, 30 July 1948, quoted in Jacalyn Duffin, "The Guru and the Godfather: Henry Sigerist, Hugh MacLean, and the Politics of Health Care Reform in 1940s Canada," *Canadian Bulletin of Medical History* 9, no. 2 (1992): 206.

27 "C.C.F. Cabinet Takes Office," *LP*, 11 July 1944, 1.

28 McLeod and McLeod, *Tommy Douglas*, 146.

29 PAS, CCF (Sask. Section) fonds, file B7 II-74, items 7553-57, typescript of Address on Medical Health Service by Dr. Hugh McLean [sic], CCF Convention, Regina, 13 July 1944 (hereafter MacLean Address to 1944 CCF Convention).

30 Henry E. Sigerist, "Socialized Medicine," *Yale Review* (1938): 463–81, reprinted in *Henry E. Sigerist on the Sociology of Medicine*, ed. Milton I. Roemer (New York: MD Publications, 1960), 39–53.

31 In fact, the SHML began preparing its own detailed plan in 1939, a plan that would go through multiple drafts before being released publicly in 1941 as *State Medicine for Saskatchewan: An Eight Point Plan*: see Aaron William Goss, "Care Regardless of the Ability to Pay: A Reconnaissance of Saskatchewan's State Hospital and Medical League" (MA thesis, University of Manitoba, 2013), 47–8. Also see Esyllt Jones, *Radical Medicine: The International Origins of Socialized Health Care in Canada* (Winnipeg: ARP Books, 2019), 138–45.

32 MacLean address to 1944 CCF Convention; Duffin, "The Guru and the Godfather," 204. To save money and to increase their power through a combined regulatory and lobbying body, the self-regulatory colleges in British Columbia, Alberta, and Saskatchewan merged with the provincial medical associations to form a single body. See David Naylor, *Private Practice, Public Payment: Canadian Medicare and the Politics of Health Insurance, 1911–1966* (Montreal and Kingston: McGill-Queen's University Press, 1986), 94–5.

33 See Gordon S. Lawson, "The Road Not Taken: The 1945 Health Services Planning Commission Proposals and Physician Remuneration in

Saskatchewan," *Canadian Bulletin of Medical History* 26, no. 2 (2009): 405–11.
34 MacLean address to 1944 CCF Convention; Duffin, "The Guru and the Godfather," 204.
35 Daniel Béland, Gregory P. Marchildon, Michele Mioni, and Klaus Petersen, "Translating Social Policy Ideas: The Beveridge Report, Transnational Diffusion, and Post-War Welfare State Development in Canada, Denmark, and France," *Social Policy & Administration* 56, no. 2 (2022): 317–21.
36 This was Sigerist's third trip to Canada: see his Canadian itineraries in Duffin, "The Guru and the Godfather," 208–9.
37 Mackenzie was one of the most activist Liberal ministers in favour of the Green Book social security proposals. Impressed by the Beveridge Report of 1942, he instructed his officials to prepare similar social security provisions for Canada. In March 1943, he presented the Marsh and Heagerty reports to the Special Committee of Social Security, of which he was also a member. See Patricia E. Roy and Peter Neary, "Ian Mackenzie," *Dictionary of Canadian Biography*, vol. 17, http://www.biographi.ca/en/bio/mackenzie_ian_alistair_17E.htm.
38 Jacalyn Duffin and Leslie A. Falk, "Sigerist in Saskatchewan: The Quest for Balance in Social and Technical Medicine" *Bulletin on the History of Medicine* 70, no. 4 (1996): 665; *House of Commons Debates*, Government of Canada (*HCD*), 19th Parliament, vol. 1, 9 Feb. 1944, 315–19. Sandy (A.M.) Nicholson was one of four new CCF members, three of whom were from Saskatchewan, elected in the 1940 election. He was a United Church minister who, liked Douglas, was attracted to the CCF because of the social gospel. Douglas had known Nicholson since the mid-1930s and travelled on his behalf to support him in his constituency (Mackenzie) in northeastern Saskatchewan. Nicholson was one of Douglas's major supporters in his bid to become president of the Saskatchewan CCF and, at Douglas's request, became treasurer for the Saskatchewan CCF after Douglas secured control of the provincial party. Betty Dyck, *Running to Beat Hell: A Biography of A.M. (Sandy) Nicholson* (Regina: Canadian Plains Research Center, University of Regina, 1988), 108–9, 126–7, 158.
39 Henry E. Sigerist, "Medical Care for All the People" *Canadian Journal of Public Health* 35, no. 7 (1944): 263–7. This piece was republished in abridged form in the *American Journal of Public Health* almost sixty years later with a commentary by Theodore M. Brown and Elizabeth Brown: "Henry E. Sigerist: Medical Historian and Social Visionary," *American Journal of Public Health* 93, no. 1 (2003): 60.
40 Duffin, "The Guru and the Godfather," 208–9.
41 Archives of Ontario (AO), A.M. Nicholson fonds, F 80, letter, A.M. (Sandy) Nicholson to Margaret Telford (CCF National Office), 20 March 1944.

42 AO, A.M. Nicholson fonds, F 80, letter, H.E. Sigerist to A.M. (Sandy) Nicholson, 13 Feb. 1944.
43 This is Elizabeth Fee's description in her foreword to the 2018 edition of Henry E. Sigerist's *Civilization and Disease* (Ithaca, NY: Cornell University Press, 2018), ix, a book that was originally published by University of Chicago Press in 1943. See also "Medicine: History in a Tea Wagon," *Time*, 30 Jan. 1939, 51.
44 Elizabeth Fee, "Henry E. Sigerist: From the Social Production of Disease to Medical Management and Scientific Socialism," *Milbank Quarterly* 67, suppl. 1 (1989): 133.
45 Henry E. Sigerist, "Trends Towards Socialized Medicine," in *Henry E. Sigerist on the Sociology of Medicine*, ed. Milton I. Roemer (1934; New York: MD Publications, 1960), 23–7.
46 Jennifer Klein, *For All These Rights: Business, Labor and the Shaping of America's Public-Private Welfare State* (Princeton, NJ: Princeton University Press, 2004), 132.
47 Alan Derickson, *Health Security for All: Dreams of Universal Health Care in America* (Baltimore, MD: Johns Hopkins University Press, 2005), 80.
48 Elizabeth Fee, "The Pleasures and Perils of Prophetic Advocacy: Henry E. Sigerist and the Politics of Medical Reform," *American Journal of Public Health* 86, no. 11 (1996): 1640.
49 For opposing views concerning these Western visitors to the Soviet Union, see Michael David-Fox, *Showcasing the Great Experiment: Cultural Diplomacy and Western Visitors to the Soviet Union, 1921–1941* (Oxford: Oxford University Press, 2012), and Ludmila Stern, *Western Intellectuals and the Soviet Union, 1920–40: From Red Square to the Left Bank* (London: Routledge, 2007). This debate is put in the context of the Soviet health system, and its perception by Sigerist and fellow scholars, by Jones in *Radical Medicine*, 41–59.
50 Henry E. Sigerist, *Socialized Medicine in the Soviet Union* (London: Victor Gollancz, 1937).
51 John F. Hutchinson, "Dances with Commissars: Sigerist and Soviet Medicine," in *Making Medical History: The Life and Times of Henry E. Sigerist*, ed. Theodore M. Brown and Elizabeth Fee (Baltimore, MD: Johns Hopkins University Press, 1997), 229.
52 See, for example, Henry E. Sigerist, "Twenty-Five Years of Health Work in the Soviet Union," *American Review of Soviet Medicine* 1, no. 1 (1943): 67–78.
53 Sigerist himself traced the development of this Bismarckian model of social health insurance, contrasting it with an approach in which benefits would be available as a matter of right through citizenship. See Henry E. Sigerist, "From Bismarck to Beveridge: Developments and Trends in Social Security Legislation," *Bulletin of the History of Medicine* 13, no. 4 (1943): 365–88.

54 Henry E. Sigerist, "Socialized Medicine," in *Henry E. Sigerist on the Sociology of Medicine*, ed. Milton I. Roemer (New York: MD Publications, 1960), 39–40; Fee, "Pleasures and Perils of Prophetic Advocacy," 1641.
55 Sigerist, "Socialized Medicine," 39.
56 Sigerist, "Socialized Medicine," 43.
57 Summarizing interview with Henry Sigerist, "Organized Medicine," *LP*, 8 Sept. 1944, 3.
58 Sigerist, "Socialized Medicine," 44–5.
59 Sigerist, "Socialized Medicine," 48–9.
60 Theodore M. Brown and Elizabeth Fee, "Henry E. Sigerist (189–1957): Medical Historian, Advocate of 'Socialized' Medicine, and Admirer of the Soviet Health System," *American Journal of Public Health* 107, no. 11 (2017): 11–12.
61 Richard E. Kerber, "A USA-USSR Experiment in Medical Journalism: The American Review of Soviet Medicine," *American Communist History* 11, no. 2 (2012): 230; Martin F. Shapiro, "Medical Aid Provided by American, Canadian and British Nationals to the Spanish Republic during the Civil War, 1936–1939," *International Journal of Health Services* 13, no. 3 (1983): 453. Also see Eric R. Smith, *American Relief Aid and the Spanish Civil War* (Columbia: University of Missouri Press, 2013).
62 "Medical War Help for Reds Studies," *Montreal Gazette*, 15 Oct. 1941, 11; "Medical Help Planned Here for Russia," *Montreal Daily Star*, 15 Oct. 1941, 2; "Russia Was Ready for Battle Even in Field of War Medicine," *Ottawa Journal*, 15 Oct. 1941, 4.
63 Michael R. Grey, *New Deal Medicine: The Rural Health Programs of the Farm Security Administration* (Baltimore, MD: Johns Hopkins University Press, 1999), 180.
64 Jones, *Radical Medicine*, 160; Duffin, "The Guru and the Godfather," 195.
65 McLeod and McLeod, *Tommy Douglas*, 147. Douglas wanted MacLean to serve at least as an advisor to Sigerist, but MacLean declined because he might embarrass the commission by adding another non-resident and a partisan CCF supporter. See Duffin "The Guru and the Godfather," 204.
66 Duffin and Falk, "Sigerist in Saskatchewan," 670.
67 "Medical Students to Hear Sigerist," *Montreal Gazette*, 8 March 1933, 17; "Medicine of Other Days in Examined," *Montreal Gazette*, 8 March 1933, 11. For the itineraries of his three 1943 and 1944 trips, see Duffin, "The Guru and the Godfather," 208–11.
68 Sigerist, *Henry E. Sigerist*, 187 (journal entry for 16 June 1944).
69 Sigerist, *Henry E. Sigerist*, 188 (journal entry for 20 July 1944).
70 PAS, Larmour history, R-8395 to R-8397, T.C. Douglas interview transcript, 4 Oct. 1982, 90.
71 PAS, Larmour history, R-8358 to R-8362, T.C. Douglas interview transcript 4, 4 Sept. 1981, 17–18.

72 Jones, *Radical Medicine*, 159.
73 Douglas provided these details concerning Sigerist's contract in answer to the opposition's question in the Saskatchewan Legislature on 10 November 1944: *Journals of the Legislative Assembly of Saskatchewan (JLAS)*, vol. 43 (1944), 71.
74 *Saskatchewan Health Services Survey Commission: Report of the Commissioner, Henry E. Sigerist* (Regina: Thomas H. McConica, King's Printer, 1944), 3.
75 Extract from journal entry for 13 September 1944, in Sigerist, *Henry E. Sigerist*, 189.
76 *Saskatchewan Health Services Survey Commission*, 3; Jones, *Radical Medicine*, 157; Duffin and Falk, "Sigerist in Saskatchewan," 672.
77 Brett Quiring, "John Michael Uhrich," in Quiring, *Saskatchewan Politicians*, 235–6.
78 McLeod and McLeod, *Tommy Douglas*, 128–9.
79 Jones, *Radical Medicine*, 190.
80 Johns Hopkins Chesney Archives (JHCA), Henry Sigerist fonds, box 25, letter, Mindel Sheps to Henry E. Sigerist, 12 Aug. 1944.
81 *Saskatchewan Health Services Survey Commission*, 3.
82 *Saskatchewan Health Services Survey Commission*, 3.
83 *Saskatchewan Health Services Survey Commission*, 4.
84 Virginia Berridge, "Polyclinics: Haven't We Been There Before," *BMJ* 336 (2008): 1161–2. On the influence of polyclinic health centres and the history of interwar polyclinics in the United Kingdom, see Jones, *Radical Medicine*, 15–36, and 91–127.
85 Jones, *Radical Medicine*, 58–9 and, on health centres–polyclinics in the United Kingdom, 103–12. On developments in the United States during the Roosevelt administration, see Grey, *New Deal Medicine*.
86 American Public Health Association, "Medical Care in a National Health Program: An Official Statement of the American Public Health Association Adopted October 4, 1944," *American Journal of Public Health* 34, no. 12 (1944): 1254.
87 Joseph Walter Mountin, Elliott Harmon Pennell, and Vane M. Hoge, *Health Service Areas: Requirements for General Hospitals and Health Centers* (Washington, DC: Federal Security Agency, US Public Health Service, 1945).
88 *Saskatchewan Health Services Survey Commission*, 4–5.
89 *Saskatchewan Health Services Survey Commission*, 12.
90 University of Saskatchewan Archives and Special Collections (USAS), Sophia Dixon fonds, MG 224, series 1, box 12, State Hospital and Medical League file, "State Medicine for Saskatchewan: An Eight Point Plan," twelve-page brochure published by the SHML in February 1941.
91 Sigerist, *Socialized Medicine in the Soviet Union*, 92.

92 *Saskatchewan Health Services Survey Commission*, 8–10.
93 Fee, "Henry E. Sigerist," 129.
94 *Saskatchewan Health Services Survey Commission*, 10.
95 *Saskatchewan Health Services Survey Commission*, 10–11.
96 JHCA, Henry Sigerist fonds, box 25, letter, Mindel Sheps to Henry E. Sigerist, 12 Aug. 1944.
97 "Separate Division of Health to Combat Venereal Disease," *LP*, 17 Oct. 1944, 3; "Capt. C. G. Sheps Made V.D. Officer for M.D. 12," *Saskatoon Star Phoenix*, 12 Oct. 1944, 6.
98 Douglas, quoted in "Separate Division of Health to Combat Venereal Disease," *LP*, 17 Oct. 1944, 3.
99 LAC, A.W. Johnson fonds, R12603, vol. 6, file 6, T.C. Douglas radio broadcasts scripts, Oct. 1945 (no exact date indicated) and 20 Nov. 1945.
100 PAS, Department of Public Health fonds, R-536, Policy Research and Management Services Branch, file 14a, "History of Public Health in Saskatchewan," prepared by the Division of Health Education, n.d. (c. 1958).
101 *Census of Saskatchewan 1946: Housing and Families* (Ottawa: Edmond Cloutier, King's Printer, 1952), 167.
102 *JLAS: Session 1945*, budget speech by C.M. Fines, 14.
103 This promise is set out in large, bold print in the CCF election brochure "Let There Be No Blackout of Health," n.d. but likely 1943: USAS, Co-operative Commonwealth Federation Pamphlets, section 1, pamphlet 16.
104 McLeod said he completed most of the drafting on the *Health Services Act*: PAS, Larmour history, R-8444 to R-8448, transcript of interview with T.H. McLeod, 25 Nov. 1981, 17.
105 Health Services Act, SS 1944, c. 51.
106 *JLAS: Second Session 1944*, 43, 60, 64.
107 The Health Services Act, SS, c. 51, *JLAS: Second Session 1944*, index, 1–2; PAS, T.C. Douglas fonds, R33.5, III, file 133b (14–24), College of Physicians and Surgeons, letter, College of Physicians and Surgeons to physicians, 27 Jan. 1945.
108 PAS, Larmour history, R-8444 to R-8448, transcript of interview with T.H. McLeod, 25 Nov. 1981, 17.
109 PAS, Larmour history, R-8444 to R-8448, transcript of interview with T.H. McLeod, 25 Nov. 1981, 21.
110 PAS, T.C. Douglas fonds, R33.1, file XIV 580 (14-31) – Reports re: Health Plans, memorandum entitled "Regional Health Services," Dec. 1944; Gordon S. Lawson, "The Co-operative Commonwealth Federation, Health Care Reform and Physician Remuneration in the Province of Saskatchewan, 1915–1949" (M.A. thesis, University of Regina, 1998), 102–5.
111 PAS, T.C. Douglas fonds, R33.1, file XIV 580 (14-31) – Reports re: Health Plans, "Report on Regional Health Services: A Proposed Plan," Health

Services Planning Commission, 15 Feb. 1945 (hereafter "Proposed Plan on Regional Health Services").

112 "Proposed Plan on Regional Health Services," Part I, 9–11.

113 C. Stuart Houston and Merle Masse, *36 Steps on the Road to Medicare: Why Saskatchewan Led the Way* (Montreal and Kingston: McGill-Queen's University Press, 2013), 25–40. C. Rufus Rorem, one of America's most prominent health economists in the interwar era, was drawn to Saskatchewan in order to study the municipal doctor system and subsequently wrote *The "Municipal Doctor" System in Rural Saskatchewan* (Chicago: University of Chicago Press, 1931), a publication of the Committee on the Costs of Medical Care.

114 Donald V. Smiley, "Local Autonomy and Central Administrative Control in Saskatchewan," *Canadian Journal of Economics and Political Science / Revue canadienne d'économique et de science politique* 26, no. 2 (1960): 299–313.

115 Rod Bantjes, "'An Imperfect Architecture of Power': Class and Local Government in Saskatchewan, 1908–1936," *Prairie Forum* 20, no. 1 (1995)" 37–62.

116 Harley D. Dickinson, "The Struggle for State Health Insurance: Reconsidering the Role of Saskatchewan Farmers." *Studies in Political Economy: A Socialist Review* 41, no. 1 (1993): 148. On this tradition, also see Mitch Diamantopoulos, "The Foundations of Agrarian Socialism: Co-operative Economic Action in Saskatchewan, 1905–1960," *Prairie Forum* 37, no. 2 (2012): 103–51, and David Laycock, *Populist and Democratic Thought in the Canadian Prairies, 1910 to 1945* (Toronto: University of Toronto Press, 1990).

117 "Proposed Plan on Regional Health Services," Part II, 1.

118 This was the central dilemma highlighted by Meyer Brownstone in "Agriculture," in *Social Purpose for Canada*, ed. Michael Oliver (Toronto: University of Toronto Press, 1961), 335.

119 Michael Owen, "Toward a New Day: The Larger School Unit in Saskatchewan, 1935–1950," in *A History of Education in Saskatchewan: Selected Readings*, ed. Brian Noonan, Dianne Hallman, and Murray Scharf (Regina: Canadian Plains Research Center, University of Regina, 2006), 33–49. Without a doubt, this experience motivated T.C. to eventually establish the Royal Commission on Agriculture and Rural Life to see if a consensual reorganization of local government could be achieved. A.W. Johnson suggests that the royal commission was Douglas's "personal idea" (*Dream No Little* Dreams, 159). The six-year long commission published fourteen report volumes, and the final report recommended major changes to the structure of local government to meet present conditions and anticipate the future: *Royal Commission on Agriculture*

*and Rural Life. Report No. 14: A Program of Improvement* (Regina: Queen's Printer, 1957). These recommendations would be rejected by SARM, creating a major political problem for the Douglas government. See Wayne Mark Skovron, "A People's Commission? High Modernism, Direct Democracy, and the Royal Commission on Agriculture and Rural Life, 1952–1957" (MA thesis, Simon Fraser University, 2011).

120 LAC, A.W. Johnson fonds, R12603, vol. 6, file 6, T.C. Douglas radio broadcast, 20 Nov. 1945, and 21 Nov. 1946.

121 PAS, Larmour history, R8444 to R-8448, transcript of interview with T.H. McLeod, 25 Nov. 1981, 19–20. On the larger school unit reform, see Owen, "Toward a New Day," 43–7.

122 PAS, Premier's Office fonds, R-191, no. 5, Thomas H. McLeod's files relating to HSPC, file 19, HSPC Minutes of Meeting of Advisory Committee to the HSPC, 2–3 March 1945 (hereafter, Minutes of HSPC Advisory Committee, 2–3 March 1945).

123 Minutes of HSPC Advisory Committee, 2–3 March 1945, 4–8.

124 J.F.C. Anderson as quoted in the minutes of the 2 September 1945 Advisory Committee meeting: Lawson, "The Co-operative Commonwealth Federation," 106.

125 *Saskatchewan Medical Quarterly* 9, no. 1 (1945): 15–16.

126 CPS resolution as quoted in *Saskatchewan Medical Quarterly* 9, no. 1 (1945): 16.

127 This meeting is well portrayed by Lawson, "The Co-operative Commonwealth Federation," 108–11.

128 Born in 1897, Clarence Francis Hames was also considerably older than Mindel Sheps and Tommy McLeod. He received his medical degree from the University of Toronto in 1924. In 1929, he moved to Saskatchewan, where he established a pediatric practice. One year later, he joined the Department of Public Health, where he "pioneered provincial 'well baby' clinics,'" where "mothers could take their children for medical checkups and care." During the Second World War, Dr. Hames was a major in the Royal Canadian Army Medical Corps. He was appointed deputy minister on 19 January 1945. When he stepped down in favour of Fred Mott on 31 December 1949, he became the medical officer of health in North Battleford. Biographical information on Hames gleaned from the page "Sapper Clarence Francis Hames," on the Canadian Great War Project website, https://canadiangreatwarproject.com/person.php?pid=141416. On his appointment and departure as deputy minister, see *Saskatchewan Executive and Legislative Directory, 1905–1970* (Regina: Government of Saskatchewan, 1971), 2.6–17.

129 Jones, *Radical Medicine*, 217; David McGrane, "Gender and Saskatchewan Social Democracy from 1900 to 2000," *Journal of Canadian Studies* 42, no. 1

(2008): 183–6; Georgina Taylor, "Review Essay: Gender and the History of the Left," *Saskatchewan History* 44, no. 1 (1992): 31–4. George Cadbury railed against such attitudes (the main victim of which was his wife, Barbara) in his letters back to his close friend in England (PAS, Larmour history, transcript R-8343 to R-8345, interview with George Cadbury, 22 Jan. 1982, 41–3), and his spouse, Barbara Cadbury, complained publicly about the scarcity of women MPs in the CCF caucus in 1947: "Canadian Women Are Not 'National' Enough," *LP*, 11 Jan. 1947, 6.

130 PAS, Larmour history, R-8444 to R-8448, transcript of interview with T.H. McLeod, 25 Nov. 1981, 17–18.
131 *Saskatchewan Medical Quarterly* 9, no. 1 (1945): 17.
132 *Saskatchewan Medical Quarterly* 9, no. 1 (1945): 17. The *Saskatchewan Medical Quarterly* was published from 1937, the year that the Saskatchewan Medical Association and the CPS merged their activities, largely to save money in the depths of the Great Depression, until 1975. The journal was remarkably transparent in relating the details of meetings between the CPS's representatives and the Douglas government. C. Stuart Houston, "The Early Years of the Saskatchewan Medical Quarterly," *Canadian Medical Association Quarterly* 188, no. 9 (1978): 1122 and 1127.
133 *Saskatchewan Medical Quarterly* 9, no. 1 (1945): 17.
134 The "disapproval of the profession was made known" to Douglas soon as they were informed of Cecil Sheps's appointment as acting chair: *Saskatchewan Medical Quarterly* 10, no. 4 (1946): 11.
135 *Saskatchewan Medical Quarterly* 9, no. 1 (1945): 20–1.
136 This is also Gordon S. Lawson's carefully drawn conclusion in "The Road Not Taken," 419–20.
137 Minutes of HSPC Advisory Committee, 2–3 March 1945, 6.
138 "Proposed Plan on Regional Health Services," Part II, 1, 6–7; Part III, 1–7.
139 By October 1945, the HSPC had received fifty-eight applications for medical care (physician) grants from fifty-eights RMs, and twenty-four from urban municipalities, and had approved twenty-two for the RMs (for grants in total of $18,588 to assist the RMs in hiring the doctors) and eleven for urban municipalities (for grants which totalled $1,624). PAS, T.C. Douglas fonds, R33.5, file III 133 (14-24), Minutes of Meeting of the Subcommittee (hereafter HSPC Advisory Committee) on Local Health Services held 20 October 1945.
140 PAS, Premier's Office fonds, R-191, no. 5, Thomas H. McLeod's files relating to HSPC, file 19, HSPC Minutes of Meeting of Advisory Committee to the HSPC, memorandum re: Meeting of HSPC with Medical Committee of CPS, 14 April 1945. This proposed model FFS contract was sent out to all municipal doctors in the province on 9

August 1945, along with a questionnaire. The results indicated that, while the majority accepted the need for a base salary in their respective municipalities, they nonetheless preferred an FFS contract as most "in the interests of patient and provider." Saskatchewan Medical Association Archives (SMA), Dr. Clarence Houston's municipal contract file, letter, Dr. R.K. Johnston to CPS, 12 Sept. 1945, found and provided by Gordon Lawson.

141 JHCA, Henry E. Sigerist Collection, letter, Mindel C. Sheps to Henry E. Sigerist, 16 Aug. 1945.

142 JHCA, Henry E. Sigerist Collection, letter, Mindel C. Sheps to Henry E. Sigerist, 16 Aug. 1945.

143 Michael R. Welton, "Conflicting Visions, Divergent Strategies: Watson Thomson and the Cold War Politics of Adult Education in Saskatchewan, 1944–6," *Labour/Le Travail* 18 (1986): 125.

144 Welton, "Conflicting Visions," 134–5. Also see Gregory P. Marchildon, "Community Clinics and Stan Rands's Struggle for the Transformation of Health Care in Canada," in Stan Rands, *Privilege and Policy: The History of Community Clinics in Canada* (Regina: Canadian Plains Research Centre, University of Regina, 2012), x–xi.

145 M.J. Coldwell (in letter to T.C. Douglas) quoted in Michael R. Welton, "'To Be and Build the Glorious World': The Educational Thought and Practice of Watson Thomson, 1899–1946" (PhD diss., University of British Columbia, 1983), 423.

146 JHCA, Henry E. Sigerist Collection, letter, Mindel C. Sheps to Henry E. Sigerist, 16 Aug. 1945.

147 JHCA, Henry E. Sigerist Collection, letter, Henry E. Sigerist to Mindel C. Sheps, 27 Aug. 1945.

148 SMA, file 6-13-6, Report to the HSPC on Proposed Medical Services Plan for Region 6 (Moose Jaw) prepared by Paul A. Dodd, 4 Nov. 1945; Paul Albert Dodd (1902–92), who had earned a PhD in economics from University of Pennsylvania in 1933, was a consulting economist to the HSPC (1945–6) while an associate professor at the University of California at Los Angeles. On Paul Dodd, see Jones, *Radical Medicine*, 211–12.

149 Joan Feather, "From Concept to Reality: Formation of the Swift Current Health Region," *Prairie Forum* 16, no. 1 (1991); 69.

150 Houston and Massie, *Road to Medicare*, 79–86.

151 This region had always been part of the Dry Belt and had suffered years of drought and land abandonment well before the collapse in the price of wheat and the prolonged and more wide-spread drought of the 1930s: see Curtis R. McManus, *Happyland: A History of the "Dirty Thirties" in Saskatchewan, 1914–1937* (Calgary: University of Calgary Press, 2011), and Gregory P. Marchildon, Jeremy Pittman, and David J. Sauchyn, "The Dry

Belt and Changing Aridity in the Palliser Triangle, 1895–2000," in *Drought and Depression: History of the Prairie West*, vol. 6, ed. Gregory P. Marchildon (Regina: University of Regina Press, 2018), 14–20.
152 Feather, "From Concept to Reality," 70.
153 Houston and Massie, *Road to Medicare*, 83.
154 In April 1945, Mindel Sheps was looking for an experiment "in at least two regions" and had already identified Swift Current as a potential candidate. PAS, T.C. Douglas fonds, R33.5, file III 121a (14-6-7), HSPC memorandum "Organization of Health Regions," 20 April 1945. Douglas, on the other hand, wanted to keep the number of "experiments" to one to avoid duelling medical care plans with differing standards and approaches and to minimize conflict with the CPS, which was highly resistant to any regional plan insuring medical care (as opposed to hospital care). While T.C. was very familiar with the similarly rapid organization of a health region in his own constituency (Weyburn-Estevan Health Region No. 3), he knew that local governments would limit coverage to hospital care.
155 Feather, "From Concept to Reality," 73; Orville Kenneth Hjertaas (1917–98) graduated from medicine at the University of Manitoba in 1942. He was a GP in rural Saskatchewan before joining the HSPC as a health region organizer on 1 September 1945. He would take over as secretary when Mindel Sheps left the HSPC on 31 January 1946 but held this position only until August, when he joined two old classmates to start a general practice in Prince Albert, Saskatchewan ( "Dr. Hjertaas New Secretary," *LP*, 30 Jan. 1946, 3). He would become the founding member of the Prince Albert Community Clinic during the doctors' strike of 1962. For a short biography of Hjertaas, see Stuart Houston and Bill Waiser, *Tommy's Team: The People Behind the Douglas Years* (Calgary: Fifth House, 2010), 60–4.
156 Houston and Waiser, *Tommy's Team*, 62–4. *LP*, advertisement by HSPC for radio broadcasts on proposed health regions (T.C. Douglas, Dr. M. Sheps, and T.H. McLeod, 20–2 Nov. 1945), 20 Nov. 1945, 13.
157 Feather, "From Concept to Reality," 74.
158 Houston and Massie, *Road to Medicare*, 84, and Feather, "Formation of the Swift Current Health Region," 75.
159 Frederick D. Mott, "A Pattern of Local Services in the Saskatchewan Health Program," *American Journal of Public Health* 30, no. 2 (1949): 217.
160 SMA, Medical Advisory Committee file, notes from meeting with premier, 30–31 Dec. 1945.
161 SMA, Medical Advisory Committee file, notes from meeting with premier, 30–31 Dec. 1945.
162 SMA, Medical Advisory Committee file, notes from meeting with premier, 30–31 Dec. 1945.

Notes to pages 125–7  535

## 5. Rise and Fall of the Green Book Proposals

1. On the depression origins of the Royal Commission on Dominion-Provincial Relations, see Robert Wardhaugh and Barry Ferguson, *The Rowell-Sirois Commission and the Remaking of Canadian Federalism* (Vancouver: UBC Press, 2021), 26–68. It should be noted that Alberta did default on its debt, although it was never put into receivership as the term "bankruptcy" implies.
2. Joan Feather, "Horse-Trading and Health Insurance: Saskatchewan and Dominion-Provincial Relations, 1937–1947," *Saskatchewan History* 39, no. 3 (1986): 95–6.
3. Beth Bilson, "William Patterson," in *Saskatchewan Premiers of the Twentieth Century*, ed. Gordon L. Barnhart (Regina: Canadian Plains Research Center, University of Regina, 2004), 149; Feather, "Horse-Trading and Health Insurance," 95; "Able Battle by Patterson, Bracken for Sirois Report," *Regina Leader-Post* (*LP*), 15 Jan. 1941, 14.
4. *Report of the Royal Commission on Dominion-Provincial Relations: Book II – Recommendations* (Ottawa: Kings Printer, 1940), 84.
5. *Report of the Royal Commission on Dominion-Provincial Relations: Book II*, 33.
6. *Report of the Royal Commission on Dominion-Provincial Relations: Book II*, 121. For a summary of the main recommendations, see Wardhaugh and Ferguson, *The Rowell-Sirois Commission*, 219–21.
7. Provincial Archives of Saskatchewan (PAS), Jean Larmour oral history of the CCF government, R-8398 to R-8402, interview with T.C. Douglas, 14 Nov. 1982, transcript 1, 77–8.
8. Feather, "Horse-Trading and Health Insurance," 97.
9. "C.C.F. Favors Sirois Report," *LP*, 8 Sept. 1944, 3.
10. Daniel Béland, Gregory P. Marchildon, Michele Mioni, and Klaus Petersen, "Translating Social Policy Ideas: The Beveridge Report, Transnational Diffusion, and Post-War Welfare State Development in Canada, Denmark, and France," *Social Policy & Administration* 56, no. 2 (2012): 315-21.
11. The tension between the two men, sharpened by the fact that Gardiner was the federal minister responsible for Saskatchewan under both Mackenzie King and St-Laurent, was permanent and palpable. In one episode in the mid-1950s, when Gardiner asked Douglas and Fines to join him in his office to talk about the South Saskatchewan River dam project, which St-Laurent had just rejected, Douglas told Gardiner to "go to hell. I don't want to discuss this with you at all." Douglas quoted in Thomas H. McLeod and Ian McLeod, *Tommy Douglas: The Road to Jerusalem* (Edmonton: Hurtig Publishers, 1987), 133.
12. T.C. Douglas, *The Making of a Socialist: The Recollections of T. C. Douglas*, ed. Lewis H. Thomas (Edmonton: University of Alberta Press, 1982), 112.

13 F.R. Scott, *Leaving the Shade of the Middle Ground: The Poetry of F.R. Scott*, selected by Laura Moss (Waterloo, ON: Wilfrid Laurier University Press, 2011), 28–9.
14 Doris French Shackleton, *Tommy Douglas: A Biography* (Toronto: McClelland & Steward, 1975), 95.
15 Mackenzie King, quoted in Robert A. Wardhaugh, *Mackenzie King and the Prairie West* (Toronto: University of Toronto Press, 2000), 247. In an interview with T.C. quoted by Shackleton in her biography, Douglas stated that he "wasn't impressed with [King] at all" and quoted Agnes Macphail, who called King "a fat man full of words." Shackleton, *Tommy Douglas*, 94.
16 Leonard Marsh, *Report on Social Security for Canada*, ed. Allan Moscovitch (1943; Montreal and Kingston: McGill-Queen's University Press, 2017); Advisory Committee on Health Insurance, *Health Insurance: Report of the Advisory Committee on Health Insurance* (Ottawa: House of Commons Special Committee on Social Security, presented by the Hon. Ian Mackenzie, 16 March 1943); Heather MacDougall, "Into Thin Air: Making National Health Policy, 1939–45," *Canadian Bulleting of Medical History / Bulletin canadien d'histoire de la médecine* 26, no. 2 (2009): 297–313.
17 Library and Archives Canada (LAC), Hon. Brooke Claxton fonds, MG 32 B5, vol. 142, file DPC, 1945 Co-ordinating and Economic Committees, *Dominion-Provincial Conference on Reconstruction: Proposals of the Government of Canada, Aug. 1945* (hereafter referred to as the Green Book Proposals).
18 LAC, Hon. Brooke Claxton fonds, MG 32 B5, vol. 185, file 13, typescript of memoirs, 674–5.
19 Green Book Proposals.
20 PAS, T.C. Douglas fonds, R-33.1, box X.395, file XXIII.745b (23-22-1) (hereafter TCD), first of seven folders, Federal-Provincial Conferences, copy of memorandum of suggestions for the agenda and procedure, Dominion-Provincial Conference, 15 May 1944.
21 Malcolm G. Taylor, *Health Insurance and Canadian Public Policy: The Seven Decisions That Created the Canadian Health Insurance System and Its Outcomes* (Montreal and Kingston: McGill-Queen's University Press, 1978), 44.
22 Winning thirty-four seats, the CCF under its new leader, Ted Joliffe, displaced the Liberal Party (fifteen seats) as the official opposition and put the Progressive Conservatives (thirty-eight seats) under leader George Drew into a minority position. Gerald L. Caplan, "The Failure of Canadian Socialism: The Ontario Experience, 1932–1945," *Canadian Historical Review* 44, no. 2 (1963): 99–103.
23 *Toronto Star* editorial, 5 Aug. 1943, quoted in Caplan, "Failure of Canadian Socialism," 103.

24 David Lewis and F.R. Scott, *Make This Your Canada: A Review of C.C.F. History and Policy* (Toronto: Central Canada Publishing Company, 1943), ix.
25 Antonia Maioni, *Parting at the Crossroads: The Emergence of Health Insurance in the United States and Canada* (Princeton, NJ: Princeton University Press, 1999), 73.
26 M.J. Coldwell, *Left Turn, Canada* (Toronto: Duell, Sloan and Pearce, 1945), 155–77.
27 Coldwell, *Left Turn, Canada*, 232–3.
28 Taylor, *Health Insurance and Canadian Public Policy*, 47.
29 Charles A. Deshaies, "The Rise and Decline of the Cooperative Commonwealth Federation in Ontario and Quebec during World War II, 1939–1945" (PhD diss., University of Maine, 2019), 347–8.
30 Deschaies, "Rise and Decline," 352–3.
31 Dean E. McHenry, *The Third Force in Canada* (Berkeley and Los Angeles: University of California Press, 1950), 135.
32 MacDougall, "Into Thin Air," 303. Also see Alvin Finkel, "Paradise Postponed: A Re-Examination of the Green Book Proposals of 1945," *Journal of the Canadian Historical Association* 4 (1993): 120–42
33 David Jay Bercuson, *True Patriot: The Life of Brooke Claxton, 1898–1960* (Toronto: University of Toronto Press, 1993), 137; Taylor, *Health Insurance and Canadian Public Policy*, 63.
34 McLeod and McLeod, *Tommy Douglas*, 136–7; Taylor, "Health Insurance," 73–6.
35 PAS, TCD, second of seven folders, Federal-Provincial Conferences, letter, F.R. Scott to T.C. Douglas, 21 July 1945.
36 *Dominion-Provincial Conference on Reconstruction: Proceedings, August 1945* (Ottawa: Edmond Cloutier, King's Printer, 1945), v–ix.
37 On the growth and quality of the federal bureaucracy, see J.L. Granatstein, *The Ottawa Men: The Civil Service Mandarins, 1935–1957* (Toronto: University of Toronto Press, 1982), and Doug Owram, *The Government Generation: Canadian Intellectuals and the State, 1900–1945* (Toronto: University of Toronto Press, 1986). On the quality of the Saskatchewan bureaucracy during the Douglas government, see A.W. Johnson with Rosemary Proctor, *Dream No Little Dreams: A Biography of the Douglas Government of Saskatchewan, 1944–1961* (Toronto: University of Toronto Press, 2004); Robert I. McLaren, *The Saskatchewan Practice of Public Administration in Historical Perspective* (New York: Edwin Mellen, 1998); and Robert I. McLaren, "George Woodall Cadbury: The Fabian Catalyst in Saskatchewan's 'Good Public Administration,'" *Canadian Public Administration* 38, no. 4 (1995): 471–80.
38 PAS, TCD, second of seven folders, Federal-Provincial Conferences, memorandum, J.W. Corman (attorney general, Government of Saskatchewan) to all ministers, 26 July 1945.

39 Robert Bothwell, Ian Drummond and John English, *Canada since 1945: Power, Politics and Provincialism*, rev. ed. (Toronto: University of Toronto Press, 1989), 75.
40 George M. Abbott, "Duff Pattullo and the Coalition Controversy of 1941," *BC Studies*, no. 102 (1994): 30–53; Jean Barman, *The West beyond the West: A History of British Columbia*, 3rd ed. (Toronto: University of Toronto Press, 2007), 278–9.
41 Gregory P. Marchildon, "Douglas versus Manning: The Ideological Battle over Medicare in Postwar Canada," *Journal of Canadian Studies* 50, no. 1 (2016): 133–4.
42 LAC, Hon. Brooke Claxton fonds, MG 32 B5, vol. 139, file Committee on Social Security, Proposals of the Government of Canada: Dominion-Provincial Conference on Reconstruction (Green Book Proposals), August 1945.
43 *Dominion-Provincial Conference on Reconstruction: Proceedings*, 5–6.
44 PAS, TCD, second of seven folders, Federal-Provincial Conferences, memorandum, J.W. Corman (attorney general, Government of Saskatchewan) to all ministers, 26 July 1945.
45 Bercuson, *True Patriot*, 141.
46 McLeod and McLeod, *Tommy Douglas*, 137.
47 Maurice Duplessis's opening remarks, quoted in Canada, *Dominion-Provincial Conference on Reconstruction: Proceedings*, 20.
48 Douglas, quoted in *Dominion-Provincial Conference on Reconstruction: Proceedings*, 35, 49.
49 *Dominion-Provincial Conference on Reconstruction: Proceedings*, 36.
50 For a balanced portrait of Duplessis's ideological orientation – in terms of both social policy and federalism – see Marcel Sarra-Bournet's entry for Duplessis in *Dictionary of Canadian Biography*, vol. 18, http://www.biographi.ca/en/bio/duplessis_maurice_le_noblet_18E.html.
51 Sean Mills, "When Democratic Socialists Discovered Democracy: The League for Social Reconstruction Confronts the Quebec Problem," *Canadian Historical Review* 86, no. 1 (2005): 8–17; Thérèse Casgrain, "The Achievements of F.R. Scott," in *On F.R. Scott: Essays on His Contributions to Law, Literature, and Politics*, ed. Sandra Djwa and R. St. J. Macdonald (Montreal and Kingston: McGill-Queen's University Press, 1983), 4.
52 Canada, *Dominion-Provincial Conference on Reconstruction: Proceedings*, 90–2.
53 Owram, *The Government Generation*, 319–21.
54 PAS, TCD, second of seven folders, Federal-Provincial Conferences, letter, T.C. Douglas to Frank R. Scott, 21 June 1945.
55 Canada, *Dominion-Provincial Conference on Reconstruction: Proceedings*, 171–2.

56 Douglas, quoted in McLeod and McLeod, *Tommy Douglas*, 137.
57 P.E. Bryden, *A Justifiable Obsession: Conservative Ontario's Relations with Ottawa, 1943–1985* (Toronto: University of Toronto Press, 2013), 23–6; McLeod and McLeod, *Tommy Douglas*, 137.
58 Alex Skelton quoted in Bryden, *A Justifiable Obsession*, 24.
59 PAS, TCD, fourth of seven folders, Federal-Provincial Conferences, letters, Brooke Claxton to T.C. Douglas, 22 Aug. 1945, and Alex Skelton to H. McLeod, 23 Aug. 1945.
60 PAS, TCD, fourth of seven folders, Federal-Provincial Conferences, letter, T.C. Douglas to M.C. Sheps, 8 Sept. 1945.
61 PAS, TCD, second of seven folders, Federal-Provincial Conferences, memorandum relating to public health services in the province of Saskatchewan together with an analysis of the proposals of the Dominion government in regard to such services as prepared for the Saskatchewan brief for the Dominion-Provincial Conference, 26 Nov. 1945
62 Blair Fraser, "Here's Plain Talk on What the Dominion-Provincial Conferences Mean to You and Why We Must Make Confederation Work," *Maclean's*, 15 March 1946.
63 "Saskatchewan Replies to the Dominion Government Proposals," 9 Jan. 1946, in *Dominion and Provincial Conference (1945): Dominion and Provincial Submissions and Plenary Conference Discussion* (Ottawa: Edmond Cloutier, King's Printer, 1946), 249–313.
64 PAS, TCD, fifth of seven folders, Federal-Provincial Conferences, "Saskatchewan's Reply," clipping from *Saskatoon Star-Phoenix*, 10 Jan. 1946.
65 Bryden, *A Justifiable Obsession*, 28–9; Bercuson, *True Patriot*, 142–3.
66 Bryden, *A Justifiable Obsession*, 31.
67 LAC, Hon. Brooke Claxton fonds, MG 32 B5, vol. 142, file Dominion-Provincial Reconstruction Conference 1945, Coordinating and Economic Committees, telegram, T.C. Douglas to W.L. Mackenzie King, 12 July 1946, and King's telegram response to T.C., 15 July 1946.
68 PAS, TCD, seven of seven folders, Federal-Provincial Conferences, T.C. Douglas to Mackenzie King, 13 Nov. 1946; LAC, Hon. Brooke Claxton fonds, MG 32 B5, vol. 142, file Dominion-Provincial Reconstruction Conference 1945, Coordinating and Economic Committees, letter, W.L. Mackenzie King to T.C. Douglas, 22 Nov. 1946.
69 PAS, TCD, seven of seven folders, Federal-Provincial Conferences, T.C. Douglas to Louis St-Laurent, 15 July 1949.
70 PAS, TCD, seven of seven folders, Federal-Provincial Conferences, T.C. Douglas to Florence, 6 Sept. 1960.
71 Bercuson, *True Patriot*, 140.
72 See Marc J. Gotlieb, "George Drew and the Dominion-Provincial Conference on Reconstruction of 1945–6," *Canadian Historical Review* 66,

540   Notes to pages 141–5

no. 1 (1985): 27–47; Bothwell, Drummond, and English, *Canada since 1945*, 74–81; Owram, *The Government Generation*, 322–5; and Finkel "Paradise Postponed."
73 Douglas, *The Making of a Socialist*, 216.

## 6. Universal Hospital Insurance in Saskatchewan

1 T.C. Douglas, quoted in Seymour Martin Lipset, *Agrarian Socialism: The Cooperative Commonwealth Federation in Saskatchewan: A Study in Political Sociology* (1950; Berkeley: University of California Press, 1971, orig. 1950), 313.
2 Von Braun, quoted in Michael J. Neufeld, *Von Braun: Dreamer of Space, Engineer of War* (New York: Alfred A. Knopf, 2007), 447.
3 Yale University Library, Manuscripts and Archives (YUA), Leonard Sidney Rosenfeld fonds (LSR), MS 1360, m-011, box 3, folder 1, "The Saskatchewan Hospital Services Plan" (unpublished manuscript, 1948), 2; Malcolm G. Taylor, *Health Insurance and Canadian Public Policy: The Seven Decisions That Created the Canadian Health Insurance System and Its Outcomes*, 2nd ed. (Montreal and Kingston: McGill-Queen's University Press, 2009), 91.
4 Since income and corporate tax had been "rented" to the federal government, Fines's options were largely limited to an increase in the provincial sales tax. When the Douglas government took office, there was already a 2 per cent sales tax on everything. In 1946, the sales tax was increased by 1 per cent, but commodities such as "grocery products, drugs, school books, farm implements, fertilizers, weed sprays, [farm] chemicals, and farm fuels" were exempted from the new tax. T.C. Douglas, *The Making of a Socialist: The Recollections of T.C. Douglas*, ed. Lewis H. Thomas (Edmonton: University of Alberta Press, 1982), 227.
5 In its first term of office, the Douglas government collected roughly 50 per cent of its own revenues, depending on the federal transfers for the rest, principally the sum allocated under the income tax transfer arrangement: A.W. Johnson with Rosemary Proctor, *Dream No Little Dreams: A Biography of the Douglas Government of Saskatchewan, 1944–1961* (Toronto: University of Toronto Press, 2004), 333.
6 Library and Archives Canada (LAC), Frederick Dodge Mott fonds, MG31 J15 (hereafter FDM), vol. 32, file 5 – Saskatchewan General, 1948–1949, memorandum entitled "Medical Care Program for Public Assistance Beneficiaries of Saskatchewan: Review and Recommendations," Milton I. Roemer (Public Health Service, Washington, DC) to F.D. Mott, 2 March 1948.
7 Provincial Archives of Saskatchewan (PAS), Jean Larmour oral history of the CCF Government (hereafter Larmour history), R-8251 to R-8352, T.C. Douglas interview, 15 June 1981, transcript, 20.

8 LAC, FDM, vol. 32, file 5 – Saskatchewan General, 1948–1949, memorandum entitled "Medical Care Program for Public Assistance Beneficiaries of Saskatchewan: Review and Recommendations," Milton I. Roemer to F.D. Mott, 2 March 1948.
9 Richard B. Saltman and Hans F.W. Dubois, "The Historical and Social Base of Social Health Insurance Systems," in *Social Health Insurance Systems in Western Europe*, ed. Richard B. Saltman, Reinhard Busse, and Josep Figueras (Maidenhead, UK: World Health Organization on behalf of the European Observatory on Health Systems and Policies, 2004), 22–5. Immediately after the release of the Beveridge Report, Henry E. Sigerist published his influential article on the history and impact of Bismarck's scheme: "From Bismarck to Beveridge: Developments and Trends in Social Security Legislation." *Bulletin of the History of Medicine* 13, no. 4 (1943): 365–88.
10 Charles Webster, *The National Health Service: A Political History* (Oxford: Oxford University Press, 2002), 10–29. On the vast literature spawned on the history of the NHS and the contrasting historical interpretations, see Martin Gorsky, "The British National Health Service 1948–2008: A Review of the Historiography," *Social History of Medicine* 21, no. 3 (2008): 437–60.
11 PAS, Department of Public Health HSPC fonds, R-326, file 159 on the New Zealand scheme. Although not implemented in the way the Labour government intended (due to the opposition of organized medicine), New Zealand was the first attempt at an NHS-style system: Guido Giarelli and Mike Saks, "Introduction – The National Health Services of Western Europe: A Historical-Comparative Perspective," In *National Health Services of Western Europe: Challenges, Reforms and Future Perspectives*, ed. Guido Giarelli and Mike Saks (Abingdon, UK: Routledge, 2023), 1–2.
12 First elected in 1935, Labour passed the social security scheme in 1938. Implementation occurred in stages beginning in 1939. Philippa Mein Smith, *A Concise History of New Zealand* (Cambridge: Cambridge University Press, 2012), 160–3. In a four-country comparison, historian Theodore Rosenoff explored the reasons why New Zealand and the United States responded to the Great Depression with major social and economic reforms, while Canada and Australia delayed initiating major reforms until after the Second World War: see Theodore Rosenoff, "The Propensity to Reform: The United States, Australia, New Zealand, and Canada Compared," *The Historian* 72, no. 1 (2010): 38–66.
13 This was evident in the articles and correspondence in the PAS, Department of Public Health HSPC fonds, R-326, file 159 on the New Zealand scheme: J.H. Gray, "The Scheme That Failed," *LP*, 17 Oct. 1945; "U.F.C. Stand on N.Z. Health Services," *Saskatchewan Commonwealth*, 24 Oct. 1945; and subsequent correspondence by Fred Mott in 1947–8 discussing the lack of cost control in the New Zealand plan.

14 David Wilson, "Social Security and Health Benefits in New Zealand," *Public Affairs* 9, no. 3 (1946): 172–7; Mein Smith, *Concise History of New Zealand*, 164–5.
15 Hugh MacLean and Dean E. McHenry: "Medical Services in New Zealand," *Milbank Memorial Fund Quarterly* 26, no. 2 (1948); 148–81, and "Medical Services in New Zealand," *Canadian Medical Association Journal* 59, no. 1 (1948): 77–80.
16 PAS, T.J. Bentley fonds, R11, file 14-6, Memorandum (no. 1) entitled "Free Hospitalization," HSPC (M. Sheps) to T.C. Douglas, 1 June 1945.
17 Hospital and equipment construction grants were modest in comparison to the cost of universal hospitalization. For the first six months, from the first grant in March 1945 ($5,000 to the Nipawin Union Hospital Board) until November 1945, the Saskatchewan government expended $27,900 in grants. *Journals of the Legislative Assembly of the Provincial of Saskatchewan (JLAS)*, vol. XLV, session 1946 (Regina: Thomas H. McConica, King's Printer, 1946), 175, 183.
18 PAS, T.J. Bentley fonds, R11, file 14-6, Memorandum (no. 1) entitled Free Hospitalization, HSPC (M. Sheps) to T.C. Douglas, 1 June 1945.
19 Duane Mombourquette, "'An Inalienable Right:' The CCF and Rapid Health Care Reform, 1944–1948," *Saskatchewan History* 43, no. 3 (1991): 106.
20 T.C. Douglas quoted in "Municipalities May Collect Fee – For Hospitalization Plan," *LP*, 19 March 1946, 8; Taylor, *Health Insurance and Canadian Public Policy*, 37, 57, and 94.
21 "Municipalities May Collect Fee – For Hospitalization Plan," *LP*, 19 March 1946, 8.
22 Taylor, *Health Insurance and Canadian Public Policy*, 95.
23 PAS, T.C. Douglas fonds, R33.5 file III 123b (14-6-33), Saskatchewan Hospitalization Act, March 1946–September 1946, and regulations under the act, 23 Aug. 1946.
24 According to the adoption announcement, Samuel Barry Sheps was born on 26 February 1945: Alan Mason Chesney Medical Archives, Johns Hopkins University (JHCA), Henry E. Sigerist Collection, adoption announcement, no date. Sam Sheps grew up in the United States, receiving a BA from Antioch College and a medical degree from Case Western Medical School. He then went on to a distinguished academic career in Canada as a clinical epidemiologist and health services researcher.
25 JHCA, Henry E. Sigerist Collection, series 3 – correspondence S, letter, C.G. Sheps to Henry E. Sigerist, 31 Dec. 1945.
26 *JLAS*, vol. XLV, session 1946, summary of debate on 11 March 1946 (Regina: King's Printer 1946), 199. That day, in response to an opposition question, Douglas informed the legislature that Dr. Mindel Sheps had

"resigned from her position" on 31 January 1946, although she could "be employed from time to time in a consultant capacity."
27 Samuel Barry Sheps was born on 26 February 1945. He was adopted by the Sheps about seven or eight months later.
28 "Dr. Hjertaas New Secretary," *LP*, 30 Jan. 1946, 3.
29 JHCA, Henry E. Sigerist Collection, series 3 – correspondence S, letter, C.G. Sheps to Henry E. Sigerist, 31 Dec. 1945.
30 JHCA, Henry E. Sigerist Collection, series 3 – correspondence S, letter, C.G. Sheps to Henry E. Sigerist, 14 May 1946.
31 T.C. Douglas quoted in "Municipalities May Collect Fee – For Hospitalization Plan," *LP*, 19 March 1946, 8.
32 "First Socialized Health Plan Step," *LP*, 12 March 1946, 1.
33 *JLAS*, vol. XLV, session 1946, Appendix: Budget Speech by C.M. Fines, 14 March 1946, 9.
34 The Saskatchewan Hospitalization Act, SS 1946, c. 82, *JLAS*, vol. XLV, session 1946, 66, 82, 107, 115, 125.
35 "Province Sets Pace Declares Douglas: Towards Full Health Services," *LP*, 16 March 1946, 9.
36 This was most evident in T.C. Douglas's article "Saskatchewan Plans for Health," *Health* 14, no. 6 (1946): 1–3. This piece was reprinted and widely distributed by the Saskatchewan Department of Public Health: PAS, T.C. Douglas fonds, R33, file 580 (14-31).
37 *JLAS*, vol. XLV, session 1946, index, Saskatchewan Hospitalization Act 1946.
38 This assertion is based on a systematic review of all questions put to T.C. Douglas by opposition MLAs during the 1946 session, as reproduced in the *JLAS* 1946.
39 The only exception was Clarence Gibson, the former administrator (what today would be the CEO) of the General Hospital in Regina, but Gibson left the HSPC on 1 September 1946, a tenure of less than twenty months: *Annual Report of the Health Services Planning Commission 1946* (Regina: Thomas H. McConica, King's Printer, 1949), 7.
40 Taylor, *Health Insurance and Canadian Public Policy*, 80–1.
41 *JLAS*, vol. XLV, session 1946, Appendix: Budget Speech by C.M. Fines, 14 March 1946.
42 LAC, FDM, vol. 32, file 5 – Saskatchewan General, 1948–1949, "Province-Wide Hospitalization in Saskatchewan," by Len Rosenfeld, spring 1947. Rosenfeld submitted a revised version of this paper to a short-lived medical journal *The Interne* in April 1947. Although the manuscript was accepted for publication many months later, it was never published, due to the demise of the journal: YUA, LSR, MS 1360, m-011, box 3, folder 1, letters: James E. Jeffries (managing editor) to Leonard S. Rosenfeld

544   Notes to pages 154–6

(vice-chairman, HSPC), 15 July 1948, and William Ruberman (editor) to Leonard S. Rosenfeld, 6 Nov. 1950, with attachments.
43 George V. Ferguson, "The Newspapers of Canada: Characteristics of the Daily Press," *Journalism Quarterly* 23, no. 3 (1946): 313. By 1946, Victor Sifton (son of Clifford Sifton) owned the *Regina Leader Post*, the *Saskatoon Star Phoenix*, and the *Winnipeg Free Press*. The most critical editorials concerning Saskatchewan's new hospital plan appeared in the *Winnipeg Free Press* in 1947. LAC, FDM, vol. 32, file 4 – Saskatchewan General 1947, "Saskatchewan Health Policy," by Isabel Atkinson, *Winnipeg Free Press* pamphlet no. 18. The pamphlet was made up of a series of Atkinson's editorials on the Saskatchewan Hospital Services Plan published in the *Free Press* in October 1947. Her last *Free Press* editorial ended on a remarkably negative, if not misleading, note: "Plans for general progress in Saskatchewan may well have been wrecked, for the time being, by the haste and improvidence with which provincial hospitalization were introduced."
44 PAS, T.C. Douglas fonds, R33.5, file III 133b (14-24), College of Physicians and Surgeons, letter, College of Physicians and Surgeons to physicians, 27 Jan. 1945.
45 PAS, T.J. Bentley fonds, R11, file 14-41, "Group Practice" radio address, Aug. 1946 (exact date not given).
46 Douglas, *Making of a Socialist*, 230.
47 Mott, quoted in J.T.H. Connor, "'One Foot on Each Side of the Border': Dr. Frederick Dodge Mott, Rural Health, and 'Socialized' Medical Care in the United States and Canada, 1930s–70s," in *Medicare's Histories: Origins, Omissions, and Opportunities in Canada*, ed. Esyllt Jones, James Hanley, and Delia Gavrus (Winnipeg: University of Manitoba Press, 2022), 59.
48 LAC, FDM, vol. 48, file 25 – biographical material, F.D. Mott's CV, 1964.
49 J.T.H. Connor, "'One Simply Doesn't Arbitrate Authorship of Thoughts': Socialized Medicine, Medical McCarthyism, and the Publishing of Rural Health and Medical Care (1948)," *Journal of the History of Medicine and Allied Sciences* 72, no. 3 (2017): 246; Frederick D. Mott, "A Public Health Program for Rural Areas," *Public Health Reports* 61, no. 17 (1946): 589–98.
50 LAC, FDM, vol. 48, file 25 – biographical material, F.D. Mott's CV, 1964; Mott, "Public Health Program."
51 Frederick D. Mott and M.I. Roemer, "A Federal Program of Public Health and Medical Services for Migratory Farm Workers," *Public Health Reports* 60, no. 9 (1945): 229–49. Also see Connor, "'One Foot on Each Side of the Border,'" 61.
52 Grey, *New Deal Medicine*, ix; Connor, "'One Foot on Each Side of the Border,'" 61.

53 Gordon R. Doss, "John R. Mott, 1865–1955: Mission Leader Extraordinaire," *Journal of Applied Christian Leadership* 4, no. 1 (2010): 72–81. Also see Connor, "'One Foot on Each Side of the Border,'" 58–60; and Grey, *New Deal Medicine*, ix.
54 LAC, FDM, vol. 45, file 8 – correspondence Do–Du, letter, F.D. Mott to T.C. Douglas, 14 Feb. 1946.
55 Grey, *New Deal Medicine*, 169.
56 LAC, FDM, vol. 45, file 8 – correspondence Do–Du, letter, F.D. Mott to T.C. Douglas, 16 March 1946.
57 LAC, FDM, vol. 45, file 8 – correspondence Do–Du, letter, F.D. Mott to T.C. Douglas, 16 March 1946.
58 Douglas, *Making of a Socialist*, 230.
59 LAC, FDM, vol. 48, file 28, Government of Saskatchewan press release (no. 2), 19 June 1946.
60 LAC, FDM, vol. 48, file 28, Government of Saskatchewan press release (no. 2), 19 June 1946.
61 "Dr. F.D. Mott named Health Chairmanship," *LP*, 19 June 1946, 3; "Dr. F. Mott Heads Health Commission," *Saskatoon Star Phoenix (SP)*, 21 June 1946, 4.
62 Editorial, "A Promising Appointment," *LP*, 21 June 1946, 13.
63 *Saskatchewan Medical Quarterly* 10, no. 4 (1946): 11.
64 LAC, FDM, MG31 J15, vol. 45, file 8 – correspondence Do–Du, letter, T.C. Douglas to F.D. Mott, 11 April 1946.
65 There was no mention of the Rosenfeld question in Mott's letter to Douglas on 15 May 1946, but he references a telephone call between the two on 26 April, in which Mott may have finally convinced Douglas that Rosenfeld's experience would be invaluable to the design and implementation of hospitalization: LAC, FDM, vol. 45, file 8 – correspondence Do–Du.
66 YUA, LSR, MS 1360, m-011, box 3, folder 1, handwritten note by L.S. Rosenfeld on Hotel Saskatchewan stationary, n.d. [1946].
67 PAS, Larmour history, R-8446 to R-8448, transcript 2 of interview with T.H. McLeod, 28 Nov. 1981, 6.
68 Frederick D. Mott and Milton I. Roemer, *Rural Health and Medical Care* (New York: McGraw-Hill, 1948); Lewis E. Weeks, *Milton I. Roemer – In First Person: An Oral History* (Chicago: American Hospital Association, 1984), 6.
69 See Connor, "'One Simply Doesn't Arbitrate Authorship of Thoughts.'" The McCarthyite right identified Mott as a member of a group of so-called communist sympathizers working in New Deal agencies: see Alan Derickson, "The House of Falk: The Paranoid Style in American Health Politics," *American Journal of Public Health* 87, no. 11 (1997): 1836–43.

70 Mott's early publications clearly reflected these values and interests. See Frederick D. Mott, "Health Services for Migrant Farm Families," *American Journal of Public Health* 35, no. 4 (1945): 308–14, and "Public Health Program for Rural Areas."
71 LAC, FDM, letter and report, M.I. Roemer to F.D. Motta, 1 March 1968.
72 Letter, M.I. Roemer to Henry Sigerist, 8 Aug. 1953, and reply, 14 Aug. 1953, in Marcel H. Bickel, *Correspondence: Henry E. Sigerist–Milton I. Roemer, 1937–1957* (Berne: Institute of the History of Medicine, University of Berne), 86–7.
73 As noted in his obituary in the *Los Angeles Times* on 10 January 2001 (https://www.latimes.com/archives/la-xpm-2001-jan-10-me-10636-story.html), Roemer (1916–2001) was a professor at Cornell, then Yale, and finally the University of California at Los Angeles in the Department of Health Services in the School of Public Health. He was the author of thirty-two books and 430 articles. He also provided health policy and systems advice in seventy-one countries in his life. His *magnus opus*, entitled *National Health Systems of the World*, was published in two volumes by Oxford University Press in 1991 and 1993.
74 Emily K. Abel, Elizabeth Fee, and Theodore M. Brown, "Milton I. Roemer: Advocate of Social Medicine, International Health and National Health Insurance," *American Journal of Public Health* 98, no. 9 (2008): 1596–7.
75 SARM Convention statement (1944), quoted in Taylor, *Health Insurance and Canadian Public Policy*, 85.
76 Taylor, *Health Insurance and Canadian Public Policy*, 102.
77 Taylor, *Health Insurance and Canadian Public Policy*, 95.
78 YUA, LSR, MS 1360, m-011, box 3, folder 1, memorandum, Edgar H. Clapp to F.D. Mott (Chair, HSPC), 7 Oct. 1946.
79 Malcolm G. Taylor, "The Saskatchewan Hospital Services Plan: A Study in Compulsory Health Insurance" (PhD diss., University of California at Berkeley, 1949), 220.
80 PAS, T.C. Douglas fonds, R 33.5, file III 123c (14-6-33), HSPC, regulations under the Saskatchewan Hospitalization Act, 1946, Order-in-Council No. 1569, 24 Sept. 1946.
81 YUA, LSR, MS 1360, m-011, box 3, folder 1, memorandum, L.D. Rosenfeld to F.D. Mott, 7 Oct. 1946, p. 4.
82 YUA, LSR, MS 1360, m-011, box 3, folder 1, memoranda: F.D. Mott's record of discussion with Jack Marshall, 23 Sept. 1946; L.S. Rosenfeld to F.D. Mott, 25 Sept. 1946; G.W. Myers (Inspection Accountant) to F.D Mott, 27 Sept. 1946; L.S. Rosenfeld to F.D. Mott, 7 Oct. 1946; and notes on meeting with F.D. Mott, L.S. Rosenfeld, Kirk, Gibson, Myers, E. Clapp and J.H.B. Gann, held in Hotel Saskatchewan on 9 Oct. 1946.
83 YUA, LSR, MS 1360, m-011, box 3, folder 1, memorandum, Edgard H. Clapp to F.D. Mott (chair, HSPC), 7 Oct. 1946.

84 YUA, LSR, MS 1360, m-011, box 3, folder 1, memorandum, Edgard H. Clapp to F.D. Mott (chair, HSPC), 7 Oct. 1946.
85 Douglas, *Making of a Socialist*, 230–1.
86 T.C. Douglas quoted in "Douglas," *SP*, 6 Nov. 1946, 5.
87 PAS, T.C. Douglas fonds, R 33.5, file III 123a (14-6-33), speaking points for HSPC presentation at SHA Convention, 5 Nov. 1946.
88 Douglas, *Making of a Socialist*, 229.
89 Carolyn Tuohy, *Remaking Policy: Scale, Pace and Political Strategy in Health Care Reform* (Toronto: University of Toronto Press, 2018), 25, 53–5; Cristóbal Cuadrado et al., "National Health Insurance: A Conceptual Framework from Conflicting Typologies," *Health Policy* 23, no. 7 (2019): 621–8.
90 PAS, Larmour history, R-8446 to R-8448, transcript 2 of interview with T.H. McLeod, 28 Nov. 1981, 21.
91 Taylor, *Health Insurance and Canadian Public Policy*, 103.
92 "Hospitalization Card No. 1 Given to Premier," *LP*, 20 Dec. 1946, 3.
93 "Hospitalization Card No. 1 Given to Premier," *LP*, 20 Dec. 1946, 3.
94 Douglas, *The Making of a Socialist*, 231; "He's First Baby," *LP*, 2 Jan. 1947, 1.
95 "Hospital Tax Payments Over $2,285,000 Mark by Thursday," *LP*, 2 Jan. 1947, 3.
96 *Annual Report of the Health Services Planning Commission 1947* (Regina: Thomas H. McConica, King's Printer, 1949), 20; *Annual Report of the Health Services Planning Commission 1948* (Regina: Thomas H. McConica, King's Printer, 1950), 16.
97 *Annual Report of the Health Services Planning Commission 1947*, 12–13; *Annual Report of the HSPC 1948*, 15.
98 *Annual Report of the Health Services Planning Commission 1947*, 14–15.
99 *Annual Report of the Health Services Planning Commission 1947*, 15–17; *Annual Report of the Health Services Planning Commission 1948*, 18–19.
100 This included residents in the Swift Current Health Region, which ceded its hospital plan in favour of the provincial plan.
101 Taylor, *Health Insurance and Canadian Public Policy*, 104.
102 PAS, Premier's Office, file 5.3, letter, Sidney Riden (British Columbia Health Insurance Commission) to Thomas H. McLeod (HSPC), 25 May 1946, reply by McLeod, 28 May 1946. British Columbia's interest in health insurance was spurred in part because it had had a social health insurance statute on the books since 1936 but the implementation of the bill "was indefinitely postponed," even after amendments were made to address the criticism of the bill by provincial manufacturers' associations and the British Columbia Medical Association. Taylor, *Health Insurance and Canadian Public Policy*, 6.
103 Taylor, *Health Insurance and Canadian Public Policy*, 163; Greg Donaghy, *Grit: The Life and Politics of Paul Martin Sr.* (Vancouver: UBC Press, 2015), 80–6.

104 In 1957, Martin jokingly told Douglas that Mott should run for the CCF in Martin's own constituency (presumably after Martin retired) so that in the future he would be "available as Minister of Health for Canada's first CCF government." LAC, Frederick Dodge Mott fonds, vol. 48, file 8, letter, T.C. Douglas to F.D. Mott, 22 May 1957.
105 Government of Canada, House of Commons Debates (HCD), 4 March 1949, 1144.
106 CCF (Sask. Section) advertisement for "Progress with Security," *LP*, 15 June 1948, 5.
107 "Tucker Sees Doubled Fees," *LP*, 1 June 1948, 18, 23; "C.C.F. Health Plan Said Inadequate," *LP*, 16 June 1948, 15. Douglas responded by warning the public that "throwing it back on the municipalities" would be tantamount to scrapping hospitalization: "Choices Defined," *LP*, 11 June 1948, 6.
108 Bill Waiser, *Saskatchewan: A New History* (Calgary: Fifth House, 2005), 350.
109 CCF (Sask. Section) advertisement, *LP*, 1 June 1948, 5, and *SP*, 1 June 1948, 5.
110 "We Stand on our Record," *LP*, 18 June 1948, 17.
111 Liberal Party of Saskatchewan advertisement, *LP*, 19 June 1948, 15.
112 "Douglas Would Quit if Land Socialized," *LP*, 4 June 1948, 5.
113 T.C. Douglas, quoted in "Douglas Weyburn Choice," *LP*, 5 June 1948, 1.
114 T.C. Douglas, quoted in "Premier Discusses," *LP*, 10 June 1948, 9.
115 CCF (Sask. Section) advertisement, *LP*, 21 June 1948, 15.
116 PAS, Larmour history, transcript R-8343 to R-8345, interview with George Cadbury, 22 Jan. 1982, 25–6.
117 Douglas told Tommy Shoyama that he would never again fight an election on the government's record – it would instead have to be based on future intentions: PAS, Larmour history, R-8457 to R-8458, transcript 1 of interview with T.K. Shoyama, 4 Nov. 1981, 28.
118 "Douglas at Weyburn," *LP*, 5 June 1948, 1, 5. On this opposition and its longer-term legacy, see Gregory P. Marchildon, "Physicians and Regionalization in Canada: Past, Present and Future," *Canadian Medical Association Journal* 189, no. 36: E1147–49.
119 This was illustrated in the case of the Swift Current Health Region, where Douglas accepted the FFS payment agreement made by the health board and the local doctors.
120 LAC, FDM, vol. 45, file 8 – correspondence Do–Du, letter, T.C. Douglas to F.D. Mott, 2 July 1952.
121 "Emphasis on Social Security," *LP*, 4 June 1948, 13. Immediately following the election, Douglas stated that introducing medical care coverage would be a priority of his government in its second term: "Douglas Pledges Five-Point Plan," *LP*, 28 June 1948, 3.

122 PAS, Larmour history, transcript R-8343 to R-8345, interview with George Cadbury, 22 Jan. 1982 (with extracts of Cadbury's letter to Lionel Elvin, principal of Ruskin College in Oxford, 24 Feb. 1947), 41–2.
123 Letter, George Cadbury to Lionel Elvin, 5 Dec. 1948, in PAS, Larmour history, transcript R-8343 to R-8345, interview with George Cadbury, 22 Jan. 1982, 54.

## 7. National Health Grants and New Frontiers

1 George Cadbury, "Planning in Saskatchewan," in *Essays on the Left: Essays in Honour of T.C. Douglas*, ed. Laurier LaPierre, Jack McLeod, Charles Taylor, and Walter Young (Toronto: McClelland and Stewart, 1971), 51.
2 Provincial Archives of Saskatchewan (PAS), T.C. Douglas fonds (TCD), R-33.1, box X.395, file XXIII.745f (23-22-1), folder 6, Federal-Provincial Conferences, telegram, Mackenzie King to Douglas, 15 July 1946.
3 PAS, TCD, R-33.1, box X.395, file XXIII.745f (23-22-1), folder 7, Federal-Provincial Conferences, letter, Douglas to Mackenzie King, 13 Nov. 1946; Library and Archives Canada (LAC), Paul Martin fonds, MG 32, B12, vol. 15, file 11, Memorandum on Health Insurance: Preliminary Steps for Cabinet Consideration, April 1948.
4 PAS, TCD, R-33.1, box X.395, file XXIII.745f (23-22-1), folder 7, Federal-Provincial Conferences, memorandum, J.W. Corman to Douglas, 4 Sept. 1947, with attached article by Chris Higginbotham for the British United Press (BUP), marked BUP, Winnipeg, and dated 22 Aug. 1947, in Regina (hereafter Higginbotham article, 22 Aug. 1947).
5 Higginbotham article, 22 Aug. 1947.
6 Malcolm G. Taylor, *Health Insurance and Canadian Public Policy: The Seven Decisions That Created the Canadian Health Insurance System and Its Outcomes* (Montreal and Kingston: McGill-Queen's University Press, 1978), 162–3.
7 Greg Donaghy, *Grit: The Life and Politics of Paul Martin Sr.* (Vancouver: UBC Press, 2015), 102.
8 PAS, T.J. Bentley fonds (TJB), file 14-6-31, letter, F.D. Mott to T.C. Douglas, 17 May 1948.
9 The decision approving the National Health Grants program was made on 13 May 1948: see Donaghy, *Grit*, 92.
10 Donaghy, *Grit*, 88.
11 Donaghy, *Grit*, 89.
12 Donaghy, *Grit*, 89–90.
13 Donaghy, *Grit*, 91.
14 This episode is recounted in detail in Donaghy, *Grit*, 91–2.

15 LAC, Paul Martin fonds, MG 32, B12, vol. 31, file 14, statement by the prime minister on Health Services and Health Insurance, House of Commons, 14 May 1948.
16 Donaghy, *Grit*, 91–2. Paul Martin was extremely grateful to the PM for his support and wrote him a glowing letter to thank him for "obtaining the concurrence of our Cabinet Colleagues with regard to our health proposals" and admitting that King's "leadership" and "influence" were "the decisive factors in bringing about the decision" in cabinet: LAC, Paul Martin fonds, vol. 15, file 11, letter, Paul Martin to Mackenzie King, 14 May 1948.
17 PAS, TJB, R-11, file 14-6-48, Dominion Health Grants – General, 1948, letter, Paul Martin to T.C. Douglas, 4 Aug. 1948.
18 This evidence was reflected in T.C. Douglas's lengthy interview with Jean Larmour of the Saskatchewan Archives conducted over various sessions in 1981 and 1982.
19 PAS, TCD, R-33.1, box X.395, file XXIII.745f (23-22-1): folders 6–7, Federal-Provincial Conferences: telegram, Douglas to Mackenzie King, 12 July 1946, and letter, Douglas to Mackenzie King, 13 Nov. 1946.
20 T.C. Douglas, *Making of a Socialist: The Recollections of T.C. Douglas*, ed. Lewis H. Thomas (Edmonton: University of Alberta Press, 1982), 127.
21 Although Paul Martin consistently used the term "National Health Program," the term generally accepted in the secondary literature and used by his own department was "National Health Grants Program." LAC, Paul Martin fonds, MG 32, B12, vol. 40, file 2, memorandum, National Health Grants Program (Main Features), 15 June 1955; Paul Martin, "A National Health Program for Canada," *Canadian Journal of Public Health / Revue canadienne de santé publique* 39, no. 6 (1948): 219–26; G.D.W. Cameron, "A New National Health Program for Canada," *American Journal of Public Health* 38, no. 12 (1948): 1643–52.
22 Between the fiscal years 1948–9 and 1956–7, the federal government transferred $16.5 million to Saskatchewan under the National Health Grants Program: LAC, Paul Martin fonds, MG 32, B12, vol. 32, file 11, memorandum, Assistance to the Province of Saskatchewan under the National Health Program, 1948–57: Expenditures by Year, February 1957. This document lists the contributions made over this same period to construct, expand, or refurbish ninety-four hospitals in the province, including the Weyburn Union Hospital ($91,145) and the Weyburn mental hospital ($133,500) in Douglas's own constituency. The single largest hospital construction grant ($492,824) went to University Hospital in Saskatoon.
23 Cameron, "New National Health Program," 1644.
24 "$5,000 Each Hour for Health," *Regina Leader-Post* (*LP*), 30 July 1949, 1.

25 Martin, "National Health Program," 220–4. The two areas in which the National Health Grants deviated from the original Green Book proposals were the addition of the grant for cancer control and the replacement of low-interest loans with outright grants for hospital construction: LAC, Paul Martin fonds, MG 32, B12, vol. 40, file 2, National Health Grants Program (Main Features), 15 June 1955.
26 PAS, TJB, R-11, file 14-6-48. Dominion Health Grants – General, 1948, memorandum, F.W. Jackson, Department of National Health and Welfare, 14 Jan. 1949; PAS, C.M. Fines fonds, F119, R-37, I-30, Specific Proposals of the Dominion Government Regarding Health Grants to the Provinces, table prepared by HSPC, n.d. (c. 1948).
27 PAS, TJB, R-11, file 14-6-10, Advisory Committee to HSPC, minutes of Advisory Committee meeting, 29 Oct. 1948.
28 Taylor would remain in this position until 1951, when he moved to Ontario to work as a health policy consultant and academic. A. Paul Williams, "In Tribute to Malcolm Gordon Taylor, 1915–1994," *Health and Canadian Society / Santé et société canadienne* 3, no. 1–2 (1995): 9.
29 Taylor, *Health Insurance*, 435n81.
30 Taylor would submit the final dissertation in March 1949 while working at HSPC. Malcolm G. Taylor, "The Saskatchewan Hospital Services Plan: A Study in Compulsory Health Insurance" (PhD diss., University of California at Berkeley, 1949). His dissertation was then mimeographed for limited distribution by the HSPC, as my own University of Toronto library copy of his dissertation attests. Stuart Houston and Bill Waiser, *Tommy's Team: The People Behind the Douglas Years* (Calgary: Fifth House, 2010), 204–8. Taylor was born in rural Alberta. A teacher during the Great Depression, he saved enough money to attend the University of California at Berkeley where he earned a BA (1942), an MA (1943), and his PhD in 1949.
31 "Singapore Job for Acker," *LP*, 21 Sept. 1956, 23. Dr. Murray Acker, a medical doctor and public health graduate originally from Toronto, was also an expert in the use of administrative and other data to better plan and manage health systems. Representative publications included "Administration and Methods of Enumeration of the Sickness Survey in Saskatchewan," *Canadian Journal of Public Health* 44, no. 4 (1953): 128–33, and (with Lloyd G. Williams) "Statistics of Medical and Hospital Care Programs: Their Use of the Coordination of Health Services," *American Journal of Public Health and the Nation's Health* 46, no. 9 (1956): 1121–9.
32 For the fiscal years 1949–51, Saskatchewan was first among the provinces in accessing the health grants available through the program: PAS, TJB, R-11, file 14-6-48, Dominion Health Grants – General, 1951–1956, memorandum, G.C. Darby to F.D. Mott, 14 Feb. 1951.

33 "Grants Proposed," *Saskatoon Star Phoenix* (*SP*), 15 March 1949, 3.
34 "Hospital X-Rays Planned in All-Out Fight on T.B.," *LP*, 19 Jan. 1948, 3; "Hospital for Handicapped," *SP*, 18 Feb. 1949, 3; "$234,571 Assistance on Cancer," *LP*, 7 March 1949, 3; "Federal Grant for Equipment," *LP*, 9 Feb. 1951, 3.
35 "Hospital Accountants to Get Short Courses," *LP*, 14 Feb. 1949, 3.
36 "Ottawa Will Grant Funds to City for Health Extension," *SP*, 24 Dec. 1948, 3.
37 "Funds Provided for Nutritionists," *SP*, 3 March 1949, 12.
38 At the ceremony opening the Foam Lake Union Hospital, for example, Douglas was listed at the second speaker after Martin: "Leaders at Foam Lake," *LP*, 10 May 1949, 2. The *Regina Leader-Post* advertised Martin's attendance the day before but made no mention of Douglas: "Martin at Opening Foam Lake Hospital," *LP*, 9 May 1949, 2.
39 LAC, Paul Martin fonds, MG 32, B12, vols 110–14, covering "National health plan" from March 1948 until December 1953.
40 Rosthern was viewed as a relatively safe Liberal seat. However, knowing that a federal general election would soon follow, the Liberal Party of Canada wanted to ensure that the CCF did not gain the seat, and both Paul Martin and Jimmy Gardiner campaigned on behalf of the new Liberal candidate, W.A. Boucher. The CCF candidate was Peter Makaroff, a Saskatoon lawyer who defended the leaders of the Regina Riot. When the votes came in on 25 October 1948, Boucher won by a large plurality of 6,255 votes to Makaroff's 3,278. As an aside, the only other by-election on that date was in Algoma East (Ontario), where Lester B. Pearson was first elected as an MP, albeit with a much smaller margin of victory. "The Rosthern By-Election," *LP*, 23 Oct. 1948, 13; "Rosthern, Algoma East Stay Liberal: W. Boucher, L.B. Pearson Win Federal By-Elections," *SP*, 26 Oct. 1948, 1; John English, *The Worldly Years: The Life of Lester Pearson, 1949–1972* (Toronto: Vintage Canada, 1992), 19.
41 "Martin, Tucker Take Issue with Policy of Social Credit; Speak at Waldheim," *SP*, 19 Oct. 1948, 3.
42 "Election of Boucher Urged by Paul Martin," *LP*, 14 Oct. 1946, 23.
43 "Liberal Victory Predicted," *LP*, 16 Oct. 1948, 3.
44 "Martin Says Health Grants 'Fundamental Prerequisite,'" *SP*, 6 April 1949, 2.
45 PAS, Political Party Pamphlets, GR 122, Co-operative Commonwealth Federation National Office, political pamphlet no. 44, "We're Covered, Why Not You? The Story of Saskatchewan Health Services," Ottawa, 1949.
46 LAC, Hon. Brooke Claxton fonds, MG 32 B5, vol. 155, file Coldwell: Opposition speakers, CBC Free Time political broadcast, M.J. Coldwell, 13 May 1949.

Notes to pages 186–9    553

47  William R. Willoughby, "Canadian Politics," *Political Science Quarterly* 66, no. 1 (1951): 112–16.
48  Malcom G. Taylor, "Government Planning: The Federal-Provincial Health Survey Reports," *Canadian Journal of Economics and Political Science / Revue canadienne d'économique et de science politique* 19, no. 4 (1953): 501–3.
49  *Annual Report of the Health Services Planning Commission 1948* (Regina: Thomas H. McConica, King's Printer, 1950), 12.
50  PAS, TCD, R33.5, III, file 133c (14-24), letter, G. Gordon Ferguson (CPS Registrar) to T.C. Douglas, 12 Nov. 1948.
51  PAS, TCD, R33.5, III, file 133c (14-24), letter, T.C. Douglas to G. Gordon Ferguson, 22 Nov. 1948.
52  Taylor, "Health Survey Reports," 503–5.
53  PAS, TCD, R33.5, III, file 133d (14-24), minutes of the meeting between the Minister of Public Health, the HSPC, and the Medical Advisory Committee of the CPS, 12 Dec. 1948.
54  PAS, TCD, R33.5, III, file 133d (14-24), letter, T.C. Douglas to G. Gordon Ferguson, 29 Dec. 1948.
55  The two final reports reflect this ambiguity, stating that they were submitted by the Health Survey Committee to the government of Saskatchewan. Although the reports were printed by the provincial government, the Health Survey Committee is listed as the author, with a collective letter of transmittal to the minister of public health (Tom Bentley rather than T.C. Douglas by this time), and Bentley's letter of transmittal to Paul Martin, minister of national health and welfare. See *Saskatchewan Health Survey Report*, vol. 1: *Health Programs and Personnel* and vol. 2: *Hospital Survey and Master Plan* (Regina: Saskatchewan Health Survey Committee, 1951).
56  C. Stuart Houston and Richard A. Rempel, "The Life and Legacy of C.J. Houston, Medicare Pioneer," *Saskatchewan History* 67, no. 2 (2015): 33.
57  Houston and Rempel, "Life and Legacy," 33.
58  Ken MacTaggart, *The First Decade: The Story of the Birth of Canadian Medicare and Its Development during the Following 10 Years* (Ottawa: Canadian Medical Association, 1973), 43.
59  "Province Backs Health Survey," *LP*, 27 March 1952, 2; "Health Survey Committee Recommends Provincial Insurance Plan," *SP*, 27 March 1952, 3. Although the report was submitted to the federal government towards the end of 1951, it was not released publicly until March 1952, at Ottawa's request: "Health Survey Took Over 2 Years," *LP*, 27 March 1962, 2.
60  *Saskatchewan Health Survey Report*, 1: 225.
61  Taylor, *Health Insurance and Canadian Public Policy*, 255.
62  C. David Naylor, *Private Practice, Public Payment: Canadian Medicare and the Politics of Health Insurance, 1911–1966* (Montreal and Kingston:

McGill-Queen's University Press, 1986), 165–6; Carolyn Tuohy, "Icon and Taboo: Single-Payer Politics in Canada and the US," *Journal of International and Comparative Social Policy* 35, no. 1 (2019): 7–8.

63 Harley D. Dickinson, *The Two Psychiatries: The Transformation of Psychiatric Work in Saskatchewan, 1905–1984* (Regina: Canadian Plains Research Center, University of Regina, 1989), 77–80. These figures are close to those provided in the *Regina Leader-Post*, which stated that 4,200 patients were crowded into two mental hospitals "built to accommodate 2,700" individuals: see "Crowded Mental Institutions Aided," 3 June 1947, 3.

64 Dickinson, *The Two Psychiatries*, 77–80.

65 John A. Mills, "Lessons from the Periphery: Psychiatry in Saskatchewan, Canada, 1944–68," *History of Psychiatry* 18, no. 2 (2007): 181.

66 In 1937, the Social Credit government of Alberta strengthened the provincial Sexual Sterilization Act by broadening its mandate and removed "the need to collect informed consent in cases where the individual was considered mentally defective": see Erika Dyck, *Facing Eugenics: Reproduction, Sterilization, and the Politics of Choice* (Toronto: University of Toronto Press, 2013), 12. In Dyck's assessment, Manning "maintained the program without further adaptations until his terms as premier ended in 1968" (116). Also see Jana Grekul, Arvey Krahn, and Dave Odynak, "Sterilizing the 'Feeble-Minded': Eugenics in Alberta, Canada, 1929–1972," *Journal of Historical Sociology* 17, no. 4 (2004): 358–84, and Amy Samson, "Eugenics in the Community: Gendered Professions and Eugenic Sterilization in Alberta, 1928–1972," *Canadian Bulletin of Medical History / Bulletin canadien d'histoire de la médecine* 31, no. 1 (2014): 153–9.

67 *LP*, 27 Nov. 1946, 3.

68 Mills, "Lessons from the Periphery," 182; "Toronto Doctor Names Provincial Psychiatrist," *LP*, 23 Nov. 1946, 13.

69 Stuart Houston and Bill Waiser, *Tommy's Team: The People behind the Douglas Years* (Calgary: Fifth House, 2010), 118. See also Gregory P. Marchildon, "The Great Divide," in *The Heavy Hand of History: Interpreting Saskatchewan's Past*, ed. Gregory P. Marchildon (Regina: Canadian Plains Research Center, University of Regina, 2005), 51–66.

70 Douglas, quoted in Colin M. Smith, "Necessity and Creativity: Innovations in Service Delivery in Saskatchewan Pre and Post War," text of unpublished speech delivered to the Saskatchewan Psychiatric Services Annual Clinical Conference, Regina, 16 Oct. 1980, obtained with permission by the author from the Canadian Mental Health Association (CMHA) Resource Centre, Regina.

71 D.G. McKerracher, "Community Psychiatric Developments in Saskatchewan," *Canadian Medical Association Journal* 59, no. 6 (1948): 546–8.

72 D.G. McKerracher, "A New Program in the Training and Employment of Ward Personnel," *American Journal of Psychiatry* 106, no. 4 (1949): 259–64.
73 Veryl Margaret Tipliski, "Parting at the Crossroads: The Emergence of Education for Psychiatric Nursing in Three Canadian Provinces, 1909–1955," *Canadian Bulletin of Medical History / Bulletin canadien d'histoire de la médecine* 21, no. 2 (2004): 265.
74 Tipliski, "Parting at the Crossroads," 266.
75 Mills, "Lessons from the Periphery," 191. I came to the same conclusion as Mills: see Gregory P. Marchildon, "A House Divided: Deinstitutionalization, Medicare and the Canadian Mental Health Association in Saskatchewan, 1944–1964," *Histoire sociale / Social History* 44, no. 88 (2011): 311–29.
76 Dickinson, *The Two Psychiatries*, 100 and 140–4.
77 Menninger, quoted in Milton I. Roemer, "Socialized Health Services in Saskatchewan," *Social Research* 25, no. 1 (1958): 95. It appears that Menninger was in Regina teaching for McKerracher's Resident Training Program as well as giving at least one public lecture on behalf of the Canadian Mental Health Association (Sask. Section) in Indian Head: Kathleen Kendall, "From Closed Ranks to Open Doors: Elaine and John Cummings' Mental Health Education Experiment in 1950s Saskatchewan," *Histoire sociale / Social History* 44, no. 88 (2011): 270.
78 Mills, "Lessons from the Periphery," 184.
79 Dickinson, *The Two Psychiatries*, 175.
80 Marchildon, "A House Divided," 312–29.
81 Mills, "Lessons from the Periphery," 182.
82 Erika Dyck, "Prairies, Psychedelics and Place: The Dynamics of Region in Psychiatric Research," *Health & Place* 15, no. 3 (2009): 659–60.
83 Erika Dyck and Alex Deighton, *Managing Madness: Weyburn Mental Hospital and the Transformation of Psychiatric Care in Canada* (Winnipeg: University of Manitoba Press, 2017), 99–100.
84 Houston and Waiser, *Tommy's Team*, 152–5.
85 See, for example, Humphrey Osmond and John Smythies, "Schizophrenia: A New Approach," *Journal of Mental Science* 98, no. 411 (1952): 309–15; Abram Hoffer, Humphrey Osmond, and John Smythies, "Schizophrenia: A New Approach II: Result of a Year's Research," *Journal of Mental Science* 100, no. 418 (1954): 29–45; and Humphrey Osmond and Abram Hoffer, "Schizophrenia: A New Approach," *Journal of Mental Science* 105, no. 440 (1959): 653–73.
86 Roemer, "Socialized Medical Services in Saskatchewan," 95.
87 Erika Dyck, *Psychedelic Psychiatry: LSD from Clinic to Campus* (Baltimore, MD: Johns Hopkins University Press, 2008).

88 Letter, Aldous Huxley to Humphrey Osmond, 30 March 1956, with Osmond's superimposed verse, in Cynthia Carson Bisbee et al., eds., *Psychedelic Prophets: The Letters of Aldous Huxley and Humphrey Osmond* (Montreal and Kingston: McGill-Queen's University Press, 2018), xx and 226.
89 Aldous Huxley, *The Doors of Perception* (New York: Harper & Row, 1954), 10–12.
90 "Francis Huxley Obituary," *Guardian*, 20 Dec. 2016, https://www.theguardian.com/science/2016/dec/20/francis-huxley-obituary.
91 McKerracher, "Community Psychiatric Developments," 546–8.
92 McKerracher, "Community Psychiatric Developments," 548.
93 Burns Roth described McKerracher as "a very quiet and persuasive man" whose greatest contribution was to use his influence to convince the members of the Saskatchewan chapter of the CMHA "to promote and accept new ideas." PAS, Jean Larmour oral history of CCF government, R-8455, recorded interview with Dr. Burns Roth, tape 2, 18 Nov. 1982.
94 Mills, "Lessons from the Periphery," 183.
95 Marchildon, "A House Divided," 309.
96 PAS, TCD, R-33.1, XIV 572 (14-26), letter, Samuel Laycock to T.C. Douglas, 9 Feb. 1951.
97 Kendall, "From Closed Ranks to Open Doors," 261.
98 Marchildon, "A House Divided," 308–9.
99 Kendall, "From Closed Ranks to Open Doors," 266–8.
100 Chris Dooley, "The End of the Asylum (Town): Community Responses to the Depopulation and Closure of the Saskatchewan Hospital, Weyburn," *Histoire sociale / Social History* 44, no. 88 (2011): 339.
101 Kendall, "From Closed Ranks to Open Doors," 267–78.
102 Elaine Cumming and John Cumming, *Closed Ranks: An Experiment in Mental Health Education* (Cambridge, MA: Harvard University Press, 1957). On this book's development, impact, and reception, see Kendall, "From Closed Ranks to Open Doors," 276–86.
103 For a short biography of Dr. Sam Lawson, see Houston and Waiser, *Tommy's Team*, 87–92.
104 PAS, Jean Larmour oral history of CCF government, R-8455, recorded interview with Dr. Burns Roth, tape 2, 18 Nov. 1982. Roth says that both he and Douglas were unhappy about Lawson's antics, but Roth resisted firing Lawson despite Douglas's dissatisfaction with the psychiatrist.
105 See Marchildon, "A House Divided," where this story is told in much more depth.
106 Dickinson, *The Two Psychiatries*, 147; Hugh G. Lafave, Alex Stewart, and Frederic Grunberg, "Community Care of the Mentally Ill: Implementation of the Saskatchewan Plan," *Community Mental Health* 4, no. 1 (1968): 37–38.

107 PAS, J. Walter Erb fonds, R-34, 172G2, letter, Sam Lawson to Thomas J. Bentley, 1 June 1955.
108 PAS, J. Walter Erb fonds, R-34, 172G2, letter, T.J. Bentley to T.C. Douglas, 5 June 1955.
109 PAS, J. Walter Erb fonds, R-34, 172G2, letter with attachments, Sam Lawson to T.J. Bentley, 14 Nov. 1955.
110 PAS, Psychiatric Unit Papers, R-999, 42, letter, McKerracher to Bentley, 2 Dec. 1955.
111 PAS, TCD, R-33.1, XIV 572 (14-26), memorandum, Sam Lawson to W.J. Erb, 22 Nov. 1956.
112 Dickinson, *The Two Psychiatries*, 154.
113 On the plans, see PAS, W.J. Erb fonds, R-34, 172 G2.
114 PAS, TCD, R-33.1, XIV 572 (14-26), memorandum, T.C. Douglas to W.J. Erb, 31 Jan. 1957, attaching *LP* article entitled "Mental Hospital Plan Discussed," 29 Jan. 1957.
115 PAS, TCD, R-33.1, XIV 572 (14-26), letter, T.C. Douglas to Mrs. M.P. Toombs, 15 March 1957, with attachment of article entitled "Mental Health Aid Criticized," morning edition of *LP*, 15 March 1957.
116 PAS, TCD, R-33.1, XIV 572 (14-26), letter, Mrs. M.P. Toombs to T.C. Douglas, 18 March 1957.
117 PAS, TCD, R-33.1, XIV 572 (14-26), letter, D.G. McKerracher to Douglas, 29 March 1957.
118 PAS, TCD, R-33.1, XIV 572 (14-26), letter, T.C. Douglas to D.G. McKerracher, 8 April 1957.
119 PAS, TCD, R-33.1, XIV 572 (14-26), clipping entitled "Mental Health Needs Neglected" (signed by Mrs. N.M. Toombs, president, and Mr. George Rohn, executive director, CMHA, Saskatchewan Section), *SP*, 13 April 1957.
120 A.W. Johnson with Rosemary Proctor, *Dream No Little Dreams: A Biography of the Douglas Government of Saskatchewan, 1944–1961* (Toronto: University of Toronto Press, 2004), 111–12.

## 8. Next-Year Country

1 Provincial Archives of Saskatchewan (PAS), T.C. Douglas fonds, R-33.1, X, 395c (10-1-1), Executive Council, T.C. Douglas Press Statement, 14 Nov. 1949.
2 PAS, T.C. Douglas fonds, R-33.1, X, 395c (10-1-1), Executive Council, T.C. Douglas Press Statement, 14 Nov. 1949. I italicized the words "and agriculture" because Douglas added these handwritten words into the typed press release.
3 Dwayne Yasinowski, "Thomas J. Bentley," in *Saskatchewan Politicians: Lives Past and Present*, ed. Brett Quiring (Regina: Canadian Plains Research Center, University of Regina, 2004), 18–19.

558   Notes to pages 206–10

4 Although Clarence Hames was still deputy minister when Bentley became minister, the real policy direction in health came from Fred Mott, the HSPC chair. This became recognized when Mott replaced Hames on 31 December 1945, first as acting deputy minister of public health, and then as deputy minister on 1 April 1951. Burns Roth was deputy minister from 1 January 1952 until 30 June 1962. *Saskatchewan Legislative Directory: Saskatchewan Executive Council, 1905–2019, Deputy Ministers*, Provincial Archives of Saskatchewan online directory, pp. 2.6–17, https://www.saskarchives.com/sites/default/files/2022-09/Legislative-Assembly-1905-2019.pdf.
5 "Deputy Health Minister to Leave at Year's End," *Regina Leader-Post* (*LP*), 23 Oct. 1951, 3; Library and Archives Canada (LAC), Frederick Dodge Mott fonds, MG31 J15, vol. 48, file 25 – biographical material, F.D. Mott's CV, 1964.
6 PAS, Jean Larmour oral history of CCF government, R-8455, recorded interview with Dr. Burns Roth, tape 2, 18 Nov. 1982.
7 Roth was appointed head of the Department of Hospital Management, the academic predecessor of the Institute of Health Policy, Management and Evaluation. Leslie A. Boehm, *Toward the Health of a Nation: The Institute of Health Policy, Management and Evaluation – the First Seventy Years* (Montreal and Kingston: McGill-Queen's University Press, 2020), 201–25.
8 This comparison of Bentley and Erb is based, in part, on the recollections of both ministers by Burns Roth. Describing Bentley as one of the three wisest men he had ever known, Roth noted that Bentley also developed a "depth of understanding" of health administration and policy never achieved by Erb, who, in Roth's view, had only a "surface understanding." PAS, Jean Larmour oral history of CCF government, R-8455, recorded interview with Dr. Burns Roth, tape 2, 18 Nov. 1982.
9 On how public revenues derived from oil and gas fuelled post-war public health spending in Alberta, see John Church and Neale Smith, *Alberta: A Health System Profile* (Toronto: University of Toronto Press, 2022), 3–4 and 10–12.
10 Bill Waiser, *Saskatchewan: A New History* (Calgary: Fifth House, 2005), 370–1.
11 Robert A. Caro, *The Years of Lyndon Johnson*, vol. 1: *The Path to Power* (New York: Alfred A. Knopf, 1982), 502–15.
12 This is based on the percentage of households with central station electricity, as determined in the annual census. See Ruth W. Sandwell, "People, Place and Power: Rural Electrification in Canada, 1890–1950," in *Transforming the Countryside: The Electrification of Rural Britain*, ed. Paul Brassley, Jeremy Burchardt, and Karen Sayer (London: Routledge, 2016), 183.

13 See Clinton O. White, *Power for a Province: A History of Saskatchewan Power* (Regina: Canadian Plains Research Center, University of Regina, 1976).
14 Debates, Legislative Assembly of Saskatchewan, 21 Feb. 1952, 15.
15 Sheri Hathaway, "Electricity Forever Changed Life on the Farm," *Western Producer*, 4 Oct. 2018.
16 The original formula based on a point system was changed in 1948 to a per diem rate based on an estimate of actual operating costs, while a further major change was made to the second formula in 1951. See Malcolm G. Taylor, "The Saskatchewan Hospital Services Plan: A Study in Compulsory Health Insurance" (PhD diss., University of California at Berkeley, 1949), 148–58, 251–7; and F. Burns Roth, Glyn W. Myers, Frederick D. Mott, and Leonard S. Rosenfeld, "The Saskatchewan Experience in Payment for Hospital Care," *American Journal of Public Health and the Nation's Health* 43, no. 6 (1953): 753–6.
17 PAS, Jean Larmour oral history of CCF Government, R-8358-62, T.C. Douglas interview transcript no. 5, 4 Sept. 1981, 18.
18 PAS, Jean Larmour oral history of CCF Government, R-8358-62, T.C. Douglas interview transcript no. 5, 4 Sept. 1981, 12. Douglas repeated this in an earlier (1973–74) interview with Doris Shackleton, which she used in her biography: Doris French Shackleton, *Tommy Douglas: A Biography* (Toronto: McClelland & Stewart, 1975), 7, 232–3. However, Joan Feather finds no clear evidence of the influence of the Swift Current Health Region on the thinking of the Hall Commission: see "Impact of the Swift Current Health Region: Experiment or Model?" *Prairie Forum* 16, no. 2 (1991): 244.
19 T.C. Douglas, "Saskatchewan Plans for Health," *Health* 14, no. 6 (1946): 3.
20 Frederick D. Mott, "A Pattern of Local Services in the Saskatchewan Health Program," *American Journal of Public Health and the Nation's Health* 39, no. 2 (1949): 217.
21 F. Burns Roth and R.D. Defries, "The Saskatchewan Department of Public Health," *Canadian Journal of Public Health / Revue canadienne de santé publique* 49, no. 7 (1958): 280–3.
22 For this reason, I resist referring to the health regions as conceived by Henry Sigerist, Mindel Sheps, and Fred Mott as the "health centre model of socialized medicine," the phrase used by Esyllt W. Jones in *Radical Medicine: The International Origins of Socialized Health Care in Canada* (Winnipeg: ARP Books, 2019), 21–34.
23 See, for example, F. Burns Roth, "The Health Officer and Hospital Regionalization," *Canadian Journal of Public Health / Revue canadienne de santé publique* 43, no. 11 (1952): 467–73.
24 *History of the Swift Current Health Region Medical Care Plan, 1946–1966* (Regina: Department of Public Health, Research and Planning Branch, June 1969), 5.

25 C. Stuart Houston, *Steps on the Road to Medicare: Why Saskatchewan Led the Way* (Montreal and Kingston: McGill-Queen's University Press, 2002), 85. On the form that regionalization took in Canada from the 1990s forward, see Gregory P. Marchildon, "Regionalization: What Have We Learned?" *Healthcare Papers* 16, no. 1 (2016): 8–14.
26 Mott, "A Pattern of Local Services," 218.
27 Malcolm G. Taylor, *Health Insurance and Canadian Public Policy: The Seven Decisions That Created the Canadian Health Insurance System and Its Outcomes* (Montreal and Kingston: McGill-Queen's University Press, 1978), 266. Also see Houston, *Steps on the Road to Medicare*, 82–3, and Stuart Houston and Bill Waiser, *Tommy's Team: The People behind the Douglas Years* (Calgary: Fifth House, 2010), 107.
28 *History of the Swift Current Health Region Medical Care Plan*, 15.
29 Mott, "A Pattern of Local Services," 218.
30 *History of the Swift Current Health Region Medical Care Plan*, 12–16.
31 Houston and Waiser, *Tommy's Team*, 104–6.
32 W.C.N. Reed, "Methods Used in the Province of Saskatchewan to Provide Vital-Statistics Information to Medical Officers of Health," *Canadian Journal of Public Health / Revue canadienne de santé publique* 42, no. 3 (1951): 101.
33 Reed, "Methods Used in the Province of Saskatchewan," 102.
34 This was Alexander D. Langmuir's definition in 1950. Langmuir promoted disease surveillance as a critical function of the newly established Communicable Diseases Center, renamed the Centers for Disease Control and Prevention (CDC) in the United States: see S. Declich and A.O. Carter, "Public Health Surveillance: Historical Origins, Methods and Evaluation," *Bulletin of the World Health Organization* 72, no. 2 (1994): 287.
35 Reed, "Methods Used in the Province of Saskatchewan," 102.
36 Mott, "A Pattern of Local Services," 219.
37 Houston, *Steps on the Road to Medicare*, 85.
38 This is also Joan Feather's assessment and the reason that the Thompson Committee did not recommend a regionalized approach in its 1961 report: see Feather, "Impact of the Swift Current Health Region," 238.
39 Douglas, quoted in Feather, "Impact of the Swift Current Health Region," 239.
40 This argument is contrary to the view put forward by Keith Brownsey in "Policy, Bureaucracy and Personality: Woodrow Lloyd and the Introduction of Medicare in Saskatchewan," *Prairie Forum* 23, no. 2 (1998): 197–210, where he suggests that Woodrow Lloyd's personal preference for centralization, in contrast to Douglas's commitment to local democracy, was the key reason that medical care insurance was administratively centralized in Saskatchewan. In fact, this plan followed the well-trod path of the hospitalization plan.

41 Milton I. Roemer, "The Saskatchewan Air Ambulance Service: Medical and Public Health Aspects," *Canadian Medical Association Journal* 75, no. 6 (1956): 530.
42 Roemer, "The Saskatchewan Air Ambulance Service," 529; Stephan A. Langford, "The Royal Flying Doctor Service of Australia: Its Foundation and Early Development," *Medical Journal of Australia* 161, no. 1 (1994): 91–4
43 PAS, Department of Public Health fonds (hereafter DPH), R-194.2, file 56 – Air Ambulance Services, 1945–1949, "Summary of Investigation and Proposals re: A Government Subsidized Air-Ambulance Service," and D.K. Malcolm's Memorandum Covering the Organization of the Government Subsidized Air-Ambulance Service of the Province of Saskatchewan, n.d., but noted as discussed with premier, 31 Dec. 1945 (hereafter D.K. Malcolm's Memorandum).
44 PAS, DPH, R-194.2, file 56 – Air Ambulance Services, 1945–1949: D.K. Malcolm's Memorandum, summary prepared for Dr. Mosley, University of Toronto re: Saskatchewan Government Air Ambulance Service, 15 Aug. 1946. For a narrative history, see Donald N. Campbell, *Wings of Mercy: A Living History of Saskatchewan's Air Ambulance Service* (North Battleford, SK: Turner-Warwick Publications, 1993).
45 PAS, DPH, R-194.2, file 56 – Air Ambulance Services, 1945–1949, memorandum, D.K. Malcolm to C.F.W. Hames, 22 Nov. 1946, on landing strips.
46 By 1949, the policy was set that only one escort could accompany the patient, and this person was charged $10 per flight. PAS, DPH, R-194.2, file 56 – Air Ambulance Services, 1945–1949, memorandum on Air Ambulance Service from D.K. Malcolm, 11 Jan. 1949.
47 PAS, DPH, R-194.2, file 56 – Air Ambulance Services, 1945–1949, summary prepared for Dr. Mosley, University of Toronto re: Saskatchewan Government Air Ambulance Service, 15 Aug. 1946.
48 PAS, DPH, R-194.2, file 56 – Air Ambulance Services, 1945–1949, summary prepared for Dr. Mosley, University of Toronto re: Saskatchewan Government Air Ambulance Service, 15 Aug. 1946. Joe Phelps, the minister of natural resources, turned this northern air service into a provincial Crown corporation – Saskatchewan Government Airlines – in 1947: Kathleen Carlisle, *Fiery Joe: The Maverick Who Lit Up the West* (Regina: University of Regina Press, 2017), 111–13; James D. Winkel, "Servant of the North: A History of Saskatchewan Government Airways," (MA thesis, University of Regina, 2006).
49 Roemer, "The Saskatchewan Air Ambulance Service," 530.
50 Roemer, "The Saskatchewan Air Ambulance Service," 529–31.
51 National Film Board of Canada, *Wings of Mercy* (Montreal: NFB, 1947), https://www.nfb.ca/film/wings_of_mercy/. PAS, DPH, R-194.2,

file 56 – Air Ambulance Services, 1945–1949, letter, Evelyn Cherry (NFB) to G.C. Darby (Department of Public Health), 14 Jan. 1948, enclosing script for documentary.
52 Roemer, "The Saskatchewan Air Ambulance Service," 529–30.
53 F. Laurie Barron, *Walking in Indian Moccasins: The Native Policies of Tommy Douglas and the CCF* (Vancouver: UBC Press, 1997), 138.
54 The standard work on this historical reconsideration is J.R. Miller's *Skyscrapers Hide the Heavens: A History of Native-Newcomer Relations in Canada*, 4th ed. (Toronto: University of Toronto Press, 2018). On the Prairie region and Saskatchewan in particular, see James Daschuk's highly influential *Clearing the Plains: Disease, Politics of Starvation, and the Loss of Indigenous Life* (Regina: University of Regina Press, 2019).
55 Barron, *Walking in Indian Moccasins*, 213.
56 David M. Quiring, *CCF Colonialism in Northern Saskatchewan: Battling Parish Priests, Bootleggers, and Fur Sharks* (Vancouver: UBC Press, 2004), 219.
57 Quiring, *CCF Colonialism*, 220.
58 Josée Lavoie, "Medicare and the Care of First Nations, Métis and Inuit," *Health Economics, Policy and Law* 13, nos. 3–4 (2018): 283–4.
59 Laura Meijer Drees, "Training Aboriginal Nurses: The Indian Health Services in Northwestern Canada, 1934–1975," in *Caregiving on the Periphery: Historical Perspectives on Nursing and Midwifery in Canada*, ed. Myra Rutherdale (Montreal and Kingston: McGill-Queen's University Press, 2010), 185–6; Lesley McBain, "Caring, Curing, and Socialization: The Ambiguities of Nursing in Northern Saskatchewan, 1944–57," in *Caregiving on the Periphery*, 284–6.
60 McBain, "Caring, Curing, and Socialization," 287.
61 Catherine Carstairs, *The Smile Gap: A History of Oral Health and Social Inequality* (Montreal and Kingston: McGill-Queen's University Press, 2022), 3–8.
62 This section is based on a previously published article: Gregory P. Marchildon, "Policy Agenda Setting in Public Health Dentistry: Implementing North America's First Universal School-Based Dental Program in Saskatchewan," *Canadian Journal of Health History* 40, no. 1 (2023): 197–222.
63 *Saskatchewan Health Services Survey Commission: Report of the Commissioner, Henry E. Sigerist* (Regina: Thomas H. McConica, King's Printer, 1944), 8.
64 Bill Waiser, *Saskatchewan: A New History* (Calgary: Fifth House, 2005), 279–340.
65 *Saskatchewan Health Survey Report*, vol. 1: *Health Programs and Personnel* (Regina: Saskatchewan Health Survey Committee, 1952), 20.
66 PAS, DPH, R-999, file XIII.71, Report on Dental Health in Saskatchewan: Present Status and Possibilities for the Future, 8 Aug. 1950.

67 PAS, DPH, R-326, file 112, letter, F.D. Mott to E. Stoner, 7 Oct. 1946, and R-194.2, file 63, letter, G. Kinneard to H.S. Doyle, 14 April 1949.
68 It was the policy of the Department of Public Health to provide provincial grants to health regions for dental plans; however, only the Swift Current Health Region set up such a program. The department provided the Swift Current Health Region with a total of $66,262 spread over four annual grants between 1946 and 1949. In the first two years (1948–50) of the National Health Grants program, the federal government transferred $65,212 to the province for use in the same dental program in Swift Current: *Saskatchewan Health Survey Report*, 1: 75.
69 In the provincial news section of the *Canadian Journal of Public Health / Revue canadienne de santé publique* 41, no. 8 (1950): 355, there is mention of Chegwin taking a short leave of absence from his position in Saskatchewan in the first half of 1950 to obtain a diploma in dental public health at the University of Toronto.
70 PAS, DPH, R-999, file XIII.7a, General Directive from the Division of Dental Health (A.E. Chegwin, author), 19 May 1949.
71 Jay W. Friedman, "The New Zealand School Dental Service: Lesson in Radical Conservatism," *Journal of the American Dental Association* 85, no. 3 (1972): 609–617; Susan M. Moffat, Lyndie A. Foster Page, and W. Murray Thompson, "New Zealand's School Dental Service over the Decades: Its Response to Social, Political, and Economic Influences, and the Effect on Oral Health Inequalities," *Frontiers in Public Health* 5, no. 177 (2017): 1–18.
72 One published evaluation of the New Zealand Dental Service in 1949–50 was conducted by the dental services advisor to the Social Security Administration, Federal Security Agency in the United States: John T. Fulton, "Experiment in Dental Care: Results of New Zealand's Use of School Dental Nurses," *Bulletin of the World Health Organization* 4, no. 1 (1951): 1–73.
73 PAS, DPH, R-999, file XIII.7b, Review of Dental Public Health in Saskatchewan (A.E. Chegwin), 24 July 1952.
74 PAS, DPH, R-999, file XIII.7c, letter, F.B. Roth to T.J. Bentley, 4 Aug. 1952.
75 PAS, DPH, R-999, file XIII.7c, memorandum. F.B. Roth to T.J. Bentley, 14 April 1953.
76 PAS, DPH, R-999, file XIII.7b, memorandum, A.E. Chegwin to G. Kinneard (Director, Regional Health Services Branch), 24 Nov. 1953.
77 PAS, DPH, R-999, file XIII.7c, memorandum, G. Kinneard to A.E. Chegwin, 8 March 1954.
78 PAS, DPH, R-999, file XIII.7c, New Zealand's Dental Nurse Program: Memorandum on the Employment of State-Trained Dental Nurses to Provide Essential Dental Services for Children in the Commonwealth of New Zealand and its Implications for Saskatchewan, Saskatchewan Department of Public Health, 30 Sept. 1954.

79 PAS, DPH, R-999, file XIII.7d, memorandum, A.E. Chegwin to F.B. Roth, 23 Nov. 1954.
80 PAS, DPH, R-999, file XIII.7d, letter, F.B. Roth to Dr. C. Lenk (regional medical health officer, Health Region No. 3, Weyburn), 21 Dec. 1959.
81 Paul Barker, "The Formulation and Implementation of the Saskatchewan Dental Plan," (PhD diss., University of Toronto, 1985), 50. It is interesting to note that Chegwin was still DDH director at this time but seemed to be working with, and perhaps under the direction of, Dr. Murray Acker, the director of the Regional Health Services Branch of the department. By this time, Chegwin felt there was a crisis in terms of oral health in rural Saskatchewan but, as usual, was much clearer on the nature of the problem rather than its solution.
82 See Gregory P. Marchildon, "Policy Agenda Setting in Public Health Dentistry: Implementing North America's First Universal School-Based Dental Program in Saskatchewan," *Canadian Journal of Health History* 40, no. 1 (2023): 207–8.
83 Allan Blakeney, *An Honourable Calling: Political Memoirs* (Toronto: University of Toronto Press, 2008), 87–8; Allan Blakeney and Sandford Borins, *Political Management in Canada* (Toronto: University of Toronto Press, 1998), 208–9; Steve Wolfson, "The Use of Paraprofessionals: The Saskatchewan Dental Plan," ed. Eleanor Glor, *Policy Innovation in the Saskatchewan Public Service, 1971–82* (Toronto: Captus Press, 1997), 126–39.

## 9. National Influence, 1948–1958

1 Douglas, quoted in Vincent Lam, *Tommy Douglas* (Toronto: Penguin Canada, 2011), ix.
2 A. Douglas Turnbull, "Memoir: Early Years of Hospital Insurance in British Columbia," *BC Studies*, no. 76 (1987/88): 60.
3 British Columbia Archives (BCA), Department of Health and Welfare fonds, GR 0117, box 6, file 11, Hospital Insurance Act, SBC 1948, c. 28.
4 Turnbull, "Memoir," 60–1; Gregory P. Marchildon and Nicole C. O'Byrne, "Bennettcare to Medicare: The Morphing of Medicare Care Insurance in British Columbia," *Canadian Bulletin of Medical History / Bulletin canadien d'histoire de la médecine* 26, no. 2 (2009): 456.
5 H.F. Angus, "Note on the British Columbia Election in June 1945," *Western Political Quarterly* 5, no. 4 (1952): 587.
6 Antonia Maioni, *Parting at the Crossroads: The Emergence of Health Insurance in the United States and Canada* (Princeton, NJ: Princeton University Press, 1999), 94.
7 Marchildon and O'Byrne, "Bennettcare to Medicare," 455–8; George M. Abbott, "Duff Pattullo and the Coalition Controversy of 1941," *BC Studies*, no. 102 (1994): 30–53.

Notes to pages 231–4    565

8   Gordon Hak, "Populism and the 1952 Social Credit Breakthrough in British Columbia," *Canadian Historical Review* 85, no. 2 (2004): 277–9. The final tally of 48 seats in the 1952 election was Social Credit 19, CCF 18, Liberals 6, PCs 4, and Labour 1. The Social Credit minority would become a majority in the 1953 election. Marchildon and O'Byrne, "Bennettcare to Medicare," 457–60.
9   Gordon S. Lawson and Andrew E. Noseworthy, "Newfoundland's Cottage Health System, 1920–1970," *Canadian Bulletin of Medical History / Bulletin canadien d'histoire de la médecine* 26, no. 2 (2009): 480–2.
10  Labrador was served by what we would today call a non-governmental organization, the International Grenfell Association. For the association's unique history, see J.T.H. Connor, "'Medicine Is Here to Stay': Rural Medical Practice, the Northern Frontier and Modernization in 1930s Newfoundland," in *Medicine in the Remote and Rural North, 1800–2000*, ed. J.T.H. Connor and Stephan Curtis (London: Routledge, 2016), 129–51; and John Matchim, "Towards a 'Total Welfare' Approach: Duncan Neuhauser, the International Grenfell Association, and Rural-Remote Health Care in Labrador and Swedish Lapland, 1950s–1970s," *Acadiensis* 49, no. 1 (2020): 172–84.
11  Lawson and Noseworthy, "Newfoundland's Cottage Health System," 479.
12  Linda Kealey and Heather Molyneaux, "On the Road to Medicare: Newfoundland in the 1960s," *Journal of Canadian Studies / Revue d'études canadiennes* 41, no. 3 (2007): 93–5.
13  Lawson and Noseworthy, "Newfoundland's Cottage Hospital System," 490.
14  Clark Banack, *God's Province: Evangelical Christianity, Political Thought, and Conservatism in Alberta* (Montreal and Kingston: McGill-Queen's University Press, 2016), 133–47.
15  Maioni, *Parting at the Crossroads*, 94.
16  Gregory P. Marchildon, "Douglas versus Manning: The Ideological Battle over Medicare in Postwar Canada," *Journal of Canadian Studies / Revue d'études canadiennes* 50, no. 1 (2016): 134–40.
17  Alvin Finkel, *The Social Credit Phenomenon in Alberta* (Toronto: University of Toronto Press, 1989).
18  Edward Bell, "Ernest C. Manning, 1943–1968," in *Alberta Premiers of the 20th Century*, ed. Bradford J. Rennie (Regina: Canadian Plains Research Center, University of Regina, 2004), 148–53.
19  David Elliott, "William Aberhart, 1935–1943," in *Alberta Premiers of the 20th Century*, 144; Bell, "Ernest C. Manning," 150–6.
20  Clark Banack, "Evangelical Christianity and Political Thought in Alberta," *Journal of Canadian Studies* 48, no. 2 (2014): 88; Marchildon, "Douglas versus Manning," 129–46.
21  Marchildon, "Douglas versus Manning," 134–7.

22 Marchildon, "Douglas versus Manning," 140. This position was partly a consequence of the Alberta Social Credit government's conflicts with the federal government in the late 1930s: see Gregory P. Marchildon, "The Prairie Farm Rehabilitation Administration: Climate Crisis and Federal-Provincial Relations during the Great Depression," *Canadian Historical Review* 90, no. 2 (2009): 275–301.
23 Provincial Archives of Saskatchewan (PAS), Jean Larmour oral history of the CCF Government, R-8387-92, interview with T.C. Douglas, 24 June 1982, transcript 1, 92–3.
24 University of Alberta Archives (UAA), E.C. Manning interviews conducted by Lydia Semotuk, 81-32 (hereafter Manning interviews), transcript 16, 23–4.
25 UAA, Manning interviews, transcript 16, 24.
26 Provincial Archives of Alberta (PAA), Premier's Office fonds, GR 1969.289, 1718, Health Insurance Digest "Alberta's New Medical Plan," 8 Nov. 1948; UAA, Manning interviews, transcript 20, 34–5.
27 PAA, Premier's Office fonds, GR 1969.289, 1718, letter, E.C. Manning to V.A. Newhall, 11 Dec. 1948. From a public administration standpoint, the Alberta hospitalization plan had many more moving parts than the Saskatchewan plan. Indeed, while providing a detailed description of the Alberta hospitalization program to Douglas, the deputy minister of public health in Saskatchewan described it as "so complicated that most people have difficulty understanding the details of what goes on: this applies to the hospitals in Alberta as well as to people outside the province." PAS, T.C. Douglas fonds (TCD), R33.1, file 575b (14-28-2), memorandum, F. Burns Roth to T.C. Douglas, 2 Feb. 1960.
28 PAA, Premier's Office fonds, GR 1969.289, 1720, letter, E.C. Manning to Archie Gillis, 4 April 1953.
29 PAA, Premier's Office fonds, GR 1969.289, 2079, letter, E.C. Manning to Mrs. Helen Clemens (High River), 1 April 1958.
30 PAS, Pamphlet Collection of Various Political Parties fonds, GR 122, Co-operative Commonwealth Federation: National Office, CCF fonds, no. 44, political pamphlet entitled "We're Covered, Why Not You? The Story of Saskatchewan Health Services," CCF National Office, Ottawa, ca. 1948 (hereafter "We're Covered,") 2.
31 "We're Covered," 2.
32 Dean E. McHenry, *The Third Force in Canada* (Berkeley: University of California Press, 1950), 135.
33 Canadian Museum of History, "Making Medicare: The History of Health Care in Canada, 1914–2007," virtual exhibit, https://www.historymuseum.ca/cmc/exhibitions/hist/medicare/medic-4h01e.html.
34 PAS, TCD, R-33.1, box X.395, file XXIII.745g (23-22-1), folder 7, Federal-Provincial Conferences, letter, T.C. Douglas to Louis St-Laurent, 15 July 1949.

35 PAS, TCD, R-33.1, box X.395, file XXIII.745g (23-22-1), folder 7, Federal-Provincial Conferences, letter, T.C. Douglas to Louis St-Laurent, 15 July 1949.
36 PAS, TCD, R-33.1, box X.395, file XXIII.745g (23-22-1), folder 7, Federal-Provincial Conferences, letter, John McNair (premier of New Brunswick) to T.C. Douglas, 13 Aug. 1949.
37 PAS, TCD, R-33.1, box X.395, file XXIII.745g (23-22-1), folder 7, Federal-Provincial Conferences, letter, Louis St-Laurent to T.C. Douglas, 18 Aug. 1949.
38 PAS, TCD, R-33.1, box X.395, file XXIII.745g (23-22-1), folder 7, Federal-Provincial Conferences, letter, T.C. Douglas to Florence (last name not provided), 6 Sept. 1960.
39 PAS, TCD, R-33.1, box X.395, file XXIII.745g (23-22-1), folder 7, Federal-Provincial Conferences, letter, T.C. Douglas to Louis St-Laurent, 22 Sept. 1949.
40 PAS, TCD, R-33.1, box X.395, file XXIII.745g (23-22-1), folder 7, Federal-Provincial Conferences, letter, T.C. Douglas to Louis St-Laurent, 22 Sept. 1949.
41 Paul Martin, *A Very Public Life*, vol. 2: *So Many Worlds* (Toronto: Deneau, 1985), 219–20.
42 Martin, *A Very Public Life*, 2: 221; Marchildon, "The Cautious Liberal: St-Laurent and National Hospitalization," in *The Unexpected Louis St-Laurent: Politics and Policies for a Modern Canada*, ed. Patrice Dutil (Vancouver: UBC Press, 2020), 284–5.
43 "Premier Points up Two Main Issues," *Regina Leader-Post* (*LP*), 1 Aug. 1953, 23; "Douglas Attacks Liberal Record," *LP*, 5 Aug. 1953, 2; "Farmer Betrayed Premier Charges," *LP*, 6 Aug. 1953, 2.
44 PAS, TCD, R-33.1, file 562 (14-16), National Health Insurance Data, letter, T.C. Douglas to J.T. Waterfield (National Old Age Pensioners' Federation, Alberta), 30 March 1954.
45 *Federal-Provincial Conference 1955: Preliminary Meeting, Ottawa, April 26th, 1955* (Ottawa: Queen's Printer, 1955), 5.
46 On Fines, Johnson, and Shoyama, see A.W. Johnson with Rosemary Proctor, *Dream No Little Dreams: A Biography of the Douglas Government of Saskatchewan, 1944–1961* (Toronto: University of Toronto Press, 2004), xvi–xxiii, 122–3, 193–5, 187–96. On Lee and his role within the Douglas government, see Gregory P. Marchildon, "The Secretary to the Cabinet in Saskatchewan: Evolution of the Role, 1944–2006," in *Searching for Leadership: Secretaries to Cabinet in Canada*, ed. Patrice Dutil (Toronto: University of Toronto Press, 2008), 162–7.
47 Gregory P. Marchildon, "Foreword," in Johnson with Proctor, *Dream No Little Dreams*, xvii–xxviii.
48 Marchildon, "Foreword," xxii. Shoyama not only supported public administration and financing of health insurance but also championed changes in the delivery of health care through his support of the community clinic movement (see chapters 12 and 13 below).

49 As Johnson put it, Ontario wanted it on the agenda "at least for talking purposes!": LAC, A.W. Johnson fonds, R12603, vol. 35, file 7, letter, A.W. Johnson to his father and mother, 4 May 1955.
50 Library and Archives Canada (LAC), A.W. Johnson fonds, R12603, vol. 35, file 7, letter, A.W. Johnson to his father and mother, 4 May 1955.
51 Louis St-Laurent quoted in *Federal-Provincial Conference 1955: Preliminary Meeting*, 8.
52 Louis St-Laurent quoted in *Federal-Provincial Conference 1955: Preliminary Meeting*, 9, 10.
53 Louis St-Laurent quoted in *Federal-Provincial Conference 1955: Preliminary Meeting*, 11–15.
54 LAC, A.W. Johnson fonds, R12603, vol. 35, file 7, letter, A.W. Johnson to his father and mother, 4 May 1955.
55 Leslie Frost quoted in *Federal-Provincial Conference 1955: Preliminary Meeting*, 19.
56 LAC, A.W. Johnson fonds, R12603, vol. 35, file 7, letter, A.W. Johnson to his father and mother, 4 May 1955.
57 Leslie Frost quoted in *Federal-Provincial Conference 1955: Preliminary Meeting*, 19.
58 P.E. Bryden, *A Justifiable Obsession: Conservative Ontario's Relations with Ottawa, 1943–1985* (Toronto: University of Toronto Press, 2013), 91.
59 *Federal-Provincial Conference 1955: Preliminary Meeting*, 23–8.
60 LAC, A.W. Johnson fonds, R12603, vol. 35, file 7, letter, A.W. Johnson to his father and mother, 4 May 1955. There is no record of Flemming's support in the public portion of the conference, but he was one "of several" premiers who voiced their support for the inclusion of health insurance for the fall meeting: LAC, Paul Martin fonds, MG 32, B12, vol. 5, file 1, Federal-Provincial Conference 1955, Preliminary Meeting, typescript summary of in-camera meetings on 27 April 1955, 3.
61 *Federal-Provincial Conference 1955: Preliminary Meeting*, 34.
62 LAC, A.W. Johnson fonds, R12603, vol. 35, file 7, letter, A.W. Johnson to his father and mother, 4 May 1955.
63 W.A.C. Bennet quoted in *Federal-Provincial Conference 1955: Preliminary Meeting*, 40. According to Johnson (LAC, A.W. Johnson fonds, R12603, vol. 35, file 7, letter, A.W. Johnson to his father and mother, 4 May 1955), Bennett's text was "solid" but his delivery "was as sparkling as a wet firecracker."
64 T.C. Douglas quoted in *Federal-Provincial Conference 1955: Preliminary Meeting*, 45, 49.
65 T.C. Douglas quoted in *Federal-Provincial Conference 1955: Preliminary Meeting*, 49.
66 PAS, TCD, R-33.4, file IX.5e, Federal-Provincial Conference – October 1955, Health and Hospital Insurance, memorandum on Health Insurance, 1 Jan. 1955.

67 The cottage hospitals – small basic-care hospitals that served the outports of Newfoundland – had been operating since the 1930s. On their history, see Lawson and Noseworthy, "Newfoundland's Cottage Health Systems." On the International Grenfell Association's and cottage hospitals in Labrador, see J.T.H. Connor, "American Aid, the International Grenfell Association, and Health Care in Newfoundland, 1920s–1930," in *The Grenfell Medical Mission and American Support in Newfoundland and Labrador, 1890s–1940s*, ed. Jennifer J. Connor and Katherine Side (Montreal and Kingston: McGill-Queen's University Press, 2018), 145–66.
68 PAS, TCD, R-33.1, file 562 (14-16), National Health Insurance Data, letter, T.C. Douglas to Ken Carlson, 17 Dec. 1953; Martin, *A Very Public Life*, 2: 221.
69 Ernest Manning quoted in *Federal-Provincial Conference 1955: Preliminary Meeting*, 52.
70 LAC, A.W. Johnson fonds, R12603, vol. 35, file 7, letter, A.W. Johnson to his father and mother, 4 May 1955.
71 Joseph R. Smallwood quoted in *Federal-Provincial Conference 1955: Preliminary Meeting*, 57 (laughter noted in text).
72 LAC, A.W. Johnson fonds, R12603, vol. 35, file 7, letter, A.W. Johnson to his father and mother, 4 May 1955.
73 LAC, A.W. Johnson fonds, R12603, vol. 35, file 7, letter, A.W. Johnson to his father and mother, 4 May 1955.
74 LAC, Paul Martin fonds, MG 32, B12, vol. 5, file 1, Federal-Provincial Conference 1955, Preliminary Meeting, typescript summary of in-camera meetings on 27 April 1955, 3–4.
75 LAC, Paul Martin fonds, MG 32, B12, vol. 5, file 1, Federal-Provincial Conference 1955, Preliminary Meeting, typescript summary of in-camera meetings on 27 April 1955, 4; Malcolm G. Taylor, *Health Insurance and Canadian Public Policy: The Seven Decisions That Created the Canadian Health Insurance System and Its Outcomes*, 2nd ed. (Montreal and Kingston: McGill-Queen's University Press, 2009), 126.
76 David M. Naylor, *Private Practice, Public Payment: Canadian Medicare and the Politics of Health Insurance, 1911–1966* (Montreal and Kingston: McGill-Queen's University Press, 1986), 152–8.
77 Louis St-Laurent, in Government of Canada, *House of Commons Debates* (*HCD*), 21st Parliament, 4th session, vol. 5, 20 Jan. 1951, 4349.
78 Stanley Knowles, in *HCD*, 21st Parliament, 4th session, vol. 5, 20 Jan. 1951, 4386.
79 Taylor, *Health Insurance*, 106.
80 Martin, *A Very Public Life*, 2: 221; Marchildon, "The Cautious Liberal," 288.
81 Taylor, *Health Insurance*, 116–18. Duplessis's sarcastic response that "my friend Mr. Frost is not going to have an election this year and did not make a speech in view of the election – I know that very well." See *Federal-Provincial Conference 1955: Preliminary Meeting*, 23. In an interview

many years later, Douglas was equally dismissive of Frost's penchant for "decrying creeping socialism" in the private portion of the first ministers' meeting and then being the first to walk out of the meeting into the press scrum and declare that "Ontario is going to introduce hospital insurance." See PAS, Jean Larmour oral history of the CCF government, R-8387-92, interview with T.C. Douglas, 24 June 1982, transcript 1, 73.
82 Taylor, *Health Insurance*, 116.
83 Taylor, *Health Insurance*, 118.
84 Bryden, *A Justifiable Obsession*, 91; Taylor, *Health Insurance*, 116.
85 Roger Graham, *Old Man Ontario: Leslie Miscampbell Frost* (Toronto: University of Toronto Press for the Ontario Historical Studies Series, 1990), 231–3.
86 In addition to writing his 1949 Berkeley doctoral dissertation on Saskatchewan hospital insurance, which he finalized while working in Regina, Taylor subsequently published a number of articles comparing provincial programs and health system initiatives, including "Some Administrative Aspects of the Integration of Health Services," *Canadian Journal of Public Health / Revue canadienne de santé publique* 42, no. 8 (1951): 329–335; "Government Planning: The Federal-Provincial Health Survey Reports," *Canadian Journal of Economics and Political Science / Revue canadienne d'économique et de science politique* 19, no. 4 (1953): 501–10; and "Social Assistance Medical Care Programs in Canada," *American Journal of Public Health* 44, no. 6 (1954): 750–9.
87 Archives of Ontario (AO), Premier Leslie M. Frost fonds, RG 3-23, Report on Health Insurance by Malcolm G. Taylor, PhD.
88 Bryden, *A Justifiable Obsession*, 91.
89 Graham, *Old Man Ontario*, 234.
90 Taylor, *Health Insurance*, 109–10.
91 Elections Ontario, 1955 General Election, https://results.elections.on.ca/en/data-explorer?fromYear=1867&toYear=2021&electionId=257&levelOfDetail=election.
92 PAS, TCD, R33.1, file 778a (23-43), Federal-Provincial Conference: Fiscal Arrangements, Unemployment Insurance, and Health Insurance, Memorandum prepared by Donald MacDonald for CCF National Executive, 23 Sept. 1955.
93 PAS, C.M. Fines fonds, F119, R-37, file IV-3, Dominion Government Health Plan, correspondence with Ottawa, memorandum, Burns Roth to A.W. Johnson, 8 July 1955. It is interesting that Roth tells Johnson of his "personal" priorities for coverage based on his experience and knowledge: 1) acute hospital care; 2) mental hospital care; 3) chronic disease care; and 4) physician services.
94 Bryden, *A Justifiable Obsession*, 91, and 254nn63 and 64.

95 PAS, C.M. Fines fonds, F119, R-37, file IV-3, Dominion Government Health Plan, correspondence with Ottawa, memorandum, T.K. Shoyama to T.C. Douglas, 24 Aug. 1955, with attached press clippings.
96 Louis St-Laurent quoted in *Federal-Provincial Conference 1955: October 3rd, 1955*, 9–10.
97 Louis St-Laurent quoted in *Federal-Provincial Conference 1955: October 3rd, 1955* (Ottawa: Edmond Cloutier, King's Printer, 1955), 10.
98 *Federal-Provincial Conference 1955: October 3rd, 1955*, 27, with full text of proposal in appendix D, 104–17. In Penny Bryden's words (*A Justifiable Obsession*, 93), the Frost proposal "moved" the first ministers "only infinitesimally closer to achieving any kind of national health insurance plan." My reading of the proceedings is that the proposal only served to muddy the waters.
99 T.C. Douglas, quoted in *Federal-Provincial Conference 1955: October 3rd, 1955*, 87.
100 T.C. Douglas, quoted in *Federal-Provincial Conference 1955: October 3rd, 1955*, 91.
101 T.C. Douglas, quoted in *Federal-Provincial Conference 1955: October 3rd, 1955*, 88.
102 Press communique, 6 Oct. 1955, in *Federal-Provincial Conference 1955: October 3rd, 1955*, 127–8.
103 PAS, C.M. Fines fonds, F119, R-37, IV.6d (2 of 2) – Dominion Government Tax Rental Agreements, Post-Conference Meeting of Saskatchewan Delegates to the Federal-Provincial Conference, Oct. 1955, 13 Oct. 1955, agenda for meeting and F.B. Roth's "Memorandum on Health Insurance Item: Federal-Provincial Conference, 1955."
104 PAS, C.M. Fines fonds, F119, R-37, IV.6d (2 of 2) – Dominion Government Tax Rental Agreements, Post-Conference Meeting of Saskatchewan Delegates to the Federal-Provincial Conference, Oct. 1955, 13 Oct. 1955, F.B. Roth's "Memorandum on Health Insurance Item: Federal-Provincial Conference, 1955," 4.
105 PAS, C.M. Fines fonds, F119, R-37, Dominion Government Health Plan, correspondence with Ottawa, letter, letters, T.J. Bentley to Paul Martin, 6 and 29 Dec. 1955.
106 PAS, C.M. Fines fonds, F119, R-37, file IV-3, Dominion Government Health Plan, correspondence with Ottawa, handwritten letter, A.W. Johnson to C.M. Fines, 20 Jan. 1956.
107 *HCD*, 22nd Parliament, 3rd session, vol. 1, 26 Jan. 1956, 555–6; AO, Deputy Minister of Health fonds, RG 10-6-0-1304, box b0254793, Memorandum on Hospital Insurance and Related Matters, 6 March 1956, Statement of the Prime Minister of Canada on Hospital Insurance in the House of Commons, 26 Jan. 1956, 32–5.

108 *HCD*, 22nd Parliament, 3rd session, vol. 1, 26 Jan. 1956, 555–6; AO, Deputy Minister of Health fonds, RG 10-6-0-1304, box b0254793, Memorandum on Hospital Insurance and Related Matters, 6 March 1956, and Summary of Statement of the Minister of Health and Welfare, the Hon. Paul Martin, at the Federal-Provincial Conference of Health, 26 Jan. 1956, 39.
109 PAS, T.J. Bentley fonds, R 11, file 17-11 – National Hospital Insurance, Statement of the Minister of Health and Welfare, 26 Jan. 1956.
110 PAS, T.J. Bentley fonds, R 11, file 17-11 – National Hospital Insurance, Statement of the Minister of Health and Welfare, 26 Jan. 1956.
111 PAS, TCD, R-33.1, file 562 (14-16), National Health Insurance Data, letter, T.C. Douglas to Betty Beeching, 21 Feb. 1956; emphasis in original.
112 Paul Martin, in *HCD*, quoted in Taylor, *Health Insurance*, 227.
113 John A. Mills, "Lessons from the Periphery: Psychiatry in Saskatchewan, Canada, 1944–68," *History of Psychiatry* 18, no. 2 (2007)" 179–201. Also see Harley D. Dickinson, *The Two Psychiatries: The Transformation of Psychiatric Work in Saskatchewan* (Regina: Canadian Plains Research Center, University of Regina, 1989), and Erika Dyck and Alex Deighton, *Managing Madness: Weyburn Mental Hospital and the Transformation of Psychiatric Care in Canada* (Winnipeg: University of Manitoba Press, 2017).
114 PAS, T.J. Bentley fonds, R 11, file 17-11 – National Hospital Insurance, letter, T.C. Douglas to R.E. Feflar (Saskatchewan Psychiatric Nurses Association), 23 Feb. 1956.
115 Sandy Nicholson, in HCD, quoted in Taylor, *Health Insurance*, 226. The result was that Douglas's government could not afford to implement the "Saskatchewan Plan" (regional, community-based psychiatric facilities) then being proposed by the Psychiatric Services Branch of the Department of Public Health: Dickinson, *The Two Psychiatries*, 133–71.
116 Taylor, *Health Insurance*, 228.
117 See Maureen Lux, *Separate Beds: A History of Indian Hospitals in Canada, 1920s–1980s* (Toronto: University of Toronto Press, 2016) and Mary Jane McCallum and Maureen Lux, "Medicare versus Medicine Chest: Court Challenges and Treaty Rights to Health Care," in *Medicare's Histories: Origins, Omissions, and Opportunities in Canada*, ed. Esyllt Jones, James Hanley, and Delia Gavrus (Winnipeg: University of Manitoba Press, 2022), 107.
118 Marchildon, "The Cautious Liberal."
119 PAS, TCD, R33.1, file 562 (14-16), letter, T.J. Bentley (Saskatchewan minister of public health) to Paul Martin, 26 March 1956.
120 PAS, C.M. Fines fonds, F119, R-37, Dominion Government Health Plan, correspondence with Ottawa, untitled assessment of the federal position in response to Paul Martin Sr.'s statement, n.d., and Walter Erb fonds, F 116, 051A – Hospital Insurance, General Correspondence, memorandum, Burns Roth to J. Walter Erb, 1 Nov. 1957.

121 PAS, TCD, R-33.1, file 562 (14-16), National Health Insurance Data, letter, T.J. Bentley to Paul Martin, 26 March 1956.
122 Taylor, *Health Insurance*, 219; PAS, T.J. Bentley fonds, R 11, file 17-22 – National Hospital Insurance, letter, T.J. Bentley to A.M. (Sandy) Nicholson, 16 May 1956.
123 Taylor, *Health Insurance*, 218.
124 PAS, TCD, R-33.1, file 562 (14-16), National Health Insurance Data, letter, T.J. Bentley to Paul Martin, 26 March 1956.
125 Taylor, *Health Insurance*, 224–5.
126 Taylor, *Health Insurance*, 225.
127 Taylor, *Health Insurance*, 230.
128 From 1935 until the election outcome of 1953, the Liberals held 47.1 per cent of the vote while the Conservatives held only 29.8 per cent, for a total two-party share of 76.7 per cent. The national vote of the CCF (11.6 per cent) and Social Credit (3.7 per cent) over these years was unable to threaten the hegemony of the two-party system: see John C. Courtney, *Revival and Change: The 1957 and 1958 Diefenbaker Elections* (Vancouver: UBC Press, 2022), table 2.1, 22.
129 Courtney, *Revival and Change*, 79.
130 LAC, Thomas Clement Douglas fonds, MG32 C28, vol. 142, file 18, T.C. Douglas, script for radio speech on national hospitalization for federal election recorded in Toronto, 16 May 1957, 2.
131 LAC, Thomas Clement Douglas fonds, MG32 C28, vol. 142, file 18, T.C. Douglas, script for radio speech on national hospitalization for federal election recorded in Toronto, 16 May 1957, 3.
132 "Martin Assails CCF, PC Tactics," and "Hospital Plan Go-Ahead is Up to Provinces – Martin," *LP*, 27 May 1957, 15.
133 "Farmers Nearly Bankrupt – Says Douglas," *LP*, 24 May 1957, 26; "1,000 Jam Melville Area to Hear Liberals Rapped," *LP*, 5 June 1957, 2; "Liberals Don't Rate Support – Says Douglas," *LP*, 10 June 1957, 2; "Premier Charges Thatcher Making False Statements," *LP*, 10 June 1957, 27
134 In Saskatchewan, the Liberals went from the five seats they had won in the 1953 election to four seats in 1957 and dropped from 37.3 per cent to 30.2 per cent of the popular vote. It should be noted, however, that the CCF came out of the 1957 election with ten seats, one less than the seats the party had won in 1953, and experienced a more dramatic fall in popular support, from 44.2 per cent to 35.8 per cent. The PCs gained at the expense of both parties, with three seats (two more than in 1953) and a jump in popular support from 11.7 per cent to 23 per cent. See Courtney, *Revival and Change*, appendix 3, 218.
135 Allan G. Priest, "Diefenbaker's 'New Frontier': Masculinity, Modernity, and Canadian Electoral Politics, 1957–58," *Canadian Journal of History* 57, no. 2 (2022): 175.

136 LAC, Thomas Clement Douglas fonds, MG32 C28, vol. 142, file 19, Premier T.C. Douglas, Report of Political Leader, 22nd Provincial Convention CCF, Saskatoon, 17 July 1957, 9.
137 John G. Diefenbaker quoted in Denis Smith, *Rogue Tory: The Life and Legend of John G. Diefenbaker* (Toronto: McFarland, Walter and Ross, 1995), 150.
138 University of Saskatchewan Archives and Special Collections (USAS), John G. Diefenbaker fonds, MG01/VI, vol. 103, file 306.1 (1957), Federal-Provincial Fiscal Arrangements, 1957, item 088390, letter, J.G. Diefenbaker to T.C. Douglas, 16 Sept. 1957.
139 Even if they did not come from Saskatchewan, some of his most trusted advisors shared Douglas's view that Diefenbaker was a welcome change to St-Laurent. Graham Spry, Saskatchewan's agent-general in the United Kingdom, who had been appointed to the post by Douglas in 1946 and remained in this position for over two decades, said Diefenbaker's "energy and directness" made a "very favourable impression" while visiting London in July 1937: Graham Spry, *Passion and Conviction: The Letters of Graham Spry*, ed. Rose Potvin (Regina: Canadian Plains Research Center, University of Regina, 1992), 182.
140 USAS, John G. Diefenbaker fonds, MG01/VI, vol. 103, file 306.1 (1957), Federal-Provincial Fiscal Arrangements, 1957, item 088412, letter, T.C. Douglas to John G. Diefenbaker, 8 Aug. 1957.
141 USAS, John G. Diefenbaker fonds, MG01/VI, vol. 103, file 306.1 (1957), Federal-Provincial Fiscal Arrangements, 1957, item 088408, letter, T.C. Douglas to John G. Diefenbaker, 10 Sept. 1957.
142 LAC, Thomas Clement Douglas fonds, MG32 C28, vol. 142, file 23, Premier T.C. Douglas Provincial Affairs Series radio broadcast entitled "The Ottawa Conference," 2 Oct. 1945, 9:45 to 10:00 p.m. MST, 7–8.
143 *Dominion-Provincial Conference 1957: Ottawa, November 25th and 26th, 1957* (Ottawa: Edmond Cloutier, Queen's Printer, 1957), 10.
144 Douglas, quoted in J.L. Granatstein, *Canada, 1957–1967: The Years of Uncertainty and Innovation* (Toronto: McClelland & Stewart, 1986), 32.
145 PAS, Jean Larmour oral history of the CCF Government, R-8387-92, interview with T.C. Douglas, 24 June 1982, transcript 1, 92–3.
146 Taylor, *Health Insurance*, 230.
147 Taylor, *Health Insurance*, 231.
148 PAS, TCD, R-33.1, file 562 (14-16), National Health Insurance Data, Canadian Press article regarding hospitalization in Alberta, 29 March 1957.
149 PAA, Premier's Office fonds, GR 1969.289, 2079, letter, E.C. Manning to Mrs. Helen Clemens (High River), 1 April 1958.
150 Taylor, *Health Insurance*, 233–4.

## 10. Setting the Political Agenda Once More

1 Provincial Archives of Saskatchewan (PAS), Jean Larmour oral history of the CCF Government, R8363-6, Interview with T.C. Douglas, 27 Nov. 1981, transcript 1.
2 The village only became a town in 1960s, after it had surpassed a population of one thousand. "Town of Birch Hills History," https://www.birchhills.ca/wp-content/uploads/2016/11/Town-History.pdf.
3 "Four Hospitals to Get Government Grants," *Regina Leader-Post* (*LP*), 13 March 1951, 2; advertisement for registered nurses, *LP*, 29 May 1951, 16.
4 Thomas H. McLeod and Ian McLeod, *Tommy Douglas: The Road to Jerusalem* (Edmonton: Hurtig Publishers, 1987), 195.
5 "Kinistino CCF Names Candidate," *LP*, 27 April 1959, 14; "Complete Health Care Program for Sask. Envisaged by Douglas," *Saskatoon Star Phoenix* (*SP*), 27 April 1959, 3; Robin F. Badgley and Samuel Wolfe, *Doctors' Strike: Medical Care and Conflict in Saskatchewan* (Toronto: Macmillan of Canada, 1967), 22.
6 A.W. Johnson with Rosemary Proctor, *Dream No Little Dreams: A Biography of the Douglas Government of Saskatchewan, 1944–1961* (Toronto: University of Toronto Press, 2004), 249.
7 These are T.K. Shoyama's recollection of the discussion at the cabinet planning session: PAS, Jean Larmour oral history of CCF Government, R-8459 to R-8462, T.K Shoyama interview transcript, 26 July 1982, 93–4. On the growing militancy of both the CPS and the CMA, see C. David Naylor, *Private Practice, Public Payment: Canadian Medicare and the Politics of Health Insurance, 1911–1966* (Montreal and Kingston: McGill-Queen's University Press, 1986), 176–91.
8 PAS, George Cadbury fonds, R880, file 2, no. 2, Memorandum from T.C. Douglas to all cabinet ministers, 6 Sept. 1950.
9 PAS, T.C. Douglas fonds (TCD), R33.5, file III, 123d (14-6-33), Sask. Hospitalization Act, March–April 1947, memorandum, T.C. Douglas to T.J. Bentley, 25 Sept. 1951.
10 PAS, TCD, R33.5, file III, 123d (14-6-33), Sask. Hospitalization Act, March–April 1947, memorandum, T.C. Douglas to T.J. Bentley, 28 Sept. 1951.
11 PAS, TCD, R33.1, file 562 (14-16) – National Health Insurance Data, memorandum, T.J. Bentley to T.C. Douglas, 6 Nov. 1951; R33.2, file 565 (14-19) – Legislation, cabinet memorandum re: medical care plan, 17 Dec. 1951.
12 PAS, TCD, R33.5, file III, 137a (14-28) – Medical Care Program, Feb. 1952–March 1960, letter, T.C. Douglas to Rev. Armand Stade (Fillmore, SK), 26 Sept. 1952.
13 PAS, TCD, R33.1, file 575c (14-28-2), "Proposals for the Medical Care Program: A Report to Cabinet by the Interdepartmental

Committee to Study a Medical Care Program," 20 Nov. 1959 (hereafter Interdepartmental Committee's Proposals for Medical Care), CPS resolution quoted at 50.

14 C. David Naylor, *Private Practice*, table 6, 179. The number of enrollees was divided by the estimate provincial population of 907,000. Interdepartmental Committee's Proposals for Medical Care, 26–7. By 1959, there was only one insurance co-operative providing medical care insurance. The Saskatoon Mutual Medical and Hospital Benefit Association Limited had 4,900 subscribers, a minor number relative to the physician carriers.

15 In his letter to Douglas on 28 April 1959 (PAS, T.C. Douglas fonds, R33.1, file 562 (14-16) – National Health Insurance Data), Peacock referred to an article in the *Saskatoon Star Phoenix*, somewhat misleadingly entitled "Complete Health Care Program Envisages for Sask. by Douglas," 27 April 1959, 3.

16 PAS, TCD, R33.1, file 562 (14-16) – National Health Insurance Data, letter, G.W. Peacock to T.C. Douglas, 28 April 1959.

17 PAS, TCD, R33.1, file 562 (14-16) – National Health Insurance Data, letter, T.C. Douglas to G.W. Peacock, 1 May 1959.

18 PAS, TCD, R33.1, file 562 (14-16) – National Health Insurance Data, letter, T.C. Douglas to G.W. Peacock, 1 May 1959.

19 From July 1948 until February 1957, Dr. Vincent L. Matthews was chief medical health officer for the Swift Current Health Region, when he moved to Regina to become director of the medical and hospital services branch in the provincial health department. He remained in this position until 1962, when he was appointed acting deputy minister of public health, a position he held for a year before he was appointed permanent associate deputy minister. Upon the change of government in 1964, he moved to the University of Saskatchewan, where he was appointed professor and head of the Department of Social and Preventive Medicine in the College of Medicine. C. Stuart Houston and Merle Masse, *36 Steps on the Road to Medicare: Why Saskatchewan Led the Way* (Montreal and Kingston: McGill-Queen's University Press, 2013), 86, 163n37.

20 PAS, Department of Public Health fonds, R-327, 1.11, College of Physicians and Surgeons, 1955–1963, memorandum prepared by Vincent L. Matthews, Department of Public Health, 21 April 1959.

21 Johnson with Proctor, *Dream No Little Dreams*, 249.

22 Johnson with Proctor, *Dream No Little Dreams*, 241.

23 Interdepartmental Committee's Proposals for Medical Care.

24 On the growth of physician-sponsored medical care insurance carriers, see Naylor, *Private Practice*, 135–75.

25 Interdepartmental Committee's Proposals for Medical Care, 50. By 1959, the municipal doctor plans were beginning to lose ground to MSI

and GMS. The number of municipal doctor plans had declined to 126 from 179 in 1943. By 1959, MSI had managed to secure contracts with sixty RMs, while MSI and GMS had a combined enrollment of 69,305 residents of local governments. Gordon S. Lawson and Luc Thériault, "Saskatchewan's Community Health Service Associations: An Historical Perspective," *Prairie Forum* 24, no. 2 (1999): 257.

26 PAS, Meyer Brownstone fonds, F 206, R-414, file IV.4a, memorandum "Organized Medicine's Official Position on Health Insurance" prepared by the Interdepartmental Committee to Study the Medical Care Insurance Program, 29 Sept. 1959. Not based on any interviews or discussions with CPS leaders, this stakeholder analysis parsed the words and resolutions of the college (which clearly showed opposition) but then used the faulty logic that, because the CPS had allowed universal coverage to occur by accepting universal plans – presumably the medical care plan in the Swift Current Health Region – then it would accept "the mandatory inclusion of the total population" in Saskatchewan. Both the premise and the conclusion of this analysis were flawed. Thus, the strength of physician opposition was identified in the final report: Interdepartmental Committee's Proposals for Medical Care, 50.

27 F. Burns Roth and R.D. Defries, "The Saskatchewan Department of Public Health," *Canadian Journal of Public Health / Revue canadienne de santé publique* 49, no. 7 (1958): 280–2.

28 This question of timing is reviewed by Malcolm Taylor in *Health Insurance and Canadian Public Policy: The Seven Decisions that Created the Canadian Health Insurance System and its Outcomes* (Montreal and Kingston: McGill-Queen's University Press, 2010, orig. 1987), 275.

29 University of Saskatchewan Archives and Special Collections (USAS), V.L. Matthews fonds, MG241, IV. Medicine/Health Care. B. 1961 – Mtgs and Min Re. Med. Plan, file 1, memorandum re: cabinet discussion of interdepartmental committee's report on proposed medical care program, M.S. Acker to F.B. Roth, 26 Nov. 1959 (hereafter Acker memorandum on cabinet discussion, 26 Nov. 1959).

30 Interdepartmental Committee's Proposals for Medical Care, 71.

31 Interdepartmental Committee's Proposals for Medical Care, 70.

32 Interdepartmental Committee's Proposals for Medical Care, 70.

33 Donald Macintyre, "Political Commentary: But Which Bastards Are on Your Side?" *Independent*, 31 July 1993, https://www.independent.co.uk/voices/political-commentary-but-which-bastards-are-on-your-side-1458580.html.

34 For a contemporary account of physician dissatisfaction with NHS salary scales in a self-described progressive magazine in the United States that was historically supportive of universal health coverage, see Anne Taylor Moore's "Medical Care in Britain," *New Republic*, 6 April 1959, 11.

35 McLeod and McLeod, *Tommy Douglas*, 197. Also see Allan M. Briens, "The 1960 Saskatchewan Provincial Election" (MA thesis, University of Regina, 2004), 27. This wave of NHS refugees had an enormous impact on the profession throughout Canada in the late 1950s and early 1960s: see Sasha Mullally and David Wright, *Foreign Practices: Immigrant Doctors and the History of Canadian Medicare* (Montreal and Kingston: McGill-Queen's University Press, 2020), 56.
36 Interdepartmental Committee's Proposals for Medical Care, 63.
37 Interdepartmental Committee's Proposals for Medical Care, 64.
38 Acker memorandum on cabinet discussion, 26 Nov. 1959.
39 The estimate of population is drawn from Statistics Canada's intercensal estimates: see *Population of Canada and the Provinces, Annual, 1926–1960* (Ottawa: Statistics Canada, 2000), table 36-10-0280-01, https://www150.statcan.gc.ca/t1/tbl1/en/tv.action?pid=3610028001
40 Interdepartmental Committee's Proposals for Medical Care, 1.
41 Indeed, this is the main thesis of Esyllt W. Jones's *Radical Medicine: The International Origins of Socialized Health Care in Canada* (Winnipeg: ARP Books, 2019).
42 This description was gleaned from the biographical information provided in the finding aid (SAFA 420) to the Meyer Brownstone fonds at PAS, R-414.
43 Donald V. Smiley, "Local Autonomy and Central Administrative Control in Saskatchewan," *Canadian Journal of Economics and Political Science / Revue canadienne d'économique et de science politique* 26, no. 2 (1960)" 301–5.
44 Led by Brownstone and Harding, this was the view expressed by the Local Government Continuing Committee: *Local Government Continuing Committee: Consultations on Local Government in Saskatchewan* (Regina: Queen's Printer, 1961), 133.
45 See, for example, Meyer Brownstone, "Agriculture," in *Social Purpose for Canada*, ed. Michael Oliver (Toronto: University of Toronto Press, 1961), 334–7.
46 Joan Feather, "Impact of the Swift Current Health Region: Experiment or Model?" *Prairie Forum* 16, no. 2 (1991): 233.
47 Feather, "Impact of the Swift Current Health Region," 233–4.
48 Interdepartmental Committee's Proposals for Medical Care, 62.
49 Acker memorandum on cabinet discussion, 26 Nov. 1959.
50 PAS, TCD, R-33.1, file 757a (14-28-2) – Medical Care Program, memorandum, M. Brownstone to T.C Douglas, 21 Dec. 1959.
51 PAS, TCD, R-33.1, file 757a (14-28-2) – Medical Care Program, memorandum, M. Brownstone to T.C Douglas, 21 Dec. 1959.
52 Acker memorandum on cabinet discussion, 26 Nov. 1959.
53 PAS, Jean Larmour oral history of the CCF Government, R8358 to-R8362, interview with T.C. Douglas, 27 Nov. 1981, transcript 5, 4 Sept. 1981, 12.

54 PAS, CPS fonds, F-696, CPS miscellaneous files, CPS draft news release, 28 Oct. 1959; "Thatcher Proposes Plebiscite," *LP*, 17 Dec. 1959, 3.
55 "No Compulsion on Doctors," *LP*, 17 Dec. 1959, 3.
56 LAC, Thomas Clement Douglas fonds, MG32 C28, vol. 142, file 47, script for Premier T.C. Douglas' Provincial Affairs radio broadcast on "Prepaid Medical Care," 16 Dec. 1959 (hereafter Douglas radio script, Prepaid Medical Care), 1–2.
57 Douglas radio script, "Prepaid Medical Care," 3–4.
58 Douglas radio script, "Prepaid Medical Care," 4.
59 Douglas radio script, "Prepaid Medical Care," 4–5.
60 Douglas radio script, "Prepaid Medical Care," 6.
61 See David U. Himmelstein, Terry Campbell, and Steffie Woolhandler, "Costs of Health Care Administration in the United States and Canada," *New England Journal of Medicine* 349, no. 8 (2003): 768–75, and "Health Care Administrative Costs in the United States and Canada, 2017," *Annals of Internal Medicine* 172, no. 2 (2020): 132–42.
62 Douglas radio script, "Prepaid Medical Care," 7.
63 Douglas radio script, "Prepaid Medical Care," 7–8.
64 David Wright, Sasha Mullally, and Mary Colleen Cordukes, "'Worse Than Being Married': The Exodus of British Doctors from the National Health Service to Canada, c. 1955–75," *Journal of the History of Medicine and Allied Sciences* 65, no. 4 (2010): 546–50.
65 Douglas radio script, "Prepaid Medical Care," 8–9.
66 Douglas, quoted in Johnson with Protor, *Dream No Little Dreams*, 251.
67 Douglas radio script, "Prepaid Medical Care," 10.
68 LAC, Thomas Clement Douglas fonds, MG32 C28, vol. 142, file 51, Premier T.C. Douglas and Mrs. Marjorie Cooper, MLA, script for provincial affairs television program on Medical Care Program, 16 Jan. 1960, 2, 6–7.
69 This was the Mossbank (a village south of Moose Jaw) debate held on 20 May 1957: see Dale Eisler, *Rumours of Glory: Saskatchewan and the Thatcher Years* (Edmonton: Hurtig Publishers, 1987), 19–32, and McLeod and McLeod, *Tommy Douglas*, 192. According to Tim (H.S.) Lee, Douglas's cabinet secretary, Thatcher and his team "out strategized" Douglas, packing the hall in advance and preparing a speech purposely putting Douglas on the defensive: PAS, Jean Larmour oral history of CCF government, R8433 to R-8435, interview with H.S. Lee, transcript, 20 Jan. 1982, 34–5.
70 PAS, W.G. Davies fonds (Public Health), R-30.1, XXVIII.7, first of five folders, clipping "Name Medical Advisory Board 'In Few Weeks,'" *LP*, 18 Dec. 1959.
71 These party positions were aptly captured in the CBC Television documentary entitled *1960 Saskatchewan Election: Tommy Douglas'*

*Medicare Plan Dominates the 1960 Election Campaign* (Ottawa: Canadian Broadcasting Corporation, 1960).
72 Michael Dupuis, "An Interview with Graham Spry, 1972," *Manitoba History*, no. 51 (2006): 40–3.
73 Upon his death in 1983, *Maclean's* magazine (5 Dec. 1983, 4) referred to Graham Spry as "the father of Canadian broadcasting."
74 As to Graham Spry and the CCF's original organization of Bethune's medical mission, see Roderick Stewart and Jesús Majada, *Bethune in Spain* (Montreal and Kingston: McGill-Queen's University Press, 2014), 13–20, and Tyler Wentzell, "Canada's *Foreign Enlistment Act* and the Spanish Civil War," *Labour/Le Travail* 90 (2017): 215–16. Also see David Rodríguez-Solás, "Remembered and Recovered: Bethune and the Canadian Blood Transfusion Unit in Málaga, 1937," *Revista Canadiense de Estudios Hispanicos* 36, no. 1 (2011): 83–97.
75 Roderick Stewart and Sharon Stewart, *Phoenix: The Life of Norman Bethune* (Montreal and Kingston: McGill-Queen's University Press, 2011), 252–368. Interestingly, one of Douglas's most determined opponents in the medicare battle in Saskatchewan between 1960 and 1962, "Staff" Barootes, subsequently wrote about Bethune's fame throughout China: E.W. Barootes, "Dr. Norman Bethune: Inspiration for a Modern China," *Canadian Medical Association Journal* 122, no. 10 (1980), 1176–84.
76 David James Smith, "Intellectual Activist: Graham Spry, a Biography" (PhD diss., York University, 2002), 308–87.
77 Smith, "Intellectual Activist," 388.
78 LAC, Graham Spry fonds, MG30 D297, vol. 54, file 12, "Notes on Trends in Saskatchewan – Opinion," by Graham Spry (marked confidential), 9 April 1960.
79 LAC, Graham Spry fonds, MG30 D297, vol. 54, file 12, "Notes on Trends in Saskatchewan – Opinion," by Graham Spry (marked confidential), 9 April 1960.
80 "Thatcher Proposes Plebiscite," *LP*, 17 Dec. 1959, 3.
81 PAS, CPS fonds, F-696, Miscellaneous College of Physicians and Surgeons files, letter to MSI subscribers from MSI, 22 Dec. 1959.
82 "Labor Scores Opponents of Gov't Medical Plan," *LP*, 12 Nov. 1959, clipping found in PAS, W.G. Davies fonds, R-301. XXVIII.7, first of five folders.
83 USAS, V.L. Matthews fonds, MG 241, IV, Medicine/Health Care. B., file 1: Interdepartmental Committee to Study Medical Care Program, memorandum, M.S. Acker to F.B. Roth re: Cabinet Discussion of Interdepartmental Committee's Report on Proposed Medical Care Program, 26 Nov. 1959.

Notes to pages 289–92    581

84 USAS, W.P. Thompson fonds (WPT), MG 17, letter (marked confidential), W.P. Thompson to T.C. Douglas, 20 Nov. 1959. This letter also reveals that Douglas had recently travelled to Europe, where he "spent considerable time re-examining the British health plan and also the health program in Israel." He concluded that the New Zealand plan and the medical care program in operation in Swift Current "would probably meet our needs better than the British or Israeli programs which are designed primarily for industrial communities. However, this is a matter for the group I have mentioned to determine when it is set up."
85 USAS, WPT, MG 17, letter (marked confidential), T.C. Douglas to W.P. Thompson, 23 Nov. 1959.
86 USAS, WPT, MG 17, letter (marked confidential), W.P. Thompson to T.C. Douglas, 27 Nov. 1959.
87 USAS, WPT, MG 17, letter (marked confidential), T.C. Douglas to W.P. Thompson, 1 Dec. 1959.
88 USAS, WPT, MG 17, letter, W.P. Thompson to F.B. Roth, 10 Dec. 1959.
89 PAS, CPS fonds, F-696, miscellaneous CPS files, letter to MSI subscribers from MSI, 22 Dec. 1959.
90 PAS, TCD, R-33.1, file 575b (14-28-2) – Medical Care Program, letter, G.W. Peacock (Registrar, CPS) to J. Walter Erb, 18 Jan. 1960.
91 PAS, TCD, R-33.1, file 575b (14-28-2) – Medical Care Program, draft letter sent to all members of the Advisory Planning Committee on Medical Care from J. Walter Erb, 30 Dec. 1959. It is interesting to note that this was a refined version of a similar draft dated 4 December 1959 (PAS, TCD, R-33.1, file 575a (14-28-2) – Medical Care Program), reflecting the careful crafting of the letter.
92 PAS, TCD, R-33.1, file 575b (14-28-2) – Medical Care Program, letter, G.W. Peacock (Registrar, CPS) to J. Walter Erb, 18 Jan. 1960.
93 *Interim Report of the Advisory Planning Committee on Medical Care to the Government of Saskatchewan, September 1961* (Regina: Lawrence Amon, Queen's Printer, 1962), 6; Lisa Dale-Burnett, "Beatrice Janet Trew," in *Saskatchewan Politicians: Lives Past and Present*, ed. Brett Quiring (Regina: Canadian Plains Research Center, University of Regina, 2004), 230–1. On Cliff H. Whiting, see the biography provided on his being awarded with an honorary doctorate at the University of Saskatchewan in May 1963, https://library.usask.ca/uasc/campus-history-databases/honorary-degrees/clifford-henry-whiting.
94 PAS, CPS fonds, F-696, miscellaneous CPS files, notes from CPS meeting with T.C. Douglas, 3 Feb. 1960 (hereafter CPS notes from meeting with T.C. Douglas).
95 CPS notes from meeting with T.C. Douglas.
96 CPS notes from meeting with T.C. Douglas (emphasis in original).

97 CPS notes from meeting with T.C. Douglas.
98 CPS notes from meeting with T.C. Douglas.
99 PAS, TCD, R-33.1, file 575b (14-28-2) – Medical Care Program, Terms of Reference for Advisory Planning Committee on Medical Care (revised), 3 Feb. 1960.
100 Efstathios William (Staff) Barootes (1918–2000), was a prominent urologist who practised in Regina until 1979. He was among the most vocal and articulate of the anti-Medicare physicians. After he retired, he became the chief fundraiser for the PC Party of Saskatchewan and was appointed to the Senate by the Mulroney government in 1984, where he remained until 1993. He also served for a time as treasurer and deputy president of the Canadian Medical Association. See Patrick Sullivan, "Dr. Efstathios (Staff) Barootes," *CMAJ* 163, no. 6 (2000): 795, and the entry in *The Encyclopedia of Saskatchewan* (Regina: Canadian Plains Research Center, University of Regina, 2005), 92.
101 "Opinions Unlimited: Program Is Sound Board on Current Events," *Canadian Broadcaster*, 5 May 1960, 11.
102 PAS, TCD, R-33.1, file 575b (14-28-2) – Medical Care Program, Premier T.C. Douglas remarks for *Opinions Unlimited*, CKCK-TV, 20 March 1960, 5–6.
103 PAS, TCD, R-33.1, file 575b (14-28-2) – Medical Care Program, Premier T.C. Douglas remarks for *Opinions Unlimited*, CKCK-TV, 20 March 1960, 4–5.
104 PAS, TCD, R-33.1, file 575b (14-28-2) – Medical Care Program, Premier T.C. Douglas remarks for *Opinions Unlimited*, CKCK-TV, 20 March 1960, 7.
105 Staff Barootes, quoted in "12 Committee Men Hinted," *LP*, 21 March 1960, 5.
106 "Government Accepts Doctors' Terms," *LP*, 30 March 1960, 1, 9; E.N. Davis, "Banks of the Wascana: A Letter for Mr. Douglas," *LP*, 30 March 1960, 21.
107 Douglas, quoted in "Government Accepts Doctors' Terms," *LP*, 30 March 1960, 1.
108 E.A. Tollefson, "The Medicare Dispute," in *Politics in Saskatchewan*, ed. Norman Ward and Duff Spafford (Toronto: Longmans Canada, 1968), 245.
109 Naylor, *Private Practice*, 185.
110 Briens, "The 1960 Saskatchewan Provincial Election," 70–1.
111 Briens, "The 1960 Saskatchewan Provincial Election," 69–70.
112 Quoted in Badgley and Wolfe, *Doctors' Strike*, 30–1.
113 PAS, CPS fonds, F-696, miscellaneous CPS files, letter, Dr. J.D. Leishman to Dr. A.J.M. Davies (CPS), 11 April 1969; Badgley and Wolfe, *Doctors' Strike*, 30. As a aside, it appears that the term "key men" was used (although perhaps with a different meaning) by the CPS as early as 1944: Gordon

S. Lawson, "The Co-operative Commonwealth Federation, Health Care Reform and Physician Remuneration in the Province of Saskatchewan, 1915–1949" (MA thesis, University of Saskatchewan, 1998), 85.

114 Dennis Gruending, *Promises to Keep: A Political Biography of Allan Blakeney* (Saskatoon: Western Producer Prairie Books, 1990), 33.

115 Allan Blakeney, "The Struggle to Implement Medicare," *Bulletin of the History of Medicine / Bulletin canadien d'histoire de la médecine* 26, no. 2 (2009): 528. The extent to which the Blakeney government operated on principles inherited from the Douglas government is clearly set out in Allan Blakeney and Sandford Borins, *Political Management in Canada* (Toronto: University of Toronto Press, 1998). The "inheritance" is further explored in Robert I. McLaren, *The Saskatchewan Practice of Public Administration in Historical Perspective* (New York: Edwin Mellen, 1998), and Gregory P. Marchildon, "The Blakeney Style of Cabinet Government: Lessons for the Twenty-First Century?" in *Back to Blakeney: Revitalizing the Democratic State*, ed. David McGrane, John D. Whyte, Roy Romanow, and Russ Singer (Regina: University of Regina Press, 2019), 33–49.

116 "Doctors Printing 'Trash' – Douglas," *LP*, 2 June 1960, 1.

117 "Alberta's Manning Gives 'Good Neighbor' Advice," *LP*, 6 June 1960, 1.

118 I explored the religious and ideological differences between the two premiers in greater depth in my article "Douglas versus Manning: The Ideological Battle over Medicare in Postwar Canada," *Journal of Canadian Studies / Revue d'études canadiennes* 50, no. 1 (2016): 129–49.

119 "Leader of CCF Foresees Victory," *LP*, 6 June 1960, 5.

120 Allan Blakeney, "The Struggle to Implement Medicare," *Bulletin of the History of Medicine / Bulletin canadien d'histoire de la médecine* 26, no. 2 (2009): 528. The extent to which the Blakeney government operated on principles inherited from the Douglas government is clearly set out in Allan Blakeney and Sandford Borins, *Political Management in Canada* (Toronto: University of Toronto Press, 1998). The "inheritance" is further explored in Robert I. McLaren, *The Saskatchewan Practice of Public Administration in Historical Perspective* (New York: Edwin Mellen, 1998), and Gregory P. Marchildon, "The Blakeney Style of Cabinet Government: Lessons for the Twenty-First Century?" in *Back to Blakeney: Revitalizing the Democratic State*, ed. David McGrane, John D. Whyte, Roy Romanow, and Russ Singer (Regina: University of Regina Press, 2019), 33–49.

121 Briens, "The 1960 Saskatchewan Provincial Election," 97.

122 According to Noel Doig, *Setting the Record Straight: A Doctor's Memoir of the 1962 Medicare Crisis* (Saskatoon: Indie Ink Publishing, 2012), the college and its members after the election recognized how counterproductive their publicity campaign had been and the damage it had done to their cause.

## 11. The Thompson Committee and the New Party

1. Library and Archives Canada (LAC), Thomas Clement Douglas fonds (TCD), MG32-C28, vol. 91, file 2, letter, T.C. Douglas to Dr. Angus H. Blair, 17 Aug. 1961.
2. "Doctors Express Opposite Views," *Regina Leader-Post* (*LP*), 10 June 1960, 1.
3. T.C. Douglas, quoted in "Doctors Express Opposite Views," *LP*, 10 June 1960, 1.
4. See account in E.A. Tollefson, *Bitter Medicine: The Saskatchewan Medicare Feud* (Saskatoon: Modern Press, 1964), 55.
5. "CMA Opposes Gov't Control: Compulsory Medical Insurance Not Ruled Out," *LP*, 15 July 1960, 1.
6. Richard A. Rempel, *Research and Reform: W.P. Thompson at the University of Saskatchewan* (Montreal and Kingston: McGill-Queen's University Press, 2013), 198–9.
7. Quoted sections from T.C. Douglas's letter to Dr. G.W. Peacock (Registrar CPS), 15 March 1960, reproduced in Appendix A in Tollefson, *Bitter Medicine*, 161.
8. *Dominion-Provincial Conference 1960: Ottawa, July 25th, 26th and 27th, 1960* (Ottawa: Roger Duhamel, Queen's Printer, 1960), 83–4.
9. University of Saskatchewan Archives and Special Collections (USAS), W.P. Thompson fonds, MG 17S1, Medical Care Correspondence (hereafter WPT correspondence), file 88, letter, W.P. Thompson to Dr. John E. Sparks, 14 Sept. 1960.
10. USAS, WPT correspondence, file 94, letter, C.J. Houston to W.P. Thompson, 9 Oct. 1960.
11. USAS, WPT correspondence, file 93, letter (marked personal and confidential), W.P. Thompson to T.C. Douglas, 7 Nov. 1960.
12. USAS, WPT correspondence, file 93, letter (marked personal and confidential), T.C. Douglas to W.P. Thompson, 9 Nov. 1960.
13. USAS, WPT correspondence, file 93, letter (marked personal and confidential), T.C. Douglas to W.P. Thompson, 9 Nov. 1960.
14. USAS, WPT correspondence, file 93, letter (marked personal and confidential), W.P. Thompson to T.C. Douglas, 15 Nov. 1960.
15. USAS, WPT correspondence, file 93, letter, T.C. Douglas to W.P. Thompson, 16 Nov. 1960.
16. USAS, WPT correspondence, file 93, letter (marked personal and confidential), T.C. Douglas to W.P. Thompson, 9 Nov. 1960.
17. David Lewis, *The Good Fight: Political Memoirs, 1909–1958* (Toronto: Macmillan of Canada, 1981), 485; John Courtney, *Revival and Change: The 1957 and 1958 Diefenbaker Elections* (Vancouver: UBC Press, 2022), 149.

18 LAC, TCD, MG32, C28, vol. 1, file 18-45: CCF-CLC Amalgamation, Part 1, TCD News Release, 24 April 1958.
19 Walter D. Young, *The Anatomy of a Party: The National CCF, 1932–1961* (Toronto: University of Toronto Press, 1969), 131–4.
20 LAC, TCD, MG32, C28, vol. 1, file 18-35, CCF Manifesto, letter, T.C. Douglas to E.D. Snyder, 1 Nov. 1956.
21 Given the enmity that soon developed between the two men, it was somewhat ironic that Hazen Argue wrote Douglas to say how much his leadership was missed at the meetings and that "had you been there I know you would have given the committee some very worthwhile leadership." LAC, TCD, MG32, C28, vol. 1, file 18-45, CCF-CLC Amalgamation, part 1, letter, Hazen Argue to T.C. Douglas, 3 Feb. 1959.
22 LAC, TCD, MG32, C28, vol. 1, file 18-45, CCF-CLC Amalgamation, part 6, T.C. Douglas to C.N. Kushner (mayor of Winnipeg), 22 Feb. 1961.
23 LAC, TCD, MG32, C28, vol. 2, file 18-48-3, Leadership of the New Party, part 3, T.C. Douglas to Dr. Sam Wolfe (New York City), 28 Feb. 1961.
24 LAC, TCD, MG32, C28, vol. 1, file 18-45, CCF-CLC Amalgamation, part 1, Douglas, quoted in Mark Harrison, "Liberals Willing but CCF Shies Away from Anti-Tory Pact," *Toronto Daily Star*, 20 Nov. 1958.
25 LAC, TCD, MG32, C28, vol. 1, file 18-45, CCF-CLC Amalgamation, part 1, letter (marked personal and confidential), T.C. Douglas to H.W. Herridge, MP, 10 Feb. 1959.
26 LAC, TCD, MG32, C28, vol. 1, file 18-45, CCF-CLC Amalgamation, part 1, T.C. Douglas to Stanley Knowles (copy to David Lewis), 4 May 1959.
27 LAC, TCD, MG32, C28, vol. 1, file 18-45, CCF-CLC Amalgamation, part 1, Stanley Knowles to T.C. Douglas, 13 July 1959
28 LAC, TCD, MG32, C28, vol. 1, file 18-45, CCF-CLC Amalgamation, part 4, Herbert W. Herridge (MP) to T.C. Douglas, 17 March 1960.
29 Thomas H. McLeod and Ian McLeod, *Tommy Douglas: The Road to Jerusalem* (Edmonton: Hurtig Publishers, 1987), 223.
30 LAC, TCD, MG32, C28, vol. 1, file 18-45, CCF-CLC Amalgamation, part 4, T.C. Douglas to Howard R. Pawley (cc. to David Lewis, Stanley Knowles, and Frank Hanson), 21 March 1960.
31 Knowles would go on to prepare a book *The New Party* (Toronto: McClelland & Stewart, 1961) that described in vivid detail how, in Walter Stewart's words, "the CCF would rise like the phoenix from the dead ashes of its former self, propelled by labour muscle, labour moxie, and labour money." Walter Stewart, *The Life and Political Times of Tommy Douglas* (Toronto: McArthur & Company, 2003), 242.
32 Susan Mann Trofimenkoff, *Stanley Knowles: The Man from Winnipeg North Centre* (Saskatoon: Western Producer Prairie Books, 1982), 155–66.
33 McLeod and McLeod, *Tommy Douglas*, 217.

34 McLeod and McLeod, *Tommy Douglas*, 217.
35 LAC, TCD, MG32, C28, vol. 1, file 18-45, CCF-CLC Amalgamation, part 5, F.A. Brewin (National Committee for the New Party) to T.C. Douglas, 26 Oct. 1960.
36 LAC, TCD, MG32, C28, vol. 1, file 18-45, CCF-CLC Amalgamation, part 5, T.C. Douglas to S.R. Laycock, 12 Oct. 1960.
37 LAC, TCD, MG32, C28, vol. 1, file 18-45, CCF-CLC Amalgamation, part 5, T.D. Douglas to F.W. Brewin, 9 Nov. 1960.
38 F. Andrew Brewin was a candidate for the leadership of the Ontario CCF in 1953 and was an NDP MP from 1962 until 1979. LAC, TCD, MG32, C28, vol. 1, file 18-45, CCF-CLC Amalgamation, part 5, T.C. Douglas to F.W. Brewin, 9 Nov. 1960.
39 LAC, TCD, MG32, C28, vol. 1, file 18-45, CCF-CLC Amalgamation, part 5, T.C. Douglas to F.W. Brewin, 9 Nov. 1960.
40 LAC, TCD, MG32, C28, vol. 2, file 1, Leadership of the New Party, T.C. Douglas to David Lewis, 16 Jan. 1961.
41 LAC, TCD, MG32, C28, vol. 1, file 18-48-1, National Seminar, Calgary, National Committee for the New Party: Policy Seminar on the Programme and Structure of the New Party: Schedule of Discussions, Calgary, 10–11 Dec. 1960.
42 Dr. John Leishman speaking to the Central Lions Club at the Hotel Saskatchewan and quoted in *LP*, 15 March 1961, 10.
43 USAS, WPT correspondence, file 93, letter, T.C. Douglas to W.P. Thompson, 16 March 1961.
44 USAS, WPT correspondence, file 93, letter (marked personal and confidential), W.P. Thompson to T.C. Douglas, 17 March 1961.
45 USAS, WPT correspondence, file 93, letter (marked personal and confidential), T.C. Douglas to W.P. Thompson, 20 March 1961.
46 A.W. Johnson with Rosemary Proctor, *Dream No Little Dreams: A Biography of the Douglas Government of Saskatchewan, 1944–1961* (Toronto: University of Toronto Press, 2004), 261.
47 Provincial Archives of Saskatchewan (PAS), W.G. Davies fonds, R-30.1, file XXVIII, no. 6 – Advisory Planning Committee on Medical Care Interim Report, letter, J. Walter Erb, to W.P. Thompson, 2 June 1961.
48 PAS, W.G. Davies fonds, R-30.1, file XXVIII, no. 6 – Advisory Planning Committee on Medical Care Interim Report, letter, J. Walter Erb, to W.P. Thompson, 2 June 1961.
49 USAS, WPT correspondence, file 94, draft letter rejected by Thompson to J. Walter Erb, 14 June 1961.
50 USAS, WPT correspondence, file 94, letter (marked personal and confidential), W.P. Thompson to J. Walter Erb, 23 Aug. 1961.
51 PAS, W.G. Davies fonds, R-30.1, XXVIII.7 (1 of 5 files), clippings from the *Leader-Post* and *Star Phoenix* (*SP*), 24 Aug. 1961.

52 "Report on Medical Care Ready in Sept.," *SP*, 24 Aug. 1961, 3.
53 Dwayne Yasinowski, "Hazen Robert Argue," in *Saskatchewan Politicians: Lives Past and Present*, ed. Brett Quiring (Regina: Canadian Plains Research Center, University of Regina, 2004), 6–7.
54 Stewart, *Life and Political Times*, 245–7; McLeod and McLeod, *Tommy Douglas*, 215–17.
55 McLeod and McLeod, *Tommy Douglas*, 217–18.
56 Both Lewis and Knowles denied any "planned attack" on Argue, but they were unarguably in favour of T.C. from the beginning and regularly made unflattering comparisons between Argue and Douglas. As early as January 1961, for example, Knowles was openly telling party members that Douglas "would make an incomparably better New Party Leader" than Argue, even though T.C. had not yet agreed to put his name forward: LAC, TCD, MG32-C28, vol. 2, file 3 (part 1), letter, Stanley Knowles to H.C. Abella, 3 Jan. 1961. Similarly, David Lewis publicly described Douglas as "the best political leader in Canada today" and defended his position against prominent pro-Argue members of the CCF: LAC, TCD, MG32-C28, vol. 2, file 3 (part 1), letter, David Lewis to Adele Pawley, 8 Feb. 1981.
57 LAC, TCD, MG32-C28, vol. 2, file 7, letter, T.C. Douglas to George R. Bothwell, 15 June 1961.
58 Walter Steward, *M.J.: The Life and Times of M.J. Coldwell* (Toronto: Stoddard, 2000), 256–7.
59 LAC, TCD, MG32-C28, vol. 2, file 7, Government of Saskatchewan news release, 28 June 1961.
60 LAC, TCD, MG32-C28, vol. 2, file 7, letter (marked personal and confidential), T.C. Douglas to E. Regier (MP), 15 June 1961.
61 LAC, TCD, MG32-C28, vol. 2, file 7, letter (marked personal and confidential), E. Regier to T.C. Douglas, 12 June 1961.
62 LAC, TCD, MG32-C28, vol. 2, file 7, Government of Saskatchewan news release, 28 June 1961.
63 Clifford Scotton, quoted in Doris French Shackleton, *Tommy Douglas: A Biography* (Toronto: McClelland & Stewart, 1975), 257.
64 Alan Whitehorn, *Canadian Socialism: Essays on the CCF-NDP* (Toronto: Oxford University Press, 1991), 53.
65 *The Federal Program of the New Democratic Party Adopted by Its Founding Convention, Ottawa, July 31–August 4, 1961 and by Its Second Federal Convention Regina, August 6–9, 1963 and Third Federal Convention, Toronto, July 12–15, 1965* (Ottawa: New Democratic Party, 1965).
66 *CAR* 1961, 76.
67 *CAR* 1961, 81; Stewart, *Life and Political Times*, 247–8.
68 LAC, TCD, MG32-C28, vol. 1, file 18-45 – New Party 1961, letter, T.C. Douglas to Marjorie Cooper, 11 July 1961.

69 LAC, TCD, MG32-C28, vol. 91, file 2, letter, T.C. Douglas to T.J. Bentley, 21 Aug. 1961.
70 LAC, TCD, MG32-C28, vol. 1, file 18-45 – New Party 1961, letter, T.C. Douglas to Marjorie Cooper, 11 July 1961.
71 LAC, TCD, MG32-C28, vol. 1, file 18-45 – New Party 1961, letter, Marjorie Cooper to T.C. Douglas, 5 July 1961.
72 Jeannie Argue, quoted in MacLeod and MacLeod, *Tommy Douglas*, 221, where this episode is recounted.
73 LAC, TCD, MG32-C28, vol. 145, New Party Founding Convention file, nomination speech, 2 Aug. 1961. The quotation includes Douglas's handwritten changes to the speech.
74 Shackleton, *Tommy Douglas*, 257.
75 Hazen Argue quoted in Stewart, *Life and Political Times*, 249.
76 LAC, TCD, MG32-C28, vol. 91, file 4, letter, T.C. Douglas to Craig N. Markle, 10 April 1961.
77 MacLeod and MacLeod, *Tommy Douglas*, 231.
78 LAC, TCD, MG32-C28, vol. 91, file 2, letter, T.C. Douglas to Dr. Louis A. Ares, 17 Aug. 1961.
79 LAC, TCD, MG32-C28, vol. 145, New Party Founding Convention file, notes for acceptance speech – national leadership, 3 Aug. 1961.
80 Douglas quoted in McLeod and McLeod, *Tommy Douglas*, 222.
81 John T. Saywell, "The New Democratic Party Convention," in *CAR* 1961, 81–6; Ramsay Cook, "The Labor-Socialist Wedding: Moderation Wins Down the Line in NDP," *Saturday Night*, 2 Sept. 1961, 9–11.
82 On 14 September, Douglas was in Oakville railing against high unemployment ("Douglas Calls Jobless Disgrace," *SP*, 15 Sept. 1961, 1). A week later, he was in Calgary arguing in favour of a policy of higher wages for workers to prevent future recessions ("Recessions Due to Low Wages, Says Douglas," *SP*, 23 Sept. 1961, 14). He then flew back east to Fort William (now Thunder Bay) and spoke on the Cold War tensions caused by the erection of the Berlin Wall ("Press Misrepresented Berlin Situation – TCD," *SP*, 25 Sept. 1961, 10).
83 Ross Thatcher, quoted in "Douglas Should Resign or Look after His Job, Liberal Leader States," *SP*, 16 Sept. 1961, 3.
84 "New but Old Philosophies," *SP*, 26 Sept. 1961, 12.
85 *Interim Report of the Advisory Planning Committee on Medical Care to the Government of Saskatchewan, September 1961* (Regina: Lawrence Amon, Queen's Printer, 1962), 118–21 (hereafter referred to as *Interim Report of the APC*).
86 *Interim Report of the APC*, 105–17.
87 *Interim Report of the APC*, 109 (emphasis in original).

88 *Interim Report of the APC*, 112 (emphasis in original).
89 *Interim Report of the APC*, 112.
90 *Interim Report of the APC*, 106.
91 A committed socialist, Stan Rands exemplified this perspective. After being forced to leave the National Film Board due to his political activity, he took up a position in the Department of Public Health in Saskatchewan, eventually becoming the deputy director of the Psychiatric Services Branch. In 1962, fed up with the compromises he felt the government had made with the doctors, he left the government to help organize and administer community clinics. See Gregory P. Marchildon, "Community Clinics and Stan Rands's Struggle for the Transformation of Health Care in Canada," in Stan Rands, *Privilege and Policy: The History of Community Clinics in Canada*, ed. Gregory P. Marchildon and Catherine Leviten-Reid (Regina: Canadian Plains Research Centre, University of Regina, 2012), vii–xiii.
92 USAS, WPT correspondence, file 93, letter, T.C. Douglas to W.P. Thompson, 12 Oct. 1961.
93 USAS, WPT correspondence, file 93, letter, W.P. Thompson to T.C. Douglas, 5 Oct. 1961
94 "Compulsory Health Plan Legislation Introduced by Erb," *SP*, 13 Oct. 1961, 3.
95 PAS, Jean Larmour oral history of CCF Government, R-8358 to R-8362, T.C. Douglas interview transcript 5, 4 Sept. 1981, 15–16.
96 He also admitted that such premiums could perhaps be dispensed with once a society was wealthy enough to have large revenues and less punishing tradeoffs involved in spending decisions. PAS, Jean Larmour oral history of CCF Government, R-8358 to R-8362, T.C. Douglas interview transcript 5, 4 Sept. 1981, 15–16
97 Allan Blakeney, *An Honourable Calling: Political Memoirs* (Toronto: University of Toronto Press, 2008), 86–7.
98 Sections 3, 4, 10, and 20 of the Saskatchewan Medical Care Insurance Act, SS 1961 (2nd), c. 1.
99 "Douglas Insists Speech 'Proper,'" *LP*, 13 Oct. 1961, 1.
100 "National Health Plan Predicted: Douglas Answers Thatcher," *LP*, 14 Oct. 1961, 1.
101 McLeod and McLeod, *Tommy Douglas*, 223.
102 In his largely negative portrait, Robert Tyre, a former journalist based in Saskatchewan, characterized Douglas as the "silver-tongued apostle of Saskatchewan-style Marxism," a "spellbinder" capable of convincing almost anyone of anything. Robert Tyre, *Douglas in Saskatchewan: The Story of a Socialist Experiment* (Vancouver: Mitchell Press, 1962), 4.

## 12. Political Repudiation

1 Advertisement for T.C. Douglas telecast entitled "The Medical Care Plan" on *Provincial Affairs Television* program: *Regina Leader-Post* (*LP*), 11 Oct. 1961, 4.
2 Library and Archives Canada (LAC), Thomas Clement Douglas fonds (TCD), MG32-C28, vol. 145, Premier T.C. Douglas Provincial Affairs telecast script entitled "Thank You Saskatchewan," 11 Oct. 1961 (hereafter Douglas Provincial Affairs telecast, 11 Oct. 1961), 5–6.
3 Douglas Provincial Affairs telecast, 11 Oct. 1961, 8.
4 Douglas Provincial Affairs telecast, 11 Oct. 1961, 8–11.
5 LAC, TCD, MG32-C28, vol. 145, Premier T.C. Douglas, *The Nation's Business* telecast script entitled "National Pride and National Purpose," 18 Oct. 1961, 11–12.
6 The was Bill No. 1 in the special fall session: "An Act to provide for Payment for Services rendered to Certain Persons by Physicians and Certain other Persons." *Journals of the Legislative Assembly of Saskatchewan* (*JLAS*), 2nd session, 1961, 43; Malcolm G. Taylor, *Health Insurance and Canadian Public Policy: The Seven Decisions That Created the Canadian Health Insurance System and Its Outcomes*, 2nd ed. (Montreal and Kingston: McGill-Queen's University Press, 2009), 285.
7 *JLAS*, 2nd session, 1961, 43. "Care Bill Provides Payment by Premius, Public Funds," *LP*, 13 Oct. 1961, 1; "Compulsory Health Plan Legislation Introduced by Erb," *LP*, 13 Oct. 1961, 3
8 "Foley's Speech Blocks Attempt to End Debate," *LP*, 24 Oct. 1961, 10; "Erb Fails to Close Debate," *LP*, 26 Oct. 1961, 26.
9 "Second Reading for Bill," *LP*, 26 Oct. 1961, 1.
10 "CCF Amends Constitution to Effect Tie-Up with NDP," *LP*, 1 Nov. 1961, 3.
11 M.J. Coldwell, quoted in "NDP Told to Go On Building on Foundation CCF Laid," *LP*, 3 Nov. 1961, 25.
12 "Douglas Presented New Car," *LP*, 3 Nov. 1961, 39; photograph of T.C. Douglas with caption title "Overwhelmed," *LP*, 3 Nov. 1961, 39.
13 "Douglas Presented New Car," *LP*, 3 November 1961, 39.
14 "Race May Shape Up for Douglas' Job," *LP*, 2 Nov. 1961, 1. Born in 1917, Olaf Turnbull was a farmer who completed a degree in agricultural economics at the University of Saskatchewan in 1943. Later, he became an active member of the Saskatchewan Farmers Union, which had been created out of the ashes of the Saskatchewan Section of the United Farmers of Canada in 1949. Although asked to be candidate by several political parties in the 1960 provincial election, Turnbull chose the CCF because of his high regard for Tommy Douglas and his support for

medicare. Brett Quiring, "Olaf Alexander Turnbull," in *Saskatchewan Politicians: Lives Past and Present*, ed. Brett Quiring (Regina: Canadian Plains Research Center, University of Regina, 2004), 234–5. On the Saskatchewan Farmers Union, see Canadian Plains Research Center, *Encyclopedia of Saskatchewan* (Regina: Canadian Plains Research Center, University of Regina, 2005), 804–5.
15 Dianne Lloyd, *Woodrow: A Biography of W.S. Lloyd* (Saskatoon: Woodrow Lloyd Memorial Fund, 1979), 106–13.
16 "Lloyd Wins: Easy Victory over Turnbull," *LP*, 3 Nov. 1961, 1, 3.
17 W.S. Lloyd as quoted in LP, "Lloyd Wins: Easy Victory over Turnbull," *LP*, 3 Nov. 1961, 5.
18 Dianne Lloyd Norton, "Woodrow S. Lloyd," in *Saskatchewan Premiers of the Twentieth Century*, ed. Gordon L. Barnhart (Regina: Canadian Plains Research Center, University of Regina, 2004), 214–17.
19 "Lloyd Takes Over Reins," *LP*, 7 Nov. 1961, 5.
20 "Lloyd Takes Over; Cabinet Sworn In," *LP*, 7 Nov. 1961, 1.
21 Lloyd, *Woodrow*, 114. Provincial Archives of Saskatchewan (PAS), Jean Larmour oral history of CCF government, R-8412, tape 2 of recorded interview with J. Walter Erb, 6 Oct. 1982. Erb's logic was that if the government "accepted their traditions," they would "over time ... move on their position." To do otherwise would inevitably result in the loss of the next election.
22 "Liberal Terms Medical Scheme 'Biggest Farce,'" *LP*, 15 Nov. 1961, 14.
23 Ross Thatcher, quoted in "Thatcher Says Plan Conscription," *LP*, 17 Nov. 1961, 28.
24 H.D. Dalgleish, quoted in "Doctors Won't Discuss Medical Act – Dalgleish," *LP*, 13 Nov. 1961, 1.
25 F.W. McClelland, president of the SFL, quoted in "SFL Raps Doctors' Position," *LP*, 14 Nov. 1961, 10.
26 On the Saskatchewan Plan, see F.S. Lawson, "The Saskatchewan Plan," *Mental Hospitals* 8, no. 3 (1957): 27–31, and Harley D. Dickinson, *The Two Psychiatries: The Transformation of Psychiatric Work in Saskatchewan* (Regina: Canadian Plains Research Center, University of Regina, 1989), 133–71.
27 See Gregory P. Marchildon, "A House Divided: Deinstitutionalization, Medicare and the Canadian Mental Health Association in Saskatchewan, 1944–1964," *Histoire sociale / Social History* 44, no. 88 (2011), 305–29, for a more comprehensive treatment of this conflict.
28 "'Saskatchewan Plan' Not for Here," *LP*, 13 Nov. 1961, 21.
29 Allan Blakeney, *An Honourable Callling: Political Memoirs* (Toronto: University of Toronto Press, 2008), 52. The description of hawks and doves is based on a two-hour-long discussion on the medicare crisis I had

with Allan Blakeney in the winter of 2007. He told me at the time that he was one of the hawks, which he confirmed in his autobiography.
30 This would come out months later when Erb resigned his cabinet position: see "Douglas Statement Surprise," *LP*, 5 May 1962, 1, 8; "Douglas Claims Erb Resentful," *LP*, 1 May 1962, 36; "Douglas Denies Erb's Statement," *LP*, 9 May 1962, 1. The episode is also recounted in a highly biased memoir of the doctors' strike by Saskatoon physician and anti-medicare activist Noel Doig in *Setting the Record Straight: A Doctor's Memoir of the 1962 Medicare Crisis* (Saskatoon: Indie Ink Publishing, 2012).
31 Originally, Walter Erb intended to become a doctor. He entered pre-medicine at the University of Manitoba in autumn 1930, the start of the Great Depression, and his parents soon became unable to pay for tuition and board. He then shifted to the arts program, where the tuition fees were substantially less. PAS, Jean Larmour oral history of CCF government, R-8411, recorded interview, tape 1, J. Walter Erb, 6 Oct. 1982.
32 McLeod and McLeod, *Tommy Douglas*, 199.
33 Blakeney, *An Honourable Calling*, 52.
34 Allan Blakeney, quoted in Cameron Smith, *Unfinished Journey: The Lewis Family* (Toronto: Summerhill Press, 1989), 294.
35 "Doctors Still Oppose New Plan," *LP*, 2 Nov. 1961, 9.
36 PAS, Jean Larmour oral history of CCF government, R-8455, recorded interview, tape 2, Dr. Burns Roth, 18 Nov. 1982.
37 "Erb, Davies Switch Jobs" and "Cabinet Switches Termed 'Matter of Reorganization,'" *LP*, 21 Nov. 1961, 1.
38 "Defeated Candidates Get Jobs – Says Staveley," *LP*, 2 Dec. 1961, 2.
39 In the 1956 election, Staveley had 41.4 per cent of the popular vote compared to T.C.'s 48.2 per cent. In 1960, Staveley's support grew slightly to 42.7 per cent, still short of T.C.'s 48.4 per cent (a slight increase due to a decline in third-party votes). Historical data drawn from Elections Saskatchewan, https://www.elections.sk.ca/reports-data/election-results/.
40 "Liberals Nominate Staveley," *LP*, 6 Nov. 1961, 27.
41 "Thatcher Outlines Election Issues," *LP*, 6 Nov. 1961, 33.
42 "Thatcher Claims Socialists Blunder," *LP*, 7 Dec. 1961, 42.
43 "People Will Welcome Medical Plan – Lloyd," *LP*, 24 Nov. 1961, 41.
44 LAC, TCD, vol. 145, T.C. Douglas message for Weyburn By-election script, filmed 28 Nov. 1961 (broadcast 30 Nov. 1961), 1.
45 LAC, TCD, vol. 145, T.C. Douglas message for Weyburn By-election script, filmed 28 Nov. 1961 (broadcast 30 Nov. 1961), 1–2.
46 "Major Issue Said Medical Care Plan," *LP*, 7 Dec. 1961, 30.
47 "Douglas Suggests Plan Start April 1," *LP*, 8 Dec. 1961, 30.
48 Advertisement, "She Knows Doctors Will Make Her Well," for Oran Reiman, *LP*, 9 Dec. 1961, 5.

49 "Tory Gov't Rapped by Argue," *LP*, 9 Dec. 1961, 32.
50 "Each Party 'Must' Win," *LP*, 11 Dec. 1961, 1, 9.
51 "Eyes of Weburn Voters," *LP*, 12 Dec. 1961, 13.
52 "Staveley Captures Douglas' Old Seat," *LP*, 14 Dec. 1961, 1.
53 "Staveley Captures Douglas' Old Seat," *LP*, 14 Dec. 1961, 1.
54 "A Two-Fold Repudiation," *LP*, 14 Dec. 1961, 29.
55 T.C. Douglas, quoted in "Medical Plan Will Go Ahead," *LP*, 14 Dec. 1961, 36.
56 As quoted in McLeod and McLeod, *Tommy Douglas*, 223.
57 Telegram (from Mike Pearson) to J.H. Staveley quoted in "Byelection Still Main Topic for Weyburn Constituency," *LP*, 15 Dec. 1961, 2.
58 Desmond Morton, *NDP: Social Democracy in Canada*, 2nd ed. (Toronto: Samuel Stevens, 1977), 34.
59 See, for example, "A Toast to Victory: Engraved Mugs for Douglas, MacDonald and Laventure," *Ottawa Citizen*, 15 Jan. 1962, 13. On Douglas's speaking on behalf of NDP provincial candidates, see "Indian Labor Vote Kenora Riding Key," *Brantford Expositor*, 15 Jan. 1962, 15; "Must Fight for Medical Plan in Ontario, Says Douglas," *North Bay Nugget*, 15 Jan. 1962, 3; and "Big Guns Boom in Kenora Byelection" and "Party Leaders Active," *Sault Star*, 15 Jan. 1962, 5, 21.
60 "Health Care in All Provinces Will Require a Fight – Douglas," *Ottawa Citizen*, 15 Jan. 1962, 13; "Douglas Criticizes Health Scheme Lack," *Windsor Star*, 15 Jan. 1962, 2.
61 "The Byelections," *Brantford Expositor*, 19 Jan. 1962, 4.
62 "Party Chiefs Have Mixed Feelings Over Results of Five Byelections," *Ottawa Citizen*, 19 Jan. 1962, 4.
63 LAC, TCD, MG32-C28, vol. 145, T.C. Douglas's *Nation's Business* telecast script entitled "Canada Needs a Health Plan," 14 Feb. 1962, 7–9.
64 "Argue Sticking with CCF-NDP," *LP*, 29 Nov. 1961, 5;
65 "Today in Ottawa" and "House Leader, Douglas Differ on Party Stands," *Windsor Star*, 16 Jan. 1962, 8.
66 Doris French Shackleton, *Tommy Douglas: A Biography* (Toronto: McClelland & Stewart, 1975), 258; McLeod and McLeod, *Tommy Douglas*, 224; "CCF Map Election Campaign," *LP*, 19 Feb. 1962, 8, and 20 Feb. 1962, 7. In fact, his NDP constituency association reminded Argue of this when they demanded his resignation through a telegram: "You strongly condemned Mr. Thatcher for his betrayal of the party which elected him and his failure to face the electors. Therefore, the executive … calls on you to resign now." "Byelection Asked for Assiniboia," *LP*, 27 Feb. 1962, 28.
67 See, for example, the *Ottawa Citizen*, "Shock Resignation: Herridge Will Replace Argue as House Leader," *Ottawa Citizen*, 19 Feb. 1962, 1; "Argue Out, Charges Tool of Labor: Schock to Party Heads: Expected to Join Liberals," *LP*, 19 Feb. 1961, 1; McLeod and McLeod, *Tommy Douglas*, 224.

68 In response to Argue's rationale for not telling Douglas (that he wanted to inform his constituency association first and could not trust Douglas to keep the news quiet), Douglas quipped, "Although he did not see fit to confide with any of his colleagues, it's rather significant that Ross Thatcher, the Liberal leader in Saskatchewan, was kept fully informed." Douglas, quoted in "No Insult Swapping," *LP*, 23 Feb. 1962, 13.
69 Shackleton, *Tommy Douglas*, 259.
70 "Argue Claims Labor Clique Runs Party," *Ottawa Citizen*, 19 Feb. 1962, 7.
71 "CCF Has Now Ceased to Exist," *Ottawa Citizen*, 19 Feb. 1962, 7; editorial, "Mr. Argue's Bold Move," *LP*, 20 Feb. 1962, 17.
72 L.B. Pearson, quoted in "CCF Has Now Ceased to Exist," *Ottawa Citizen*, 19 Feb. 1962, 7; Diefenbaker, quoted in "Shock Resignation: Herridge Will Replace Argue as House Leader," *Ottawa Citizen*, 19 Feb. 1962, 1.
73 "Argue and Douglas Share Silent Flight, Loud Landing," *Globe and Mail*, 20 Feb. 1962, 1.
74 Douglas, quoted in "Argue Out, Charges Tool of Labor: Schock to Party Heads: Expected to Join Liberals," *LP*, 19 Feb. 1961, 1.
75 "Argue Calling to Socialists," *LP*, 21 Feb. 1962, 1.
76 Excerpts from various Canadian newspaper editorials in "Argue's Departure Seen as NDP Blow," *LP*, 24 Feb. 1962, 17.
77 The *Leader Post* conducted a small (n = 24) telephone opinion survey in the Assiniboia constituency to determine how Argue might fare as a Liberal. The poll showed that he could pull at least some of the people who had voted for him before. In a separate question where he would be pitted against Douglas as the NDP candidate, the poll showed an even split between the two in terms of support. "Poll Indicates Voters Will Swing with Argue," *LP*, 27 Feb. 1962, 2.
78 "Argue Told to Resign Seat Immediately," *LP*, 21 Feb. 1962, 15.
79 "Change of Seat Asked by Argue," *LP*, 22 Feb. 1962, 23.
80 "Manitoba's NDP Headed by Transcona Railwayman," *LP*, 6 Nov. 1961, 23.
81 PAS, Jean Larmour oral history of CCF government, R-8412, recorded interview, tape 2, J. Walter Erb, 6 Oct. 1982. Erb would run as a Liberal candidate in the 1964 provincial election, only to be defeated.
82 The actual quote by Vladimir Lenin, which he made while living in exile before the 1917 revolution was "There are decades when nothing happens; and there are weeks when decades happen."
83 PAS, W.G. Davies fonds, R-30.1, file XXVIII, no. 10 – CPS, 1959–May 1962, memorandum to file by W.G. Davies re: conversation (28 Nov. 1961) with Dr. H. Dalgleish, 29 Nov. 1961.
84 Letter, W.G. Davies to H.D. Dalgleish, 4 Dec. 1961, reproduced in Appendix B of E.A. Tollefson's *Bitter Medicine: The Saskatchewan Medicare Feud* (Saskatoon: Modern Press, 1964), 164–5.

85 Letter, W.G. Davies to H.D. Dalgleish, 28 Dec. 1961, reproduced in Appendix B of Tollefson, *Bitter Medicine*, 165.
86 Robin F. Badgley and Samuel Wolfe, *Doctors' Strike: Medical Care and Conflict in Saskatchewan* (Toronto: Macmillan of Canada, 1967), 42–3.
87 Letter, W.G. Davies to H.D. Dalgleish, 5 Jan. 1962, reproduced in Appendix B of Tollefson, *Bitter Medicine*, 166.
88 Edwin A. Tollefson, "The Medicare Dispute," in *Politics in Saskatchewan*, ed. Norman Ward and Duff Spafford (Toronto: Longmans Canada, 1968), 250.
89 W.G. Davies, quoted in McLeod and McLeod, *Tommy Douglas*, 201 n18, 323.
90 This was a personal anecdote that Tansley shared with me on 30 April 2004 during a symposium on the Douglas government at the University of Regina.
91 Archives of Ontario (AO), A.M. Nicholson fonds, F-80, item 10-169, transcript of A.M. (Sandy) Nicholson interview with Dr. Sam Wolfe, 29 Sept. 1976, 26–7, on Wolfe's work with the government on the medical care bill.
92 Tolleson, "Medicare Dispute," 251.
93 Johnson, *Dream No Little Dreams*, 275.
94 Letter, W.G. Davies to H.D. Dagliesh, 2 March 1962, reproduced in Appendix B of Tollefson, *Bitter Medicine*, 170; "Gov't Makes Bid for Medicare Talks," *LP*, 3 March 1962, 9.
95 Letter, W.G. Davies to H.D. Dalgleish, 2 March 1962, reproduced in Appendix B of Tollefson, *Bitter Medicine*, 170; "Gov't Makes Bid for Medicare Talks," *LP*, 3 March 1962, 9.
96 "Medicare Program Off until July 1," *LP*, 3 March 1962, 1; "Saskatchewan Medical Care Program Effective on April 1," *Saskatoon Star Phoenix* (*SP*), 3 March 1962, 1.
97 SLD, 3rd Session, 14th Legislature, 1 March 1962, 30; Tollefson, "Medicare Dispute," 250–1.
98 Quotations from Hansard in "Medical Care Starts July 1," *LP*, 3 March 1962, 8.
99 McLeod and McLeod, *Tommy Douglas*, 201–2.
100 AO, A.M. Nicholson fonds, F-80.1, oral history transcripts, A.M. (Sandy) Nicholson interview with T.C. Douglas, 15 June 1980. A portion of this interview is also quoted in McLeod and McLeod, *Tommy Douglas*, 203.
101 McLeod and McLeod, *Tommy Douglas*, 203.
102 Advertisement in *LP*, 7 May 1962, 2.
103 "Text of Erb's Resignation," *LP*, 3 May 1962, 1, 3.
104 Indeed, Lloyd accused Erb of talking to "certain leaders" of the CPS, an accusation that Erb said was "utter nonsense," although he readily

admitted that he did have doctor friends with whom he had "been associated for many years."
105 "Milestone CCF Ask Erb to Resign," *LP*, 7 May 1962, 1.
106 Letter, W.S. Lloyd to H.D. Dalgleish, 4 April 1962, reproduced in Appendix B of Tollefson, *Bitter Medicine*, 172; Johnson with Proctor, *Dream No Little Dreams*, 274.
107 "Doctors, Cabinet Fail to Agree on Medicare," *LP*, 12 April 1962, 1.
108 Johnson with Proctor, *Dream No Little Dreams*, 274–5.
109 "Lloyd Thinks Many Doctors Will Agree," *LP*, 12 April 1962, 3.
110 Badgley and Wolfe, *Doctors' Strike*, 47. The *Leader Post* counted 534 doctors in the room when Lloyd gave his address: "Plan Will Go Ahead," *LP*, 3 May 1962, 1.
111 "Erb Quits Govt' Over Medicare," *LP*, 3 May 1962, 1.
112 Woodrow Lloyd's speech to CPS, quoted in Badgley and Wolfe, *Doctors' Strike*, 48.
113 Woodrow Lloyd's speech to CPS, quoted in Badgley and Wolfe, *Doctors' Strike*, 48–9.
114 Woodrow Lloyd's speech to CPS, quoted in Badgley and Wolfe, *Doctors' Strike*, 49.
115 Quoted in Badgley and Wolfe, *Doctors' Strike*, 49; "Loud Applause for Barrotes," *LP*, 3 May 1962, 1.
116 "Loud Applause for Barootes" and "Plan Will Go Ahead," *LP*, 3 May 1962, 1.
117 "Good Slogan Worth Thousand Speeches," *Ottawa Citizen*, 6 June 1962, 7.
118 LAC, Thomas K. Shoyama fonds (TKS), R10881, vol. 5, file 5, clipping from the *Winnipeg Tribune*, "He Makes Bullets for NDP," by Don McGillivray, 25 Nov. 1961, 4.
119 PAS, Jean Larmour oral history of CCF Government, R-8459 to R-8462, T.K Shoyama interview transcript, 26 July 1982, 80.
120 PAS, Jean Larmour oral history of CCF Government, R-8459 to R-8462, T.K Shoyama interview transcript, 26 July 1982, 86; "Lack of Funds Hampers NDP Campaign – Douglas," *Ottawa Citizen*, 11 June 1962, 5; "Mr. Douglas's Campaign," *Ottawa Citizen*, 15 Jan. 1962, 6.
121 "Douglas to Hit Six Cities," *Ottawa Journal*, 11 June 1961, 21; "'Hoax' Charge by Douglas," *Ottawa Citizen*, 13 June 1962, 17.
122 "Election Candidates State Nuclear Arms Policies," *LP*, 2 June 1962, 6.
123 "Douglas Campaigns in Saskatchewan," *LP*, 25 May 1962, 3.
124 This is Tommy Shoyama's memory of the words used by Douglas: PAS, Jean Larmour oral history of CCF Government, R-8459 to R-8362, transcript of T.K Shoyama interview, 26 July 1982, 80.
125 Quotation form W.S. Lloyd's "Progress Report on Medical Care," transcript of a radio and television address, 9 May 1962, reproduced

in Ahmed Mohiddin Mohamed, "Keep Our Doctors Committees in the Saskatchewan Medicare Controversy" (MA thesis, University of Saskatchewan, 1963), 46.
126 PAS, Jean Larmour oral history of CCF Government, R-8459 to R-8462, T.K Shoyama interview transcript, 26 July 1982, 84; "Douglas Presses Job Plan," *Ottawa Citizen*, 28 May 1962.
127 "NDP Speakers Making Medicare a Big Issue," *LP*, 8 June 1962, 2.
128 This brochure combined the New Party's position on health care that delegates to the founding convention decided the summer before with additional policy detail and arguments prepared by Tommy Shoyama (Research Office, NDP): LAC, TKS, vol. 5, file 5, "Social Security," 24 March 1962, section on health insurance, 3–5.
129 LAC, TKS, vol. 5, file 5, NDP 1962 election brochure "The Right to Health."
130 Douglas quoted in "Medicare Issue Biggest – Douglas," *Ottawa Citizen*, 18 May 1962, 5.
131 Portion of petition from the Mothers Committee of Regina quoted in Mohamed, "Keep Our Doctors Committees," 55.
132 Tollefson, "The Medicare Dispute," 263–4, 275n 121, and 277n131. Tollefson established that "many prominent Liberals [were] holding high offices in the K.O.D." and "that efforts were made by certain Liberals to use the K.O.D. as a means of consolidating the anti-C.C.F. vote behind the Liberal Party at the next provincial election," based in part upon an interview conducted with Hans Taal in 1966. Taal had been the president of the Saskatoon KOD committee as well as vice-president of the provincial KOD.
133 Doig, quoted in "KOD Delegate in London," *LP*, 19 July 1962, 2. Doig used these same words as the title in his privately published account of the doctors' strike: Doig, *Setting the Record Straight*. Later, Doig became the long-serving chair of the CMA's Ethics Committee, and was later succeeded by his daughter (and eventual CMA president) Anne Doig (personal communication with Bill Tholl, 15 Oct. 2023).
134 Jacalyn Duffin and Joseph L. Pater, "Mrs Robinson's Revenge: Peter Seeger, Earl Robinson and the Medicare Protest Song," *Canadian Bulletin of Medical History / Bulletin canadien d'histoire de la médecine* 35, no. 2 (2018): 424.
135 McLeod and McLeod, *Tommy Douglas*, 220.
136 Mohamed, "Keep Our Doctors Committees," Appendix C, iv.
137 "400 Cars Reported Arriving in Regina," *LP*, 30 May 1962, 1.
138 Mohamed, "Keep Our Doctors Committees," 69–76.
139 Mohamed, "Keep Our Doctors Committees," 81.
140 "Tyranny or Integrity" advertisement by KOD, *LP*, 8 June 1962, 8 (and repeated on 9 June 1962); Mohamed, "Keep Our Doctors Committees," 83.

141 Second advertisement for David (Ed) Mahood authorized by Saskatchewan NDP, *SP*, 15 June 1962, 2.
142 LAC, TKS, vol. 5, file 5, separately typed copy of article in *Toronto Star Weekly*, "Medical Plan Is Wanted," 7 April 1962, with emphasis on certain sentences and paragraphs for use by NDP candidates in 1962 election campaign.
143 First advertisement for David (Ed) Mahood authorized by Saskatchewan NDP, *SP*, 15 June 1962, 2.
144 Diefenbaker, quoted in "PM's Wit Hits Sharply," *LP*, 25 May 1962, 3.
145 *Getting Things Done for Canada and Canadians: An Outline of Progressive Conservative Government Action 1957–1962* (Ottawa: Progressive Conservative Party of Canada, 1962).
146 *The Liberal Programme: General Election 1962* (Ottawa: National Liberal Federation, 1962), 11.
147 Pearson quoted in "Medical Care Conditions Listed by Liberal Leader," *LP*, 5 May 1962, 6. This episode was also recounted in the *Canadian Annual Review* (*CAR*) 1962, 13, but with the wrong date.
148 Tom Kent, *A Public Purpose: An Experience of Liberal Opposition and Canadian Government* (Montreal and Kingston: McGill-Queen's University Press, 1988), 90–1.
149 *The Liberal Programme*, 11.
150 "Prime Minister and Pearson Trade Thrusts with Hecklers," *LP*, 29 May 1962, 1.
151 Charles Lynch, "Medicare – Tory Obstacle," *Ottawa Citizen*, 29 May 1962, 7.
152 Advertisement "The Right to Health," *LP*, 1 June 1962, 2.
153 Some candidates, such as Liberal Fred Johnson, who was running against Douglas in Regina, concluded that medicare would draw voters away from, and not to, Douglas. "Medicare Said Voting Issue," *LP*, 9 June 1962, 3.
154 Pat O'Dwyer, "Medical Crisis Arouses Voters: Threat to NDP," *Ottawa Journal*, 15 June 1962, 7.
155 PAS, Jean Larmour oral history of CCF Government, R-8459 to R-8462, T.K Shoyama interview transcript, 26 July 1982, 85.
156 Don McGillivray, "Rising Medicare Fever Grips Saskatchewan," *Ottawa Citizen*, 5 June 1962, 7.
157 Don McGillivray, "Rising Medicare Fever Grips Saskatchewan," *Ottawa Citizen*, 5 June 1962, 7.
158 "Douglas Levels Broadside at Doctors," *Ottawa Citizen*, 7 June 1962, 13; "Douglas Says Doctors United in the Battle," *Ottawa Citizen*, 9 June 1962, 7.
159 Shackleton, *Tommy Douglas*, 265.
160 Douglas, quoted in "NDP Speakers Making Medicare a Big Issue," *LP*, 8 June 1962, 2.
161 "Douglas Stirring Up Class Hatred – Liberal MLA Says," *LP*, 2 June 1992, 18.

162 Eleanor McKinnon, quoted in Shackleton, *Tommy Douglas*, 265.
163 "Douglas Win Not Assured – Blakeney," *LP*, 9 June 1962, 10.
164 "Canvassers Said Rudely Treated," *LP*, 9 June 1962, 10.
165 "Heckler Gets Bloody Nose," *Ottawa Citizen*, 9 June 1962, 22.
166 "Sign of the Times," *LP*, 16 June 1962, 1.
167 "Douglas Windup," *Ottawa Journal*, 14 June 1962, 1; "Douglas Charges Liberal Rowdyism," *Ottawa Journal*, 14 June 1962, 7.
168 "The Election," *LP*, 14 June 1962, 3; KOD ad, *LP*, 15 June 1962, 12.
169 McLeod and McLeod, *Tommy Douglas*, 229.
170 "3,000 Cheer Douglas' Defence of Medicare," *LP*, 16 June 1962, 24; "NDP Chief Flays Govt. on TCA, CBC," *Ottawa Citizen*, 16 Jan. 1962, 16.
171 "Douglas Winds Up Campaign in His Old Weyburn Riding," *LP*, 18 June 1962, 2; "New Deal Is Due," *Ottawa Citizen*, 18 June 1962, 11.
172 Shackleton, *Tommy Douglas*, 268.
173 PAS, Jean Larmour oral history of the CCF government, R-8329 to R-8402, T.C. Douglas interview, transcript 1, 14 Nov. 1982, 70.
174 *CAR* 1962, 25–7.
175 McLeod and McLeod, *Tommy Douglas*, 227.
176 McLeod and McLeod, *Tommy Douglas*, 225.
177 McLeod and McLeod, *Tommy Douglas*, 227.
178 Quoted "'Worst Kind of Deadlock,'" *LP*, 20 June 1962, 35.
179 British and American newspaper election coverage in "'Worst Kind of Deadlock,'" 20 June 1962, 35.
180 This was very much understood at the time in the NDP party establishment: "NDP Party Caucus Plans to Map Commons Strategy," *LP*, 9 July 1962, 13.
181 LAC, TKS, vol. 5, file 5, handout for 1962 federal election entitled "Political Duplicity … The Enemy of Democracy: An Internationally Known Journalist Looks at the Case of Hazen Argue," by John A Stevenson. This handout, authorized by the Saskatchewan CCF Section of the NDP stated at the end, "in Assiniboia, you can support the principles and policies of the New Democratic Party by working for Cecil Bailey the candidate who is a member of the T.C. Douglas team!"
182 Hazen Argue came out on top with 7,739 votes, only slightly more than the PC's Lawrence Watson (7,386 votes) but well above the NDP's Cecil Bailey vote count of 5,153, with Social Credit only getting 1,009 votes. Data from Canadian Elections Database, University of Calgary, https://canadianelectionsdatabase.ca/PHASE5/?p=0&type=election&ID=521#page_1=saskatchewan&page_2=constituency_3012. What worked for Argue in the 1962 election, however, would not work in the 1963 and 1965 federal elections, when he was defeated. In 1966, Argue was appointed by Pearson to the Senate: Shackleton, *Tommy Douglas*, 259.
183 *CAR* 1962, 22.

184 Results for Regina City federal electoral district obtained from the Canadian Elections Database, University of Calgary, https://canadianelectionsdatabase.ca/PHASE5/?p=0&type=election&ID=521#page_1=saskatchewan&page_2=constituency_3174.
185 "Liberals Jubilant over Ken More's Victory," *LP*, 19 June 1962, 3.
186 "Four City Candidates Comment on Elections," *LP*, 19 July 1962, 8.
187 David Lewis, quoted in the *Ottawa Journal*, 19 July 1962, 4.
188 Allan Blakeney, "The Struggle to Implement Medicare," *Bulletin of the History of Medicine / Bulletin canadien d'histoire de la médecine* 26, no. 2 (2009): 530.
189 Douglas, quoted in "Confidence Turns to Gloom for Regina NDP Supporters," *LP*, 19 June 1962, 3.
190 McLeod and McLeod, *Tommy Douglas*, 229.
191 This is recounted by both Shackleton, *Tommy Douglas*, 269, and Walter Stewart, *The Life and Political Times of Tommy Douglas* (Toronto: McArthur & Company, 2003), 252. It was also repeated by Eleanor McKinnon, Douglas's long-time administrative assistant, who was present: PAS, Jean Larmour oral history of CCF Government, R-8441 to R-8443, Eleanor McKinnon interview, partial transcript, 14 Nov. 1982, 8.
192 Lewis, quoted in interview in Shackleton, *Tommy Douglas*, 270.
193 This is exactly how Douglas's old friend Grace MacInnis described it in her interview with Shackleton in, *Tommy Douglas*, 270. MacInnis, who was a CCF MLA in British Columbia from 1941 to 1945 and an NDP MP from 1965 until 1974, was the daughter of J.S. Woodsworth and wife of Angus MacInnis (one of the original group of MPs in the tiny CCF caucus of which Douglas was a member from 1935 until he became premier).
194 This is evident in Jane Roberts's carefully constructed examination of the psychological impact of political defeat in the United Kingdom: *Losing Political Office* (London: Palgrave Macmillan, 2017). For a more anecdotal but similar study of political defeat in Canada, see Steven Paikin, *The Dark Side: The Personal Price of a Political Life* (Toronto: Viking Canada, 2003).
195 Shackleton, *Tommy Douglas*, 270; "Douglas Planning Move to Ottawa," *LP*, 14 July 1962, 1.
196 Douglas, quoted in "Four City Candidates Comment on Elections," *LP*, 19 July 1962, 8; "'We Are Still the Government,'" *LP*, 19 June 1962, 15.
197 "Four City Candidates Comment on Elections," *LP*, 19 July 1962, 8; "'We Are Still the Government,'" *LP*, 19 June 1962, 15.
198 Douglas, quoted in "Douglas Getting Bit Tired of Speculation," *LP*, 22 June 1962, 39. The word "exploded" was used by the newspaper in the article.

## 13. The Doctors' Strike and the Cost of Peace

1 Robin F. Badgley, "The Public and Medical Care in Saskatchewan," *American Journal of Public Health* 53, no. 5 (1963): 720.
2 Provincial Archives of Saskatchewan (PAS), W.G. Davies fonds, R-30.1, XXVIII.1, 181A – Medical Care Insurance – General, "The Ministry of Reconciliation" (a sermon preached in Lakeview United Church, Regina, on 15 July 1962, by Rev. Reid E. Vipond).
3 Athol Murray, quoted in "Hatred Sweeping Province Because of Crisis – Murray," *Saskatoon Star Phoenix* (*SP*), 7 July 1962, 2–3; Ahmed Mohiddin Mohamed, "Keep Our Doctors Committees in the Saskatchewan Medicare Controversy" (MA thesis, University of Saskatchewan, 1963), 166–9.
4 Athol Murray, quoted in David Spurgeon, "Anti-Communist Speeches and Professional Ostracism: The Ugly Side of the Doctor's Strike against Medicare in Saskatchewan," *Globe and Mail*, 9 July 1962, 7.
5 "Douglas Won't Attend NDP Executive Meeting," *Regina Leader-Post* (*LP*), 25 June 1962, 3.
6 His constituency association voted 165 to 11 in favour of giving Regier the authority to resign: "National Executive of NDP to Meet in Toronto Thursday," *LP*, 23 June 1962, 8; "Douglas Likely to Run in BC," *LP*, 27 June 1962, 1; "B.C. Seat Voted Open to Douglas," *LP*, 27 June 1962, 27; "NDP Executive Meets in Toronto," *LP*, 28 June 1962, 1; "Douglas Chances Believed Strong," *LP*, 30 June 1962, 5.
7 E.A. Tollefson, *Bitter Medicine: The Saskatchewan Medicare Feud* (Saskatoon: Modern Press, 1964), 107–10, appendix B (180–8) with letters, W.S. Lloyd to Dr. H.D. Dalgleish, 26 June 1962, and W.S. Lloyd to G.W. Peacock, 26 June 1962.
8 "Lloyd Raps Doctors' Conditions for Meet to Discuss Solution of Medical Care Crisis: Dalgleish Accepts Lloyd Invite; Says Present Act Must Change Substantially," *SP*, 21 June 1964, 3.
9 Tollefson, *Bitter Medicine*, 109.
10 Library and Archives Canada (LAC), Thomas Clement Douglas fonds (TCD), MG 32 C28, vol. 2, file 2 (no. 5), letters, Sam Wolfe to T.C. Douglas, 28 Feb. 1961, and Douglas to Wolfe, 7 March 1961.
11 Archives of Ontario (AO), Sandy Nicholson fonds, F 80, 10-169, transcript of interview with Dr. Sam Wolfe, Part I: 29 Sept. 1976, 29–31
12 Thomas H. McLeod and Ian McLeod, *Tommy Douglas: The Road to Jerusalem* (Edmonton: Hurtig Publishers, 1987), 181. Joan Douglas Tulchinsky, who was adopted in 1945, was six years younger than Shirley: Doris French Shackleton, *Tommy Douglas: A Biography* (Toronto: McClelland & Stewart, 1975), 134; AO, Sandy Nicholson fonds, F 80,

10–169, transcript of interview with Dr. Sam Wolfe, Part I: 29 Sept. 1976, 8–24.
13 While the secondary literature is silent on the issue, the primary sources reveal a major conflict between Spry and Wolfe, particularly on the issue of temporary versus permanent recruitment and the perception of their relative contributions. LAC, Graham Spry fonds, MG 30 D297, vol. 61, file 9, draft letter, Graham Spry to Don Tansley, July 1962.
14 LAC, Graham Spry fonds, MG 30 D297, vol. 61, file 9, draft letters, Graham Spry to the editors of the *Times* and the *Guardian*, n.d., but first sometime in first week of July 1962, and file 12, standard form letter, W.C.A. Knights (executive assistant to Graham Spry), to doctors, n.d., setting out alternative methods of remuneration and amounts doctors could expect: 1) payment on FFS – not less than $10,000 gross earnings in their first year; 2) FFS with experience bonuses – $12,000 to $16,000 gross earnings; and 3) salary – $14,000 to $18,000, based on experience. Doctors also could receive an advance of $2,000 upon arrival in Saskatchewan. The government paid for economy (tourist) class air tickets for the doctor and their spouse plus all children under the age of twelve. The contracts (file 13) made it clear that the choice of payment was up to the physician.
15 As noted earlier, T.C. stated this publicly during the 1948 provincial election: "Douglas at Weyburn," *LP*, 5 June 1948, 1, 5. Both Tommy McLeod and Al Johnson felt that Douglas was almost deluded in this optimistic view of the doctors in the province.
16 Thomas and McLeod, *Tommy Douglas*, 199.
17 London School of Economic and Political Science Archives (LSE), Richard Titmuss fonds, Titmuss/7/68, letters: Graham Spry to R.M. Titmuss, 9 Sept. 1960; T.C. Douglas to R.M. Titmuss, 19 Sept. 1960; and telegram, Dr. A. (Sandy) Robertson to B. Abel-Smith, 8 Sept. 1960. While in London in September 1960, T.C. wanted to meet with Richard Titmuss and Brian Abel-Smith concerning both the medical care plan and the Thompson Committee (the terms of reference were sent in advance). Since Abel-Smith was not in London at the time, Spry arranged for T.C. and Titmuss to have dinner together at Saskatchewan House on 13 September 1960. The term "high priest of the welfare state" was used by Sir Edmund Leach to describe Titmuss: see revised entry for Richard Morris Titmuss by A.H. Halsey in the online edition of the *Oxford Dictionary of National Biography*, www.oxforddnb.com.
18 LAC, Graham Spry fonds, MG 30 D297, vol. 61, file 12, 2nd draft of letter (private and confidential), Graham Spry to Lord Taylor and Richard Titmuss, 1 July 1962.
19 LAC, Graham Spry fonds, MG 30 D297, vol. 61, file 12, memorandum to News Editors from the Secretary, Saskatchewan House, 3 July 1962.

20 Gregory P. Marchildon, "Policy Lessons from Physicians' Strikes," *Israel Journal of Health Policy Research* 2, no. 1 (2013): 1. There is a limited literature on the history physician strikes: Robin F. Badgeley, "Health Worker Strikes: Social and Economics Bases of Conflict," *International Journal of Health Services* 5, no. 1 (1975): 9–17; David G. Green, "The 1918 Strike of the Medical Profession against the Friendly Societies in Victoria," *Labour History*, no. 46 (1984): 72–87; Stephen L. Thompson and J. Warren Salmon, "Strike by Physicians: A Historical Perspective Toward an Ethical Evaluation," *International Journal of Health Services* 36, no. 2 (2006): 331–54; and Gregory P. Marchildon and Klaartje Schrijvers, "Physician Resistance and the Forging of Public Health Care: A Comparative Analysis of Doctors' Strikes in Canada and Belgium in the 1960s," *Medical History* 55, no. 2 (2011): 203–22.

21 Sasha Mullally and Gregory P. Marchildon, "Striking a Chord: Physician-Publics, Citizen-Audiences and a Half Century of Health-Care Debates in Canada," in *Communicating the History of Medicine: Perspectives on Audiences and Impact*, ed. Solveign Jülich and Sven Widmalm (Manchester: Manchester University Press, 2020), 107–37.

22 The top story as voted by the wire editors of Canadian newspapers: William Thomson, "Press Coverage of the Medicare Dispute in Saskatchewan: II," *Queen's Quarterly* 70, no. 3 (1963): 363. William Thomson was a *Regina Leader-Post* editor at the time of the strike.

23 "Expert Offers Aid," *Globe and Mail*, 4 July 1962, 8.

24 LAC, Graham Spry fonds, MG 30 D297, vol. 61, file 9, key points for press conference, 5 July 1962.

25 "Saskatchewan Sends Circulars to U.K. Doctors," *Globe and Mail*, 4 July 1962, 8.

26 PAS, MCIC Executive Branch, R-576, box 3, file 16 – Emergency Services: Special Problems re: Temporary Physicians, six-page list of temporary doctors, length of contracts, and place of practice.

27 This is the view taken by Gordon S. Lawson and Luc Thériault, "Saskatchewan's Community Health Service Associations: An Historical Perspective," *Prairie Forum* 24, no. 2 (1999): 256–7.

28 The legislation under which the community clinics were established was the Municipal Medical and Hospital Association Act of 1938: Lawson and Thériault, "Saskatchewan's Community Health Service Associations," 256. On the co-operative movement and its relationship with the CCF, see Mitch Diamantopoulos, "The Foundations of Agrarian Socialism: Co-operative Economic Action in Saskatchewan, 1905–1960," *Prairie Forum* 37, no. 2 (2012): 103–51; Jean Larmour, "The Douglas Government's Changing Emphasis on Public, Private, and Co-operative Development," in *Building the Co-operative Commonwealth: Essays on the*

*Democratic Socialist Tradition in Canada*, ed. J. William Brennan (Regina: Canadian Plains Research Center, University of Regina, 1985), 161–80; and Ian MacPherson, "The CCF and the Co-operative Movement in the Douglas Years: An Uneasy Alliance," in Brennan, *Building the Co-operative Commonwealth*, 181–203.

29 Stanley Knowles, quoted in Ormond K. McKague, "Socialist Education in Saskatchewan, 1942–1948" (PhD diss., University of Oregon, 1981), 264.
30 Gregory P. Marchildon, "Community Clinics and Stan Rands's Struggle for the Transformation of Health Care in Canada," in Stan Rands, *Privilege and Policy: The History of Community Clinics in Canada* (Regina: Canadian Plains Research Centre, University of Regina, 2012), vii–xiii.
31 Stan Rands, "The CCF in Saskatchewan," in *Western Canadian Politics: The Radical Tradition*, ed. D.C. Kerr (Edmonton: NeWest Institute for Western Canadian Studies, 1981), 60–1.
32 University of Regina Archives, Stan Rands fonds, letter, W.M. Harding to Stan Rands, 29 Nov. 1962
33 Rands, "The CCF in Saskatchewan," 62–3; Rands, *Privilege and Policy*, 1–36.
34 Dennis Gruending, *The First Ten Years: A Brief History of the Community Health Services (Saskatoon) Association* (Saskatoon: Community Health Services Association, 1974), 4-5, 23.
35 Gruending, *The First Ten Years*, 25.
36 PAS, Meyer Brownstone fonds, F 206, R-414, file IV.4c – Medical Care Advisory Planning Committee, letter marked personal and confidential, Graham Spry to Meyer Brownstone, 17 Oct. 1962; LAC, Graham Spry fonds, MG 30 D297, vol. 60, file 39, and vol. 61, file 6, files on community clinics.
37 David James Smith, "Intellectual Activist: Graham Spry, a Biography" (PhD diss., York University, 2002), 390; Lord (Stephen) Taylor, "Saskatchewan Adventure: A Personal Record. Part I, Background to the Story," *Canadian Medical Association Journal* 110, no. 6 (1974): 726.
38 "Doctors Reject Further Talks until Saskatchewan Kills Act: Premiers Seeks Third-Party Medication," *Globe and Mail*, 3 July 1962, 1; "Outside Mediation Rejected by Doctors," *Globe and Mail*, 6 July 1962, 4.
39 Taylor, "Saskatchewan Adventure: Part I," 726–7.
40 Smith, "Intellectual Activist," 389–91.
41 LAC, Thomas K. Shoyama fonds (TKS), R 10881, vol. 6, file 2 – Medical Care, "Report of Staff Committee to the Strategy Committee," n.d., but during doctors' strike.
42 Taylor, "Saskatchewan Adventure: Part I," 727.
43 LAC, TKS, R 10881, vol. 6, file 3, letters, G. Cadbury to T.K. Shoyama, 13 July 1962 and 19 July 1962.

44 Robin F. Badgley and Samuel Wolfe, *Doctors' Strike: Medical Care and Conflict in Saskatchewan* (Toronto: Macmillan of Canada, 1967), 64.
45 Mohammed, "Keep Our Doctors Committees," 178; Badgley and Wolfe, *Doctors' Strike*, 67; Tollefson, "The Medicare Dispute," in *Politics in Saskatchewan*, ed. Norman Ward and Duff Spafford (Toronto: Longmans Canada, 1968), 276n125.
46 Given the extent to which Jewish doctors from other parts of Canada, from Mindel and Cecil Sheps to Sam Wolfe as well as new arrivals at the community clinics, had been a thorn in the side of the college while the CCF was in power, the "garbage of Europe" may have been intended to refer to Jews as well.
47 PAS, W.G. Davies Fonds, R-30.1, XXVIII.14, 181J – Resolutions and Submissions, KOD petition to the provincial government, 11 July 1962.
48 PAS, W.G. Davies fonds, R-30.1, XXVIII.1, folder no. 5 of 9, press statement by W.S. Lloyd, 11 July 1962.
49 Douglas quoted in "Douglas Planning Move to Ottawa," *LP*, 14 July 1962, 1.
50 Badgley and Wolfe, *Doctors' Strike*, 67,
51 Badgley and Wolfe, *Doctors' Strike*, 67–8. By 16 July 1962, the recruitment figures were as follows: 32 doctors placed and working; 28 doctors awaiting registration and allocation; 5 doctors scheduled to arrive the next day; 15 in the next 3 days; and a further 15 to arrive within 7 days. LAC, TKS, R10881, vol. 6, file 3, Daily Situation Report – Confidential, 16 July 1962.
52 "Dalgleish to Go Before CCF-NDP," *LP*, 17 July 1962, 1.
53 PAS, W.G. Davies fonds, R-30.1, XXVIII.1, folder no. 2 of 9, letter, F.D. Mott to W.G. Davies, 3 July 1962 (repeating what was in telegram).
54 PAS, W.S. Lloyd fonds, R-61.6, II, 14d, text of W.S. Lloyds' speech at CCF-NDP convention, Saskatoon, 18 July 1962 (hereafter Lloyd 1962 CCF-NDP convention speech).
55 Lloyd 1962 CCF-NDP convention speech, 5–6.
56 Lloyd 1962 CCF-NDP convention speech, 12. Also see Malcolm G. Taylor, *Health Insurance and Canadian Public Policy: The Seven Decisions That Created the Canadian Health Insurance System and Its Outcomes*, 2nd ed. (Montreal and Kingston: McGill-Queen's University Press, 2009), 321.
57 PAS, Jean Larmour oral history of CCF Government, R-8398 to R-8402, T.C. Douglas interview transcript 1, 14 Nov. 1982, 70.
58 That was how it was understood by others at the time. PAS, W.G. Davies fonds, R-30.1, XXVIII.1, 181A – Medical Care Insurance – General, letter John W. Wood (Administrative Assistant for CCF Leader of the Opposition in British Columbia) to W.G. Davies, 16 July 1962: "We were pleased to hear about the [Woods] Royal Commission and we hope that

perhaps enough evidence will come out to give you grounds to take away licensing from the doctors."
59 LAC, TCD, MG32 C28, vol. 145, notes for T.C. Douglas address at CCF-NDP convention, Saskatoon, 18 July 1962.
60 "Bitter Douglas' [sic] Attack," *Ottawa Citizen*, 19 July 1962, 40.
61 Douglas, quoted in Thomson, "Press Coverage during the Medicare Dispute," 367. In this piece, Thomson argued that his newspaper, the *Regina Leader-Post* had tried to be impartial before and during the strike, a position vehemently rebutted by CCF government minister Allan E. Blakeney in "Press Coverage of the Medicare Dispute in Saskatchewan: I," *Queen's Quarterly* 70, no. 3 (1963): 354–61.
62 Nor did he back down when asked to clarify his statement. "Douglas Raps Two Papers for Medicare Coverage," *SP*, 23 July 1962, 1.
63 Douglas, quoted in "Bitter Douglas' [sic] Attack," *Ottawa Citizen*, 19 July 1962, 40.
64 Douglas, quoted in "Bitter Douglas' [sic] Attack," *Ottawa Citizen*, 19 July 1962, 40.
65 Of course, this is speculation on my part, but there is no doubt that Lloyd did everything he could to dampen emotions during the crisis including restraining the actions of some CCF supporters. See Dianne Lloyd, *Woodrow: A Biography of W. S. Lloyd* (Saskatoon: Woodrow Lloyd Memorial Fund, 1979), 126–7.
66 This was certainly Lord Taylor's judgment. He says that Kelly and Wigle helped the Saskatchewan doctors see sense during his negotiations, "especially when feelings were running high and common sense was disappearing out the window," although Kelly is referred to more often by the other participants. See Lord (Stephen) Taylor, "Saskatchewan Adventure: A Personal Record, Part II: Making Contact," *Canadian Medical Association Journal* 110, no. 7 (1974): 834.
67 This description is drawn from Lloyd, *Woodrow*, 133–4.
68 Dr. A.D. Kelly, quoted in Taylor, *Health Insurance and Canadian Public Policy*, 321–2.
69 Lord (Stephen) Taylor, "Saskatchewan Adventure: A Personal Record, Part III: Drafting the Saskatoon Agreement," *Canadian Medical Association Journal* 110, no. 8 (1974): 982.
70 "Douglas Raps Two Papers for Medicare Coverage," *SP*, 23 July 1962, 1.
71 LAC, TKS, R 10881, vol. 6, file 2 – Medical Care, marked up document with TKS's writing at top, "Proposal from College of Physicians & Surgeons," 25 June 1962.
72 LAC, TKS, R 10881, vol. 6, file 2 – Medical Care, "Report of Staff Committee to the Strategy Committee," n.d., but during doctors' strike.

73 Johnson completed his PhD in 1963, and a substantially revised version of the thesis was published as *Dream No Little Dreams: A Biography of the Douglas Government of Saskatchewan, 1944–1961* (University of Toronto Press, 2004). Douglas was enthusiastic and, in Johnson's words (p. xxxiv), promised "to assist me in any way he could, subject to one condition: that I was to 'write it as I saw it,' unaffected by the fact that I was in the employ of the government of Saskatchewan (albeit on leave without pay at that point). Need I say how indebted I felt and still feel?" I first read Johnson's thesis early in 1997 to help me better understand the machinery of government in Saskatchewan. At the time, as cabinet secretary and deputy minister to the premier, I was trying to improve cabinet and cabinet committee structures and processes. I was so impressed with his thesis that I urged Johnson to consider turning the thesis into a book and, subsequently, wrote the book's foreword.
74 LAC, TKS, R 10881, vol. 6, file 4 – Medical Care, series of annotated drafts with Shoyama's written notes and changes on what would become the Saskatoon Agreement.
75 PAS, A.E. Blakeney fonds, R-12.2, file 21-5-1, Memorandum of Agreement, Government of Saskatchewan and the College of Physicians and Surgeons of Saskatchewan, 23 July 1962 (hereafter Saskatoon Agreement), clauses 16–17.
76 C. David Naylor, *Private Practice, Public Payment: Canadian Medicare and the Politics of Health Insurance, 1911–1966* (Montreal and Kingston: McGill-Queen's University Press, 1986), 210.
77 Over the years, Douglas debated the demerits of extra billing with all comers, including Saskatoon surgeon, member of the Hall Commission, and CMA president-elect (1983), Marc Baltzan, on CBC's *Sunday Morning*, the transcript of which was printed in the *CMAJ*: "Politics: Dr. Marc Baltzan and Tommy Douglas Debate Medicare," *Canadian Medical Association Journal* 126, no. 3 (1982): 290, 295, and 300.
78 Saskatoon Agreement, clauses 6–7.
79 Saskatoon Agreement, clause 14.
80 T. Kue Young, "Lay-Professional Conflict in a Canadian Community Health Center: A Case Report," *Medical Care* 13, no. 11 (1975): 898.
81 Taylor, "Saskatchewan Adventure: Part I," 727.
82 At the time, Spry kept a thick file on the development of the community clinics, which he saw as an important counterbalance to the influence of the CPS and its defence of the status quo. LAC, Graham Spry fonds, MG 30 D297, vol. 60, file 39 and vol. 61, files 6 and 7.
83 LAC, TKS, R 10881, vol. 5, file 13, letters, brochures and receipts for Community Health Services Association (Regina) Ltd. Shoyama was

thanked for his donations to the clinic in a letter from J.R. Lane to Mr. and Mrs. Tom Shoyama, 20 Jan. 1966.
84 Saskatoon Agreement, clause 11.
85 LAC, TCD, MG 32 C28, vol. 130, file 12 – Saskatchewan provincial government correspondence – part I, letter, T.C. Douglas to J.H. Brocklebank, 13 Aug. 1962.
86 Roy J. Romanow, "My Experience in the Medicare Battle and the Woods Commission," *Canadian Bulletin of Medical History / Bulletin canadien d'histoire de la médecine* 26, no. 2 (2009): 538–41; LAC, Graham Spry fonds, vol. 63, file 19, the Report of the Honourable Mr. Justice Mervyn Woods on Hospital Staff Appointments, 11 Dec. 1963.
87 Young, "Lay-Professional Conflict," 899–900; Gruending, *The First Ten Years*, 16–17. On the outcome of the Woods Commission, see Lawson and Thériault, "Saskatchewan's Community Health Service Associations," 258. Following the recommendations of the Woods Commission in December 1963, the Lloyd government passed the Hospital Standards Act. This legislation provided doctors who had been denied, or delayed in obtaining, hospital privileges with the right of an appeal; however, the law was repealed by the Thatcher government after it gained office in 1964.
88 There was also a belief among community clinic activists that the government had, above and beyond the Saskatoon Agreement, quietly agreed to the college's demand that it not directly assist the community clinics financially or in obtaining medical personnel. I do not address this question, as I could find no documentary or oral interview evidence supporting this belief.
89 Douglas, along with Fred Mott and Sam Wolfe, spoke on the potential of community health centres and community clinics at a Medicare conference sponsored by the CLC in Sault Ste. Marie, Ontario, on 2–4 December 1969: LAC, TCD, MG32 C28, vol. 147, file 54, "Community Health Centres" Reference Material, 1968–69. Other examples of speeches in the LAC, TCD, MG32 C28 include: vol. 149, file 13, notes for speech by TCD entitled "Health Insurance and Beyond" to Association of University Programs in Hospital Administration, Carleton University, 14 June 1973; vol. 150, file 11, address by T.C. Douglas to the Canadian College of Health Service Executives, 15 June 1976; and vol. 150, file 31, notes for T.C. Douglas speech "Measuring Performance of Primary Health Services," 4 March 1977.

## 14. The Hall Commission and the Leftward Tilt of Canadian Politics

1 Emmett M. Hall, quoted in letter sent to T.C. Douglas in April 1971, in Doris French Shackleton, *Tommy Douglas: A Biography* (Toronto: McClelland & Stewart, 1975), 241–2.

2 Tom Kent, *A Public Purpose: An Experience of Liberal Opposition and Canadian Government* (Montreal and Kingston: McGill-Queen's University Press, 1988), 201.
3 On the mixed liberal and social democratic nature of the Canadian welfare state as originally categorized by Esping-Andersen, see Gregory P. Marchildon: "Social Democratic Solidarity and the Welfare State: Health Care and Single-Tier Universality in Sweden and Canada," *Canadian Bulletin of Medical History / Bulletin canadien d'histoire de la médecine* 38, no. 1 (2021): 177–96; "The Single-Tier Universality of Canadian Medicare," in *Universality and Social Policy in Canada*, ed. Daniel Béland, Gregory P. Marchildon and Michael J. Prince (Toronto: University of Toronto Press, 2019), 49–62; and "Canadian Medicare as a Policy Success," in *Policy Success in Canada: Cases, Lessons, Challenges*, ed. Evert A. Lindquist, Michael Howlett, Grace Skogstad, Geneviève Tellier, and Paul 'T Hart (Oxford: Oxford University Press, 2022), 17–35.
4 On the nature and implications of this cultural shift in Canada, see Doug Owram, *Born at the Right Time: A History of the Baby-Boom Generation* (Toronto: University of Toronto Press, 1996).
5 Tom Kent himself described his health proposal at the Kingston conference as "a limited kind of Medicare." Library and Archives Canada (LAC), Peter Stursberg fonds, vol. 29, file 1, transcript of interview with Tom Kent on Pearson government, 30 March 1977, 14 (hereafter Stursberg-Kent interview, 30 March 1977).
6 This transition is documented by Kenneth C. Dewar, *Frank Underhill and the Politics of Ideas* (Montreal and Kingston: McGill-Queen's University Press, 2015), 127–58.
7 Frank H. Underhill, *In Search of Canadian Liberalism* (Toronto: Macmillan of Canada, 1960).
8 John English, *The Worldly Years: The Life of Lester Pearson, 1949–1972* (Toronto: Vintage Canada, 1992), 276.
9 Kent, *A Public Purpose*, 88. This point is emphasized by Kenneth C. Dewar in "Liberalism, Social Democracy, and Tom Kent," *Journal of Canadian Studies* 53, no. 1 (2019): 188.
10 Robert Bothwell, Ian Drummond, and John English, *Canada since 1945: Power, Politics and Provincialism*, rev. ed. (Toronto: University of Toronto Press, 1989), 240.
11 English, *The Worldly Years*, 234–6.
12 English, *The Worldly Years*, 235.
13 LAC, Liberal Party of Canada fonds, MG 28 IV 3, vol. 692, file Pre-Campaign Strategy, 1961–62, Pre-Campaign Strategy (no. 1), n.d.
14 Douglas told his supporters that the federal election of 1957 was "the first step" in this "realignment of political forces in Canada." According to a speech he delivered to the CCF provincial convention in 1957, he stated

publicly as early as 1954 (in a CBC forum entitled "Are the Liberals in to Stay?") that "eventually the Liberal Party would disintegrate with the right wing joining the Conservatives and their political allies, and the left wing Liberals would find their way into a movement headed by the CCF and comprising farmer, labour and progressive groups right across Canada." LAC, Thomas Clement Douglas fonds (TCD), MG32 C28, vol. 142, file 19, Premier T.C. Douglas, report of political leader at the 22nd provincial convention of the CCF, Saskatoon, 17 July 1957, 13.
15 Mark A. Noll, "What Happened to Christian Canada?" *Church History* 75, no. 2 (2006): 249–52; Gregory P. Marchildon, "Douglas versus Manning: The Ideological Battle over Medicare in Postwar Canada," *Journal of Canadian Studies / Revue d'études canadiennes* 50, no. 1 (2016): 131–2.
16 Government of Canada, *House of Commons Debates* (*HCD*), 21 December 1960, 1023–4.
17 *HCD*, 21 Dec. 1960, 1024–5. Paul Martin Sr. spoke on behalf of the Liberals in the role of health critic, while Hazen Argue spoke on behalf of the CCF in his capacity as party leader.
18 LAC, Cabinet Conclusions, R62, Privy Council Office, Series A-5-a, vol. 6176, cabinet conclusions on Royal Commission on Health Services, 5 Jan. 1961, 2–3.
19 "Judge to Study Health Services," *Ottawa Journal*, 5 Jan. 1961; "Helped Draft Hospital Plan," *Ottawa Journal*, 7 Jan. 1961, 3; Frederick Vaughn, *Aggressive in Pursuit: The Life of Justice Emmett Hall* (Toronto: University of Toronto Press, 2004), 112–13. According to Vaughn, Diefenbaker made the announcement after he has asked Hall but before he had received Hall's final decision on whether or not to accept the position.
20 "Saskatchewan Chief Justice to Head Royal Commission to Study Health Plan Need," *Saskatoon Star Phoenix* (*SP*), 5 Jan. 1961, 1.
21 Dennis Gruending, *Emmett Hall: Establishment Radical* (Markham, ON: Fitzhenry & Whiteside, 2005), 63–72.
22 Douglas, quoted in Vaughn, *Aggressive in Pursuit*, 115.
23 Gruending, *Emmett Hall*, 36–40.
24 Gruending, *Emmett Hall*, 79.
25 Provincial Archives of Saskatchewan (PAS), T.C. Douglas fonds (TCD), R-33.1, XXIII.797 (23-60) – Royal Commission on Health Services: Hall Commission, H.S. Lee, cabinet minute no. 607, 8 March 1961.
26 Letter, Diefenbaker to Hall, 27 May 1961, extracts quoted in Vaughn, *Aggressive in Pursuit*, 118.
27 PAS, TCD, R-33.1, XXIII.797 (23-60) – Royal Commission on Health Services: Hall Commission, federal cabinet order-in-council (P.C. 1961-883), 20 June 1961. The mandate of the Hall Commission was remarkably broad, well beyond investigating and reporting on "the methods of financing any new or extended programs" of health coverage. Although

no deadline was established for the final report, the commission was expected to report to cabinet "with all reasonable despatch."
28 Although Baltzan agreed with many of the views of the College of Physicians and Surgeons of Saskatchewan, he also counted himself Douglas's friend and may have helped convince him to get his government to cooperate with the Hall Commission when it was first established. Verne Clemence, *David M. Baltzan, Prairie Doctor* (Markham, ON: Fitzhenry & Whiteside, 1995), 18–22, 63–73.
29 Gruending, *Emmett Hall*, 108–9.
30 "The Medical Care Study," *Ottawa Citizen*, 22 June 1961, 6.
31 Quoted in Vaughn, *Aggressive in Pursuit*, 120.
32 PAS, TCD, R-33.1, XXIII.797 (23-60), Royal Commission on Health Services file, letter, T.C. Douglas to E.M. Hall, 31 Aug. 1961.
33 PAS, TCD, R-33.1, XIII.714 (23-1), Prime Minister file, letter, J.G. Diefenbaker to T.C. Douglas, 28 Dec. 1960. Mary Diefenbaker fell ill in 1957 and was subsequently hospitalized for many months at University Hospital. She died in 1961. Clemence, *David M. Baltzan*, 66, 70.
34 PAS, TCD, R-33.1, XXIII.797 (23-60) – Royal Commission on Health Services: Hall Commission, letter attaching hearing schedule, E.M. Hall to T.C. Douglas, 28 July 1961.
35 "Expect 30 Briefs at Hall Hearings," *Regina Leader-Post* (*LP*), 12 Jan. 1962, 3.
36 "Inquiry Not Favoring Doctors or Province," *LP*, 22 Jan. 1962, 1.
37 "Inquiry Not Favoring Doctors or Province," *LP*, 22 Jan. 1962, 1, 5; "Effective Control of Docttors Noted," *LP*, 23 Jan. 1962, 1, 5.
38 Heward Grafftey (MP for Brome-Missisquoi), quoted in *HCD*, 19 Feb. 1962, 997. "MPs Amiable after Tension," *Ottawa Citizen*, 20 Feb. 1962, 4; Don McGillivray, "NDP Names Herridge as Argue Successor," *Calgary Herald*, 19 Feb. 1962, 1.
39 *HCD*, 18 Feb. 1982, 999; Greg Connolley, "Successor to Argue as a Renegade, Too" and "Parliament," *Ottawa Citizen*, 20 Feb. 1962, 4.
40 "Shuffle Seen Preparing for New Election" and "'Kennedy's Got McNamara, I've Got McCutcheon' Exults Diefenbaker," *Montreal Gazette*, 10 Aug. 1962, 1; "Firm Financial Reputation," *Ottawa Citizen*, 10 Aug. 1962. Nothing was mentioned in this media coverage about his departure from the Hall Commission.
41 Douglas, quoted in Peter Stursberg, *Diefenbaker: Leadership Lost, 1962–67* (Toronto: University of Toronto Press, 1976), 64. Douglas's position stood in stark contrast to that of Ernest Manning, who pushed national Social Credit leader Robert Thompson to insist on Diefenbaker's resignation as part of any deal for Social Credit support of the PC government on the vote: see Peter C. Newman, *Renegade in Power: The Diefenbaker Years* (1963; Toronto: McClelland & Stewart, 2008), 368–9.
42 Douglas, quoted in Stursberg, *Diefenbaker*, 64.

43 Douglas, quoted in Stursberg, *Diefenbaker*, 68–9.
44 Douglas's campaign team had changed somewhat as well. Having returned to the government of Saskatchewan, Tom Shoyama was no longer with him. However, he still had Eleanor McKinnon managing the office at home, while, as in the 1962 federal election campaign, Cliff Scotton travelled with him everywhere: "New Backroom Boys Hit Campaign Trail," *Red Deer Advocate*, 4 March 1963, 12.
45 Keith Davey went on to say that "most of us were determined to move the party to the left, but no matter how far we went, Kent wanted us to go further." Davey, quoted in Dewar, "Liberalism, Social Democracy," 188; "Liberals Nominate Tom Kent," *Vancouver Province*, 26 Feb. 1963, 2.
46 Tom Kent, quoted in Charles Lynch, "'Grey Eminence' of Liberals Tackles Douglas in Burnaby," *Calgary Herald*, 2 March 1963, 42.
47 "Liberals' Lust Blamed for Election Bill," *Vancouver Province*, 27 Feb. 1963, 17.
48 The *Vancouver Sun* first announced Kent's candidature two weeks after Parliament ended on 6 February, when the parties began campaigning: "Top Liberal Due to Fight Douglas," 20 Feb. 1963, 3. The Liberal Party saw the NDP as its main opponent in British Columbia: "Liberals' Main Target: NDP," *Vancouver Province*, 20 Feb. 1963, 3.
49 "Unionists Back Liberal Campaign," *Vancouver Sun*, 6 March 1963, 6; "4 Unionists Join in Liberal Cause," *Vancouver Province*, 6 March 1963, 2.
50 Kent, *A Public Purpose*, 201–2.
51 P.E. Bryden, *Planners and Politicians: Liberal Politics and Social Policy, 1957–1968* (Montreal and Kingston: McGill-Queen's University Press, 1997), 76; Owen Carrigan, *Canadian Party Platforms, 1867–1968* (Toronto: Copp Clark, 1968), 294.
52 "Change on A-Arms 'to Maintain Respect,'" *Vancouver Province*, 7 March 1963, 2.
53 Carrigan, *Canadian Party Platforms*, 299.
54 *New Democratic Party Program* (Ottawa: New Democratic Party of Canada, 1963).
55 "Berger Raps Kent as Liberal 'Boy,'" *Vancouver Sun*, 23 Feb. 1963, 6.
56 T.C. Douglas, quoted in "Medical Plan Hit by NDP," *Vancouver Province*, 26 Feb. 1963, 2.
57 John Saywell, "Parliament and Politics," in *Canadian Annual Review* (*CAR*), 1963, 30.
58 P.E. Bryden, "Prescience, Prudence and Procrastination: National Social Policies in the Pearson Era," in *Pearson: The Unlikely Gladiator*, ed. Norman Hillmer (Montreal and Kingston: McGill-Queen's University Press, 1999), 100. Also see English, *The Worldly Years*, 263. Kent, *A Public Purpose*, 206, on the sixty days of decision.

59 "Drama in 4 Lively, Noisy Acts," *Vancouver Sun*, 23 March 1963, 2. Ironically, Kent fundamentally disagreed with Pearson's position, which contradicted the resolution at the Liberal Rally of 1961 "that Canada should not 'acquire, manufacture or use' nuclear weapons either under Canadian control or under joint US-Canadian control." See Kent, *A Public Purpose*, 187.
60 Kent, *A Public Purpose*, 203.
61 "Called Backward," *Vancouver Province*, 25 March 1963, 21.
62 The NDP's share of the popular vote declined slightly (by 0.35 per cent) to 13.22 per cent.
63 This is the title ("Victory, of a Sort") of Tom Kent's chapter on the 1963 election in *A Public Purpose*.
64 Douglas, quoted in Stursberg, *Diefenbaker*, 89.
65 The options available to a minority government are many: it can govern as if it were a majority; it can seek, on an ad hoc basis, support for every vote from different combinations of the opposition parties; it can reach an implicit understand with one of the parties (informal agreement); it can enter into a formal agreement that falls short of a coalition; it can create a coalition government with another party; and finally willing political parties can merge their identities into a single party. There was at least some history of these various arrangements at the provincial level: Gregory P. Marchildon, "Provincial Coalition Governments in Canada: An Interpretive Survey," in *Continuity and Change in Canadian Politics: Essays in Honour of David E. Smith*, ed. Hans J. Michelmann and Christine de Clercy (Toronto: University of Toronto Press, 2006), 170–94
66 LAC, Peter Stursberg fonds, vol. 28, file 18, transcript of Stursberg interview with T.C. Douglas on the Pearson Government, Ottawa, 3 Sept. 1976 (hereafter Stursberg-Douglas interview, 3 Sept. 1976), 31–3.
67 "Liberals Change Structure in Step toward NDP Merger," *Vancouver Sun*, 4 June 1964, 4.
68 LAC, TCD, MG32 C28, vol. 12, file 3, letter, Grace MacInnis to T.C. Douglas, 5 June 1964.
69 LAC, TCD, MG32 C28, vol. 12, file 3, letter, T.C. Douglas to Grace MacInnis, 9 June 1964.
70 LAC, TCD, MG32 C28, vol. 12, file 3, letter (marked personal and confidential), Thérèse Casgrain to T.C. Douglas, 13 June 1964, and reply by Douglas to Casgrain, 15 June 1964.
71 P.E. Bryden, "The Liberal Party and the Achievement of National Medicare," *Canadian Bulletin of Medical History / Bulletin canadien d'histoire de la médecine* 26, no. 2 (2009): 322.
72 Bryden, *Planners and Politicians*, 83–4.
73 Judy LaMarsh, quoted in Bryden, *Planners and Politicians*, 84.

74 Tom Kent, quoted in Stephen Azzi, *Walter Gordon and the Rise of Canadian Nationalism* (Montreal and Kingston: McGill-Queen's University Press, 1999), 102.
75 Bryden, *Planners and Politicians*, 85–6; Azzi, *Walter Gordon*, 92–110.
76 John English notes that Gordon, "a novice in the House," performed very poorly in response to Fisher's questions: *The Worldly Years*, 273.
77 Stursberg-Douglas interview, 3 Sept. 1976, 24–7. In this same interview (p. 28), Douglas also said that Gordon's lack of political experience made him a poor choice for "the no. 2 spot in cabinet," a position that is too important "to be handed to a complete newcomer who has no experience with Parliament, who has no experience in cabinet administration or in departmental administration."
78 Azzi, *Walter Gordon*, 95–106.
79 Bryden, *Planners and Politicians*, 87.
80 I also discuss Al Johnson's departure and its implications in the transition from the Lloyd CCF government to the Thatcher Liberal government in April 1964 in my foreword to A.W. Johnson with Rosemary Proctor's *Dream No Little Dreams: A Biography of the Douglas Government of Saskatchewan, 1944–1961* (Toronto: University of Toronto Press, 2004), xxi.
81 At the NDP National Convention in Regina in August 1963, delegates called for a single, comprehensive public pension that would mark "a radical departure from free enterprise welfare practice." Bryden, *Planners and Politicians*, 94.
82 Judy LaMarsh, quoted in Bryden, *Planners and Politicians*, 93 (emphasis in original).
83 This remained his view more than a decade later: Stursberg-Douglas interview, 3 Sept. 1976, 81.
84 LAC, RG2, Privy Council Office, Series A-5-a, vol. 6265, cabinet conclusions on Royal Commission on Health Services, 16 June 1964. The conclusions indicate that there was discussion concerning whether it would be better to study the report and figure out what the government's "policy on the report should be" before releasing, or to "table it at once and indicate that the government had not yet had an opportunity to study it." However (and unusually so for cabinet conclusions at this time), the cabinet secretary did not reveal "the remarks of the Prime Minister and other Ministers concerning the report of the Royal Commission on Health Services."
85 *Royal Commission on Health Services*, vol. 1 (Ottawa: King's Printer, 1964), 10.
86 CMA spokesperson quoted in "Doctors Warn against Arbitrary Health Plan," *Ottawa Citizen*, 20 June 1964, 3.
87 Don McGillivray, "Medicare for all Canada Urged by Commission: Ottawa Would Pay Half Cost," *Ottawa Citizen*, 19 June 1964, 1.

88 *Royal Commission on Health Services*, 1: 19.
89 *Royal Commission on Health Services*, 1: 28: "the next essential service to be organized is care provided by physicians and surgeons and some ancillary services all of which we refer to as 'medical services.'"
90 *Royal Commission on Health Services*, 1: 19.
91 *Royal Commission on Health Services*, 1: Part V on "Future Health Costs and the Canadian Economy," 749–879.
92 Don McGillivray, "Canada Lines Up Best but Costliest Welfare," *Ottawa Citizen*, 20 June 1964, 3; *Royal Commission on Health Services*, 1: 879.
93 *Royal Commission on Health Services*, 1: 11. On Emmett Hall's personal stamp on the health charter, see Jack Boan, "A Brief Retrospective on the Royal Commission on Health Services," *Canadian Bulletin of Medical History / Bulletin canadien d'histoire de la médecine* 26, no. 2 (2009): 543. Boan was employed as a research office in the Hall Commission. Bernard Blishen, the research director of the Hall Commission, confirmed that the health charter was very much Hall's personal initiative: PAS, Dennis Gruending fonds, BF22, file I.46 (1 of 2) – Hall biography interviews, Gruending interview with Bernard Blishen, transcript, 24 April 1984, 2.
94 Don McGillivray, "Canada Lines Up Best but Costliest Welfare," *Ottawa Citizen*, 20 June 1963, 3.
95 According to Douglas, Hall told him how valuable the Swift Current Health Region data were to his royal commission: PAS, Jean Larmour oral history of CCF government, R-8358 to R-8362, T.C. Douglas interview transcript, tape 3, p. 1.
96 *Royal Commission on Health Services*, 1: 62–83.
97 T.C. Douglas, quoted in "Canadians Being Offered Biggest Health Package in History at Extra $20 a Year," *SP*, 20 June 1964, 1; LAC, TCD, MG32 C28, vol. 8, file 12, letter, T.C. Douglas to Hugh Bushore (UMWA, Sydney Mines, Nova Scotia), 29 June 1964.
98 T.C. Douglas, quoted in "Canadians Being Offered Biggest Health Package in History at Extra $20 a Year," *SP*, 20 June 1964, 1.
99 Gruending, *Emmett Hall*, 111.
100 Gregory P. Marchildon, "Douglas versus Manning: The Ideological Battle over Medicare in Postwar Canada," *Journal of Canadian Studies / Revue d'études canadiennes* 50, no. 1 (2016): 133–41.
101 Provincial Archives of Alberta (PAA), Premier's Office (E.C. Manning) fonds, GR 1977.173, 239, Alberta Medical Plan, 1962 (no month or day indicated).
102 Cam Traynor, "Manning against Medicare," *Alberta History* 43 (1995): 7–19
103 This was Bill 163 on the Medical Services Insurance Program.
104 Malcolm G. Taylor, *Health Insurance and Canadian Public Policy: The Seven Decisions That Created the Canadian Health Insurance System and Its*

616  Notes to pages 422–5

*Outcomes* (Montreal and Kingston: McGill-Queen's University Press, 1978), 340.
105 P.E. Bryden, *A Justifiable Obsession: Conservative Ontario's Relations with Ottawa, 1943–1985* (Toronto: University of Toronto Press, 2013), 134; Taylor, *Health Insurance*, 340.
106 Archives of Ontario (AO), Premier John P. Robarts fonds, RG 3-26, B440099, Medicare, Nov. 1961–Dec. 1962 file, clipping from the *Globe and Mail*, "Ontario Studying Medicare Plan, No Decision Yet, Premier Says," 17 Oct. 1962, 1–2.
107 Like Douglas, Robert Strachan had immigrated to Canada from Glasgow and was a lifelong devotee of Robbie Burns. A messenger boy in Glasgow, he then became a carpenter in Canada. Eventually, he became head of the BC chapter of the Brotherhood of Carpenters and Joiners of America. First elected as a CCF member of the BC Legislative Assembly in 1952, he became leader of the provincial CCF in 1956 and remained in that position until 1969, the longest service leader of the official opposition in the history of the province. British Columbia Archives (BCA), Robert Martin Strachan fonds, PR-0322, MS-1291, box 891000-0001, folders 11–12 – Robbie Burns speeches and correspondence, and folder 16 – biographical notes.
108 BCA, Robert Martin Strachan fonds, PR-0322, MS-1291, box 891000-00013, folder 24, Royal Commission on Health Services Brief, Robert M. Strachan, MLA, Leader of the Opposition, Leader of the New Democratic Party of British Columbia, Victoria, 19 Feb. 1962, summary of submissions, i.
109 BCA, Department of Health and Welfare (Deputy Minister) fonds, GR 117, box 2, file7, Hon. Eric Martin as quoted in speech, CBC transcript, 13 Sept. 1963.
110 Walter D. Young, "British Columbia," *CAR*, 1963, 139.
111 W.A.C. Bennett, quoted in Young, "British Columbia," *CAR*, 1963, 140.
112 Gregory P. Marchildon and Nicole C. O'Byrne, "Bennettcare to Medicare: The Morphing of Medicare Care Insurance in British Columbia," *Canadian Bulletin of Medical History / Bulletin canadien d'histoire de la médecine* 26, no. 2 (2009): 216–19.
113 James A. Dosman, "The Medical Care Issue as a Factor in the Electoral Defeat of the Saskatchewan Government in 1964" (MA thesis, University of Saskatchewan, 1969), 123–4.
114 "Lord Taylor versus U.K. Medicare," *SP*, 1 April 1964.
115 Bryden, *Planners and Politicians*, 130.
116 The CCF-NDP tried to bait the Liberals into making medicare the major issue in the campaign, but the Liberals refused to bite: Dosman, "The Medical Care Issue," 134–5.
117 Douglas, quoted in "Secret Talks on Issue," *Vancouver Province*, 22 June 1964, 2.

118 *Royal Commission on Health Services*, 1: 91–2.
119 *HCD*, 19 June 1964, 4598; "Health Plan Talks Likely within Six Months – PM," *Ottawa Citizen*, 24 June 1964, 34.
120 Pearson, quoted in English, *The Worldly Years*, 305.
121 Bryden, *Planners and Politicians*, 134–5.
122 LAC, Privy Council Office, RG2, Series A-5-1, vol. 6271, cabinet conclusions on Royal Commission on Health Services, 26 Jan. 1965, 8.
123 C. David Naylor, *Private Practice, Public Payment: Canadian Medicare and the Politics of Health Insurance, 1911–1966* (Montreal and Kingston: McGill-Queen's University Press, 1986), 232; *Royal Commission on Health Services*, vol. 2 (Ottawa: King's Printer, 1965), 2–12.
124 Emmett Hall, quoted in Vaughn, *Aggressive in Pursuit*, 126.
125 The final report was dated 7 December 1964, though it would not be published until 1965: LAC, Privy Council Office, RG2, Series A-5-1, vol. 6271, cabinet conclusions on Royal Commission on Health Services, 9 Feb. 1965, 10.
126 Emmett Hall, quoted in Gruending, *Emmett Hall*, 115.
127 This one paragraph was called an "Addendum by Dr. D.M. Baltzan" rather than a dissent and was dated 8 January 1965. *Royal Commission on Health Services*, 2: 300.
128 Gruending, *Emmett Hall*, 119.
129 "Doctors Renew Attack on Plan," *Ottawa Citizen*, 19 Feb. 1965, 38; "CMA Renews Attack: Opposes System 'Defended' in Report," *Ottawa Journal*, 19 Feb. 1965, 2; "Recommendations of Hall Report," *Ottawa Journal*, 19 Feb. 1965, 7. Volume 2 was tabled in the House of Commons on 18 February 1965, with no response from Douglas or any other member of his NDP caucus: *HCD*, 18 Feb. 1965, 11458–9.
130 Judy LaMarsh, *Memoirs of a Bird in a Gilded Cage* (Toronto: McClelland & Stewart, 1969), 120; *Royal Commission on Health Services*, 1: 10–11, 91–2. According to Gruending (*Emmett Hall*, 117), Hall subsequently claimed that, despite LaMarsh's views, Pearson himself had "invited Hall to go public in defence of his report."
131 Taylor, *Health Insurance*, 353.
132 Speech from the Throne, *HCD*, 5 April 1965, 1–3.
133 *HCD*, 6 April 1965, 49. NDP MP W.D. Howe followed up the next day with a speech on Liberal inaction on the Hall Commission recommendations: *HCD*, 7 April 1965, 80–1.
134 Bryden, *Planners and Politicians*, 136.
135 *HCD*, 3 May 1965, 840.
136 On this migration and the Saskatchewan Mafia in Ottawa, see Gregory P. Marchildon, "Foreword," in Johnson with Proctor, *Dream No Little Dreams*, xxi–xxiii. A smaller contingent also went to work for reforming Liberal premier Louis Robichaud in New Brunswick. See Lisa Pasolli,

"Bureaucratizing the Atlantic Revolution: The 'Saskatchewan Mafia' in the New Brunswick Civil Service, 1960–1970," *Acadiensis* 38, no. 1 (2009): 133–47.
137 Bryden, *Planners and Politicians*, 136–7.
138 Johnson was not only the primary interlocuter for Quebec but he was also working closely with Ontario's chief officials on both medicare and federal-provincial tax restructuring: Bryden, *A Justifiable Obsession*, 147–8.
139 "The Premiers Say …," *Ottawa Citizen*, 21 July 1965, 17.
140 Kent, *A Public Purpose*, 366; also see Bryden, *Planners and Politicians*, 141–3.
141 Marchildon, "Douglas versus Manning," 144.
142 This is based on a series of conversations I had with A.W. Johnson between 2000 and 2003, where he pointed to Douglas's 1959 speech as his inspiration for the idea: LAC, TCD, MG32 C28, vol. 42, file 147, text of T.C. Douglas speech on "Prepaid Medical Care" for Provincial Affairs Series radio broadcast, 16 Dec. 1959.
143 Bryden, "Prescience, Prudence and Procrastination," 101.
144 "PM Lays Down Medicare Rules" and "'Real Fight' in Autumn," *Ottawa Citizen*, 19 July 1965, 1.
145 *Federal-Provincial Conference: Ottawa, July 19–22, 1965* (Ottawa: Privy Council Office, 1968), appendix A on federal and provincial representatives and advisers, 119–29.
146 J. Graham Clarkson would be hired by Donald Tansley to be deputy minister of health in New Brunswick a couple of years later: see Gregory P. Marchildon and Nicole C. O'Byrne, "Last Province Aboard: New Brunswick and National Medicare," *Acadiensis* 42, no. 1 (2013): 162–7.
147 Opening statement by L.B. Pearson, *Federal-Provincial Conference: Ottawa, July 19–22, 1965*, 15–16.
148 Opening statement by L.B. Pearson, *Federal-Provincial Conference: Ottawa, July 19–22, 1965*, 16–17.
149 While the word "criteria" was purposely used by Pearson to downplay the notion of the federal government setting national standards, he nonetheless called these "standards" when he met with cabinet immediately before he opened the Federal-Province Conference. LAC, Privy Council Office, RG2, Series A-5-1, vol. 6271, cabinet conclusions on Provision of Health Services – Medicare, 19 July 1965, 5.
150 Opening statement by L.B. Pearson, *Federal-Provincial Conference: Ottawa, July 19–22, 1965*, 16, and communique of the Federal-Provincial Conference, 22 July 1965, 115.
151 "Robarts Killed Election Issue?" *Ottawa Citizen*, 21 July 1965, 17.
152 As early as March, the Pearson Liberals were tempted to call a "snap election on medicare" to "offset clear signs of increasing NDP strength." The 10 March Gallup poll showed that, in two months, the Liberals had fallen 2 per cent to 45 per cent, the PCs showed a 3 per cent drop to 29

per cent, and the NDP increased from 12 to 15 per cent. John Saywell, "Parliament and Politics," in *CAR*, 1965, 66.
153 "Gordon Pleased with Reaction," *Ottawa Citizen*, 21 July 1965, 17.
154 Walter Gordon and Lester B. Pearson, quoted in "Pearson Says Medicare No Springboard to Vote," *Ottawa Journal*, 23 July 1965, 21.
155 "Medicare Is Ready to Go: Could Start within a Year," *Ottawa Journal*, 20 July 1965, 17.

## 15. National Medicare

1 Jack Wasserman column, *Vancouver Sun*, 8 Sept. 1965, 37; "Ponder Medicare, Manning Warns," *Vancouver Sun*, 9 Sept. 1965, 7.
2 Provincial Archives of Alberta (PAA), E.C. Manning fonds, GR1977.173, box 22, file 2416, text of E.C. Manning's television broadcast "National Medicare: Let's Look Before We Leap," 8 Sept. 1965 (hereafter referred to as Manning, "National Medicare").
3 Manning, "National Medicare."
4 Manning, "National Medicare."
5 Since the PCs under Diefenbaker had set up the Hall Commission, the campaign team felt they had little to gain by campaigning against medicare: P.E. Bryden, *Planners and Politicians: Liberal Politics and Social Policy, 1957–1968* (Montreal and Kingston: McGill-Queen's University Press, 1997), 147.
6 T.C. Douglas, quoted in John Saywell, "Parliament and Politics," *Canadian Annual Review* (*CAR*), 1965, 71.
7 Douglas interview in Peter Stursberg, *Diefenbaker: Leadership Lost, 1962–67* (Toronto: University of Toronto Press, 1976), 139.
8 Jean Marchand, quoted in Robert Bothwell, Ian Drummond, and John English, *Canada Since 1945: Power, Politics and Provincialism*, rev. ed. (Toronto: University of Toronto Press, 1989), 275.
9 *The Way Ahead for Canada* (Ottawa: New Democratic Party of Canada, 1965), 12.
10 Owen Carrigan, *Canadian Party Platforms, 1867–1968* (Toronto: Copp Clark, 1968), 320.
11 University of Toronto Archives (UTA), Desmond Morton fonds, B1999005316, box 23, file 16 – 1965 speeches and releases for T.C. Douglas, longer statement for T.C. Douglas during 1965 election campaign (n.d.).
12 In 1968, he would be appointed assistant deputy minister of finance just as Johnson was leaving that department to become Pierre Trudeau's economic advisor on the constitution. Entry for Thomas Kunito Shoyama in *The Encyclopedia of Saskatchewan* (Regina: Canadian Plains Research Center, University of Regina, 2005).

13 UTA, Desmond Morton fonds, B1999005316, box 23, file 16 – 1965 speeches and releases for T.C. Douglas: Desmond Morton, "Travelling with Tommy: Memories of the 1965 Election," *NeWest Review* 12, no. 9 (May 1987), proof pages (no page numbers).
14 UTA, Desmond Morton fonds, B1999005316, box 23, file 16 – 1965 speeches and releases for T.C. Douglas: Desmond Morton, "Travelling with Tommy: Memories of the 1965 Election," *NeWest Review* 12, no. 9 (May 1987), proof pages (no page numbers).
15 "Douglas Predicts Major NDP Gains," *Ottawa Citizen*, 8 Nov. 1965, 5; "No Coalition – Douglas," *Ottawa Citizen*, 9 Nov. 1965, 25. This momentum was real, based on Gallup Polls results: the NDP went from 12 per cent popular support in January 1965 to 15 per cent by March. This held steady until the campaign, when support increased to 16 per cent in early October and then 18 per cent by early November. Saywell, "Parliament and Politics," *CAR*, 1965, 109.
16 Saywell, "Parliament and Politics," 85.
17 Douglas, quoted in Peter Stursberg, transcript of interview with T.C. Douglas on his memories of Prime Minister Pearson in the Pearson Government, Ottawa, 3 Sept. 1976, 17.
18 Walter Steward, "Tommy Douglas: Strong Man in the Middle," *Star Weekly*, 8 Jan. 1966, 1–7.
19 "No Coalition – Douglas," *Ottawa Citizen*, 9 Nov. 1965, 25.
20 UTA, Desmond Morton fonds, 1597, box 23, file 16 – 1965 speeches and releases for T.C. Douglas, statement by Douglas on Liberal minority, 8 Nov. 1965.
21 G. Ross Langley and Joanne M. Langley, "'A Tense and Courageous Performance': The Role of the Honourable Allan J. MacEachen in the Creation, Passage and Implementation of Legislation for Medicare (Medical Care Act 1966, Bill C-227)," *Journal of the Nova Scotia Historical Society* 18 (2015): 10.
22 Bryden, *Planners and Politicians*, 80–123; John English, *The Worldly Years: The Life of Lester Pearson, 1949–1972* (Toronto: Vintage Canada, 1992), 284–8. As for LaMarsh, while she was ready to admit that a different cabinet ministers "might have done" the pension plan "better or more easily," she quite correctly points out that she was not the cause of the insurance industry's hostility to the policy, Ontario's opposition, or Quebec's determination to have its own pension plan: see Judy LaMarsh, *Memoirs of a Bird in a Gilded Cage* (Toronto: McClelland & Stewart, 1969), 98-9.
23 Malcolm G. Taylor, *Health Insurance and Canadian Public Policy: The Seven Decisions That Created the Canadian Health Insurance System and Its Outcomes*, 2nd ed. (Montreal and Kingston: McGill-Queen's University Press, 2009), 369.

24 P.E. Bryden, *A Justifiable Obsession: Conservative Ontario's Relations with Ottawa, 1943–1985* (Toronto: University of Toronto Press, 2013), 144.
25 Library and Archives Canada (LAC), Thomas Clement Douglas fonds (TCD), MG32 C28, vol. 146, T.C. Douglas speech in House of Commons, 20 Jan. 1966.
26 "Provinces Balk at Medicare," *Ottawa Citizen*, 1 Feb. 1966, 1.
27 Dr. Donovan Ross, quoted in "Final Medicare Lineup of Provinces Not Ready," *Ottawa Citizen*, 1 Feb. 1966, 5.
28 This conference, and the positions taken by the federal and provincial ministers, was described in a ten-page detailed summary by the delegation from British Columbia: British Columbia Archives (BCA), British Columbia Department of Health, GR 0678, box 21, file 21, Meetings re: Health Resources Fund held in West Block, Ottawa, 31 Jan. 1966.
29 BCA, British Columbia Department of Health, GR 0678, box 21, file 21, Meetings re: Health Resources Fund held in West Block, Ottawa, 31 Jan. 1966, 7–9.
30 Davey Steuart had been "instrumental" in Thatcher's bid for the provincial Liberal leadership in 1958. First elected in 1962, he was re-elected in 1964 and appointed by Thatcher as minister of health. He was responsible both for the retention of the existing medicare plan and for the introduction of deterrence fees in 1968. Steven Lloyd, "David Gordon Steuart," in *Saskatchewan Politicians: Lives Past and Present*, ed. Brett Quiring (Regina: Canadian Plains Research Center, University of Regina, 2004), 217–18.
31 BCA, British Columbia Department of Health, GR 0678, box 21, file 21, Meetings re: Health Resources Fund held in West Block, Ottawa, 31 Jan. 1966, attachment C, Communique of the Federal-Provincial Conference of the Ministers of Health, Ottawa, 1 Feb. 1966.
32 "MacEachen Encouraged on Medicare," *Ottawa Journal*, 2 Feb. 1966, 2.
33 Don McGillivray, "Grits May Apply Tactic Dief Used," *Ottawa Citizen*, 2 February 1966, 44.
34 LAC, Privy Council Office (PCO), RG2, Series A-5-1, vol. 6321, cabinet conclusions on medicare, 1 March 1966, 7–8.
35 MacEachen telegram to CMA, quoted in C. David Naylor, *Private Practice, Public Payment: Canadian Medicare and the Politics of Health Insurance, 1911–1966* (Montreal and Kingston: McGill-Queen's University Press, 1986), 237.
36 Government of Canada, *House of Commons Debates (HCD)*, 12 July 1966, 7544–5.
37 *HCD*, 12 July 1966, 7548.
38 *HCD*, 12 July 1966, 7547.

39 *HCD*, 12 July 1966, 7557.
40 *HCD*, 12 July 1966, 7557.
41 *HCD*, 12 July 1966, 7557.
42 *HCD*, 12 July 1966, 7558.
43 *HCD*, 12 July 1966, 7559.
44 Taylor, *Health Insurance*, 369.
45 *HCD*, 23 July 1966, 7559. Such differences in administrative overhead have contributed significantly to the lower per capita cost of health care in Canada relative to the United States since the 1960s: see two articles by David U. Himmelstein, Terry Campbell, and Steffie Woolhandler: "Costs of Health Care Administration in the United States and Canada," *New England Journal of Medicine* 349, no. 8 (2003): 768–75, and "Health Care Administrative Costs in the United States and Canada, 2017," *Annals of Internal Medicine* 172, no. 2 (2020): 132–42.
46 *HCD*, 12 July 1966, 7560.
47 T.C. Douglas, *HCD*, 12 July 1966, 7560–1.
48 Langley and Langley, "'A Tense and Courageous Performance,'" 15.
49 T.C. Douglas, *HCD*, 12 July 1966, 7561.
50 *HCD*, 12 July 1966, 7592.
51 HCD, 12 July 1966, 7594. John Munro was first elected as an MP in 1962. Not a cabinet minister at the time of this debate, he was appointed minister of health and welfare by Pierre Trudeau on 6 July 1968 and held this portfolio until 26 November 1972. He was forced to resign from cabinet in 1978 after evidence emerged that he had contacted a judge to give a character reference for a man facing an assault conviction. Parliament of Canada, Parlinfo, profile of John Carr Munro, https://lop.parl.ca/sites/ParlInfo/default/en_CA/People/Profile?personId=11640.
52 *HCD*, 13 July 1968, 7619–20 and 14 July 1968, 7660–1.
53 LAC, PCO, RG2, series A-5-1, vol. 6321, cabinet conclusions on medicare, 3 Aug. 1966, 9.
54 "Medicare: Inflation Victim?" *Montreal Gazette*, 8 Sept. 1966, 1.
55 Charles Lynch, "An Unexpected Budget Speech," *Ottawa Citizen*, 9 Sept. 1966, 7.
56 P.E. Bryden, "The Liberal Party and the Achievement of National Medicare," *Canadian Bulletin of Medical History / Bulletin canadien d'histoire de la médecine* 26, no. 2 (2009): 327.
57 John Robarts and Dr. R.K.C. Thomson, president of the CMA, quoted in "Robarts Happy with Delay," *Regina Leader-Post* (*LP*), 9 Sept. 1966, 13.
58 T.C. Douglas, quoted in the "Anti-Inflation Measures Branded Incomprehensible," *Vancouver Sun*, 10 Sept. 1966, 16; "Bennett's Technique 'Hitlerian,'" *Vancouver Province*, 10 Sept. 1966, 2; "Douglas Sharply Critical," *LP*, 10 Sept. 1966, 36.

59 "Sharp v. the Radicals: Courage in a Bad Cause," *Ottawa Citizen*, 10 Sept. 1966, 6.
60 "Sharp v. the Radicals: Courage in a Bad Cause," *Ottawa Citizen*, 10 Sept. 1966, 6.
61 Walter Gordon suspected that Mitchell Sharp was responsible for the leaks. See Bryden, *Planners and Politicians*, 158.
62 Peter C. Newman, *The Distemper of Our Times* (1968; Toronto: McClelland & Stewart, 1978), 413.
63 Langley and Langley, "'A Tense and Courageous Performance,'" 16.
64 Langley and Langley, "'A Tense and Courageous Performance,'" 16–18.
65 Entitled "Medicare Now!" Douglas's House of Commons debate speech was circulated to NDP constituency offices throughout the country. LAC, TCD, MG32 C28, vol. 147, T.C. Douglas speech in House of Commons, 19 Oct. 1966, 1–8 (hereafter referred to as "Medicare Now!").
66 LAC, TCD, MG32 C28, vol. 147, notes for T.C. Douglas speech in House of Commons, Oct. 1966, indicates that Douglas was originally going to raise other issues, as well as more explicit criticism of Mitchell Sharp, but he did not do so in the speech as delivered in Parliament.
67 Douglas, "Medicare Now!" 5–6.
68 Douglas, "Medicare Now!" 8.
69 S. Heiber and Raisa Deber, "Banning Extra-Billing in Canada: Just What the Doctors Didn't Order," *Canadian Public Policy* 13, no. 1 (1987): 62–74.
70 Exchange between Douglas and MacEachen in *HCD*, 6 Dec. 1966, 10770.
71 Douglas, "Medicare Now!" 8.
72 Taylor, *Health Insurance*, 373; *HCD*, 8 Dec. 1966, 10872–82.
73 Medical Care Act, 1966–67, c. 64. The long title was "An Act to authorize the payment of contributions by Canada towards the cost of insured medical care services incurred by provinces pursuant to provincial medical care insurance plans."
74 LAC, A.W. Johnson fonds (AWJ), R12603, vol. 35, file 15, letter, Eric W. Kierans (Quebec minister of health) to A.W. Johnson, 4 Feb. 1966. The Lesage government had already insisted on contracting out other social programs such as HIDSA and the National Health Grants program, with fiscal compensation through a transfer of federal tax points. In April 1965, the federal government passed the Established Programs (Interim Arrangements) Act, 1965 to provide a legal basis for this arrangement: see Richard Simeon, *Federal-Provincial Diplomacy: The Making of Recent Policy in Canada* (1972; Toronto: University of Toronto Press, 2006), 177.
75 Medical Care Act, 1966–67, c. 64, s. 8.
76 LAC, AWJ, R12603, vol. 9, file 1, memorandum entitled "A Suggested Approach to Fiscal and Economic Aspects of Federal-Provincial Relations," A.W. Johnson to R.B. Bryce, 1 Sept. 1964.

77 Simeon, *Federal-Provincial Diplomacy*, 68.
78 LAC, AWJ, R12603, vol. 9, file 1, memorandum, A.W. Johnson to W.L. Gordon and R.B. Bryce, 10 Nov. 1965, and attached seventy-six-page paper (not including appendices), "An Approach to Federal-Provincial Relations in the Fields of Fiscal and Economic Policy," classified secret, 8 Nov. 1965 (hereafter Johnson, Federal-Provincial Fiscal proposal, 10 Nov. 1965).
79 Simeon, *Federal-Provincial Diplomacy*, 72.
80 Johnson, Federal-Provincial Fiscal proposal, 10 Nov. 1965, 44–5.
81 LAC, AWJ, R12603, vol. 8, file 20, Statement by the Hon. M.W. Sharp, Minister of Finance, to the Federal-Provincial Tax Structure Committee, Ottawa, 14 Sept. 1966.
82 Gregory P. Marchildon and Nicole C. O'Byrne, "Last Province Aboard: New Brunswick and National Medicare," *Acadiensis* 42, no. 1 (2013): 157–8.
83 LAC, TCD, MG32 C28, vol. 8, file 12, letter, T.C. Douglas to R.W. Trollope, 29 Jan. 1968. The MacEachen estimate of $885 million involved a $805 transfer from the private sector (private health insurance plus individual out-of-pocket payment) to the public sector (federal and provincial government revenues) and $80 million of additional public money.
84 LAC, TCD, MG32 C28, vol. 147, T.C. Douglas's notes for speech on medicare in the House of Commons, 20 Nov. 1967.
85 "N.B. Opts Out of Medicare," *Ottawa Citizen*, 4 Jan. 1968, 3; "Provinces Could Stall Medicare," *Ottawa Citizen*, 5 Jan. 1968, 5; "Ontario Demands a Decision on Fate of Medicare," *Ottawa Citizen*, 22 Jan. 1968, 21; "Medicare Fight Stiffens," *Ottawa Citizen*, 12 Jan. 1968, 1.
86 LAC, TCD, MG32 C28, vol. 8, file 12, letter, T.C. Douglas to H. Spraggs, chair, United Packinghouse Food and Allied Workers, Winnipeg, 26 Jan. 1968.
87 LAC, TCD, MG32 C28, vol. 8, file 12, letter from Normand Belliveau, president of the CMA, to Lester B. Pearson, with a c.c. to all cabinet ministers, 17 Jan. 1968.
88 LAC, TCD, MG32 C28, vol. 8, file 13: letter, Maynard Woollard, executive assistant to T.C. Douglas, to Roy Atkinson, president, National Farmers Union, 19 Jan. 1968; card from Anita Strong to T.C. Douglas and reply, 12 Feb. 1968; letter, Maynard Woollard, executive assistant to T.C. Douglas, to Ben A.R. Morley, Building Services Employees International Union, Vancouver, 14 Feb. 1968.
89 LAC, PCO, RG2, Series A-5-a, vol. 6338, cabinet conclusions on "Meeting of Federal and Provincial Ministers of Finance – Federal Position on Medicare," 10 Oct. 1968, 8–9.
90 "PM Fretting Over Cabinet Rifts," *Montreal Gazette*, 16 Jan. 1968, 2.

91 Douglas quoted in "NDP Chief Vows Medicare in '68," *Vancouver Sun*, 15 Jan. 1968, 3; "Douglas Demands Medicare Now," *Montreal Gazette*, 16 Jan. 1968, 2.
92 LAC, PCO, RG2, Series A-5-a, vol. 6338, cabinet conclusions on "Medicare," 18 Jan. 1968, 3–6.
93 LAC, PCO, RG2, Series A-5-a, vol. 6338, cabinet conclusions on "Medicare," 23 Jan. 1968, 3–4.
94 LAC, PCO, RG2, Series A-5-a, vol. 6338, cabinet conclusions on "Medicare," 30 Jan. 1968, 6–9.
95 LAC, PCO, RG2, Series A-5-a, vol. 6338, cabinet conclusions on "Medicare," 1 Feb. 1968, 4.

**16. Defender of Medicare**

1 Douglas, quoted in Michael Rachlis, Robert G. Evans, Patrick Lewis, and Morris L. Barrer, *Revitalizing Medicare: Shared Problems, Public Solutions* (Toronto: Tommy Douglas Research Institute, 2001), x.
2 See Paul Litt, *Trudeaumania* (Vancouver: UBC Press, 2016); Robert Wright, *Trudeaumania: The Rise to Power of Pierre Elliott Trudeau* (Toronto: HarperCollins, 2016); and the chapter by Paul Litt, "Bobby and Pierre," in *1968 in Canada: A Year and Its Legacies*, ed. Christopher Kirkey, Andrew C. Holman, and Michael K. Hawes (Ottawa: University of Ottawa Press, 2021), 9–31.
3 Douglas's statement to Canadian Press in "Martin Hard One to Beat: Douglas Thinks," *Regina Leader-Post* (*LP*), 15 Jan. 1968, 16.
4 "Congratulates Trudeau," *Ottawa Journal*, 8 April 1968, 26. By this time, Douglas appeared not to be shocked at the outcome, perhaps because he had seen Trudeau in action during the nomination campaign.
5 Joe Greene, quoted in "From the Heart," *Montreal Gazette*, 6 April 1968, 8.
6 Thomas H. McLeod and Ian McLeod, *Tommy Douglas: The Road to Jerusalem* (Edmonton: Hurtig Publishers, 1987), 279.
7 Donald MacDonald, quoted in McLeod and McLeod, *Tommy Douglas*, 268.
8 Stephen Lewis, quoted in Cameron Smith, *Unfinished Journey: The Lewis Family* (Toronto: Summerhill Press, 1989), 414–15.
9 David Lewis, quoted in Doris French Shackleton, *Tommy Douglas: A Biography* (Toronto: McClelland & Stewart, 1975), 286.
10 Walter Stewart, *The Life and Political Times of Tommy Douglas* (Toronto: McArthur & Company, 2003), 271; University of Regina Archives (URA), Walter Stewart fonds, 2013-23, box 29, file 370, email, Robin Sears to Walter Stewart, 19 April 2001.
11 URA, Walter Stewart fonds, 2013-23, box 29, file 370, email, Robin Sears to Walter Stewart, 23 April 2001.

12 This expression is taken from the title of Gerd-Rainer Horn's transnational study *The Spirit of '68: Rebellion in Western Europe and North America, 1956–1976* (Oxford: Oxford University Press, 2007).
13 John English, *Just Watch Me: The Life of Pierre Elliott Trudeau, 1968–2000* (Toronto: Vintage Canada, 2010), 11–16.
14 Litt, *Trudeaumania*, 272–3.
15 *Liberal Party Policy Statement: Election 1968* (Ottawa: Liberal Federation, 1968), https://www.poltext.org/sites/poltext.org/files/plateformesV2/Canada/CAN_PL_1968_LIB_en.pdf.
16 R.G. Beck and J.M. Horne, "Utilization of Publicly Insured Health Services in Saskatchewan before, during and after Copayment," *Medical Care* 18, no. 8 (1980): 787; "NDP Leader Attempts to Halt Deterrent Fees," *LP*, 10 April 1968, 1; "Lloyd Attempts to Put off Fees," *LP*, 10 April 1968, 4; "Smishek Urges Session on Utlization Fees," *LP*, 10 April 1968, 4.
17 Douglas, quoted in "Many Problems Facing New PM," *LP*, 20 April 1968, 2.
18 Gordon S. Lawson and Luc Thériault, "Saskatchewan's Community Health Service Associations: An Historical Perspective," *Prairie Forum* 24, no. 2 (1999): 258.
19 Berton was sponsored by the Community Health Services Association of Regina, a community clinic whose board of directors was made up of prominent community activists: "Overflow Crowd Hears Berton Criticize Deterrent Fees," *LP*, 11 April 1968, 3. On the composition of the clinic board, see T. Kue Young, "Lay-Professional Conflict in a Canadian Community Health Center: A Case Report," *Medical Care* 13, no. 11 (1975): 899.
20 "MP Says Insurance Plan Deterrent Fees Unfair: Private Bill Talked Out," *Ottawa Journal*, 10 Oct. 1968, 31.
21 Gregory P. Marchildon and Nicole C. O'Byrne, "Bennettcare to Medicare: The Morphing of Medicare Care Insurance in British Columbia," *Canadian Bulletin of Medical History / Bulletin canadien d'histoire de la médecine* 26, no. 2 (2009): 460–70.
22 "Medicare Monday: Only Two Provinces Participating," *Ottawa Citizen*, 29 June 1968, 53.
23 *Progressive Conservative Policy Handbook: 1968 – General Election* (Ottawa: Progressive Conservative National Headquarters, 1970), 3, https://www.poltext.org/sites/poltext.org/files/plateformesV2/Canada/CAN_PL_1968_PC.pdf.
24 Gregory P. Marchildon, "Douglas versus Manning: The Ideological Battle over Medicare in Postwar Canada," *Journal of Canadian Studies / Revue d'études canadiennes* 50, no. 1 (2016): 141–4.
25 New Democratic Party's "1968 Speakers' Notes," section 16 on Medicare, https://www.poltext.org/sites/poltext.org/files/plateformesV2/Canada/CAN_PL_1968_NDP.pdf.

26 Some within the NDP saw the advent of television as a major shift in the way that parties campaigned in the 1960s. Commenting on the successful election of an NDP government in Manitoba in 1969, Frank R. Scott wrote in his diary: "Once again it seems to be the leader quite as much as the party program which makes the difference between success & failure in our media-dominated society." Library and Archives Canada (LAC), Frank Reginald Scott fonds, MG 30 D211, vol. 114, 1969 diary, entry for 6 July 1969.
27 Stewart, *The Life and Political Times*, 273.
28 Litt, *Trudeaumania*, 286.
29 Peter Newman, quoted in Litt, *Trudeaumania*, 276.
30 T.C. Douglas, quoted in Paul Stevens and John Saywell, "Parliament and Politics" in *CAR*, 1968, 57.
31 Douglas was so impressed with Mel Watkins's report on foreign investment tabled in Parliament in mid-February 1968, that he asked Watkins to tour with him during the 1968 election. However, Watkins had promised Walter Gordon (who was aware that Watkins was an NDP member) that he would not be involved in politics for one year after the release of his task force report: Stephen Azzi, "The Nationalists of 1968 and the Search for Canadian Independence," in Kirkey, Holman, and Hawes, *1968 in Canada*, 82.
32 Even though, as Ian McKay wrote in his study of the intellectual history of socialism in Canada, Douglas was one of the two "most revered figures in the Canadian socialist tradition" (the other being J.S. Woodsworth), there has been no major study of Douglas's relationship with the New Left and the Waffle. Ian McKay, *Rebels, Reds, Radicals: Rethinking Canada's Left History* (Toronto: Between the Lines, 2005), 235n14.
33 *Federal Elections: 1968 Leaders' Debate* (Ottawa: Canadian Broadcasting Corporation, 1968), https://www.cbc.ca/player/play/1842543948; English, *Just Watch Me*, 17.
34 Jennifer Ditchburn "Ruffled Feathers, Power Plays: Canada's First TV Election Debate Was also a Headache," CBC, 25 May 2015. https://www.cbc.ca/news/politics/ruffled-feathers-power-plays-canada-s-first-tv-election-debate-was-also-a-headache-1.3086026.
35 From a low of 34 per cent popularity in October 1967, the Liberals under Trudeau climbed to a peak of 50 per cent popular support by May 1968. By election day, 19 June, it had dropped slightly to 47 per cent. According to the same Gallup poll, the NDP was sitting at 16 per cent popular support in May 1968 but climbed to 18 per cent by election day, a bump partially due to the television debate. See table 1 in Stevens and Saywell, "Parliament and Politics," in *CAR*, 1968, 62.
36 Charles Lynch, "The Nation," *Calgary Herald*, 10 June 1968, 6. The actions and statements of Woodrow Lloyd and the NDP opposition in

Saskatchewan were covered in the *Regina Leader-Post* at the time: "NDP Leader Attempts to Halt Deterrent Fees" and "Smishek urges Session on Utilization Fees," 10 April 1968, 1, 4.
37 James Ferrebee, "The Debate: Who Won? Who Lost? Well, Guess ...," *Montreal Gazette*, 10 June 1968, 10.
38 Jim Hayes, quoted in McLeod and McLeod, *Tommy Douglas*, 272.
39 Stevens and Saywell, "Parliament and Politics" in *CAR*, 1968, 41–2, T.C. quoted on 60.
40 Pierre Trudeau, quoted in English, *Just Watch Me*, 4. On Trudeau's complicated relationship with, and gradual distancing from, the CCF-NDP, see Christo Aivalis, *The Constant Liberal: Pierre Trudeau, Organized Labour, and the Canadian Social Democratic Left* (Vancouver: UBC Press, 2018), 22–65.
41 LAC, Thomas Clement Douglas fonds (TCD), MG32 C32, vol. 147, file 27, transcript of national television debate, 9 June 1968.
42 McLeod and McLeod, *Tommy Douglas*, 272.
43 The 1968 election results are in tables 2 and 3 in Stevens and Saywell, "Parliament and Politics," *CAR*, 1968, 63.
44 Desmond Morton, *NDP: Social Democracy in Canada*, 2nd ed. (Toronto: Samuel Stevens, 1977), 89.
45 "Douglas Loses Burnaby by 93," *LP*, 26 June 1968, 1; "Will NDP's Tommy Douglas Rise to Fight Again? Leader's Defeat Shakes Party to Its Roots," *Ottawa Journal*, 26 June 1968, 3; "Only Slim Chance Douglas Will Regain Lost Seat: Successor to Be Named Next July?" *Ottawa Journal*, 27 June 1968, 35; "Tommy Down – and Out Too?" *Ottawa Citizen*, 26 June 1966, 1; Stevens and Saywell, "Parliament and Politics," *CAR*, 1968, 67.
46 This is based on the official vote recount number in which Douglas lost by 138 votes, not the 152 votes tabulated before the recount. "Douglas Loses Burnaby by 93," *LP*, 26 June 1968, 1; "Lead Cut in Recount," *Ottawa Journal*, 12 July 1968, 5; McLeod and McLeod, *Tommy Douglas*, 273. The issue that likely contributed most to these gains in Saskatchewan was the negative reaction to the imposition of deterrent fees on hospital and medical care by Thatcher's provincial Liberal government. Lorne Nystrom, the twenty-two-year-old candidate for Yorkton-Melville, credited deterrent fees for the large margin of his victory: "Generation Gap Problem for MP," *Ottawa Citizen*, 11 Sept. 1968, 84. The *Regina Leader-Post* also concluded that deterrent fees contributed to the NDP seat gains and vote counts: "PCs Lose Grip in Sask.; NDP Get 6, Liberals 2," 26 June 1968, 1. This was an assessment contested by Ross Thatcher in the immediate aftermath of the election: "Thatcher Blames Split Vote, Not Fees," *LP*, 26 June 1968, 1.
47 Morton, *NDP*, 86.

48 "Backroom Party Adviser Future Role for Douglas?" *Vancouver Province*, 27 June 1968, 1; "Douglas Unlikely to Seek New Seat Elsewhere," *Vancouver Province*, 27 June 1968, 2; "Tommy Stays NDP Head Unit '69," *Ottawa Journal*, 2 July 1968, 10; "Wanted: Young Man to Lead NDP," *Ottawa Citizen*, 8 July 1968, 15.
49 Headline quoted in McLeod and McLeod, *Tommy Douglas*, 273.
50 Charles Lynch, "Tommy's Just Fading Away," *Vancouver Province*, 2 July 1968, 2.
51 Stewart, *Life and Political Times*, 275.
52 In his biography of the Lewis family, Cameron Smith repeats a story told him by Robin Sears, the grandson of Colin Cameron. At the first caucus meeting following the 1968 election, Cameron offered to nominate David Lewis as parliamentary leader if Lewis would nominate Cameron as caucus chair. The deal was conditional on Lewis not using the "position as a jumping-off post for the party leadership" or Cameron would do everything to end Lewis's career – a viable threat, given Cameron stature among the left wingers within the party. Lewis agreed, but Cameron died a few weeks later, thereby removing the threat. See Smith, *Unfinished Journey*, 416.
53 McLeod and McLeod, *Tommy Douglas*, 274.
54 John Bird, "Now It's Turn of NDP to Plan for Leadership," *Financial Post*, 19 Oct. 1968, 7.
55 These were among several younger candidates Douglas himself identified in a press conference following his decision to remain beyond 1969: "Douglas to Seek Final Term," *Albertan*, 6 May 1969, 1.
56 McLeod and McLeod, *Tommy Douglas*, 274.
57 University of Toronto Archives (UTA), Desmond Morton fonds, box B1999-0023/023, file 19, 1969 byelection brochure entitled "Tommy Douglas: A Special Kind of Canada," the backside of which stated: "February 10: a special kind of by-election … elect Tommy Douglas to strengthen your Parliament."
58 McLeod and McLeod, *Tommy Douglas*, 274.
59 Stewart, *Life and Political Times*, 278.
60 T.C. Douglas, quoted in "Douglas to Seek Leadership Last Time," *Saskatoon Star Phoenix (SP)*, 5 May 1969, 2.
61 "Douglas to Seek Leadership Last Time," *SP*, 5 May 1969, 1.
62 Stewart, *Life and Political Times*, 278.
63 "Douglas to Seek Final Term," *Albertan*, 8 May 1969, 1.
64 W.A. Wilson, "Persuasions of Time: NDP Leadership," *Montreal Star*, 6 May 1969, 9.
65 "NDP Leader's Daughter Charged in Grenade Buying," *Ottawa Journal*, 4 Oct. 1969, 1.

66 "Medicare's Scrappy Defender," *Zoomer*, 1 Jan. 2006, https://www.everythingzoomer.com/style/home-garden/2006/01/01/medicares-scrappy-defender-2/.

67 Shirley Sutherland (as she was then known), quoted in Shackleton, *Tommy Douglas*, 295.

68 Lanre Bakare, "How Hollywood Feted the Black Power Movement – and Fell Foul of the FBI," *Guardian*, 5 Dec. 2019, https://www.theguardian.com/film/2019/dec/05/how-hollywd-feted-the-black-power-movement-and-fell-foul-of-the-fbi.

69 This FBI program (known by the acronym Cointelpro) remained secret until 1971. See John Drabble, "Fighting Black Power–New Left Coalitions: Covert FBI Media Campaigns and American Cultural Discourse," *European Journal of American Culture* 27, no. 2 (2008): 65–91.

70 Donald Sutherland, quoted in John Patterson, "Donald Sutherland: Total Recall," *Guardian*, 3 Sept. 2005, https://www.theguardian.com/world/2005/sep/03/usa.film.

71 Stewart, *Life and Times of Tommy Douglas*, 276–7.

72 T.C. Douglas from an interview with the *Toronto Star*, quoted in Shackleton, *Tommy Douglas*, 295.

73 "Douglas's Daughter 'Buying Poor Food,'" *Ottawa Citizen*, 6 Oct. 1969, 3.

74 Stewart, *Life and Times of Tommy Douglas*, 277. A thirty-second clip of Douglas's televised encounter with journalists has been preserved on YouTube: https://www.youtube.com/watch?v=iTVh55J6dCs.

75 McLeod and McLeod, *Tommy Douglas*, 254. This association with the Black Panthers destroyed the career of Jean Seberg: Lanre Bakare, "How Hollywood Feted the Black Power Movement – and Fell Foul of the FBI," *Guardian*, 5 Dec. 2019, https://www.theguardian.com/film/2019/dec/05/how-hollywood-feted-the-black-power-movement-and-fell-foul-of-the-fbi.

76 LAC, Canadian Security Intelligence Service fonds, RCMP files on T.C. Douglas, A201100233201, vol. 6, Oct. 1969. This RCMP file shows that informers were tracking Douglas concerning the indictment of his daughter and her alleged affiliation with the Black Panthers, but two pages were withheld and key passages redacted in the material I received under an Access to Information request.

77 For many in the Waffle, the word "socialist" seemed self-evident, implying an updated (New Left) Marxian class analysis. Frank R. Scott, for one, was upset by this shift: "When I used to be asked whether I was a Socialist, I would answer, 'Tell me what the word means to you, and I will tell you if I am one' … Today it seems to mean some kind of Marxist, either Communist or Maoist. This is quite wrong." LAC, Frank Reginald Scott fonds, MG 30 D211, vol. 114, 1969 diary, entry for 11 July 1969.

78 LAC, CCF and NDP fonds, MG 28 IV 1, vol. 446, file 3 – Correspondence re: The Waffle, 1969–1972, "For an Independent Socialist Canada." This document, along with some contextual historical analysis, is available online: see Roberta Lexier, "'For an Independent Socialist Canada': Rediscovering the Waffle Manifesto," in Findings: The Champlain Society (May 2017), https://champlainsociety.utpjournals.press/findings-trouvailles/for-an-independent-socialist-canada-rediscovering-the-waffle-manifesto.

79 Azzi, "The Nationalists of 1968," 74–84.

80 *Foreign Ownership and the Structure of Canadian Industry: Report of the Task Force on the Structure of Canadian Industry* (Ottawa: Queen's Printer, 1968); "Left-Wing NDP Group Issues Radical Socialism Manifesto," *Edmonton Journal*, 5 Sept. 1969, 54; editorial, "Radicalizing the NDP," *Vancouver Sun*, 6 Sept. 1969, 4.

81 David Lewis, quoted in "NDP Group Unveils 'Ottawa Manifesto': Lewis Raps Strident Criticism of U.S.," *Saskatoon Star Phoenix*, 5 Sept. 1969, 29.

82 LAC, TCD, MG32 C28, file 18-35, CCF Manifesto, letter, T.C. Douglas to E.D. Snyder, 1 Nov. 1956.

83 Carlyle King, quoted in McLeod and McLeod, *Tommy Douglas*, 278. King was an English literature professor at the University of Saskatchewan (1929–79), president of the Saskatchewan CCF from 1945 until 1960, and a well-known pacifist who opposed Douglas on Canada's entry into the Second World War. There was always some tension between the two, due to Douglas's pragmatism in getting CCF policies and programs put into practice and King's emphasis on the ideal. It seems to me that this tension was constructive for Douglas, even if he viewed individuals such as King as armchair politicians. According to King, from 1945 until 1960, he and Douglas met every second Saturday afternoon to discuss the issues of the day from the party's and the government's perspectives: Carlyle King, "Recollections: The CCF in Saskatchewan," in *Western Canadian Politics: The Radical Tradition*, ed. Donald C. Kerr (Edmonton: NeWest Press, 1981), 40–1. Also see Donald C. Kerr and Stan Hanson, "Pacifism and the CCF at the Outbreak of World War II," *Prairie Forum* 23, no. 2 (1998): 21–43, and Carlyle King, "Recollections and Reminiscences: A Beginning in Politics: Saskatoon CCF, 1938–1943," *Saskatchewan History* 36, no. 3 (1983): 102–14. King was also the author of *What Is Democratic Socialism?* (Ottawa: Co-operative Commonwealth Federation, 1943).

84 "Leadership Race Out, Says Lewis," *SP*, 5 Sept. 1969, 29.

85 In Charles Taylor's view, Lewis was the only NDP MP at the time "with a real grasp of the Quebec scene." Taylor, quoted in Alan Whitehorn, *Canadian Socialism: Essays on the CCF-NDP* (Toronto: Oxford University Press, 1991), 165.

86 "It's Premier Schreyer in Surprised Manitoba," *Ottawa Citizen*, 26 June 1969, 21.
87 LAC, Stanley Knowles fonds, MG 32 C-59, vol. 45, file 92-A-Resignation, declaration of resignation by Ed Schreyer, 9 June 1969; "Schreyer Resigns as MP to Lead Manitoba NDP," *SP*, 9 June 1969, 12.
88 Gregory P. Marchildon and Ken Rasmussen, "Edward Schreyer, 1969–1977," in *Manitoba Premiers of the 19th and 20th Centuries*, ed. Barry Ferguson and Robert Wardhaugh (Regina: Canadian Plains Research Center, University of Regina, 2010), 286–90; "Schreyer's a Conservative," *Montreal Star*, 9 June 1969, 29.
89 Ed Schreyer, quoted in an editorial by Charles King, "Two Routes to the New Jerusalem," *Ottawa Citizen*, 29 Oct. 1969, 6. King's column examined what he called the "contrast of style and approach" of Schreyer and Douglas.
90 Ed Schreyer, quoted in a column by W.A. Wilson, "Ambivalence in NDP," *Montreal Star*, 30 Oct. 1969, 13.
91 Quoted in McLeod and McLeod, *Tommy Douglas*, 279.
92 Charles Lynch, "Gentlemen, the Main Bout: NDP vs. Left-Wing," *Vancouver Province*, 17 Oct. 1969, 4.
93 "Clash with New Left to Bring NDP Sparks," *Edmonton Journal*, 27 Oct. 1965, 5.
94 Bert Bargrave of the Steelworkers Union, quoted in "NDP's Douglas Threatens to Quit if Anti-U.S. Manifesto Approved," *Vancouver Sun*, 28 Oct. 1969, 7.
95 T.C. Douglas, quoted in McLeod and McLeod, *Tommy Douglas*, 280.
96 William Tetley, *The October Crisis, 1970: An Insider's View* (Montreal and Kingston: McGill-Queen's University Press, 2006), 6.
97 Malcolm G. Taylor, *Health Insurance and Canadian Public Policy: The Seven Decisions That Created the Canadian Health Insurance System and Its Outcomes*, 2nd ed. (Montreal and Kingston: McGill-Queen's University Press, 2009), 394.
98 Taylor, *Health Insurance*, 396.
99 "CMA Critical, but Doctors Going Back," *Montreal Star*, 17 Oct. 1970, 1–2.
100 Taylor, *Health Insurance*, 406–8.
101 There is a large literature on the October Crisis; for a comprehensive yet succinct summary, see Dominique Clément, "The October Crisis of 1970: Human Rights Abuses under the War Measures Act," *Journal of Canadian Studies* 42, no. 2 (2008): 160–86.
102 T.C. Douglas, quoted in Tetley, *The October Crisis*, 108.
103 McLeod and McLeod, *Tommy Douglas*, 263–4.
104 McLeod and McLeod, *Tommy Douglas*, 263–4.
105 LAC, TCD, MG32 C28, vol. 31, file 7, letter, Edna A. Hibbitt to T.C. Douglas, 17 Oct. 1970.

106 Eric Kierans, *Remembering* (Toronto: Stoddart, 2001), 184.
107 LAC, TCD, MG32 C28, vol. 147, file 44, report of the federal leader, T.C. Douglas, NDP Federal Leadership Convention, Ottawa, 21 April 1971.
108 McLeod and McLeod, *Tommy Douglas*, 283.
109 The Hatfield PC government brought in New Brunswick, the final province, on 1 January 1970: see Gregory P. Marchildon and Nicole C. O'Byrne, "Last Province Aboard: New Brunswick and National Medicare," *Acadiensis* 42, no. 1 (2013): 150–67. The two territorial programs began on 1 April 1971 (Northwest Territories) and 1 April 1972 (Yukon): Taylor, *Health Insurance*, 375.
110 "Welfare, Wage Rates Hiked, Health Premiums Abolished," *LP*, 22 Sept. 1973, 1.
111 Allan Blakeney, *An Honourable Calling: Political Memoirs* (Toronto: University of Toronto Press, 2008), 86.
112 Provincial Archives of Saskatchewan (PAS), Jean Larmour oral history of the CCF government, R-8358 to R-8362, T.C. Douglas interview, transcript no. 5, 4 Sept. 1981, 14–15; Gregory P. Marchildon, "Private Finance and Canadian Medicare: Learning from History," in *Is Two-Tier Health Care the Future?* ed. Colleen M. Flood and Bryan Thomas (Ottawa: University of Ottawa Press, 2020), 29–32.
113 Marchildon and O'Byrne, "Bennettcare to Medicare," 468–70.
114 "Medicare: MacEachen Confident," *Halifax Chronicle Herald*, 19 April 1967, 2. The Liberal opposition also agreed with the arrangement: "Regan Sees System for Medicare Plan," *Halifax Chronicle Herald*, 8 May 1967, 6.
115 This remains the arrangement, with Medavie (the renamed company) continuing to contract with the Nova Scotia government to administer the medical care insurance plan. Katherine Fierlback, *Nova Scotia: A Health System Profile* (Toronto: University of Toronto Press, 2018), 38.
116 Marchildon, "Private Finance and Canadian Medicare," 19–26.
117 "Trudeau Proposes Cash Payments," *Ottawa Journal*, 14 June 1976, 1.
118 LAC, Privy Council Office, RG2, Series A-5-a, vol. 6495, cabinet conclusions, 27 May 1976, 14–16.
119 André Lecours, Daniel Béland, and Gregory P. Marchildon, "Fiscal Federalism: Pierre Trudeau as an Agent of Decentralization," *Supreme Court Law Review* 99 (2020): 81–3.
120 As late as November 1962, Douglas was still asking Shoyama to join him in Ottawa. Although his reasons for staying in Regina are not revealed in the correspondence, the decision to stay appears to have been a very difficult one for Shoyama: LAC, Thomas K. Shoyama fonds (TKS), R 10881, vol. 5, file 17 – correspondence (file 2 of 2), letters: David Lewis to Shoyama, 27 Aug. 1962; T.C. Douglas to T.K. Shoyama, 31 Oct. 1962; Michael Oliver to Shoyama, 20 Nov. 1962; and Terrence Grier to Shoyama, 21 Nov. 1962.

121 LAC, TKS, R 10881: vol. 9, files 23–5, Shoyama's New Democratic Party files from the 1960s. Shoyama also continued to contribute money to the Saskatchewan CCF-NDP: vol. 5, file 18, letter, Woodrow Lloyd to Shoyama, 25 Jan. 1965.

122 LAC, TKS, R 10881, vol. 7, file 14 – Federal-Provincial Fiscal Arrangements. I could find no record of contact between Douglas and Shoyama at this time, although there was some back and forth between Al Johnson and Shoyama concerning Johnson's concerns about the potential impact of Established Programs Financing: LAC, TKS, R 10881, vol. 10, file 10, phone messages and notes that show a long call from Johnson on 18 April 1975 concerning an offending paragraph in the draft legislation and a subsequent call from Johnson on 21 April 1975. These differences were confirmed in my personal discussions with Johnson in 2001 and 2002, when I asked him for advice during my time as executive director of the Royal Commission on the Future of Health Care in Canada.

123 Marc Lalonde, *A New Perspective on the Health of Canadians: A Working Document* (Ottawa: National Health and Welfare, 1974). On the history of the report, see Heather MacDougall, "Challenging Medicare's Dominance: New Paradigms in Health Promotion and Population Health, 1970–2018," in *Medicare's Histories: Origins, Omissions, and Opportunities in Canada*, ed. Esyllt Jones, James Hanley, and Delia Gavrus (Winnipeg: University of Manitoba Press, 2022), 346–9, and Carolyn Tuohy, *Remaking Policy: Scale, Pace and Political Strategy in Health Care Reform* (Toronto: University of Toronto Press, 2018), 142–5.

124 LAC, TCD, vol. 150, file 12, letter, T.C. Douglas to constituents enclosing speech in House of Commons, 17 June 1976.

125 Robert G. Evans, "A Retrospective on the 'New Perspective,'" *Journal of Health Politics, Policy and Law* 7, no. 2 (1982): 329–31.

126 This was Bill C-68, introduced by John Turner as minister of finance in July 1975. LAC, TCD, MG32 C28, vol. 149, file 62, notes for speech by T.C. Douglas on Bill C-68 – Medical Care Act, 30 Jan. 1976; "NDP Fails to Kill Spending Bill," *Montreal Gazette*, 19 June 1976, 9.

127 LAC, Privy Council Office, RG2, series A-5-a, vol. 6495, cabinet conclusions, "Major Shred-Cost Programs – The Elaborated Foundation Financing Proposal," 27 May 1976, 14–24.

128 LAC, TCD, MG32 C28, vol. 150, file 12, speech in House of Commons, 17 June 1976.

129 LAC, TCD, MG32 C28, vol. 150, file 12, speech in House of Commons, 17 June 1976; "Keep 50-50 Plan for Health Care, Douglas Urges," *Ottawa Citizen*, 18 June 1976, 13.

130 T.C. Douglas quoted in "Douglas See Dangers for Canada," *Ottawa Citizen*, 27 March 1971, 7; also see Shackleton, *Tommy Douglas*, 297.

131 T.C. Douglas, quoted in "Douglas See Dangers for Canada," *Ottawa Citizen*, 27 March 1971, 7.
132 *Working Paper on Social Security in Canada* (Ottawa: Minister of National Health and Welfare, 1973), commonly known as the Orange Paper because of the colour of its cover. Gregory P. Marchildon, "Foreword," in A.W. Johnson with Rosemary Proctor, *Dream No Little Dreams: A Biography of the Douglas Government of Saskatchewan, 1944–1961* (Toronto: University of Toronto Press, 2004), xxii–xxiv.
133 This was noted at the time (but without recognizing the policy conflicts) by Fred Harrison, the Ottawa bureau chief for the *Regina Leader-Post*: see "Ottawa Review," 31 Jan. 1976, 29. Tansley's name was forwarded to Pierre Trudeau by Tommy Shoyama and his minister, Donald Macdonald. Ed Broadbent, who took over the leadership of the NDP in 1975, demanded Tansley's dismissal and described one of his decisions as "an act of unbelievable perversity." Dan Turner, "Confessions of a Self-Styled S.O.B.," *Saturday Citizen*, 22 Jan. 1977, 18–19. On the contributions of Douglas's Saskatchewan Mafia, including Don Tansley, to the Robichaud administration in New Brunswick, see Lisa Pasolli, "Bureaucratizing the Atlantic Revolution: The 'Saskatchewan Mafia' in the New Brunswick Civil Service, 1960–1970," *Acadiensis* 38, no. 1 (2009): 126–50.
134 Taylor, *Health Insurance*, 424.
135 LAC, TCD, MG32 C28, vol. 92, file 11, letter, T.C. Douglas to Iain Gow, 18 April 1979.
136 Monique Bégin, *Ladies, Upstairs! My Life in Politics and After* (Montreal and Kingston: McGill-Queen's University Press, 2019), 241–2.
137 According to Monique Bégin, the appointment "was a clever move by Crombie, giving himself at least a year of breathing space" to figure out exactly what to do about the erosion of medicare. Bégin, *Ladies, Upstairs*, 246. Crombie also needed an answer to the allegation made by Bégin as health critic that the "provinces were diverting federal health payments to roads, schools and other projects." Dennis Gruending, *Emmett Hall: Establishment Radical* (Markham, ON: Fitzhenry & Whiteside, 2005), 250.
138 "Labor Congress Asks New Medicare Deal," *Montreal Gazette*, 1 May 1979, 16; "Coalition to Save Medicare," *Kingston Whig-Standard*, 21 Aug. 1979, 6.
139 A transcript of T.C. Douglas' speech can be found in Shirley Douglas, "SOS Medicare: A (Cautionary) Tale of Two Conferences," in *Medicare: Facts, Myths, Problems, and Promise*, ed. Bruce Campbell and Greg Marchildon (Toronto: Lorimer, 2007), 22–4.
140 Douglas, "SOS Medicare," 22–3.
141 Douglas, "SOS Medicare," 23.
142 In the House of Commons, Bégin said that Crombie lacked "the guts" to protect medicare: Gruending, *Emmett Hall*, 253.

143 *Canada's National-Provincial Health Program for the 1980's* (Ottawa: Health and Welfare Canada, 1980); "Medicare Report: Abolish Extra-Billing," *Ottawa Citizen*, 3 Sept. 1980, 1.
144 Taylor, *Health Insurance*, 428–9; Gruending, *Emmett Hall*, 249–57.
145 Hall, quoted in Taylor, *Health Insurance*, 430.
146 Milan Korcok, "Medicare's Pioneers Rally to the Cause," *Canadian Medical Association Journal* 128, no. 4 (1983): 469.
147 LAC, Douglas-Coldwell Foundation fonds, vol. 3, file 9, T.C. Douglas speech on medicare for CCPA Conference in Montreal, 1982 (no month or day indicated).
148 Stewart, *The Life and Political Times*, 7.
149 Monique Bégin, *Medicare: Canada's Right to Health* (Montreal: Optimum Publishing, 1988).
150 LAC, Stanley Knowles fonds, MG 32 C-59, vol. 502, file 26, Bill Blaikie's Statements and Questions concerning Medicare, 26 January 1982 to 15 July 1982.
151 LAC, Stanley Knowles fonds, MG 32 C-59, vol. 502, file 57-66 Medicare, letter, Monique Bégin to John C. Eull, cc'd to Stanley Knowles, 22 July 1983.
152 "Douglas Badly Hurt but Condition Stable," *LP*, 21 June 1984, A1; "Douglas Stable after Accident," *Ottawa Citizen*, 21 June 1984, 1.
153 "Douglas 'Will Miss It,'" *LP*, 23 June 1984, A1.
154 "Tommy Douglas Dies at 81," *Ottawa Citizen*, 24 February 1986, A1.
155 These were Tory MP Ted Schellenberg's words: *HCD*, 24 Feb. 1986, 10875.
156 "Parliamentarians Pay Tribute to Tommy Douglas," *Ottawa Citizen*, 25 Feb. 1986 (unrevised version), A1; LAC, Douglas-Coldwell Foundation fonds, vol. 3, file 4, *HCD*, 24 Feb. 1986, 10871–5.
157 *HCD*, 24 Feb. 1986, 10871.
158 John Harney, "Medicare Best Tribute to Tommy Douglas," *Ottawa Citizen*, 1 March 1986, B4.
159 "Tommy's Legacy," *Ottawa Citizen*, 25 Feb. 1986, 8.
160 Frank Scott, quoted in Doris Shackleton, "Remembering Tommy Douglas – Fondly," *Ottawa Citizen*, 1 March 1986, B1.

## Conclusion

1 T.C. Douglas, as quoted in Jeffrey Simpson, "Saskatchewan and the Difficult Birth of Medicare," *Queen's Quarterly* 119, no. 2 (2012): 283. I was unable to discover the provenance of this statement and or the date it was made.
2 See Carolyn Tuohy, "Icon and Taboo: Single-Payer Politics in Canada and the US," *Journal of International and Comparative Social Policy* 35, no. 1

(2019): 7–13, and Gregory P. Marchildon, "The Douglas Legacy and the Future of Medicare," in *Medicare: Facts, Myths, Problems, and Promise*, ed. Bruce Campbell and Greg Marchildon (Toronto: Lorimer, 2007), 36–41.

3  I have had some personal experience with this. In October 2017, Danielle Martin (then at Women's College Hospital) and I (representing the University of Toronto) co-sponsored a visit to Toronto by US senator Bernie Sanders. During our conversation over dinner and in his speech the next day at my university's Convocation Hall, he raised Tommy Douglas's example multiple times as an illustration of how it was possible to achieve universal health coverage. See Steve Kupperman, "Some Takeaways from Bernie Sanders' Speech at the University of Toronto," *Toronto Life*, 30 Oct. 2017, https://torontolife.com/city/takeaways-bernie-sanders-speech-university-toronto/.

4  Some prominent examples of this literature include Jeffrey Simpson, *Chronic Condition: Why Canada's Health-Care System Needs to Be Dragged into the 21st Century* (Toronto: Penguin Canada, 2013); David Gratzer, *Code Blue: Reviving Canada's Health Care System* (Toronto: ECW Press, 1999); and Michael Bliss, *Critical Condition: A Historian's Prognosis on Canada's Aging Healthcare System* (Toronto: C.D. Howe Institute, 2010).

5  See, for example, Gregory P. Marchildon, "Canadian Medicare as a Policy Success," in *Policy Success in Canada: Cases, Lessons, Challenges*, ed. Evert A. Lindquist et al. (Oxford: Oxford University Press, 2022), 17–32.

6  I was asked to prepare two expert reports for the court, one of which concerned the history of Medicare as it related to the issues in contention.

7  *Cambie Surgeries Corporation v. British Columbia (Attorney General)*, 2020 BCSC 1310; Colleen M. Flood, "Two-Tier Healthcare after Cambie," *Healthcare Management Forum* 34, no. 4 (2021): 221–4.

8  *Cambie Surgeries Corporation v. British Columbia (Attorney General)*, 2022 BCCA 245.

9  CBC News, "Supreme Court Dismisses B.C. Doctor's Appeal in Challenge over Access to Private Health Care," 6 April 2023, https://www.cbc.ca/news/canada/british-columbia/private-health-care-dr-brian-day-supreme-court-appeal-dismissed-1.6803463.

10  Gregory P. Marchildon, "The Single-Tier Universality of Canadian Medicare," in *Universality and Social Policy in Canada*, ed. Daniel Béland, Gregory P. Marchildon, and Michael J. Prince (Toronto: University of Toronto Press, 2019), 49–62.

11  Jonathan Eig, *King: A Life* (New York: Farrar, Strauss and Giroux, 2023), 7.

# Bibliography

**Archival and Special Collection Sources**

Archives of Manitoba, Winnipeg, MB
Archives of Ontario (AO), Toronto, ON
British Columbia Archives (BCA), Royal BC Museum, Victoria, BC
Johns Hopkins Chesney Archives (JHCA), Johns Hopkins University, Baltimore, MD
Library and Archives Canada (LAC), Ottawa, ON
London School of Economics and Political Science (LSE), London, UK
Provincial Archives of Alberta (PAA), Edmonton, AB
Provincial Archives of Saskatchewan (PAS), Regina, SK
Queen's University Archives (QUA), Kingston, ON
University of Alberta Archives (UAA), Edmonton
University of Regina Archives (URA), Regina
University of Saskatchewan Archives and Special Collections, Saskatoon (USAS)
University of Toronto Archives (UTA)
Yale University Library, Manuscripts and Archives (YUA)

**Published Government and Political Party Documents (Listed Chronologically)**

**Canada, Government of**

*Report of the Royal Commission on Dominion-Provincial Relations: Book I – Canada 1867–1939*. Ottawa: King's Printer, 1940.
*Report of the Royal Commission on Dominion-Provincial Relations: Book II – Recommendations*. Ottawa: Kings Printer, 1940.

Advisory Committee on Health Insurance. *Health Insurance: Report of the Advisory Committee on Health Insurance*. Ottawa: House of Commons Special Committee on Social Security, presented by the Hon. Ian Mackenzie, 16 March 1943.

*Dominion-Provincial Conference on Reconstruction: Proceedings, August 1945*. Ottawa: Edmond Cloutier, King's Printer, 1945.

*Dominion and Provincial Conference (1945): Dominion and Provincial Submissions and Plenary Conference Discussion*. Ottawa: Edmond Cloutier, King's Printer, 1946.

*Census of the Prairie Provinces 1946*. Ottawa: Department of Trade and Commerce / Dominion Bureau of Statistics, 1949.

*Census of Saskatchewan 1946: Housing and Families*. Ottawa: Edmond Cloutier, King's Printer, 1952.

*Federal-Provincial Conference 1955: Preliminary Meeting, Ottawa, April 26th, 1955*. Ottawa: Edmond Cloutier, Queen's Printer, 1955.

*Federal-Provincial Conference 1955: Ottawa, October 3rd, 1955*. Ottawa: Edmond Cloutier, Queen's Printer, 1955.

*Dominion-Provincial Conference 1957: Ottawa, November 25th and 26th, 1957*. Ottawa: Edmond Cloutier, Queen's Printer, 1958.

*Dominion-Provincial Conference 1960: Ottawa, July 25th, 26th and 27th, 1960*. Ottawa: Roger Duhamel, Queen's Printer, 1960.

*Royal Commission on Health Services*, vol. 1. Ottawa: King's Printer, 1964.

*Royal Commission on Health Services*, vol. 2. Ottawa: King's Printer, 1965.

*Foreign Ownership and the Structure of Canadian Industry: Report of the Task Force on the Structure of Canadian Industry*. Ottawa: Queen's Printer, 1968.

*Federal-Provincial Conference: Ottawa, July 19–22, 1965*. Ottawa: Privy Council Office, 1968.

*Working Paper on Social Security in Canada*. Ottawa: Minister of National Health and Welfare, 1973.

*Canada's National-Provincial Health Program for the 1980's*. Ottawa: Health and Welfare Canada, Emmett M. Hall, 1980.

*Building on Values: The Future of Health Care in Canada*. Ottawa: Commission on the Future of Health Care in Canada, Commissioner Roy J. Romanow, 2002.

**Co-operative Commonwealth Federation (CCF), Saskatchewan Section**

*Let There Be No Blackout of Health*. Regina: CCF Sask., n.d. (c. 1943).

*The CCF Program for Saskatchewan*. Regina: CCF Sask., November 1943; reprinted April 1944.

*The CCF Program for Saskatchewan: Condensed Summary*. Regina: Canadian Co-operative Federation, Saskatchewan Section, 1944.

## Liberal Party of Canada

*The Liberal Programme: General Election 1962.* Ottawa: National Liberal Federation, 1962.
*Liberal Party Policy Statement: Election 1968.* Ottawa: Liberal Federation, 1968. https://www.poltext.org/sites/poltext.org/files/plateformesV2/Canada/CAN_PL_1968_LIB_en.pdf.

## New Democratic Party of Canada (NDP)

*The Federal Program of the New Democratic Party* (Adopted by Its Founding Convention, Ottawa, July 31–August 4, 1961 and by Its Second Federal Convention Regina, August 6-9, 1963 and Third Federal Convention, Toronto, July 12–15, 1965).
*The Way Ahead for Canada.* Ottawa: New Democratic Party of Canada, 1965.
*T.C. Douglas: A Biographical Essay.* Ottawa: New Democratic Party, 1971.

## Progressive Conservative Party of Canada (PC)

*Getting Things Done for Canada and Canadians: An Outline of Progressive Conservative Government Action 1957–1962.* Ottawa: Progressive Conservative Party of Canada, 1962.
*Progressive Conservative Policy Handbook: 1968 – General Election.* Ottawa: Progressive Conservative National Headquarters, 1970. https://www.poltext.org/sites/poltext.org/files/plateformesV2/Canada/CAN_PL_1968_PC.pdf.

## Saskatchewan Farmer-Labor Group (CCF)

*Handbook for Speakers: Compiled from Reports of Conferences Held in Saskatoon and Regina, January 7 and February 11 Respectively, 1933.* Saskatoon: Farmer-Labor Group (CCF), 1933.

## Saskatchewan, Government of

*Saskatchewan Health Services Survey Commission: Report of the Commissioner, Henry E. Sigerist.* Regina: Thomas H. McConica, King's Printer, 1944.
*Annual Report of the Health Services Planning Commission 1946.* Regina: Thomas H. McConica, King's Printer, 1949.
*Annual Report of the Health Services Planning Commission 1947.* Regina: Thomas H. McConica, King's Printer, 1949.
*Annual Report of the Health Services Planning Commission 1948.* Regina: Thomas H. McConica, King's Printer, 1950.

*Annual Report of the Health Services Planning Commission 1949 and Final Quarter of the Fiscal Year, 1949–50*. Regina: Thomas H. McConica, King's Printer, 1951.
*Saskatchewan Health Survey Report*, vol. 1: *Health Programs and Personnel*. Regina: Saskatchewan Health Survey Committee, 1952.
*Saskatchewan Health Survey Report*: vol. 2: *Hospital Survey and Master Plan*. Regina: Saskatchewan Health Survey Committee, 1952.
*Royal Commission on Agriculture and Rural Life. Report No. 14: A Program of Improvement* Regina: Queen's Printer, 1957.
*Local Government Continuing Committee: Consultations on Local Government in Saskatchewan*. Regina: Queen's Printer, 1961.
*Interim Report of the Advisory Planning Committee on Medical Care to the Government of Saskatchewan, September 1961*. Regina: Lawrence Amon, Queen's Printer, 1962.
*History of the Swift Current Health Region Medical Care Plan, 1946–1966*. Regina: Department of Public Health, Research and Planning Branch, 1969.
*Saskatchewan Executive and Legislative Directory, 1905–1970*. Regina: Government of Saskatchewan, 1971.

**Radio, Film, and Television Documentaries**

*1960 Saskatchewan Election: Tommy Douglas' Medicare Plan Dominates the 1960 Election Campaign*. Ottawa: Canadian Broadcasting Corporation, 1960.
*Wings of Mercy*. Montreal: National Film Board of Canada, 1947. https://www.nfb.ca/film/wings_of_mercy/.

**Secondary Sources**

Abbott, George M. "Duff Pattullo and the Coalition Controversy of 1941." *BC Studies*, no. 102 (1994): 30–53.
Abel, Emily K., Elizabeth Fee, and Theodore M. Brown, "Milton I. Roemer: Advocate of Social Medicine, International Health and National Health Insurance." *American Journal of Public Health* 98, no. 9 (2008): 1596–7.
Acker, Murray S. "Administration and Methods of Enumeration of the Sickness Survey in Saskatchewan." *Canadian Journal of Public Health* 44, no. 4 (1953): 128–33.
Acker, Murray S., and Lloyd G. Williams, "Statistics of Medical and Hospital Care Programs: Their Use of the Coordination of Health Services." *American Journal of Public Health and the Nation's Health* 46, no. 9 (1956): 1121–9. https://doi.org/10.2105/ajph.46.9.1121.
Aivalis, Christo. *The Constant Liberal: Pierre Trudeau, Organized Labour, and the Canadian Social Democratic Left*. Vancouver: UBC Press, 2018.

American Public Health Association. "Medical Care in a National Health Program: An Official Statement of the American Public Health Association Adopted October 4, 1944." *American Journal of Public Health* 34, no. 12 (1944): 1252–6.

Andrews, Ken. "'Progressive' Counterparts of the CCF: Social Credit and the Conservative Party in Saskatchewan, 1935–1938." *Journal of Canadian Studies* 17, no. 3 (1982): 58–74.

Angel, William A. *The International Law of Youth Rights*. Leiden, NL: Brill Nijhoff, 2015.

Angus, H.F. "Note on the British Columbia Election in June 1945." *Western Political Quarterly* 5, no. 4 (1952): 585–91.

Azzi, Stephen. "The Nationalists of 1968 and the Search for Canadian Independence." In *1968 in Canada: A Year and Its Legacies*, edited by Christopher Kirkey, Andrew C. Holman, and Michael K. Hawes, 71–94. Ottawa: University of Ottawa Press, 2021.

– *Walter Gordon and the Rise of Canadian Nationalism*. Montreal and Kingston: McGill-Queen's University Press, 1999.

Badgeley, Robin F. "Health Worker Strikes: Social and Economics Bases of Conflict." *International Journal of Health Services* 5, no. 1 (1975): 9–17.

– "The Public and Medical Care in Saskatchewan." *American Journal of Public Health* 53, no. 5 (1963): 720–4. https://doi.org/10.2105/ajph.53.5.720.

Badgley, Robin F., and Samuel Wolfe. *Doctors' Strike: Medical Care and Conflict in Saskatchewan*. Toronto: Macmillan of Canada, 1967.

Banack, Clark. "Evangelical Christianity and Political Thought in Alberta." *Journal of Canadian Studies* 48, no. 2 (2014): 70–99. https://doi.org/10.3138/jcs.48.2.70.

– *God's Province: Evangelical Christianity, Political Thought, and Conservatism in Alberta*. Montreal and Kingston: McGill-Queen's University Press, 2016.

Banner, Lois W. "Biography as History." *American Historical Review* 114, no. 3 (2009): 579–86. https://doi.org/10.1086/ahr.114.3.579.

Bantjes, Rod. "'An Imperfect Architecture of Power': Class and Local Government in Saskatchewan, 1908–1936." *Prairie Forum* 20, no. 1 (1995): 37–62.

Barker, Paul. "The Formulation and Implementation of the Saskatchewan Dental Plan." PhD diss., University of Toronto, 1985.

Barman, Jean. *The West beyond the West: A History of British Columbia*, 3rd ed. Toronto: University of Toronto Press, 2007.

Barman, Roderick J. "Biography as History." *Journal of the Canadian Historical Association* 21, no. 2 (2010): 61–75. https://doi.org/10.7202/1003088ar.

Barron, F. Laurie. *Walking in Indian Moccasins: The Native Policies of Tommy Douglas and the CCF*. Vancouver: UBC Press, 1997.

Baum, Gregory. *Catholics and Canadian Socialism: Political Thought in the Thirties and Forties*. Toronto: Lorimer, 1980.

Beardsall, Sandra. "'One Here Will Constant Be': The Christian Witness of T.C. 'Tommy' Douglas." In *Baptists and Public Life in Canada*, edited by Gordon L. Heath and Paul R. Wilson, 143–66. Hamilton: McMaster Divinity College Press, 2012.

Beck, R.G., and J.M. Horne. "Utilization of Publicly Insured Health Services in Saskatchewan before, during and after Copayment." *Medical Care* 18, no. 8 (1980): 787–806. https://doi.org/10.1097/00005650-198008000-00001.

Bégin, Monique. *Ladies, Upstairs! My Life in Politics and After*. Montreal and Kingston: McGill-Queen's University Press, 2019.

– *Medicare: Canada's Right to Health*. Montreal: Optimum Publishing, 1988.

Béland, Daniel, Gregory P. Marchildon, Michele Mioni, and Klaus Petersen. "Translating Social Policy Ideas: The Beveridge Report, Transnational Diffusion, and Post-War Welfare State Development in Canada, Denmark, and France." *Social Policy & Administration* 56, no. 2 (2012): 315–28. https://doi.org/10.1111/spol.12755.

Bell, Edward. "Ernest C. Manning, 1943–1968." In *Alberta Premiers of the 20th Century*, edited by Bradford J. Rennie, 147–82. Regina: Canadian Plains Research Center, University of Regina, 2004.

– *Social Classes and Social Credit in Alberta*. Montreal and Kingston: McGill-Queen's University Press, 1993.

Bercuson, David Jay. *True Patriot: The Life of Brooke Claxton, 1898–1960*. Toronto: University of Toronto Press, 1993.

Berridge, Virgina. "Polyclinics: Haven't We Been There Before." *BMJ* 336 (2008): 1161–2. https://doi.org/10.1136/bmj.39583.414572.AD.

Bickel, Marcel H. *Correspondence: Henry E. Sigerist–Milton I. Roemer, 1937–1957*. Berne: Institute of the History of Medicine, University of Berne. https://www.img.unibe.ch/e40437/e40444/e153944/section154575/files154580/CorrespondenceHenryE.Sigerist-MiltonI.Roemer_ger.pdf.

Bilson, Beth. "William Patterson." In *Saskatchewan Premiers of the Twentieth Century*, edited by Gordon L. Barnhart, 139–60. Regina: Canadian Plains Research Center, University of Regina, 2004.

Bisbee, Cynithia Carson, Paul Bisbee, Erika Dyck, Patrick Farrell, James Sexton, and James W. Spisak. *Psychedelic Prophets: The Letters of Aldous Huxley and Humphrey Osmond*. Montreal and Kingston: McGill-Queen's University Press, 2018.

Blakeney, Allan E. *An Honourable Calling: Political Memoirs*. Toronto: University of Toronto Press, 2008.

– "Press Coverage of the Medicare Dispute in Saskatchewan: I." *Queen's Quarterly* 70, no. 3 (1963): 352–61.

– "The Struggle to Implement Medicare." *Bulletin of the History of Medicine / Bulletin canadien d'histoire de la médecine* 26, no. 2 (2009): 527–32. https://doi.org/10.3138/cbmh.26.2.527.

Blakeney, Allan E., and Sandford Borins. *Political Management in Canada*. Toronto: University of Toronto Press, 1998.

Bliss, Michael. *Critical Condition: A Historian's Prognosis on Canada's Aging Healthcare System*. Toronto: C.D. Howe Institute, 2010.
Boan, Jack. "A Brief Retrospective on the Royal Commission on Health Services." *Canadian Bulletin of Medical History / Bulletin canadien d'histoire de la médecine* 26, no. 2 (2009): 541–5.
Boehm, Leslie A. *Toward the Health of a Nation: The Institute of Health Policy, Management and Evaluation – the First Seventy Years*. Montreal and Kingston: McGill-Queen's University Press, 2020.
Bothwell, Robert, Ian Drummond and John English. *Canada since 1945: Power, Politics and Provincialism*. Rev. ed. Toronto: University of Toronto Press, 1989.
Bothwell, Robert, John English, and Ian M. Drummond. *Canada, 1900–1945*. Toronto: University of Toronto Press, 1987.
Brennan, J. William. "From 'Honest Connie' to 'Rockpile Rink': The Political Rise and Fall of Cornelius Rink in 1930s Regina." *Urban History Review / Revue d'histoire urbaine* 40, no. 2 (2012): 29–44. https://doi.org/10.7202/1009195ar.
Briens, Allan M. "The 1960 Saskatchewan Provincial Election." MA thesis, University of Regina, 2004.
Brown, Lorne. "Unemployed Struggles in Saskatchewan and Canada, 1930–1935." In *Drought and Depression: History of the Prairie West Series*, vol. 6, edited by Gregory P. Marchildon, 109–37. Regina: University of Regina Press, 2018.
Brown, Theodore M., and Elizabeth Brown. "Henry E. Sigerist: Medical Historian and Social Visionary." *American Journal of Public Health* 93, no. 1 (2003): 60. https://doi.org/10.2105/ajph.93.1.60.
Brownsey, Keith. "Policy, Bureaucracy and Personality: Woodrow Lloyd and the Introduction of Medicare in Saskatchewan." *Prairie Forum* 23, no. 2 (1998): 197–210.
Brownstone, Meyer. "Agriculture." In *Social Purpose for Canada*, edited by Michael Oliver, 302–39. Toronto: University of Toronto Press, 1961.
Bryden, P.E. *A Justifiable Obsession: Conservative Ontario's Relations with Ottawa, 1943–1985*. Toronto: University of Toronto Press, 2013.
– "The Liberal Party and the Achievement of National Medicare." *Canadian Bulletin of Medical History / Bulletin canadien d'histoire de la médecine* 26, no. 2 (2009): 315–32. https://doi.org/10.3138/cbmh.26.2.315.
– *Planners and Politicians: Liberal Politics and Social Policy, 1957–1968*. Montreal and Kingston: McGill-Queen's University Press, 1997.
– "Prescience, Prudence and Procrastination: National Social Policies in the Pearson Era." In *Pearson: The Unlikely Gladiator*, edited by Norman Hillmer, 92–103. Montreal and Kingston: McGill-Queen's University Press, 1999.
Cadbury, George. "Planning in Saskatchewan." In *Essays on the Left: Essays in Honour of T.C. Douglas*, edited by Laurier LaPierre, Jack McLeod, Charles Taylor, and Walter Young, 51–64. Toronto: McClelland & Stewart, 1971.
Cameron, G.D.W. "A New National Health Program for Canada." *American Journal of Public Health* 38, no. 12 (1948): 1643–52.

Campbell, Donald N. *Wings of Mercy: A Living History of Saskatchewan's Air Ambulance Service*. North Battleford, SK: Turner-Warwick Publications, 1993.
Campbell, R.H. *Carron Company*. Edinburgh: Oliver and Boyd, 1961.
– "The Industrial Revolution: A Revision Article." *Scottish Historical Review* 46, no. 141 (1961): 106–16.
Canadian Plains Research Centre. *Encyclopedia of Saskatchewan*. Regina: Canadian Plains Research Center, University of Regina, 2005.
Caplan, Gerald L. "The Failure of Canadian Socialism: The Ontario Experience, 1932–1945." *Canadian Historical Review* 44, no. 2 (1963): 93–121.
Carlisle, Kathleen. *Fiery Joe: The Maverick Who Lit Up the West*. Regina: University of Regina Press, 2017.
Carlyle, King. "A Beginning in Politics: Saskatoon CCF, 1938–1943." *Saskatchewan History* 36, no. 3 (1983): 102–13.
Caro, Robert A. *The Years of Lyndon Johnson*, vol. 1: *The Path to Power*. New York: Alfred A. Knopf, 1982.
Carstairs, Catherine. *The Smile Gap: A History of Oral Health and Social Inequality*. Montreal and Kingston: McGill-Queen's University Press, 2022.
Casgrain, Thérèse. "The Achievements of F.R. Scott." In *On F.R. Scott: Essays on His Contributions to Law, Literature, and Politics*, edited by Sandra Djwa and R. St. J. Macdonald, 3–5. Montreal and Kingston: McGill-Queen's University Press, 1983.
Chariandy, David. "Canadians of Tomorrow: J.S. Woodsworth and the New Ethnicities." In *Human Welfare, Rights, and Social Activism: Rethinking the Legacy of J.S. Woodsworth*, edited by Jane Pulkingham, 266–86. Toronto: University of Toronto Press, 2016.
Church, John, and Neale Smith. *Alberta: A Health System Profile*. Toronto: University of Toronto Press, 2022.
Clemence, Verne. *David M. Baltzan, Prairie Doctor*. Markham, ON: Fitzhenry & Whiteside, 1995.
Clément, Dominique. "The October Crisis of 1970: Human Rights Abuses under the War Measures Act." *Journal of Canadian Studies* 42, no. 2 (2008): 160–86. https://doi.org/10.3138/jcs.42.2.160.
Coldwell, M.J. *Left Turn, Canada*. Toronto: Duell, Sloan and Pearce, 1945.
Connor, J.T.H. "American Aid, the International Grenfell Association, and Health Care in Newfoundland, 1920s–1930." In *The Grenfell Medical Mission and American Support in Newfoundland and Labrador, 1890s–1940s*, edited by Jennifer J. Connor and Katherine Side, 145–66. Montreal and Kingston: McGill-Queen's University Press, 2018.
– "'Medicine Is Here to Stay': Rural Medical Practice, the Northern Frontier and Modernization in 1930s Newfoundland." In *Medicine in the Remote and Rural North, 1800–2000*, edited by J.T.H. Connor and Stephan Curtis, 129–51. London: Routledge, 2016.

- "'One Foot on Each Side of the Border': Dr. Frederick Dodge Mott, Rural Health, and 'Socialized' Medical Care in the United States and Canada, 1930s–70s." In *Medicare's Histories: Origins, Omissions, and Opportunities in Canada*, edited by Esyllt Jones, James Hanley, and Delia Gavrus, 57–78. Winnipeg: University of Manitoba Press, 2022.
- "'One Simply Doesn't Arbitrate Authorship of Thoughts': Socialized Medicine, Medical McCarthyism, and the Publishing of Rural Health and Medical Care (1948)." *Journal of the History of Medicine and Allied Sciences* 72, no. 3 (2017): 245–71. https://doi.org/10.1093/jhmas/jrx004.

Conway, J.F. *The Prairie Populist: George Hara Williams and the Untold Story of the CCF*. Regina: University of Regina Press, 2018.

Cook, Ramsay. "The Labor-Socialist Wedding: Moderation Wins Down the Line in NDP." *Saturday Night*, 2 September 1961: 9–11.

Cook, Tim. *Lifesavers and Body Snatchers: Medical Care and the Struggle for Survival in the Great War*. Toronto: Allen Lane, 2022.

Courtney, John C. *Revival and Change: The 1957 and 1958 Diefenbaker Elections*. Vancouver: UBC Press, 2022.

Crowley, Terry. *Agnes Macphail and the Politics of Equality*. Toronto: Lorimer, 1990.

Cuadrado, Cristóbal, Francisca Crispi, Matías Libuy, Gregory Marchildon, and Camilo Cid. "National Health Insurance: A Conceptual Framework from Conflicting Typologies." *Health Policy* 23, no. 7 (2019): 621–9. https://doi.org/10.1016/j.healthpol.2019.05.013.

Cumming, Elaine, and John Cumming. *Closed Ranks: An Experiment in Mental Health Education*. Cambridge, MA: Harvard University Press for the Commonwealth Fund, 1957.

Dale-Burnett, Lisa. "Beatrice Janet Trew." In *Saskatchewan Politicians: Lives Past and Present*, edited by Brett Quiring, 230–1. Regina: Canadian Plains Research Center, University of Regina, 2004.

Daschuk, James. *Clearing the Plains: Disease, Politics of Starvation, and the Loss of Indigenous Life*. Regina: University of Regina Press, 2019.

David-Fox, Michael. *Showcasing the Great Experiment: Cultural Diplomacy and Western Visitors to the Soviet Union, 1921–1941*. Oxford: Oxford University Press, 2012.

Davies, Thomas R. "Internationalism in a Divided World: The Experience of the International Federation of League of Nations Societies, 1919–1939." *Peace & Change* 37, no. 2 (2012): 227–52. https://doi.org/10.1111/j.1468-0130.2011.00744.x.

DeClercy, Cristine. "Women and the Public Sphere in Saskatchewan, 1905–2005." *Prairie Forum* 32, no. 2 (2007): 357–82.

Declich, S., and A.O. Carter. "Public Health Surveillance: Historical Origins, Methods and Evaluation." *Bulletin of the World Health Organization* 72, no. 2 (1994): 285–304.

Deighton, Alex. "The Nature of Eugenic Thought and Limits of Eugenic Practice in Interwar Saskatchewan." In *Eugenics at the Edges of Empire: New Zealand, Australia, Canada, and South Africa*, edited by Diane B. Paul, John Stenhouse, and Hamish G. Spencer, 63–84. Cham, CH: Palgrave Macmillan, 2018.

Dennis, Robert H. "Beginning to Restructure the Institutional Church: Canadian Social Catholics and the CCF, 1931–1944." CCHA *Historical Studies* 74 (2008): 51–74.

– "Faith on the Prairies: Social Catholics and the CCF in the Generation before Vatican II." CCHA *Historical Studies* 85 (2019): 7–32.

Derickson, Alan. *Health Security for All: Dreams of Universal Health Care in America*. Baltimore, MD: Johns Hopkins University Press, 2005.

– "The House of Falk: The Paranoid Style in American Health Politics." *American Journal of Public Health* 87, no. 11 (1997): 1836–43. https://doi.org/10.2105/ajph.87.11.1836.

Deshaies, Charles A. "The Rise and Decline of the Cooperative Commonwealth Federation in Ontario and Quebec during World War II, 1939–1945." PhD diss., University of Maine, 2019.

Devine, T.M. *The Scottish Nation, 1700–2000*. London: Penguin, 2000.

Dewar, Kenneth C. *Frank Underhill and the Politics of Ideas*. Montreal and Kingston: McGill-Queen's University Press, 2015.

– "Liberalism, Social Democracy, and Tom Kent." *Journal of Canadian Studies* 53, no. 1 (2019): 178–96. https://doi.org/10.3138/jcs.2018-0011.

Diamantopoulos, Mitch. "The Foundations of Agrarian Socialism: Co-operative Economic Action in Saskatchewan, 1905–1960." *Prairie Forum* 37, no. 2 (2012): 103–51.

Dickinson, Harley D. "The Struggle for State Health Insurance: Reconsidering the Role of Saskatchewan Farmers." *Studies in Political Economy: A Socialist Review* 41, no. 1 (1993): 133–56.

– *The Two Psychiatries: The Transformation of Psychiatric Work in Saskatchewan*. Regina: Canadian Plains Research Center, University of Regina, 1989.

Diefenbaker, John G. *One Canada: Memoirs of the Right Honourable John G. Diefenbaker*, vol. 1: *The Crusading Years, 1895–1956*. Toronto: Macmillan of Canada, 1975.

Doig, Noel. *Setting the Record Straight: A Doctor's Memoir of the 1962 Medicare Crisis*. Saskatoon: Indie Ink Publishing, 2012.

Donaghy, Greg. *Grit: The Life and Politics of Paul Martin Sr.* Vancouver: UBC Press, 2015.

Dooley, Chris. "The End of the Asylum (Town): Community Responses to the Depopulation and Closure of the Saskatchewan Hospital, Weyburn." *Histoire sociale / Social History* 44, no. 88 (2011): 331–54. https://doi.org/10.1353/his.2011.0015.

Dosman, James A. "The Medical Care Issue as a Factor in the Electoral Defeat of the Saskatchewan Government in 1964." MA thesis, University of Saskatchewan, 1969.

Doss, Gordon R. "John R. Mott, 1865–1955: Mission Leader Extraordinaire." *Journal of Applied Christian Leadership* 4, no. 1 (2010): 72–81.

Douglas, Shirley. "SOS Medicare: A (Cautionary) Tale of Two Conferences." In *Medicare: Facts, Myths, Problems, and Promise*, edited by Bruce Campbell and Greg Marchildon, 19–24. Toronto: Lorimer, 2007.

Douglas, T.C. "The Highlights of the Dirty Thirties." In *The Dirty Thirties in Prairie Canada: 11th Western Canada Studies Conference*, edited by R.D. Francis and H. Ganzevoort, 163–73. Vancouver: Tantalus Research, 1980.

– *The Making of a Socialist: The Recollections of T.C. Douglas*. Edited by Lewis H. Thomas. Edmonton: University of Alberta Press, 1982.

– "The Problems of the Subnormal Family." MA thesis, McMaster University, 1934.

– "Saskatchewan Plans for Health." *Health* 14, no. 6 (1946): 1–3. Reprinted and distributed by Saskatchewan Department of Health with the permission of the Health League of Canada, PAS, T.C. Douglas fonds, R33.1-580, Saskatchewan Hospitalization Act folder.

Drabble, John. "Fighting Black Power–New Left Coalitions: Covert FBI Media Campaigns and American Cultural Discourse." *European Journal of American Culture* 27, no. 2 (2008): 65–91.

Drees, Laura Meijer. 2010. "Training Aboriginal Nurses: The Indian Health Services in Northwestern Canada, 1934–1975." In *Caregiving on the Periphery: Historical Perspectives on Nursing and Midwifery in Canada*, edited by Myra Rutherdale, 181–209. Montreal and Kingston: McGill-Queen's University Press.

Duffin, Jacalyn. "The Guru and the Godfather: Henry Sigerist, Hugh MacLean, and the Politics of Health Care Reform in 1940s Canada." *Canadian Bulletin of Medical History / Bulletin canadien d'histoire de la médecine* 9, no. 2 (1992): 191–218. https://doi.org/10.3138/cbmh.9.2.191.

Duffin, Jacalyn, and Leslie A. Falk. "Sigerist in Saskatchewan: The Quest for Balance in Social and Technical Medicine." *Bulletin on the History of Medicine* 70, no. 4 (1996): 658–83. https://doi.org/10.1353/bhm.1996.0174.

Duffin, Jacalyn, and Joseph L. Pater. "Mrs Robinson's Revenge: Peter Seeger, Earl Robinson and the Medicare Protest Song." *Canadian Bulletin of Medical History / Bulletin canadien d'histoire de la médecine* 35, no. 2 (2018): 413–36. https://doi.org/10.3138/cbmh.243-122017.

Dunn, Christopher. *The Institutionalized Cabinet: Governing the Western Provinces*. Montreal and Kingston: McGill-Queen's University Press, 1995.

Dupuis, Michael. "An Interview with Graham Spry, 1972." *Manitoba History*, no. 51 (2006): 40–3.

Dyck, Betty. *Running to Beat Hell: A Biography of A.M. (Sandy) Nicholson*. Regina: Canadian Plains Research Center, University of Regina, 1988.
Dyck, Erika. *Facing Eugenics: Reproduction, Sterilization, and the Politics of Choice*. Toronto: University of Toronto Press, 2013.
– "Prairies, Psychedelics and Place: The Dynamics of Region in Psychiatric Research." *Health & Place* 15, no. 3 (2009): 657–63. https://doi.org/10.1016/j.healthplace.2009.02.005.
– *Psychedelic Psychiatry: LSD from Clinic to Campus*. Baltimore, MD: Johns Hopkins University Press, 2008.
Dyck, Erika, and Alex Deighton. *Managing Madness: Weyburn Mental Hospital and the Transformation of Psychiatric Care in Canada*. Winnipeg: University of Manitoba Press, 2017.
Eig, Jonathan. *King: A Life*. New York: Farrar, Strauss and Giroux, 2023.
Eisler, Dale. *Rumours of Glory: Saskatchewan and the Thatcher Years*. Edmonton: Hurtig Publishers, 1987.
Elliott, David. "William Aberhart, 1935–1943." In *Alberta Premiers of the 20th Century*, edited by Bradford J. Rennie, 125–46. Regina: Canadian Plains Research Center, University of Regina, 2004.
Endicott, Stephen. *Bienfait: The Saskatchewan's Miners' Struggle of 1931*. Toronto: University of Toronto Press, 2002.
English, John. *Just Watch Me: The Life of Pierre Elliott Trudeau, 1968–2000*. Toronto: Vintage Canada, 2010.
– *The Worldly Years: The Life of Lester Pearson, 1949–1972*. Toronto: Vintage Canada, 1992.
Evans, Chris. "The Industrial Revolution in Iron in the British Isles." In *The Industrial Revolution in Iron: An Introduction*, edited by Chris Evans and Göran Rydén, 15–27. London: Routledge, 2004.
Evans, Robert G. "A Retrospective on the 'New Perspective.'" *Journal of Health Politics, Policy and Law* 7, no. 2 (1982): 325–44.
Feather, Joan. "From Concept to Reality: Formation of the Swift Current Health Region." *Prairie Forum* 16, no. 1 (1991): 59–80.
– "Horse-Trading and Health Insurance: Saskatchewan and Dominion-Provincial Relations, 1937–1947." *Saskatchewan History* 39, no. 3 (1986): 94–106.
– "Impact of the Swift Current Health Region: Experiment or Model?" *Prairie Forum* 16, no. 2 (1991): 225–48.
Fee, Elizabeth. "Henry E. Sigerist: From the Social Production of Disease to Medical Management and Scientific Socialism." *Milbank Quarterly* 67, suppl. 1 (1989): 127–50.
– "The Pleasures and Perils of Prophetic Advocacy: Henry E. Sigerist and the Politics of Medical Reform." *American Journal of Public Health* 86, no. 11 (1996): 1637–47. https://doi.org/10.2105/ajph.86.11.1637.

Fenwick, C. Marie. "'Building the Future in a Steady but Measured Pace': The Respectable Feminism of Marjorie Cooper." *Saskatchewan History* 54, no. 1 (2002): 18–34.

Ferguson, George V. "The Newspapers of Canada: Characteristics of the Daily Press." *Journalism Quarterly* 23, no. 3 (1946): 310–14.

Fierlbeck, Katherine. *Nova Scotia: A Health System Profile*. Toronto: University of Toronto Press, 2018.

Fines, C.M. "The Impossible Dream: An Account of People and Events Leading to the First CCF Government, Saskatchewan, 1944." Unpublished manuscript, Trinity College, Toronto, 1982.

Finkel, Alvin. "Obscure Origins: The Confused Early History of the CCF in Alberta." In *Building the Co-operative Commonwealth: Essays on the Democratic Socialist Tradition in Canada*, edited by J. William Brennan, 99–122. Regina: Canadian Plains Research Center, University of Regina, 1985.

– "Paradise Postponed: A Re-Examination of the Green Book Proposals of 1945." *Journal of the Canadian Historical Association / Revue de la Société historique du Canada* 4, no.1 (1993): 120–42. https://doi.org/10.7202/031059ar.

– *The Social Credit Phenomenon in Alberta*. Toronto: University of Toronto Press, 1989.

Flood, Colleen M. "Two-Tier Healthcare after Cambie." *Healthcare Management Forum* 34, no. 4 (2021): 221–4. https://doi.org/10.1177/0840470421994304.

Friedman, Jay W. "The New Zealand School Dental Service: Lesson in Radical Conservatism." *Journal of the American Dental Association* 85, no. 3 (1972): 609–17. https://doi.org/10.14219/jada.archive.1972.0388.

Fudge, Judy, and Eric Tucker. *Labour before the Law: The Regulation of Workers' Collective Action in Canada, 1900–1948*. Toronto: University of Toronto Press, 2004.

Fulton, John T. "Experiment in Dental Care: Results of New Zealand's Use of School Dental Nurses." *Bulletin of the World Health Organization* 4, no. 1 (1951): 1–73.

Giarelli, Guido, and Mike Saks. "Introduction – The National Health Services of Western Europe: A Historical-Comparative Perspective." In *National Health Services of Western Europe: Challenges, Reforms and Future Perspectives*, edited by Guido Giarelli and Mike Saks, 1–22. Abingdon, UK: Routledge, 2023.

Glassford, Larry A. *Reform and Reaction: The Politics of the Conservative Party under R.B. Bennett, 1927–1938*. Toronto: University of Toronto Press, 1992.

Goldman, Lawrence. "History and Biography." *Historical Research* 89, no. 245 (2016): 399–411. https://doi.org/10.1111/1468-2281.12144.

Gorsky, Martin. "The British National Health Service 1948–2008: A Review of the Historiography." *Social History of Medicine* 21, no. 3 (2008): 437–60. https://doi.org/10.1093/shm/hkn064.

Goss, Aaron William. "Care Regardless of the Ability to Pay: A Reconnaissance of Saskatchewan's State Hospital and Medical League." MA thesis, University of Manitoba, 2013.

Gotlieb, Marc J. "George Drew and the Dominion-Provincial Conference on Reconstruction of 1945–6." *Canadian Historical Review* 66, no. 1 (1985): 27–47.

Gourluck, Russ. *The Mosaic Village: A History of Winnipeg's North End*. Winnipeg: Great Plains Publications, 2010.

Green, David G. "The 1918 Strike of the Medical Profession against the Friendly Societies in Victoria." *Labour History*, no. 46 (1984): 72–87.

Grekul, Jana, Arvey Krahn and Dave Odynak, "Sterilizing the 'Feeble-Minded': Eugenics in Alberta, Canada, 1929–1972." *Journal of Historical Sociology* 17, no. 4 (2004): 358–84. https://doi.org/10.1111/j.1467-6443.2004.00237.x.

Graham, Roger. *Old Man Ontario: Leslie Miscampbell Frost*. Toronto: University of Toronto Press for the Ontario Historical Studies Series, 1990.

Granatstein, J.L. *Canada, 1957–1967: The Years of Uncertainty and Innovation*. Toronto: McClelland & Stewart, 1986.

– *The Ottawa Men: The Civil Service Mandarins, 1935–1957*. Toronto: University of Toronto Press, 1982.

Gratzer, David. *Code Blue: Reviving Canada's Health Care System*. Toronto: ECW Press, 1999.

Grauer, A.E. "Canada's Program of Social Security: The Marsh Report and the Report of the Advisory Committee on Health Insurance." *Public Affairs* 6, no. 4 (1943): 181–7.

Grey, Michael R. *New Deal Medicine: The Rural Health Programs of the Farm Security Administration*. Baltimore, MD: Johns Hopkins University Press, 1999.

Gruending, Dennis. *The First Ten Years: A Brief History of the Community Health Services (Saskatoon) Association*. Saskatoon: Community Health Services (Saskatoon) Association, 1974.

– *Emmett Hall: Establishment Radical*. Markham, ON: Fitzhenry & Whiteside, 2005.

– "Paternalism on the Prairies." In *Canadian Newspapers: The Inside Story*, edited by Walter Stewart, 139–56. Edmonton: Hurtig Publishers, 1980.

– *Promises to Keep: A Political Biography of Allan Blakeney*. Saskatoon: Western Producer Prairie Books, 1990.

Hak, Gordon. "Populism and the 1952 Social Credit Breakthrough in British Columbia." *Canadian Historical Review* 85, no. 2 (2004): 277–96. https://doi.org/10.3138/CHR.85.2.277.

Hall, D.J. *Clifford Sifton*, vol. 2: *The Lonely Eminence, 1901–1929*. Vancouver: UBC Press 1985.

Hathaway, Sheri. "Electricity Forever Changed Life on the Farm." *Western Producer*, 4 October 2018. https://www.producer.com/news/electricity-forever-changed-life-on-the-farm/.

Heagerty, J.J. "The Proposed Canadian National Health Bill." *American Journal of Public Health* 34, no. 2 (1943): 117–22.
Heiber, S., and Raisa Deber. "Banning Extra-Billing in Canada: Just What the Doctors Didn't Order." *Canadian Public Policy* 13, no. 1 (1987): 62–74. https://doi.org/10.2307/3550545.
Hewitt, Steve. "September 1931: A Re-interpretation of the Royal Canadian Mounted Police's Handling of the 1931 Estevan Strike and Riot." *Labour/Le Travail* 39 (1997): 159–78. https://doi.org/10.2307/25144110.
Hiebert, Daniel, "Class, Ethnicity and Residential Structure: The Social Geography of Winnipeg, 1901–1921." *Journal of Historical Geography* 17, no. 1 (1991): 56–86. https://doi.org/10.1016/0305-7488(91)90005-G.
Himmelstein, David U., Terry Campbell, and Steffie Woolhandler. "Costs of Health Care Administration in the United States and Canada." *New England Journal of Medicine* 349, no. 8 (2003): 768–75. https://doi.org/10.1056/nejmsa022033.
– "Health Care Administrative Costs in the United States and Canada, 2017." *Annals of Internal Medicine* 172, no. 2 (2020): 132–42. https://doi.org/10.7326/m19-2818.
Hoffer, Abram, Humphrey Osmond, and John Smythies. "Schizophrenia: A New Approach II: Result of a Year's Research." *Journal of Mental Science* 100, no. 418 (1954): 29–45. https://doi.org/10.1192/bjp.100.418.29.
Hoffman, George. "The Entry of the United Farmers of Canada Saskatchewan Section into Politics: A Reassessment." *Saskatchewan History* 30, no. 3 (1977): 99–109.
– "Frank Eliason: A Forgotten Founder of the CCF." *Saskatchewan History* 58, no. 1 (2006): 18–31.
– "The Saskatchewan Farmer-Labour Party, 1932–1934: How Radical Was Its Origin?" *Saskatchewan History* 28, no. 2 (1975): 52–64.
– "The 1934 Saskatchewan Provincial Election Campaign." *Saskatchewan History* 36, no. 2 (1983): 41–57.
Holroyd, Michael. "The Case against Biography." In *Works on Paper: The Craft of Biography and Autobiography*, edited by Michael Holroyd, 3–9. London: Counterpoint, 2002.
Holt, Arthur E. "Social Justice and the Present Duty of the Church." *Biblical World* 54, no. 2 (1920): 136–39.
Horn, Gerd-Rainer. *The Spirit of '68: Rebellion in Western Europe and North America, 1956–1976*. Oxford: Oxford University Press, 2007.
Horn, Michiel. "Frank Underhill's Early Draft of the Regina Manifesto, 1933." *Canadian Historical Review* 54, no. 4 (1973): 393–418.
– *The League for Social Reconstruction: Intellectual Origins of the Democratic Left in Canada, 1930–1942*. Toronto: University of Toronto Press, 1980.
– "The LSR, the CCF, and the Regina Manifesto." In *Building the Co-operative Commonwealth: Essays on the Democratic Socialist Tradition in Canada*, edited

by J. William Brennan, 25–41. Regina: Canadian Plains Research Center, University of Regina, 1985.

Houston, C. Stuart. "The Early Years of the Saskatchewan Medical Quarterly." *Canadian Medical Association Quarterly* 188, no. 9 (1978): 1122, 1127–8.

Houston, C. Stuart, and Merle Masse. *36 Steps on the Road to Medicare: Why Saskatchewan Led the Way*. Montreal and Kingston: McGill-Queen's University Press, 2013.

Houston, C. Stuart, and Richard A. Rempel. "The Life and Legacy of C.J. Houston, Medicare Pioneer." *Saskatchewan History* 67, no. 2 (2015): 32–41.

Houston, Stuart, and Bill Waiser. *Tommy's Team: The People behind the Douglas Years*. Calgary: Fifth House, 2010.

Humphries, Mark Osborne. *A Weary Road: Shell Shock in the Canadian Expeditionary Force, 1914–1918*. Toronto: University of Toronto Press, 2018.

Hutchinson, John F. "Dances with Commissars: Sigerist and Soviet Medicine." In *Making Medical History: The Life and Times of Henry E. Sigerist*, edited by Theodore M. Brown and Elizabeth Fee, 229–58. Baltimore, MD: Johns Hopkins University Press, 1997.

Huxley, Aldous. *Brave New World*. London: Harper Perennial Modern Classics, 2006, orig. 1932.

– *The Doors of Perception*. New York: Harper & Row, 1954.

Ibbitson, John. *The Duel: Diefenbaker, Pearson, and the Making of Modern Canada*. Toronto: Signal, 2023.

Idiong, Uduak, "Third Force: Returned Soldiers in the Winnipeg General Strike of 1919." *Manitoba History*, no. 34 (Fall 1997): 15–22.

Johnson, A.W., with Rosemary Proctor. *Dream No Little Dreams: A Biography of the Douglas Government of Saskatchewan, 1944–1961*. Toronto: University of Toronto Press, 2004.

Johnston, Charles M. *McMaster University: The Toronto Years*, vol. 1. Toronto: University of Toronto Press, 1976.

Jones, Edgar. "Terror Weapons: The British Experience of Gas and Its Treatments in the First World War." *War in History* 2, no. 3 (2014): 355–75. https://doi.org/10.1177%2F0968344513510248.

Jones, Esyllt W. *Radical Medicine: The International Origins of Socialized Health Care in Canada*. Winnipeg: ARP Books, 2019.

Kealey, Linda, and Heather Molyneaux. "On the Road to Medicare: Newfoundland in the 1960s." *Journal of Canadian Studies / Revue d'études canadiennes* 41, no. 3 (2007): 90–111.

Kendall, Kathleen. "From Closed Ranks to Open Doors: Elaine and John Cummings' Mental Health Education Experiment in 1950s Saskatchewan." *Histoire sociale / Social History* 44, no. 88 (2011): 257–86. https://doi.org/10.1353/his.2011.0012.

Kent, Tom. *A Public Purpose: An Experience of Liberal Opposition and Canadian Government*. Montreal and Kingston: McGill-Queen's University Press, 1988.

Kerber, Richard E. "A USA-USSR Experiment in Medical Journalism: The American Review of Soviet Medicine." *American Communist History* 11, no. 2 (2012): 229–35. https://doi.org/10.1080/14743892.2012.705988.

Kerr, Donald C., and Stan Hanson. "Pacifism and the CCF at the Outbreak of World War II." *Prairie Forum* 23, no. 2 (1998): 21–43.

Kierans, Eric. *Remembering*. Toronto: Stoddart, 2001.

King, Carlyle. "Recollections: The CCF in Saskatchewan." In *Western Canadian Politics: The Radical Tradition*, edited by Donald C. Kerr, 31–41. Edmonton: NeWest Press, 1981.

– "Recollections and Reminiscences: A Beginning in Politics: Saskatoon CCF, 1938–1943." *Saskatchewan History* 36, no. 3 (1983): 102–14.

– *What Is Democratic Socialism?* Ottawa: Co-operative Commonwealth Federation, 1943.

Kisby, Ben. "'Politics Is Ethics Done in Public': Exploring Linkages and Disjunctions between Citizen Education and Character Education in England." *Journal of Social Science Education* 16, no. 3 (2017): 8–21. https://doi.org/10.4119/jsse-835.

Klein, Jennifer. *For All These Rights: Business, Labor and the Shaping of America's Public-Private Welfare State*. Princeton, NJ: Princeton University Press, 2005.

Knowles, Stanley. *The New Party*. Toronto: McClelland & Stewart, 1961.

Korcok, Milan. "Medicare's Pioneers Rally to the Cause." *Canadian Medical Association Journal* 128, no. 4 (1983): 469–75.

Kramer, Reinhold, and Tom Mitchell, "'Daniel DeLeon Drew up the Diagram': Winnipeg's Seditious-Conspiracy Trials of 1919–20." In *Canadian State Trials*, vol. 4: *Security, Dissent, and the Limits of Toleration in War and Peace, 1914–1939*, edited by Barry Wright, Eric Tucker, and Susan Binns, 217–60. Toronto: University of Toronto Press for the Osgood Society for Canadian Legal History, 2015.

– *When the State Trembled: How A.J. Andrews and the Citizen's Committee Broke the Winnipeg General Strike*. Toronto: University of Toronto Press, 2010.

Kupperman, Steve. "Some Takeaways from Bernie Sanders' Speech at the University of Toronto." *Toronto Life*, 30 October 2017. https://torontolife.com/city/takeaways-bernie-sanders-speech-university-toronto/

Kyba, Patrick. "Ballots and Burning Crosses." In *Politics in Saskatchewan*, edited by Norman Ward and Duff Spafford, 105–23. Toronto: Longmans Canada, 1968.

– "J.T.M. Anderson." In *Saskatchewan Premiers of the Twentieth Century*, edited by Gordon L. Barnhart, 109–38. Regina: Canadian Plains Research Center, University of Regina, 2004.

Lafave, Hugh G., Alex Stewart, and Frederic Grunberg. "Community Care of the Mentally Ill: Implementation of the Saskatchewan Plan." *Community Mental Health* 4, no. 1 (1968): 37–45.

Lalonde, Marc. *A New Perspective on the Health of Canadians: A Working Document*. Ottawa: National Health and Welfare, 1974.
Lam, Vincent. *Tommy Douglas*. Toronto: Penguin Canada, 2011.
LaMarsh, Judy. *Memoirs of a Bird in a Gilded Cage*. Toronto: McClelland & Stewart, 1969.
Langford, Stephan A. "The Royal Flying Doctor Service of Australia: Its Foundation and Early Development." *Medical Journal of Australia* 161, no. 1 (1994): 91–4. https://doi.org/10.5694/j.1326-5377.1994.tb127334.x.
Langley, G. Ross, and Joanne M. Langley. "'A Tense and Courageous Performance': The Role of the Honourable Allan J. MacEachen in the Creation, Passage and Implementation of Legislation for Medicare (Medical Care Act 1966, Bill C-227)." *Journal of the Nova Scotia Historical Society* 18 (2015): 1–29.
Larmour, Jean. "The Douglas Government's Changing Emphasis on Public, Private, and Co-operative Development." In *Building the Co-operative Commonwealth: Essays on the Democratic Socialist Tradition in Canada*, edited by J. William Brennan, 161–80. Regina: Canadian Plains Research Center, University of Regina, 1985.
Lavery, Kevin P. "'Youth of the World, Unite So That You May Live': Youth, Internationalism, and the Popular Front in the World Youth Congress Movement, 1936–1939." *Peace & Change* 46, no. 3 (2021): 269–85. https://doi.org/10.1111/pech.12476.
Lavoie, Josée. "Medicare and the Care of First Nations, Métis and Inuit." *Health Economics, Policy and Law* 13, nos. 3–4 (2018): 280–98. https://doi.org/10.1017/S1744133117000391.
Lawson, F.S. "The Saskatchewan Plan." *Mental Hospitals* 8, no. 3 (1957): 27–31.
Lawson, Gordon S. "The Co-operative Commonwealth Federation, Health Care Reform and Physician Remuneration in the Province of Saskatchewan, 1915–1949." MA thesis, University of Regina, 1998.
– "The Road Not Taken: The 1945 Health Services Planning Commission Proposals and Physician Remuneration in Saskatchewan." *Canadian Bulletin of Medical History / Bulletin canadien d'histoire de la médecine* 26, no. 2 (2009): 395–427. https://doi.org/10.3138/cbmh.26.2.395.
Lawson, Gordon S., and Andrew E. Noseworthy. "Newfoundland's Cottage Health Systems: 1920–1970." *Canadian Bulletin of Medical History / Bulletin canadien d'histoire de la médecine* 26, no. 2 (2009): 477–98. https://doi.org/10.3138/cbmh.26.2.477.
Lawson, Gordon S., and Luc Thériault. "Saskatchewan's Community Health Service Associations: An Historical Perspective." *Prairie Forum* 24, no. 2 (1999): 251–68.
Laycock, David. *Populist and Democratic Thought in the Canadian Prairies, 1910 to 1945*. Toronto: University of Toronto Press, 1990.

League for Social Reconstruction. *Social Planning for Canada*. Edited by Michael Bliss. 1935; Toronto: University of Toronto Press, 1975.

Lecours, André, Daniel Béland, and Gregory P. Marchildon. "Fiscal Federalism: Pierre Trudeau as an Agent of Decentralization." *Supreme Court Law Review* 99 (2020): 77–100.

Lepore, Jill. "Historians Who Love Too Much: Reflections on Microhistory and Biography." *Journal of American History* 88, no. 1 (2001): 129–44. https://doi.org/10.2307/2674921.

Lewis, David. *The Good Fight: Political Memoirs, 1909–1958*. Toronto: Macmillan of Canada, 1981.

Lewis, David, and F.R. Scott. *Make This Your Canada: A Review of C.C.F. History and Policy*. Toronto: Central Canada Publishing Company, 1943.

Lexier, Roberta. "'For an Independent Socialist Canada': Rediscovering the Waffle Manifesto." In *Findings: The Champlain Society* (May 2017). https://champlainsociety.utpjournals.press/findings-trouvailles/for-an-independent-socialist-canada-rediscovering-the-waffle-manifesto

Lipset, Seymour Martin. *Agrarian Socialism: The Cooperative Commonwealth Federation in Saskatchewan – A Study in Political Sociology*. 1950; Berkeley: University of California Press, 1971.

Litt, Paul. "Bobby and Pierre." In *1968 in Canada: A Year and Its Legacies*, edited by Christopher Kirkey, Andrew C. Holman, and Michael K. Hawes, 9–31. Ottawa: University of Ottawa Press, 2021.

– *Trudeaumania*. Vancouver: UBC Press, 2016.

Lloyd, Dianne. *Woodrow: A Biography of W.S. Lloyd*. Saskatoon: Woodrow Lloyd Memorial Fund, 1979.

Lloyd Norton, Dianne. "Woodrow S. Lloyd." In *Saskatchewan Premiers of the Twentieth Century*, edited by Gordon L. Barnhart, 213–36. Regina: Canadian Plains Research Center, University of Regina, 2004.

Lloyd, Steven. "David Gordon Steuart." In *Saskatchewan Politicians: Lives Past and Present*, edited by Brett Quiring, 217–18. Regina: Canadian Plains Research Center, University of Regina, 2004.

Lovick, L.D. *Tommy Douglas Speaks: Till Power Is Brought to Pooling*. Lantzville, BC: Oolichan Books, 1979.

Lux, Maureen. *Separate Beds: A History of Indian Hospitals in Canada, 1920s–1980s*. Toronto: University of Toronto Press, 2016.

MacDougall, Heather. "Challenging Medicare's Dominance: New Paradigms in Health Promotion and Population Health, 1970–2018." In *Medicare's Histories: Origins, Omissions, and Opportunities in Canada*, edited by Esyllt Jones, James Hanley, and Delia Gavrus, 343–65. Winnipeg: University of Manitoba Press, 2022.

– "Into Thin Air: Making National Health Policy, 1939–45." *Canadian Bulleting of Medical History / Bulletin canadien d'histoire de la médecine* 26, no. 2 (2009): 283–313. https://doi.org/10.3138/cbmh.26.2.283.

MacLean, Hugh, and Dean E. McHenry. "Medical Services in New Zealand." *Milbank Memorial Fund Quarterly* 26, no. 2 (1948): 148–81.
– "Medical Services in New Zealand." *Canadian Medical Association Journal* 59, no. 1 (1948): 77–80.
Macpherson, C.B. *Democracy in Alberta: Social Credit and the Party System*. 1953. Toronto: University of Toronto Press, 2013.
MacPherson, Ian. "The CCF and the Co-operative Movement in the Douglas Years: An Uneasy Alliance." In *Building the Co-operative Commonwealth: Essays on the Democratic Socialist Tradition in Canada*, edited by J. William Brennan, 181–203. Regina: Canadian Plains Research Center, University of Regina, 1985.
MacTaggart, Ken. *The First Decade: The Story of the Birth of Canadian Medicare and Its Development during the Following 10 Years*. Ottawa: Canadian Medical Association, 1973.
Maioni, Antonia. *Parting at the Crossroads: The Emergence of Health Insurance in the United States and Canada*. Princeton, NJ: Princeton University Press, 1999.
Manley, John. "'Communists Love Canada!' The Communist Party of Canada, the 'People' and the Popular Front, 1933–1939." *Journal of Canadian Studies* 36, no. 4 (2002): 59–86. https://doi.org/10.3138/jcs.36.4.59.
Marchildon, Gregory P. "The Blakeney Style of Cabinet Government: Lessons for the Twenty-First Century?" In *Back to Blakeney: Revitalizing the Democratic State*, edited by David McGrane, John D. Whyte, Roy Romanow, and Russ Singer, 33–49. Regina: University of Regina Press, 2019.
– "Canadian Medicare as a Policy Success." In *Policy Success in Canada: Cases, Lessons, Challenges*, edited by Evert A. Lindquist, Michael Howlett, Grace Skogstad, Geneviève Tellier, Paul 'T Hart, 17–35. Oxford: Oxford University Press, 2022. https://doi.org/10.1093/oso/9780192897046.003.0002.
– "The Cautious Liberal: St-Laurent and National Hospitalization." In *The Unexpected Louis St-Laurent: Politics and Policies for a Modern Canada*, edited by Patrice Dutil, 281–95. Vancouver: UBC Press, 2020.
– "Community Clinics and Stan Rands's Struggle for the Transformation of Health Care in Canada." In Stan Rands, *Privilege and Policy: The History of Community Clinics in Canada*, edited by Gregory P. Marchildon and Catherine Leviten-Reid. Regina: Canadian Plains Research Centre, University of Regina, 2012, vii–xii.
– "The Douglas Legacy and the Future of Medicare." In *Medicare: Facts, Myths, Problems, and Promise*, edited by Bruce Campbell and Greg Marchildon, 36–41. Toronto: Lorimer, 2007.
– "Douglas versus Manning: The Ideological Battle over Medicare in Postwar Canada." *Journal of Canadian Studies / Revue d'études canadiennes* 50, no. 1 (2016): 129–49. https://doi.org/10.3138/jcs.2016.50.1.129.
– "Foreword." In Johnson with Proctor, *Dream No Little Dreams*, xv–xxxi.

- "The Great Divide." In *The Heavy Hand of History: Interpreting Saskatchewan's Past*, edited by Gregory P. Marchildon, 51–66. Regina: Canadian Plains Research Center, University of Regina, 2005.
- "A House Divided: Deinstitutionalization, Medicare and the Canadian Mental Health Association in Saskatchewan, 1944–1964." *Histoire sociale / Social History* 44, no. 88 (2011): 305–29. https://doi.org/10.1353/his.2011.0014.
- "Physicians and Regionalization in Canada: Past, Present and Future." *Canadian Medical Association Journal* 189, no. 36 (2017): E1147–49. https://doi.org/10.1503/cmaj.170164.
- "Policy Agenda Setting in Public Health Dentistry: Implementing North America's First Universal School-Based Dental Program in Saskatchewan." *Canadian Journal of Health History* 40, no. 1 (2023): 197–222. https://doi.org/10.3138/cjhh.618-112022.
- "Policy Lessons from Physicians' Strikes." *Israel Journal of Health Policy Research* 2, no. 1 (2013). https://doi.org/10.1186/2045-4015-2-34.
- "The Prairie Farm Rehabilitation Administration: Climate Crisis and Federal-Provincial Relations during the Great Depression." *Canadian Historical Review* 90, no. 2 (2009): 275–301. http://dx.doi.org/10.3138/chr.90.2.275.
- "Private Finance and Canadian Medicare: Learning from History." In *Is Two-Tier Health Care the Future?* edited by Colleen M. Flood and Bryan Thomas, 15–35. Ottawa: University of Ottawa Press, 2020.
- "Provincial Coalition Governments in Canada: An Interpretive Survey." In *Continuity and Change in Canadian Politics: Essays in Honour of David E. Smith*, edited by Hans J. Michelmann and Christine de Clercy, 170–94. Toronto: University of Toronto Press, 2006. https://doi.org/10.3138/9781442657083-009.
- "Regionalization: What Have We Learned?" *Healthcare Papers* 16, no. 1 (2016): 8–14. https://doi.org/10.12927/hcpap.2016.24766.
- "The Secretary to the Cabinet in Saskatchewan: Evolution of the Role, 1944–2006." In *Searching for Leadership: Secretaries to Cabinet in Canada*, edited by Patrice Dutil, 161–84. Toronto: University of Toronto Press, 2008.
- "The Single-Tier Universality of Canadian Medicare." In *Universality and Social Policy in Canada*, edited by Daniel Béland, Gregory P. Marchildon, and Michael J. Prince, 49–62. Toronto: University of Toronto Press, 2019.
- "Social Democratic Solidarity and the Welfare State: Health Care and Single-Tier Universality in Sweden and Canada." *Canadian Bulletin of Medical History / Bulletin canadien d'histoire de la médecine* 38, no. 1 (2021): 177–96. https://doi.org/10.3138/cbmh.443-052020.
- "Thomas Clement Douglas." *Dictionary of Canadian Biography*, vol. 21 (2021): http://www.biographi.ca/en/bio/douglas_thomas_clement_21E.html.
- "War, Revolution and the Great Depression in the Global Wheat Trade, 1917–39." In *A Global History of Trade and Conflict since 1500*, edited by Lucia

Coppolaro and Francine McKenzie, 142–62. London: Palgrave Macmillan, 2013. http://dx.doi.org/10.1057/9781137326836_8.

Marchildon, Gregory P., and Carl Anderson, "Robert Weir: Forgotten Farmer-Minister in R.B. Bennett's Depression-Era Cabinet." In *Drought and Depression: History of the Prairie West*, vol. 6, edited by Gregory P. Marchildon, 261–90. Regina: University of Regina Press, 2018.

Marchildon, Gregory P., and Don Black, "Henry Black, the Conservative Party and the Politics of Relief." *Saskatchewan History* 58, no. 1 (2006): 4–17.

Marchildon, Gregory P., Suren Kulshreshtha, Elaine Wheaton, and David J. Sauchyn. "Drought and Institutional Adaptation in Alberta and Saskatchewan, 1914–1939." *Natural Hazards* 45, no. 3 (2008): 391–411. https://doi.org/10.1007/s11069-007-9175-5.

Marchildon, Gregory P., and Nicole C. O'Byrne. "Bennettcare to Medicare: The Morphing of Medicare Care Insurance in British Columbia." *Canadian Bulletin of Medical History / Bulletin canadien d'histoire de la médecine* 26, no. 2 (2009): 453–75. https://doi.org/10.3138/cbmh.26.2.453.

– "Last Province Aboard: New Brunswick and National Medicare." *Acadiensis* 42, no. 1 (2013): 150–67.

Marchildon, Gregory P., Jeremy Pittman, and David J. Sauchyn. "The Dry Belt and Changing Aridity in the Palliser Triangle, 1895–2000." In *Drought and Depression: History of the Prairie West*, vol. 6, edited by Gregory P. Marchildon, 13–25. Regina: University of Regina Press, 2018.

Marchildon, Gregory P., and Ken Rasmussen. "Edward Schreyer, 1969–1977." In *Manitoba Premiers of the 19th and 20th Centuries*, edited by Barry Ferguson and Robert Wardhaugh, 283–305. Regina: Canadian Plains Research Center, University of Regina, 2010.

Marchildon, Gregory P., and Klaartje Schrijvers. "Physician Resistance and the Forging of Public Health Care: A Comparative Analysis of Doctors' Strikes in Canada and Belgium in the 1960s." *Medical History* 55, no. 2 (2011): 203–22. https://doi.org/10.1017%2Fs0025727300005767.

Margoshes, Dave. *Tommy Douglas: Building the New Society*. Toronto: XYZ Publishing, 1999.

Marier, Patrik. "A Swedish Welfare State in North America? The Creation and Expansion of the Saskatchewan Welfare State, 1944–1982." *Journal of Policy History* 25, no. 4 (2013): 614–37. https://doi.org/10.1017/S0898030613000328.

Marsh, Leonard. *Report on Social Security for Canada*. 1943. Edited by Allan Moscovitch. Montreal and Kingston: McGill-Queen's University Press, 2017.

Martin, Paul. "A National Health Program for Canada." *Canadian Journal of Public Health / Revue canadienne de santé publique* 39, no. 6 (1948): 219–26.

Martin, Paul. *A Very Public Life*, vol. 2: *So Many Worlds*. Toronto: Deneau, 1985.

Matchim, John. "Towards a 'Total Welfare' Approach: Duncan Neuhauser, the International Grenfell Association, and Rural-Remote Health Care in

Labrador and Swedish Lapland, 1950s–1970s." *Acadiensis* 49, no. 1 (2020): 172–84.

McBain, Lesley. "Caring, Curing, and Socialization: The Ambiguities of Nursing in Northern Saskatchewan, 1944–57." In *Caregiving on the Periphery: Historical Perspective on Nursing and Midwifery in Canada*, edited by Myra Rutherdale, 278–308. Montreal and Kingston: McGill-Queen's University Press, 2010.

McCallum, Mary Jane, and Maureen Lux, "Medicare versus Medicine Chest: Court Challenges and Treaty Rights to Health Care." In *Medicare's Histories: Origins, Omissions, and Opportunities in Canada*, edited by Esyllt Jones, James Hanley, and Delia Gavrus, 103–30. Winnipeg: University of Manitoba Press, 2022.

McGrane, David. "Gender and Saskatchewan Social Democracy from 1900 to 2000." *Journal of Canadian Studies* 42, no. 1 (2008): 179–203. https://doi.org/10.3138/jcs.42.1.179.

McHenry, Dean E. *The Third Force in Canada*. Berkeley: University of California Press, 1950.

McKay, Ian. *Rebels, Reds, Radicals: Rethinking Canada's Left History*. Toronto: Between the Lines, 2005.

McKerracher, D.G. "Community Psychiatric Developments in Saskatchewan." *Canadian Medical Association Journal* 59, no. 6 (1948): 546–8.

– "A New Program in the Training and Employment of Ward Personnel." *American Journal of Psychiatry* 106, no. 4 (1949): 259–64.

McKillop, A.B. "Engaging History: Historians, Storytelling, and Self." In *Thinkers and Dreamers: Historical Essays in Honour of Carl Berger*, edited by Gerald Friesen and Douglas Owram, 33–52. Toronto: University of Toronto Press, 2011.

McLaren, Angus. *Our Own Master Race: Eugenics in Canada, 1885–1945*. Toronto: McClelland & Stewart, 1990.

McLaren, Robert I. "George Woodall Cadbury: The Fabian Catalyst in Saskatchewan's 'Good Public Administration.'" *Canadian Public Administration* 38, no. 3 (1995): 471–80.

– *The Saskatchewan Practice of Public Administration in Historical Perspective*. New York: Edwin Mellen, 1998.

McLeman, Robert A., Juliette Dupre, Lea Berrang Ford, James Ford, Konrad Gajewski, and Gregory Marchildon. "What We Learned from the Dust Bowl: Lessons in Science, Policy, and Adaptation." *Population and Environment* 35, no. 4 (2014): 417–40. https://doi.org/10.1007/s11111-013-0190-z.

McLeod, Thomas H., and Ian McLeod. *Tommy Douglas: The Road to Jerusalem*. Edmonton: Hurtig Publishers, 1987.

McManus, Curtis R. *Happyland: A History of the "Dirty Thirties" in Saskatchewan, 1914–1937*. Calgary: University of Calgary Press, 2011.

McNaught, Kenneth. *A Prophet in Politics: A Biography of J.S. Woodsworth*. Toronto: University of Toronto Press, 2001.

Mein Smith, Philippa. *A Concise History of New Zealand*. Cambridge: Cambridge University Press, 2012.

Miller, J.R. *Skyscrapers Hide the Heavens: A History of Native-Newcomer Relations in Canada*, 4th ed. Toronto: University of Toronto Press, 2018.

Mills, John A. "Lessons from the Periphery: Psychiatry in Saskatchewan, Canada, 1944–68." *History of Psychiatry* 18, no. 2 (2007): 179–201. https://doi.org/10.1177/0957154x06073011.

Mills, Sean. "When Democratic Socialists Discovered Democracy: The League for Social Reconstruction Confronts the Quebec Problem." *Canadian Historical Review* 86, no. 1 (2005): 1–17.

Mishler, Paul C. *Raising Reds: The Young Pioneers, Radical Summer Camps, and Communist Political Culture in the United States*. New York: Columbia University Press, 1999.

Mohamed, Ahmed Mohiddin. "Keep Our Doctors Committees in the Saskatchewan Medicare Controversy." MA thesis, University of Saskatchewan, 1963.

Moffat, Susan M., Lyndie A. Foster Page, and W. Murray Thompson, "New Zealand's School Dental Service over the Decades: Its Response to Social, Political, and Economic Influences, and the Effect on Oral Health Inequalities." *Frontiers in Public Health* 5, no. 177 (2017): 1–18. https://doi.org/10.3389/fpubh.2017.00177.

Mombourquette, Duane. "'An Inalienable Right:' The CCF and Rapid Health Care Reform, 1944–1948." *Saskatchewan History* 43, no. 3 (1991): 101–16.

Morgan, Kenneth O. *Keir Hardie: Radical and Socialist*. London: Weidenfeld & Nicolson, 1975.

– *Kenneth O. Morgan: My Histories*. Cardiff: University of Wales Press, 2015.

Morton, Desmond. *NDP: Social Democracy in Canada*. 2nd ed. Toronto: Samuel Stevens, 1977.

Mott, Frederick D. "Health Services for Migrant Farm Families." *American Journal of Public Health* 35, no. 4 (1945): 308–14.

– "A Pattern of Local Services in the Saskatchewan Health Program." *American Journal of Public Health and the Nation's Health* 39, no. 2 (1949): 216–20. https://doi.org/10.2105/ajph.39.2.216.

– "A Public Health Program for Rural Areas." *Public Health Reports* 61, no. 17 (1946): 589–98.

Mott, Frederick D., and M.I. Roemer. "A Federal Program of Public Health and Medical Services for Migratory Farm Workers." *Public Health Reports* 60, no. 9 (1945): 229–49.

– *Rural Health and Medical Care*. New York: McGraw-Hill, 1948.

Mott, Frederick D., Leonard S. Rosenfeld, Malcolm G. Taylor. "Health Services for the Aging in Saskatchewan." *Public Health Reports* 67, no. 2 (1952): 136–7.

Mountin, Joseph Walter, Elliott Harmon Pennell, and Vane M. Hoge. *Health Service Areas: Requirements for General Hospitals and Health Centers*. Washington, DC: Federal Security Agency, US Public Health Service, 1945.

Mullally, Sasha, and Gregory P. Marchildon. "Striking a Chord: Physician-Publics, Citizen-Audiences and a Half Century of Health-Care Debates in Canada." In *Communicating the History of Medicine: Perspectives on Audiences and Impact*, edited by Solveign Jülich and Sven Widmalm, 107–37. Manchester: Manchester University Press, 2020.

Mullally, Sasha, and David Wright. *Foreign Practices: Immigrant Doctors and the History of Canadian Medicare*. Montreal and Kingston: McGill-Queen's University Press, 2020.

Naylor, C. David. *Private Practice, Public Payment: Canadian Medicare and the Politics of Health Insurance, 1911–1966*. Montreal and Kingston: McGill-Queen's University Press, 1986.

Naylor, James. "'Pacifism or Anti-Imperialism?' The CCF Response to the Outbreak of World War II." *Journal of the Canadian Historical Association / Revue de la Société historique du Canada* 8, no. 1 (1997): 213–37. https://doi.org/10.7202/031123ar.

– "Socialism for a New Generation: CCF Youth in the Popular Front Era." *Canadian Historical Review* 94, no. 1 (2013): 55–79. https://doi.org/10.3138/chr.1164.

Neatby, Blair. "The Saskatchewan Relief Commission, 1931–34." In *Historical Essays on the Prairie Provinces*, edited by Donald Swainson, 267–88. Montreal and Kingston: McGill-Queen's University Press, 1978.

Neufeld, Michael J. *Von Braun: Dreamer of Space, Engineer of War*. New York: Alfred A. Knopf, 2007.

Newman, Peter C. *The Distemper of Our Times*. Toronto: McClelland & Stewart, 1978.

Noll, Mark A. "What Happened to Christian Canada?" *Church History* 75, no. 2 (2006): 245–73. https://doi.org/10.1017/S000964070011131X.

Norton, Dianne. "Woodrow S. Lloyd." In *Saskatchewan Premiers of the Twentieth Century*, edited by Gordon L. Barnhart, 213–36. Regina: Canadian Plains Research Center, University of Regina, 2004.

Osmond, Humphrey, and Abram Hoffer. "Schizophrenia: A New Approach." *Journal of Mental Science* 105, no. 440 (1959): 653–73. https://doi.org/10.1192/bjp.105.440.653.

Osmond, Humphrey, and John Smythies. "Schizophrenia: A New Approach." *Journal of Mental Science* 98, no. 411 (1952): 309–15. https://doi.org/10.1192/bjp.98.411.309.

Oussoren, Jan. *From Baptist Preacher to Social Gospel Politician: T.C. Douglas's Transition*. Vancouver: Vancouver School of Theology, Chalmers Institute, 1998.

Owen, Michael. "Toward a New Day: The Larger School Unit in Saskatchewan, 1935–1950." In *A History of Education in Saskatchewan: Selected Readings*, edited by Brian Noonan, Dianne Hallman, and Murray Scharf, 33–49. Regina: Canadian Plains Research Center, University of Regina, 2006.

Owram, Doug. *Born at the Right Time: A History of the Baby-Boom Generation*. Toronto: University of Toronto Press, 1996.

– *The Government Generation: Canadian Intellectuals and the State, 1900–1945*. Toronto: University of Toronto Press, 1986.

Paikin, Steven. *The Dark Side: The Personal Price of a Political Life*. Toronto: Viking Canada, 2003.

Pasolli, Lisa. "Bureaucratizing the Atlantic Revolution: The 'Saskatchewan Mafia' in the New Brunswick Civil Service, 1960–1970." *Acadiensis* 38, no. 1 (2009): 126–50.

Patrias, Carmella. "Socialists, Jews and the 1947 Saskatchewan Bill of Rights." *Canadian Historical Review* 87, no. 2 (2006): 265–92.

Petrou, Michael. *Renegades: Canadians in the Spanish Civil War*. Vancouver: UBC Press, 2008.

Pitsula, James M. *Keeping Canada British: The Ku Klux Klan in 1920s Saskatchewan*. Vancouver: UBC Press, 2013.

Priest, Allen G. "Diefenbaker's 'New Frontier': Masculinity, Modernity, and Canadian Electoral Politics, 1957–58." *Canadian Journal of History* 57, no. 2 (2022): 169–90. https://doi.org/10.3138/cjh-57-2-2021-0103.

Quiring, Brett. "Carlyle King." In *Saskatchewan Politicians: Lives Past and Present*, edited by Brett Quiring, 119–20. Regina: Canadian Plains Research Center, University of Regina, 2004.

– "John Michael Uhrich." In *Saskatchewan Politicians: Lives Past and Present*, edited by Brett Quiring, 135–6. Regina: Canadian Plains Research Center, University of Regina, 2004.

– "Olaf Alexander Turnbull." In *Saskatchewan Politicians: Lives Past and Present*, edited by Brett Quiring, 234–5. Regina: Canadian Plains Research Center, University of Regina, 2004.

Quiring, David M. *CCF Colonialism in Northern Saskatchewan: Battling Parish Priests, Bootleggers, and Fur Sharks*. Vancouver: UBC Press, 2004.

Rachlis, Michael, Robert G. Evans, Patrick Lewis, and Morris L. Barrer, *Revitalizing Medicare: Shared Problems, Public Solutions*. Toronto: Tommy Douglas Research Institute, 2001. https://www.michaelrachlis.com/2001/01/29/revitalizing-medicare-shared-problems-public-solutions/.

Rands, Stan. "The CCF in Saskatchewan." In *Western Canadian Politics: The Radical Tradition*, edited by D.C. Kerr, 58–61. Edmonton: NeWest Institute for Western Canadian Studies, 1981.

Rands, Stan. *Privilege and Policy: The History of Community Clinics in Canada*, edited by Gregory P. Marchildon and Catherine Leviten-Reid. Regina: Canadian Plains Research Centre, University of Regina, 2012.

Rasmussen, Ken, and Gregory P. Marchildon. "Saskatchewan's Executive Decision-Making Style: The Centrality of Planning." In *Executive Styles in Canada: Cabinet Structures and Leadership Practices in Canadian Government*, edited by Luc Bernier, Keith Brownsey, and Michael Howlett, 184–207. Toronto: University of Toronto Press, 2005.

Reed, W.C.N. "Methods Used in the Province of Saskatchewan to Provide Vital-Statistics Information to Medical Officers of Health." *Canadian Journal of Public Health / Revue canadienne de santé publique* 42, no. 3 (1951): 101–2.

Reid, Escott. "The Saskatchewan Liberal Machine before 1929." In *Politics in Saskatchewan*, edited by Norman Ward and Duff Spafford, 93–104. Toronto: Longmans Canada, 1968.

Rempel, Richard A. *Research and Reform: W.P. Thompson at the University of Saskatchewan*. Montreal and Kingston: McGill-Queen's University Press, 2013.

Riall, Lucy. "The Shallow End of History? The Substance and Future of Political Biography." *Journal of Interdisciplinary History* 40, no. 3 (2010): 375–97. https://doi.org/10.1162/jinh.2010.40.3.375.

Richards, John, and Larry Pratt. *Prairie Capitalism: Power and Influence in the New West*. Toronto: McClelland & Stewart, 1979.

Roberts, Jane. *Losing Political Office*. London: Palgrave Macmillan, 2017.

Roemer, Milton I. *National Health Systems of the World*, vol.1: *The Countries*. New York: Oxford University Press, 1991.

– *National Health Systems of the World*, vol. 2: *The Issues*. New York: Oxford University Press, 1993.

– "The Saskatchewan Air Ambulance Service: Medical and Public Health Aspects." *Canadian Medical Association Journal* 75, no. 6 (1956): 529–33.

– "Socialized Health Services in Saskatchewan." *Social Research* 25, no. 1 (1958): 87–101.

Romanow, Roy J. "My Experience in the Medicare Battle and the Woods Commission." *Canadian Bulletin of Medical History / Bulletin canadien d'histoire de la médecine* 26, no. 2 (2009): 538–41. https://doi.org/10.3138/cbmh.26.2.538.

Rorem, C. Rufus. *The "Municipal Doctor" System in Rural Saskatchewan*. Chicago: University of Chicago Press, 1931.

Rosenoff, Theodore. "The Propensity to Reform: The United States, Australia, New Zealand, and Canada Compared." *The Historian* 72, no. 1 (2010): 38–66. https://doi.org/10.1111/j.1540-6563.2009.00256.x.

Rotberg, Robert I. "Biography and Historiography: Mutual Evidentiary and Interdisciplinary Considerations." *Journal of Interdisciplinary History* 40, no. 3 (2010): 305–20. https://doi.org/10.1162/jinh.2010.40.3.375.

Roth, F. Burns. "The Health Officer and Hospital Regionalization." *Canadian Journal of Public Health / Revue canadienne de santé publique* 43, no. 11 (1952): 467–73.

Roth, F. Burns, and R.D. Defries. "The Saskatchewan Department of Public Health." *Canadian Journal of Public Health / Revue canadienne de santé publique* 49, no. 7 (1958): 276–85.

Roth, F. Burns, Glyn W. Myers, Frederick D. Mott, and Leonard S. Rosenfeld. "The Saskatchewan Experience in Payment for Hospital Care." *American Journal of Public Health and the Nation's Health* 43, no. 6 (1953): 752–6. https://doi.org/10.2105%2Fajph.43.6_pt_1.752.

Saltman, Richard B., and Hans F.W. Dubois. "The Historical and Social Base of Social Health Insurance Systems." In *Social Health Insurance Systems in Western Europe*, edited by Richard B. Saltman, Reinhard Busse, and Josep Figueras, 21–32. Maidenhead, UK: World Health Organization on behalf of the European Observatory on Health Systems and Policies, 2004.

Samson, Amy. "Eugenics in the Community: Gendered Professions and Eugenic Sterilization in Alberta, 1928–1972." *Canadian Bulletin of Medical History / Bulletin canadien d'histoire de la médecine* 31, no. 1 (2014): 143–63. https://doi.org/10.3138/cbmh.31.1.143.

Sandwell, Ruth W. "People, Place and Power: Rural Electrification in Canada, 1890–1950." In *Transforming the Countryside: The Electrification of Rural Britain*, edited by Paul Brassley, Jeremy Burchardt, and Karen Sayer, 178–204. London: Routledge, 2016.

Sangster, Joan. *Dreams of Equality: Women on the Canadian Left, 1920–1950*. Toronto: McClelland & Stewart, 1989.

– "The Role of Women in the Early CCF, 1933–1940." In *Beyond the Vote: Canadian Women and Politics*, edited by Linda Kealey and Joan Sangster, 118–138. Toronto: University of Toronto Press, 1989.

Sarra-Bournet, Marcel. "Maurice Le Noblet Duplessis." *Dictionary of Canadian Biography*, vol. 18. http://www.biographi.ca/en/bio/duplessis_maurice_le_noblet_18E.html.

Scott, F.R. *Leaving the Shade of the Middle Ground: The Poetry of F.R. Scott*, selected by Laura Moss. Waterloo, ON: Wilfrid Laurier University Press, 2011.

Scott, F.R., Leonard Marsh, Graham Spry, J. King Gordon, Eugene Forsey, and J.F. Parkinson, "Introduction." In League for Social Reconstruction, *Social Planning for Canada*, edited by Michael Bliss, vi–xxiv. 1935; Toronto: University of Toronto Press, 1975.

Shackleton, Doris French. *Tommy Douglas: A Biography*. Toronto: McClelland & Stewart, 1975.

Shapiro, Martin F. "Medical Aid Provided by American, Canadian and British Nationals to the Spanish Republic during the Civil War, 1936–1939." *International Journal of Health Services* 13, no. 3 (1983): 443–58. https://doi.org/10.2190/66uf-txre-t50h-ay1b.

Shevell, Michael. "A Canadian Paradox: Tommy Douglas and Eugenics." *Canadian Journal of Neurological Sciences* 39, no. 1 (2012): 35–9. https://doi.org/10.1017/s0317167100012658.
- "Tommy Douglas, the Young Eugenicist." *National Post*, 24 March 2012. https://nationalpost.com/opinion/michael-shevell-tommy-douglas-the-young-eugenicist
Sigerist, Henry E. "From Bismarck to Beveridge: Developments and Trends in Social Security Legislation." *Bulletin of the History of Medicine* 13, no. 4 (1943): 365–88.
- *Civilization and Disease*. 1943; Ithaca, NY: Cornell University Press, 2018.
- *Henry E. Sigerist: Autobiographical Writings*. Edited by Nora Beeson. Montreal and Kingston: McGill-Queen's University Press, 1966.
- "Medical Care for All the People." *Canadian Journal of Public Health* 35, no. 7 (1944): 263–7.
- *Socialized Medicine in the Soviet Union*. London: Victor Gollancz, 1937.
- "Socialized Medicine." *Yale Review* (1938): 463–81. Reprinted in *Henry E. Sigerist on the Sociology of Medicine*, edited by Milton I. Roemer, 39–53. New York: MD Publications, 1960.
- "Trends Towards Socialized Medicine." In *Henry E. Sigerist on the Sociology of Medicine*, edited by Milton I. Roemer, 1934; New York: MD Publications, 1960.
- "Twenty-Five Years of Health Work in the Soviet Union." *American Review of Soviet Medicine* 1, no. 1 (1943): 67–78.
Simeon, Richard. *Federal-Provincial Diplomacy: The Making of Recent Policy in Canada*. 1972. Toronto: University of Toronto Press, 2006.
Simpson, Jeffrey. *Chronic Condition: Why Canada's Health-Care System Needs to Be Dragged into the 21st Century*. Toronto: Penguin Canada, 2013.
- "Saskatchewan and the Difficult Birth of Medicare." *Queen's Quarterly* 119, no. 2 (2012): 270–83.
Sinclair, Peter R. "The Saskatchewan CCF: Ascent to Power and the Decline of Socialism." *Canadian Historical Review* 54, no. 4 (1973): 419–33.
Skovron, Wayne Mark. "A People's Commission? High Modernism, Direct Democracy, and the Royal Commission on Agriculture and Rural Life, 1952–1957." MA thesis, Simon Fraser University, 2011.
Smiley, Donald V. "Local Autonomy and Central Administrative Control in Saskatchewan." *Canadian Journal of Economics and Political Science / Revue canadienne d'économique et de science politique* 26, no. 2 (1960): 299–313.
Smith, Cameron. *Unfinished Journey: The Lewis Family*. Toronto: Summerhill Press, 1989.
Smith, David E. "James G. Gardiner." In *Saskatchewan Premiers of the Twentieth Century*, edited by Gordon L. Barnhart, 89–108. Regina: Canadian Plains Research Center, University of Regina, 2004.

– *Prairie Liberalism: The Liberal Party in Saskatchewan, 1905–71.* Toronto: University of Toronto Press, 1975.
Smith, David James. "Intellectual Activist: Graham Spry, a Biography." PhD diss., York University, 2002.
Smith, Denis. *Rogue Tory: The Life and Legend of John G. Diefenbaker.* Toronto: McFarland, Walter and Ross, 1995.
Smith, Eric R. *American Relief Aid and the Spanish Civil War.* Columbia: University of Missouri Press, 2013.
Spencer, Dick. *Singing the Blues: The Conservatives in Saskatchewan.* Regina: Canadian Plains Research Center, University of Regina, 2007.
Spry, Graham. *Passion and Conviction: The Letters of Graham Spry.* Edited by Rose Potvin. Regina: Canadian Plains Research Center, University of Regina, 1992.
Stebner, Eleanor J. "The Education of Stanley Howard Knowles." *Manitoba History*, no. 36 (1998): 41–51.
Stern, Ludmila. *Western Intellectuals and the Soviet Union, 1920–40: From Red Square to the Left Bank.* London: Routledge, 2007.
Stewart, Roderick, and Jesús Majada. *Bethune in Spain.* Montreal and Kingston: McGill-Queen's University Press, 2014.
Stewart, Walter. *The Life and Political Times of Tommy Douglas.* Toronto: McArthur & Company, 2003.
– *M.J.: The Life and Times of M.J. Coldwell.* Toronto: Stoddard, 2000.
Stone, Charles M., and F. Joan Garnett, *Brandon College: A History, 1899–1967.* Brandon, MB: Brandon University, 1969.
Struthers, James. *No Fault of Their Own: Unemployment and the Canadian Welfare State, 1914–1941.* Toronto: University of Toronto Press, 1983.
Stursberg, Peter. *Diefenbaker: Leadership Lost, 1962–67.* Toronto: University of Toronto Press, 1976.
Sullivan, Patrick. "Dr. Efstathios (Staff) Barootes." *CMAJ* 163, no. 6 (2000): 795.
Taylor, Georgina. "Review Essay: Gender and the History of the Left, 1992." *Saskatchewan History* 44, no. 1 (1992): 31–4.
Taylor, Lord (Stephen). "Saskatchewan Adventure: A Personal Record. Part I: Background to the Story." *Canadian Medical Association Journal* 110, no. 6 (1974): 720–8.
– "Saskatchewan Adventure: A Personal Record. Part II: Making Contact." *Canadian Medical Association Journal* 110, no. 7 (1974): 829–36.
– "Saskatchewan Adventure: A Personal Record. Part III: Drafting the Saskatoon Agreement." *Canadian Medical Association Journal* 110, no. 8 (1974): 978–83.
Taylor, Malcolm G. "Government Planning: The Federal-Provincial Health Survey Reports." *Canadian Journal of Economics and Political Science / Revue canadienne d'économique et de science politique* 19, no. 4 (1953): 501–10. https://doi.org/10.2307/138297.

- "Health Insurance: The Roller-Coaster in Federal-Provincial Relations." In *Federalism and Political Community: Essays in Honour of Donald Smiley*, edited by David P. Shugarman and Reginald Whitaker, 73–92. Peterborough, ON: Broadview Press, 1989.
- *Health Insurance and Canadian Public Policy: The Seven Decisions That Created the Canadian Health Insurance System and Its Outcomes*, 2nd ed. Montreal and Kingston: McGill-Queen's University Press, 2009.
- "The Saskatchewan Hospital Services Plan: A Study in Compulsory Health Insurance." PhD diss., University of California at Berkeley, 1949.
- "Social Assistance Medical Care Programs in Canada." *American Journal of Public Health* 44, no. 6 (1954): 750–9.
- "Some Administrative Aspects of the Integration of Health Services." *Canadian Journal of Public Health / Revue canadienne de santé publique* 42, no. 8 (1951): 329–35.
Tetley, William. *The October Crisis, 1970: An Insider's View*. Montreal and Kingston: McGill-Queen's University Press, 1970.
Thompson, Stephen L., and J. Warren Salmon. "Strike by Physicians: A Historical Perspective Toward an Ethical Evaluation." *International Journal of Health Services* 36, no. 2 (2006): 331–54.
Thomson, William. "Press Coverage of the Medicare Dispute in Saskatchewan: II." *Queen's Quarterly* 70, no. 3 (1963): 362–71.
Thorpe, Andrew. *A History of the British Labour Party*. Basingstoke, UK: Palgrave Macmillan, 2008.
Tipliski, Veryl Margaret. "Parting at the Crossroads: The Emergence of Education for Psychiatric Nursing in Three Canadian Provinces, 1909–1955." *Canadian Bulletin of Medical History / Bulletin canadien d'histoire de la médecine* 21, no. 2 (2004): 253–79. https://doi.org/10.3138/cbmh.21.2.253.
Tollefson, E.A *Bitter Medicine: The Saskatchewan Medicare Feud*. Saskatoon: Modern Press, 1964.
- "The Medicare Dispute." In *Politics in Saskatchewan*, edited by Norman Ward and Duff Spafford, 238–79. Toronto: Longmans Canada, 1968.
Traynor, Cam. "Manning against Medicare." *Alberta History* 43 (1995): 7–19.
Trofimenkoff, Susan Mann. *Stanley Knowles: The Man from Winnipeg North Centre*. Saskatoon: Western Producer Prairie Books, 1982.
Tuohy, Carolyn. *The Dynamics of Change in the Health Care Arena in the United States, Britain, and Canada*. New York: Oxford University Press, 1999.
- "Icon and Taboo: Single-Payer Politics in Canada and the US." *Journal of International and Comparative Social Policy* 35, no. 1 (2019): 5–24. https://doi.org/10.1080/21699763.2018.1550010.
- *Remaking Policy: Scale, Pace and Political Strategy in Health Care Reform*. Toronto: University of Toronto Press, 2018.
Turnbull, A. Douglas. "Memoir: Early Years of Hospital Insurance in British Columbia." *BC Studies*, no. 76 (1987/88): 58–81.

Tyre, Robert. *Douglas in Saskatchewan: The Story of a Socialist Experiment*. Vancouver: Mitchell Press, 1962.
Underhill, Frank H. *In Search of Canadian Liberalism*. Toronto: Macmillan of Canada, 1960.
Vaughn, Frederick. *Aggressive in Pursuit: The Life of Justice Emmett Hall*. Toronto: University of Toronto Press for the Osgoode Society for Canadian Legal History, 2004.
Wagner, Jonathan F. "Heim Ins Reich: The Story of Loon River's Nazis." *Saskatchewan History* 24, no. 2 (1976): 41-50.
Waiser, Bill. *All Hell Can't Stop Us: The On-to-Ottawa Trek and Regina Riot*. Calgary: Fifth House, 2003.
– *Saskatchewan: A New History*. Calgary: Fifth House, 2005.
– "Wiping Out the Stain: The On-to-Ottawa Trek, the Regina Riot, and the Search for Answers." In *Canadian State Trials*, vol. 4: *Security, Dissent, and the Limits of Toleration in War and Peace, 1914–1939*, edited by Barry Wright, Eric Tucker, and Susan Binnie, 402–35. Toronto: University of Toronto Press for the Osgoode Society for Canadian Legal History, 2015.
Ward, Norman. "The Politics of Patronage: James Gardiner and Federal Appointments in the West, 1935–57." *Canadian Historical Review* 58, no. 3 (1977): 294–10. https://doi.org/10.3138/CHR-058-03-03.
Ward, Norman, and David E. Smith. *Jimmy Gardiner: Relentless Liberal*. Toronto: University of Toronto Press, 1990.
Wardhaugh, Robert A. *Mackenzie King and the Prairie West*. Toronto: University of Toronto Press, 2000.
Wardhaugh, Robert A., and Barry Ferguson. *The Rowell-Sirois Commission and the Remaking of Canadian Federalism*. Vancouver: UBC Press, 2021.
Webster, Charles. *The National Health Service: A Political History*. Oxford: Oxford University Press, 2002.
Weeks, Lewis E. *Milton I. Roemer – In First Person: An Oral History*. Chicago: American Hospital Association, 1984. https://www.aha.org/system/files/media/file/2022/03/Milton-L-Roemer.pdf.
Weinberg, Robert. "The Pogrom of 1905 in Odessa: A Case Study." In *Pogroms: Anti-Jewish Violence in Modern Russian History*, edited by John D. Klier and Shlomo Lambroza, 248–89. Cambridge: Cambridge University Press, 1992.
Welton, Michael R. "Conflicting Visions, Divergent Strategies: Watson Thomson and the Cold War Politics of Adult Education in Saskatchewan, 1944–6." *Labour/Le Travail* 18 (1986): 111–38.
– "'To Be and Build the Glorious World': The Educational Thought and Practice of Watson Thomson, 1899–1946." PhD diss., University of British Columbia, 1983.

Wentzell, Tyler. "Canada's *Foreign Enlistment Act* and the Spanish Civil War." *Labour/Le Travail* 90 (2017): 213–46.
Whatley, Christopher A. *The Industrial Revolution in Scotland*. Cambridge: Cambridge University Press, 1997.
Whelan, Ed, and Pemrose Whelan. *Run It by Jack: Tommy Douglas' First Attorney General, J.W. Corman*. Regina: Whelan Publications, 2002.
White, Clinton O. *Power for a Province: A History of Saskatchewan Power*. Regina: Canadian Plains Research Center, University of Regina, 1976.
Whitehorn, Alan. *Canadian Socialism: Essays on the CCF-NDP*. Toronto: Oxford University Press, 1991.
Williams, A. Paul. "In Tribute to Malcolm Gordon Taylor, 1915–1994." *Health and Canadian Society / Santé et société canadienne* 3, nos. 1–2 (1995): 9–12.
Willoughby, William R. "Canadian Politics." *Political Science Quarterly* 66, no. 1 (1951): 104–19. https://doi.org/10.2307/2145387.
Wilson, David. "Social Security and Health Benefits in New Zealand." *Public Affairs* 9, no. 3 (1946): 172–7.
Winkel, James D. "Servant of the North: A History of Saskatchewan Government Airways." MA thesis, University of Regina, 2006.
Wiseman, Nelson. "Ethnicity, Religion, and Socialism in Canada: The Twenties through the War." *Canadian Ethnic Studies* 47, no. 2 (2015): 1–19. https://doi.org/10.1353/ces.2015.0015.
– *Social Democracy in Manitoba: A History of the CCF/NDP*. Winnipeg: University of Manitoba Press, 1983.
Wiseman, Nelson, and Benjamin Isitt. "Social Democracy in Twentieth Century Canada: An Interpretive Framework." *Canadian Journal of Political Science* 40, no. 3 (2007): 567–89.
Woodsworth, J.S. *Strangers within Our Gates: Or, Coming Canadians*. Toronto: Missionary Society of the Methodist Church, Canada, 1909.
Wolfson, Steve. "The Use of Paraprofessionals: The Saskatchewan Dental Plan." *Policy Innovation in the Saskatchewan Public Service, 1971–82*, edited by Eleanor Glor, 126–39. Toronto: Captus Press, 1997.
Wright, David, Sasha Mullally, and Mary Colleen Cordukes, "'Worse than Being Married': The Exodus of British Doctors from the National Health Service to Canada, c. 1955–75." *Journal of the History of Medicine and Allied Sciences* 65, no. 4 (2010): 546–75. https://doi.org/10.1093/jhmas/jrq013.
Wright, Robert. *Trudeaumania: The Rise to Power of Pierre Elliott Trudeau*. Toronto: HarperCollins Publishers, 2016.
Yasinowski, Dwayne. "Hazen Robert Argue." In *Saskatchewan Politicians: Lives Past and Present*, edited by Brett Quiring, 6–7. Regina: Canadian Plains Research Center, University of Regina, 2004.

- "Thomas J. Bentley." In *Saskatchewan Politicians: Lives Past and Present*, edited by Brett Quiring, 18–19. Regina: Canadian Plains Research Center, University of Regina, 2004.
Young, T. Kue. "Lay-Professional Conflict in a Canadian Community Health Center: A Case Report." *Medical Care* 13, no. 11 (1975): 897–904. https://doi.org/10.1097/00005650-197511000-00002.
Young, Walter D. *The Anatomy of a Party: The National CCF, 1932–1961*. Toronto: University of Toronto Press, 1969.

# Index

Abel-Smith, Brian, 602n1
Aberhart, William, 67–70, 233–4
Abott, Doug, 179–80
Acker, Dr. Murray S., 182, 271, 551n31, 564n81
Advisory Planning Committee on Medical Care. *See* Thompson Committee
air ambulance services. *See* Saskatchewan Air Ambulance Service
Alberta, 108, 126, 208, 210, 417, 421–2, 429, 433–4; Alberta hospital insurance plan, 232–7, 246, 248, 250, 255–7, 263–5, 268, 492–3; CCF-NDP in, 66–8, 324; eugenics and policy of sterilization, 44, 190, 554n66; impact of Great Depression in, 34–5, 120, 125; Manningcare (medical care insurance plan), 413–14, 419, 422, 433, 439–41, 444, 460, 476
All Peoples' Mission, 26
American Medical Association (AMA), 18, 98, 100, 297, 361, 368; Operation Coffee Cup, 361
American Public Health Association, 106
American Soviet Medical Society, 160

Anderson, Dr. J.F.C. (Jack), 114–16, 296, 303
Anderson, J.T.M. (James), 40, 49
Anglican Church, 220, 222, 376
Anti-Tuberculosis League, 22
Argue, Eugenia, 321–2
Argue, Hazen, 309–10, 344, 346–7, 365, 370, 372, 585n21, 599n182; background, 316; contesting T.C. Douglas for NDP leadership, 315–19, 321–2, 587n56; defection from the NDP, 347–50, 410, 593n66, 594n77, 599n181
Argus Corporation, 412
Assiniboia, SK, 349, 373, 594n77
Atlee, Clement, 130
Australia, 21, 218, 541n12

Baltimore, MD, 93, 151
Baltzan, Dr. David, 407–10, 611n28; dissenting view in Hall Commission report, 427, 617n127
Baptist Church, 7–8, 25, 30–4, 55–6, 74; Baptist preachers (other than T.C.), 6, 28, 70; Baptist Union of Scotland, 31; Beulah Baptist Church, Winnipeg, 31; Calvary Baptist Church (Weyburn), 21, 34, 37–9; progressives versus

fundamentalists in, 31–2; Western Canadian Baptist Union, 62
Barootes, Dr. Efstathios W. (Staff), 294–6, 303, 356, 580n75, 582n100
Batten, Mary, 368
Beechwood Cemetery. *See* Ottawa
Bégin, Monique, 482, 484–6, 635n137, 635n142; and NDP criticism, 486
Benjamin, Leslie Gordon (Les), 459
Bennett, Richard Bedford (R.B.), 58, 60–1, 63–4, 72
Bennett, W.A.C., 231, 245, 247, 423, 432, 459
Bennett buggy, 63, 513n39
Bennettcare. *See* British Columbia
Benson, Jacob (Jake), 70
Bentley, Thomas J. (Tom), 188, 198–9, 199, 205–7, 225–7, 254–5, 268, 272, 340, 558n8
Berton, Pierre, 459, 626n19
Bevan, Aneurin, 146
Beveridge, Sir William, 79–80, 101
Beveridge Report, 78–80, 95, 127–8, 146
Bienfait, SK, 38–9
Biggar, SK, 69
biography, nature of, 5–6
Birch Hills, SK, 267, 340, 575n2
Bismarck, Otto von, 146, 333, 526n53
Black Panthers, 467–9. *See also* Shirley Douglas
Blaikie, William Alexander (Bill), 485–6
Blakeney, Allan E., 228, 298, 312, 331, 338, 341, 354, 368–9, 372, 475, 485, 498n6, 583n115, 591n29
block transfers. *See* Established Programs Financing
blood tests. *See* diagnostic services
blood transfusion, 285
Blue Cross (insurance carrier), 232, 235, 248–9
Blum, Léon, 74
Bourassa, Robert, 472–3

Bracken, John, 126
Brando, Marlon, 467
Brandon College, 31–4, 37, 42, 55, 90, 507n114
Brandon, MB, 31–4
Britain. *See* United Kingdom
British Columbia, 58, 134, 138, 489–90; Bennettcare and medical care insurance, 298, 421–3, 432, 440–1, 459, 475; burden of relief spending during Great Depression, 125; *Cambie Surgeries* case, 489–90; CCF-NDP in, 129, 134, 168, 178, 230–1, 371–2, 376, 410, 414, 446, 463; hospital insurance, 140, 168, 230–1, 233, 239–40, 246–7, 250–1, 254, 263–5, 492; provincial health survey, 187
British Medical Association, 14, 384
Britnell, George, 137
Broadbent, John Edward (Ed), 465–6, 474, 482, 486, 635n133
Brockelbank, John H., 81, 88–9, 337, 457
Brownstone, Meyer, 271, 274–7, 578n44
Buffalo Narrows, SK, 223
Burnaby, BC, 376, 410–12, 436, 455, 461, 463–4
Burton, Richard, 467
Bryden, Penny, 417–18
Burak, William J., 121

Cadbury, George, 137–8, 164, 173, 175, 178, 243, 275, 384–5, 395, 399, 531n129
Calgary, AB, 47
*Cambie Surgeries* case. *See* British Columbia
Cameron, Colin, 464, 629n52
Cameron, G.D.W. (Donald), 180
Camp, Dalton, 463
Campbell, Douglas, 243, 245

Index 675

Canada, Government of:
– Department of National Defence, 58
– Department of National Health and Welfare, 75, 128, 177, 181, 222, 242, 252, 265, 416, 438, 478, 482; Indian Health Services (division), 222
– Department of Pensions and National Health, 79
Canada Health Act, 4, 455–6
Canada Pension Plan, 415–20, 426, 429, 438; preceding medical care plan, 417
Canadian Broadcasting Corporations (CBC), 3, 104, 285, 445, 461
Canadian Charter of Rights and Freedoms, 490
Canadian Club, 80, 104
Canadian Expeditionary Force, 28
Canadian Federation of Agriculture, 131
Canadian Federation of Nurses Unions, 482
Canadian Health Coalition, 482–3
Canadian Labour Congress (CLC), 131, 308–9, 482
Canadian League Against War and Fascism, 53, 73, 511n161
Canadian Manufacturers' Association, 452
Canadian Medical Association (CMA), 94, 325, 361, 365, 490, 499n9, 597n133; *Canadian Medical Association Journal*, 394, 484; Hall Commission and, 364, 405, 407–8, 410, 419, 426–7; hospital insurance preferences, 233, 248, 252, 268, 281; Medical Care Act (1966), 441, 446, 448, 451–2; provincial health surveys, 187–9; Saskatchewan doctors' strike, role in, 384, 388–9, 392–3; T.C.'s criticism of, 368; universal medical care insurance, opposition to, 14–15, 18, 281, 297, 302, 379, 388, 410
Canadian Mental Health Association (CMHA), 189, 198; National Committee for Mental Hygiene (predecessor), 189; Saskatchewan Division, 196–201, 339
Canadian Press, 416
Canadian Public Health Association, 95
Canadian Sickness Survey Report (Government of Canada, 1951), 20, 279
cancer, treatment and control, 81, 93, 104, 181, 183, 220, 237, 281, 491; free cancer treatment in Saskatchewan, 111, 143, 145, 168, 229, 294, 327, 335, 389, 491
Canora, SK, 119
Caouette, Réal, 461
Carberry, MB, 33
Caribbean, 156
Carlyle Lake, SK, 87
Caro, Robert, 208
Carron Company, Scotland, 24–5
Casgrain, Thérèse, 416
Cassidy, Harry, 177–8
Castonguay, Claude, 484
Catholics. *See* Roman Catholic Church
CCF-NDP, 7, 11, 235, 263
– national: 56, 58–80, 129–32, 184–6, 237–41, 248, 258–63; *Canada Through C.C.F. Glasses* (1934), 66; efforts to draft T.C. Douglas as national leader, 309–11; formation of CCF, 40–2, 45–6; leftist CCF activists, 13, 48, 82, 94, 152, 172, 229, 235, 272–4, 288, 293, 325, 329, 378, 381, 399, 458; merger discussion between

676   Index

NDP and Liberals (1964), 415–16; NDP's founding convention (1961), 319–24; National Health Plan for Canada, 319–20, 323–4; New Party movement, 306–12, 324; ongoing hostility to, 345–6, 348; position on war, 75; relationship with communists, 119; Winnipeg Declaration, 307, 319, 470
– provincial. *See* individual provinces
cerebral palsy, 183
chambers of commerce (Canada), 493
Chegwin, A.E., 225–8, 563n69, 564n81
Cherniak, Fana (née Goldwin), 103
Cherniak, Joseph Alter, 103
Cherniak, Saul, 103
Chicago, IL, 37–8
chief medical officer of health. *See* physicians
children's dental care, 9, 204, 224–228, 413; state of oral health in Saskatchewan, 225
Christianity, 30, 33, 56
Churchill, Winston, 286
Citizen's Defence Movement, 62
Citizens' Emergency Committee (CEC), 59–60
Citizen's Legal Defence Committee, 62
Clapp, Edgar, 161–2
Clark, Joe, 482
Clarkson, Dr. J. Graham, 395–7, 430, 618n146
Claxton, Brooke, 128, 136, 139–40, 142, 168, 177
Clement, Andrew, 28
Cliche, Robert, 463–4
Cold War, 96
Coldwell, M.J., 40–2, 46, 50–4, 59–60, 62, 69–70, 72–3, 75–7, 80–1, 88, 119, 130–1, 184–5, 299, 306, 316, 336, 464, 488, 507n110; *Left Turn Canada*, 129–30, 520n148
College of Dental Surgeons of Saskatchewan, 187, 227
College of Physicians and Surgeons of Saskatchewan (CPS), 94, 101, 104, 368; campaign in 1960 Saskatchewan election, 277, 297–300; doctors' strike, 383–4, 388–9, 391, 398–400, 409 (*see also* Saskatchewan doctors' strike; Saskatoon Agreement); dual role as regulatory and political entity, 94, 297, 302, 499n9; fee-for-service versus salary payment, 115–16, 154, 214, 281–2; health regions, opposition to, 114, 122–3; insurance carriers (*see* Group Medical Services; Medical Services Incorporated); opposition to Saskatchewan Medical Care Insurance Plan, 12–18, 269–73, 282, 287–98, 301–5, 313–15, 325–7, 329, 331, 334, 339–40, 350–2, 354–6, 361–2, 368, 374–80; provincial health survey, 186–9; relationship with HSPC staff, 111, 115–17, 122–3, 157–8; relationship with ministers of health, 111–16, 206; and Saskatchewan Hospital Services Plan, 145–6, 149, 152–3, 162
Columbia University, 80, 378; Presbyterian–Columbia Medical Center, 156
Commission on the Future of Health Care in Canada, vii–viii
Commonwealth Fund, 197
Communist Party of Canada (CPC), 48, 53–4, 74, 119, 131, 468, 516n89
Communist Party, Soviet Union, 48, 52, 74

community clinics (Saskatchewan), 381–3; Community Health Services Association (provincial umbrella), 382; influence of US-based non-profit group practices, 382; Prince Albert community clinic, 383; reasons established and objectives, 381; Regina community clinic, 459; Saskatoon community clinic, 383
Community Health Association (Detroit, MI), 389
comprehensive health coverage. *See* universal health coverage
Connel, Dr. J.L., 101
Connor, J.T.H. (Jim), 159
Conservative Party of Canada, 64
Conservative Party of Saskatchewan, 49
constitution. *See* federalism
Cooper, Marjorie, 13–14, 282, 320–1, 523n19
Co-operative Commonwealth Federation (CCF). *See* CCF-NDP
Co-operative Commonwealth Youth Movement (CCYM), 53, 59, 62, 73, 359
cooperatives, 28, 40, 46, 91, 381; cooperative health clinics, 381, 399, 483 (*see also* community clinics); cooperative health insurance carriers, 459; cooperative movement, 204, 221, 291; relationship with CCF-NDP, 46, 91, 113, 204–5, 221, 307
Corman, John (Jack), 88, 92, 522n13
cottage hospital plan. *See* Newfoundland
Cripps, Stafford, 285
Crombie, David, 482
Cronkite, Frederick, 135, 137
Cumberland House, SK, 223

Cumming, John and Elaine, 197; *Closed Ranks: An Experiment in Mental Health Education* (1957), 197

Dalgleish, Dr. Harold, 339, 350–1, 357, 377, 389–94
Dauphin, MB, 359
Davey, Keith, 412, 415–16, 612n45
Davies, Dr. Alan, 302
Davies, William G. (Bill), 341, 350–2, 354, 410
Day, Dr. Brian, 490
DeMolay, Order of, 31
dental nurses, 224, 226–8,
dental programs. *See* children's dental care
dental therapists. *See* dental nurses
dentists, 21, 66, 81–2, 108, 110, 131, 201, 215, 224–8, 460
deterrent fees. *See* Medicare; user charges
Deutscher Bund Canada, 74
diagnostic services, 8, 66, 79, 94, 99, 106, 110–11, 129, 145, 147, 150, 166, 183, 195, 213–14, 217, 238, 253, 255–7, 263, 274, 382, 491, 494; blood tests, 136, 161; as first step in national health insurance, 253; laboratory services, 66, 94, 106, 136, 253; X-ray (radiological services), 129, 136, 161, 166, 267, 378
*Dictionary of Canadian Biography*, 6
Diefenbaker, John G., 35, 306, 348–9, 358, 402–5, 414–15, 434–5, 437, 441, 461, 463, 466, 479, 523n25; election of 1962, 345, 364–5, 367, 371–2; election sweep of 1958, 309–10, 316; and Hall Commission, 303, 364, 405–8, 410–12, 419, 427; removal of double-majority requirement for national hospital insurance, 261–4, 283–4, 439

doctors' strike. *See* Saskatchewan doctors' strike
Dodd, Paul A., 120, 533n148
Doig, Dr. Noel, 361, 583n122, 597n133
Dominion-Provincial Reconstruction Conference, 8, 124–9, 131–44, 151, 154, 176–7, 180, 239–40, 254; Green Book proposals, 8, 124, 128, 134–6, 138–42, 144, 149–50, 171, 176–80, 229, 239–40, 244–5, 360, 425, 492, 536n17; historical debate concerning, 141; impact of failure, 141–2
Douglas, Annie (née Clement), 24, 29–31, 93
Douglas, C.H. (Major), 68
Douglas, Irma (née Dempsey), 37–8, 71–2, 83, 92–3, 320, 436, 467, 481, 486; impact of doctors' strike and 1962 election loss, 369, 373, 376; marriage to T.C., 33–4
Douglas, Shirley, 71–2, 83, 92–3, 229; friends of the Black Panthers organization, 467–9
Douglas, T.C. (Thomas Clement): belief in Liberal Party's eventual demise, 307, 404, 415, 438, 609n14; boxer and instructor, 30, 36; on communist organizations and members, 38, 53–4, 73–4, 119, 171, 468; on democratic socialism and socialist ideology, 7, 30, 33, 38, 54, 74, 89, 134, 321–2, 371, 456, 488, 627n32; on eugenics (master's thesis), 42–5; illness and death, 484–7; on health regions, 212–13, 217, 277, 534n154; on immigrants, 8, 25–7; and Minister of Public Health portfolio, 91–2, 204–5, 207, 524n26; on nature of democracy, 22, 57, 155, 320; organized medicine, attacks on, 361, 368, 370, 375, 388, 391–2; pragmatic idealist, 6–7, 30, 113, 402, 470, 488, 495; prominence after death, 3–4, 489, 494; on public fiscal management and deficits, 21, 144, 154, 204; on Quebec, 323, 463, 631n85; radio broadcasts, use of, 81, 114, 121–2, 154–5, 261, 264, 277–82, 288, 490; and Regina Manifesto, 45, 66, 307 (*see also* Winnipeg Declaration); relationship with Indigenous peoples, 220–3; and Ross Thatcher, 18–20; selecting and managing cabinet, 86–92; Social Credit support (1934), 68–71; television appearances, 282, 293–5, 334–5, 353, 360, 367, 461–2; on "tin cup medicare," 14, 414, 447; on two phases for Medicare, 483; on women in government, 89–90, 531n129
Douglas, Tom (T.C.'s father), 25, 29–30, 71
Douglas (Tulchinsky), Joan, 379, 601n12
Douglas-Coldwell Foundation, 482
Drew, George, 129, 131, 133–5, 140, 536n22
Dry Belt. *See* Great Depression
Dunning, Charles, 72
Duplessis, Maurice, 133–6, 140, 245–7, 254, 265
Dyck, Erika, 194; *Psychedelic Psychiatry*, 194

Eaglesham, Dr. Hugh, 49–50, 510n14
Eastwood, Clint, 467–8
Economic Council of Canada, 436, 477
Eden, Anthony, 74
Edinburgh, Scotland, 24
Eig, Jonathan, 6, 495

Index    679

elections, federal:
- 1935, 56, 64–70
- 1945, 135, 185, 237–8; Liberal platform on health insurance, 240
- 1949, 184–5, 237–8; CCF platform on health insurance, 238–9; Liberal platform, 237–9; results, 238–9
- 1953, 241
- 1957, 19, 261–2, 573n134
- 1958, 19, 309
- 1962, 347, 357–74; Liberal strategy and concerns, 404; NDP platform on national medical care insurance, 353, 366–7; PC and Liberal platforms on national medical care insurance, 365–6; result, 371–2; Saskatchewan Medical Care Plan as issue, 352–3, 359–70, 386; T.C.'s campaign in Regina, 357–8, 369–70; T.C.'s defeat and impact of election, 371–4
- 1963, 412–15; health insurance platforms, 412–14; NDP's role in precipitating election, 412; results, 414–15
- 1965, 426, 435–8; Hall Commission report, 436; Liberal recruitment of leftist candidates in Quebec, 435; Manning's televised attack on national medical care plan, 433–4; result and portrayal of T.C., 438
- 1968, 456–64; first televised leaders' debate, 461–2; implementation of national medicare as issue, 459–60; Liberal's portrayal of T.C. Douglas and NDP, 456, 461; NDP criticism of Liberals' approach to medicare, 460; result, including T.C.'s loss of seat, 463–4. *See also* Trudeaumania
emergency services. *See* air ambulance

equalization. *See* federalism
Erb, J. Walter, 11–13, 199, 205, 207, 289, 303, 314–15, 336, 338–41, 350, 410, 558n8; allegations that T.C. prevented deal with CPS, 353–6; demotion as Saskatchewan health minister, 341–2; departure from Saskatchewan CCF-NDP, 350, 354–5; resignation, 356
Established Programs Financing (EPF), 476–82, 483–4, 623n74, 634n122; impact, 481–2; negotiations with provinces, 476–81; origins of, 449–50, 455; T.C.'s antipathy to, 477–80
Estevan Coal Strike, 38–9, 58–9
Eston, SK, 104
Ethiopia, invasion of, 75
eugenics, 42–4
evidence-based medicine, 107
extra billing (physician). *See* user fees

Falkirk, Scotland, 24, 26
Farmer-Labor Group (CCF), 41–2, 46–52, 67, 171
farm organizations. *See* organized farm groups
Farm Security Administration (FSA). *See* New Deal
fascism, 53, 73–5, 98–9, 136, 392
Federal Bureau of Investigation (FBI), 273, 467–9
Federal Emergency Relief Administration (FERA). *See* New Deal
federalism (Canada):
- conditional versus unconditional social transfers, 79, 246, 256, 448–9
- constitution (division of powers), 126, 135–6, 234, 246; Douglas's and Manning's interpretation of, 234;

health as provincial jurisdiction, 133, 136, 234, 253, 449; watertight interpretation, 234, 246
- equalization, 126, 139, 449–50
- federal health transfers to provinces: change to block transfer (*see* Established Programs Financing); double-majority rule, 253–4, 256–8, 260–4; eligibility requirements for, 9, 150, 248, 254, 256–7, 265, 419, 422–3, 430–1, 433, 475–6; impact of tax transfer replacing cash transfer, 479 (*see also* Established Programs Financing)
- federal spending power, 234, 251, 421, 491
- first ministers' conferences: 1941 Dominion-Provincial Conference, 127; 1945–6 (*see* Dominion-Provincial Reconstruction Conference); 1950 Conference of Federal and Provincial Governments, 241; 1955 Federal-Provincial Conference, 230, 242–55; 1957 Dominion-Provincial Conference, 263–4; 1960 Dominion-Provincial Conference, 303; 1965 Federal-Provincial Conference, 425, 430–2; 1976 Federal-Provincial Conference, 477
- health ministers' conferences: 1956 Federal-Provincial Conference of Health Ministers, 256; 1966 Federal-Provincial Conference of the Ministers of Health, 440
- shared-cost social programs, 246, 449, 455, 476, 478; Pearson on why Medical Care Act transfers not shared cost, 431; Quebec's opposition to, 133, 245, 319, 429; T.C.'s support of, 8, 230, 480–1
- tax-rental agreements, 8, 12, 135, 138–40, 145, 176, 208, 242, 244, 338
federal-provincial conferences. *See* federalism
field ambulance, 28
Fines, Clarence, 47, 59, 62, 81, 87–9, 92, 144–5, 154, 168–9, 183, 204, 242–3, 252, 254, 338, 512n22
Firestone, O.J., 408–9
First Baptist Church, Winnipeg, 34
Fisher, Doug, 415–16
Flemming, Hugh John, 245, 568n60
Flin Flon, MB, 358–9
Fonda, Jane, 457
foreign ownership, in Canada, 417, 461, 470, 474
Forsey, Eugene, 65
France, 75, 96
Franco, Francisco, 73–5
Front de Libération du Québec (FLQ), 472–3
Frost, Leslie, 243–5, 247–55, 259, 569n81, 571n98; loss of private health insurance, 249; role in getting hospital insurance onto national agenda, 242, 249

Gaelic, 25
Gallup poll, 84, 129, 435, 620n15, 627n35
Gardiner, James G. (Jimmy), 47–9, 84, 127, 184, 238, 406, 523n25, 535n11
Gatineau Hills, 72
Geneva, 73–4, 285
Germany, 53, 65, 96
Gibson, Clarence, 101, 543n39
Girard, Alice, 408–9
Glasgow, Scotland, 24–5, 28, 61; Clydeside, 28
Glebe Collegiate, Ottawa, 95
Godbout, Joseph-Adélard, 80

Goldman, Lawrence, 5
Gordon, King, 65, 285
Gordon, Walter, 403, 415–18, 426, 439, 450, 623n61, 627n31; support for a national medical care plan, 432; T.C. on Gordon's descent, 417–18
Great Depression, 4, 34–9, 63–5, 97; drought, 34–5, 40, 49, 64, 72, 120, 173, 204, 217; impact on children and teenagers, 36; impact on Ernest Manning, 235; impact of farms and farm families, 21, 35, 47, 63–4, 67, 157; impact on oral hygiene, 224–5; relief (payments and vouchers), 35–6, 39–40, 49, 97, 125, 227; relief camps (federal), 58–60; relief costs (provinces and municipalities), 125, 505n82; Saskatchewan Relief Commission, 36
Green Book proposals. *See* Dominion-Provincial Reconstruction Conference
Grey, Michael, 156
Grier, Terry, 457
Group Medical Services (GMS), 153, 268–9, 271–2, 283, 288, 291, 293, 394, 397–8, 576n25
Gull Lake, SK, 205

Hall Commission (1961–4), 9, 19, 213, 303, 364, 422–3, 428, 432, 435–6, 439, 441–2, 460
– appointment of chair, 405–6
– members of, 407–8
– origins of, 405–6
– public hearings, 408–10; government of Saskatchewan presentation, 410
– Saskatchewan Hospital Services Plan, influence of, 421

– Swift Current Health Region, influence of, 420–1
– T.C. approving report as blueprint for Medicare, 435–6
– volume 1 of final report and recommendations (June 1964), 419–21, 425, 430; CMA's negative reaction, 419; financing, 420; Health Charter for Canadians, 420; national medical care program as next essential step, 420; single-payer design, 424–5, 447; T.C.'s reaction, 421, 428
– volume 2 of final report (January 1965), 426; dissent by Dr. David Baltzan, 427; rejection of physician extra-billing, 427

Hall, Emmett (Justice), 5, 19, 213, 401; appointment to Supreme Court of Canada, 427; background and ideology, 406–7; defending report and attacking organized medicine, 427; Judy LaMarsh and, 427; insistence on Health Charter for Canadians, 420, 615n93; second review and report, Medicare (1979–80), 482, 484; report's conclusions, 484; and SOS Medicare Conference, 482–3
Hames, Clarence Francis, 115, 122–3, 531n128
Hardie, Keir, 30
Harding, William M., 271, 274–5, 578n44
Harney, John Paul, 486
Hart, John, 134, 230
Harvard University, 197, 381, 395
Heagerty, J.J., 79, 142, 177
Heagerty Report, 78–80, 84, 95, 115, 128, 171, 174, 177
health centres, 99
health promotion. *See* public health

health regions, 9, 11, 93–4, 99, 107–23, 141, 143, 147–8, 155, 168, 172, 184, 195, 203, 210–17, 224–8, 268, 272, 274, 276–7, 282, 295, 491, 559n22
- Assiniboia-Gravelbourg (No. 2), 211
- dental programs in, 225–7
- map of proposed health regions (1945), 118
- Meadow Lake (No. 14), 211
- Moose Jaw Health Region (No. 6), 117, 211
- North Battleford Health Region (No. 13), 211, 225
- Prince Albert (no. 12), 211,
- Swift Current Health Region (No. 1), 117, 121–2, 211–17, 227, 270, 274, 282, 389, 420, 534n154, 563n68, 577n26, 615n95; and decline in infant mortality, 217; dental care in, 215, 217, 226; district health centres within region (Leader, Maple Creek, Shaunavon), 214; health coverage, 212–14; health data collection, 213–15; infant and pre-school programs, 216; model for future socialized health system, 213–14; payment of physicians, 214; as pilot project for Saskatchewan, 212–13; provincial government's frustrations with, 217; public health surveillance, 215–16; Swift Current Union Hospital (tertiary care provider for region), 214; usefulness to Hall Commission, 213; user fees after 1953, 214–15, 217
- Weyburn–Estevan Health Region (No. 3), 117, 121–2, 211, 224, 534n154

Health Resources Fund, 432
Health Survey Committee (Saskatchewan), 176, 181, 186–9, 211, 553n55
Heeney, Arnold, 285
Heffel, Ann, 101
Herridge, H.W. (Bert), 389
Hicks, Henry, 245
Higginbotham, Chris, 176
Hincks, Dr. Clarence, 189–90, 196
Hippocratic Oath, 61
Hitler, Adolf, 73–4, 517n102
Hjertaas, Dr. Orville Kenneth, 121, 151, 351, 383, 534n157
Hoffer, Abram, 193–5, 198
home care, 136, 253, 274, 276, 419, 478
Hong Kong, defence of, 77
Hoover, J. Edgar, 273
Hoover mobiles, 63
Hopkins, Harry, 97
hospital insurance, national, 230, 256–66, 492–3; debate on, 259; exclusion of mental hospitals, 258, 260; federal cost sharing with provinces, 144, 230; First Nations, coverage of "registered Indians," 258–60; implementation by provincial governments, 265; legislation (see Hospital Insurance and Diagnostic Services Act); national unifier, 264; single-payer and single-tier, 265; user charges, 265
Hospital Insurance and Diagnostic Services Act (1957), 256, 259–60, 262–3, 265, 421, 431, 439, 444, 448–9, 478, 623n73
hospitals, 112
- hospital construction, 111, 149, 167; National Health Grants Program, 180–3, 232, 550n22, 551n25

– mental (psychiatric) hospitals: Saskatchewan (general), 105, 111–12, 130, 189–95, 198–9, 282, 339, 382, 491, 554n63; exclusion from federal cost-sharing, 200, 251, 258, 260, 463, 570n93; North Battleford mental hospital (Saskatchewan Hospital North Battleford), 104, 152, 189–91, 198, 201; Weyburn mental hospital (Saskatchewan Hospital Weyburn), 42–4, 104, 189–91, 193, 195, 197–8, 378, 550n22
– ratio of hospital beds to population, standard, 112
– role in health system, 148
– training in hospital accounting, 183–4
House of Commons. *See* Canada, Government of
Houston, Dr. Clarence, 114–17, 188, 296, 303
Houston, Stuart, 188
Howard, Frank, 410
Huxley, Aldous, 194–5; *Brave New World* (1932), 194; *The Doors of Perception* (1954), 195
Huxley, Francis, 194–5

Île-a-la-Crosse, SK, 223
illness prevention. *See* public health
Ilsley, J.L. (James Lorimer), 139
Independent Labour Party (ILP), 40–2, 46–7, 56–7
Indian Head, SK, 197
Indian hospitals, 221–2, 258, 260
Institute of the History of Medicine, Johns Hopkins University, 96
Interdepartmental Committee to Study the Medical Care Insurance Program (1959), 270–7; centralized versus decentralized administration (debate), 274–7; coverage recommendations, 273–4; health regions, role of, 276–7; physician payment options, 273, 276
International Woodworkers of America, 412
Isumi, Kiyoshi, 194
Italy, 53

Japan, 75, 77
Jewish (ethnicity), 48, 74, 102–3, 157, 274, 309, 378, 504n64; anti-Semitism, 115, 157, 309, 605n46
Johns Hopkins University, 93, 96, 151
Johnson, A.W. (Al), 164, 242–3, 252, 254–5, 271, 403, 477, 530n119, 607n73; doctors' strike strategy committee, 395–6; national medicare negotiations with provinces, 428–33, 618n142; observations at Federal-Provincial Conference of 1955, 244–7, 568n50, 568n63; recruitment in federal government by Walter Gordon, 418; tax transfer (social programs) proposal, 448–50, 477, 480, 634n122
Johnson, Lyndon B., 208–9, 273
Jones, Esyllt, 101
just society, 435, 462–3

Kamsack, SK, 119, 359
Keep Our Doctors (KOD) movement, 361–3, 368, 370, 376; KOD provincial rally in Regina, 385–8; effigies of T.C. and Woodrow Lloyd, 386–7
Kelly, Dr. Arthur D., 302, 384, 389, 393, 606n66
*Kelly's Heroes* (film), 467

Index 683

684    Index

Kennedy, John F., 403–4; influence of Theodore White's *The Making of the President, 1960*, 404
Kent, Tom, 401, 403, 413, 417–18, 429–30, 433, 456, 609n5, 612n45, 613n59; background, 412; as Liberal candidate against T.C. (1963), 412–15; Plan for Health proposal at National Liberal Rally (1961), 365
Keynes, John Maynard, 138
Keynesian economics, 132, 307
Kierans, Eric, 474, 623n74
King, Carlyle, 77, 80
King, Jack, 59–60, 62, 510n16, 513n32
King, Martin Luther, Jr., 6, 495
King, William Lyon Mackenzie, 64, 72, 75, 77–80, 84, 229, 238, 425, 492; on CCF, 64; Dominion-Provincial Reconstruction Conference, 124, 127–9, 131–5, 138, 140–2; National Health Grants Program, 175–80; perception of T.C., 128
Kingston Conference (1960), 403, 609n5
Kingston, ON, 394
Kipling, A.V., 383
Knowles, Stanley, 32–4, 55, 306, 381, 428, 445, 474, 485, 518n106, 585n31, 587n56; and national health insurance, 248, 256–7; and New Party, 308–11, 316–17
Kronau, SK, 60
Ku Klux Klan, 48

laboratory tests. *See* diagnostic services
Labour Party (UK), 30
Labour-Progressive Party. *See* Communist Party of Canada
Labour Zionist, 103
Lac La Ronge, SK, 223

Lalonde, Marc, 478
Lalonde Report (1974), 478
La Loche, SK, 223
LaMarsh, Judy, 403, 416–18, 429; and Emmett Hall's defence of his report, 427, 617n130; replaced as minister of health, 438, 620n22
*Lancet, The*, 384
Langmuir, Alexander, 216, 500n34
LaPierre, Laurier, 464, 466
Laporte, Pierre, 473
larger school unit, Saskatchewan, 85, 88, 114, 144, 171, 530n119; act, 114
Lawson, Dr. Sam, 198–202
Laxer, James, 469, 474
Laycock, Samuel, 196
Leader, SK, 358
League for Social Reconstruction (LSR), 45–6, 65–6, 79, 128, 285, 403; *Social Planning for Canada* (1935), 65–6, 79
League of Nations, 73–5, 285
Lee, Tim, 242–3, 396, 579n69
Lennon, John, 458
Lesage, Jean, 265, 429–30, 432, 438, 444, 449, 623n74
Lewis, David, 306, 308–11, 316, 348, 372–3, 415–16, 448, 457–8, 470–2, 474, 477, 587n56; leadership of NDP, 466–7, 474; *Make This Your Canada* (1943), 129; parliamentary leader of NDP (1968–9), 465–7
Lewis, Stephen, 456–7
Liberal Party: of British Columbia, 168, 230, 240; of Canada, 9, 18, 64–9, 72, 78, 84, 95, 127, 128–9, 131, 177, 179, 184, 186, 235, 238, 248, 261–3, 268, 307, 319, 349, 359, 365–8, 372, 401–4, 406, 412–19, 435, 438, 441, 445–7, 456–62, 482, 486, 493; of Manitoba, 134, 471;

of New Brunswick, 134, 430, 450; of Newfoundland, 432; of Nova Scotia, 245; of Ontario, 252, 345–7; of Prince Edward Island, 134; of Quebec, 80, 265, 444, 473; of Saskatchewan, 16–20, 47–52, 78, 82, 84, 92–3, 125, 170–1, 261, 277, 283, 287, 300, 336, 338–9, 342–5, 352, 361, 391–2, 475, 494; in United Kingdom, 30, 415

Lloyd Brown, Dr. J., 101

Lloyd, Woodrow, 88, 119, 312, 341, 345, 347, 350–2, 354–7, 360, 363, 368–9, 372–3, 394–5, 398, 400, 418, 423–4, 427, 477, 560n40; background, 338; becoming premier, 337–8; biography, 382; leadership during doctors' strike, 375–8, 380–2, 384, 386–92

local government. *See* municipalities

London School of Economics, 79, 380

long-term care and nursing home residency, 44, 104–5, 136, 148–9, 478

Los Angeles, 92

Lynch, Charles, 367, 464, 471

MacArthur, (General) Douglas, 431

Macdonald, Angus, 134

MacDonald, Donald C., 251

MacEachen, Allan J., 5, 403, 417, 456, 459, 475–6, 624n83; appointment as minister of national health and welfare, 438; negotiating national medical care plan, 438–41; preparing and passing Medical Care Act (Bill C-227), 441–8; struggle over medicare's implementation date, 450–4

MacInnis, Grace, 416, 600n193

Mackenzie, Ian, 95, 525n37

MacLean, Dr. Hugh, 60–2, 65–6, 92–5, 100, 102, 107, 147, 521n6, 524n26, 527n65

MacLeod, A.A., 53

MacMillan, Alexander S., 134

MacNeil, Harris Lachlan, 32

Mahood, Dr. Ed, 363–4

Malcolm, Keith, 218

Manchuria, invasion of, 75

Manitoba: CCF-NDP in, 70, 102–3, 108, 414, 465, 470–1; hospital insurance, 243, 255, 265; impact of Great Depression in, 35, 125–6; medical care insurance, 432

Manningcare. *See* Alberta

Manning, Ernest C., 133–4, 190, 247, 298–9, 554n66; hospital insurance, alternative, 232–7, 246–7, 252, 255, 265; medical care insurance, 413, 421–2, 429, 432–5, 448

Maple Creek, SK, 121, 214

Maple Leaf Gardens, Toronto, 437

Marchand, Jean, 435–7, 453–4

Marsh, Leonard, 65, 79–80

Marsh Report, 79–80, 95, 128

Martin, Paul, Sr., 5, 142, 168, 196, 307, 443, 456, 548n104; National Health Grants Program, 177–85, 441, 550n16; national hospital insurance, 241–2, 248–9, 252, 255–61, 265; national medical care insurance, 443, 452, 456; relationship with T.C., 73–5, 517n105; and St-Laurent's position on hospital insurance, 248–9

Martin, William Melville, 92

Marx, Karl, 297

Marxism, 7, 30, 53, 56, 382, 589n102, 630n77

Massey, Denton, 73–4

Matthews, Dr. Vincent L. (Vince), 215–16, 270–1, 274, 291, 576n19

686   Index

Mayo Clinic, 220
McClelland, F.W., 339
McClung, Nellie, 44
McCutcheon, Wallace, 407, 409–12
McGillivray, Don, 368, 420
McGill University, 45, 80, 137, 155, 488
McKerracher, Dr. Donald Griffith (Griff), 190–3, 195–9, 201–2, 222, 378, 556n92; background, 190; Canadian Mental Health Association, establishing Saskatchewan branch, 196–7; psychiatric nursing, establishment of, 191–2; Psychiatric Services Branch, establishment and use of, 196–7
McKinnon, Eleanor, 358, 369, 612n44
McLarty, Robert, 430
McLeod, Ian, 352
McLeod, Thomas H. (Tommy), 37, 102, 109, 135, 138–9, 164, 352; health policy functions, 102, 109, 111–12, 121–3, 139, 151, 158, 160; organizational role in government, 90–1; on T.C.'s relationship with organized medicine, 111–12
McMaster University, 31, 42, 507n114
McNab, Archibald, 93
measles. *See* public health
medical appliances, 136
Medical Care Act (Canada), 438–50
– Bill C-227 introduced in House of Commons (June 1966), 441–4
– criteria, 431, 448–9; comprehensiveness, 429, 431; portability, 429, 431, 441; public administration, 441, 443–4; universality, 433, 442, 447–8, 460
– delay of start date from 1 July 1967 to 1 July 1968, 445–6
– extra-billing (user fees), 441, 448
– limited to coverage for physician services, 443, 447
– passage of Bill C-277 (December 1966), 448
– provinces, meeting eligibility requirements, 474–6
– provincial opposition to, 439–40, 446, 450, 452–3
– split in Pearson cabinet, 447, 451–4
– tax transfer provision, 449–50
– timing of Bill C-227 after first reading, 444–7
medical care insurance (medicare), national: federal proposal, 430–2; legislation (*see* Medical Care Act); negotiations with provinces for national plan, 429–30, 433–41; Quebec, influence of, 429–30, 440, 449–50, 472–3, 475
Medical Care Insurance Commission (MCIC). *See* Saskatchewan Medical Care Insurance Plan
medical health officer. *See* physicians
Medical Council of Canada, 155
Medical Services Incorporated (MSI), 153, 235, 268–9, 271, 283, 287–9, 291, 293, 394, 397–8, 576n25
medicare, defined, 11; as distinguished from Medicare, 298; T.C. on "tin cup" medicare, 14, 41, 447
Medicare, defined, 455. *See also* universal health coverage
Melfort, Saskatchewan, 199, 358, 362
Menninger, Carl, 192
mental health reform, 9, 43–4, 111, 176, 181, 186, 189–202; community psychiatry and clinics, 192–3 (*see also* Saskatchewan Plan); LSD, research in, and therapeutic use of, 194–5; Mental Health Act (Saskatchewan, 1950), 193; mental

health education and changing public perceptions, 196–7; mental health research, 176, 186, 193–7; psychiatric hospital reform, 189–93, 195; psychiatric nursing program, 191–2; Saskatchewan Plan (regional psychiatric facilities), 194, 198–201, 339–40
Methodist Church, 26, 33
Mexico, 156
Mikkelson, Peter, 60
Milbank Memorial Fund, 97
Mills, John A., 190
Monteith, Waldo, 364
Montreal, 80, 137, 316, 437, 458, 461; Montreal Stock Exchange, 472
*Montreal Gazette*, 461, 471
*Montreal Star*, 466
Moose Jaw, SK, 19, 58, 104, 110, 117, 120, 183, 302, 347, 362, 368–9, 504n75
More, Ken, 365, 372
Morin, Claude, 429–30
Morton, Desmond, 436–7
Mossbank, SK, debate between T.C. and Ross Thatcher, 283–4
Mott, Frederick D. (Fred), 9, 182, 202, 213, 225, 280, 389, 548n104; deputy minister, 182, 205–7, 211; health regions and, 210–11, 216; hiring of as chair of HSPC, 123, 155–8; implementing hospital insurance, 159–66, 168, 170, 172–3, 352; and National Health Grants Program, 177, 181; provincial health survey, 186–8; *Rural Health and Medical Care* (1948), 159
Mott, John R., 156
municipal doctor plans. *See* municipalities
municipalities (Saskatchewan), 36, 84, 93, 111–13, 116–17, 149–50, 160, 167, 183, 218, 225, 269, 272, 276; collection of health taxes (premiums), 149–50, 160, 164; municipal doctor plans, 93, 110, 113, 116, 117, 121, 180, 232, 269, 290–1; rural municipalities (RMs), 36, 113, 117, 120–2, 275, 532n139; Saskatchewan Association of Rural Municipalities (SARM), 113–14, 151, 160; Saskatchewan Urban Municipalities Association (SUMA), 113–14, 151, 160; union hospital districts, 93, 112–13, 121, 149, 166–7; union hospitals, 104, 149, 167, 183, 214, 267, 542n17, 550n22, 552n38; urban municipalities, 36, 113, 122, 532n139
Murray, Father Athol, 376

Nanaimo–Cowichan–The Islands (federal constituency), 464–5, 481
National Committee for Mental Hygiene. *See* Canadian Mental Health Association
National Film Board (NFB), 220, 589n91
National Health Council (United States), 158
National Health Grants Program, 167, 175–89, 199, 225, 230, 232, 240–1, 244, 246, 262, 421, 441, 550n21, 550n22, 551n25, 563n68; categories of grants, 181; formula for distribution to provinces, 181; hospital construction grants, 181–3; name of, 180; origins of, 177–80; provincial health surveys, 176, 181, 186–9, 553n55; quantum of spending, 180–1, 183; ribbon-cutting events, 184

688 Index

national health insurance system, 163
National Health Service (NHS). *See* United Kingdom
national health service system, 163, 261, 541n11
National Liberal Rally (1961), 403
National Old Age Pensioners' Federation, 241
Nazi Germany, 74–5, 99–100
Naylor, C. David, xi
New Brunswick, 25, 125, 134–5, 184; hospital insurance, 245, 265; medical care insurance, 430, 440, 450, 617n136, 618n146, 635n133
New Deal (US), 9, 64, 67, 72, 97–8, 123, 156–8; Farm Security Administration (FSA), Health Services Branch, 156–9; Federal Emergency Relief Administration (FERA), 97; migrant farm workers, health programs for, 156; national health insurance, 157; rural health initiatives, 106, 159
New Democratic Party (NDP). *See* CCF-NDP
Newfoundland, 225, 231
– hospital insurance, 246–7, 255, 265; cottage hospital scheme, 231–2, 246, 565n10, 560n67
– medical care insurance, 440
New Haven, CT, 151
New Jerusalem, 56
New Left, 402, 461, 467, 469–71, 627n32, 630n77
Newman, Paul, 467
New Party. *See* New Democratic Party
New York City, 25, 80, 97, 151, 155, 197, 378
New York State, 156
New York University, 158

New Zealand, 86, 229, 541n12; children's school-based dental plan, 224, 226–8, 563n72; New Zealand Labour Party, 86, 147, 541n11; universal health coverage plan, 21, 146–7, 521n6, 541n11, 541n13, 581n84
Nicholson, A.M. (Sandy), 95, 258, 525n38
North American Air Defense Command (NORAD), 347
North Atlantic Treaty Organization (NATO), 347
North Battleford, SK, 104, 199, 201, 211, 339
North Battleford mental hospital. *See* hospitals
North End (Winnipeg). *See* Winnipeg
Nova Scotia, 125, 134, 139, 359
– hospital insurance, 245, 265
– medical care insurance, 432, 475–6; Maritime Medical Care Incorporation, 475, 633n115
– Nova Scotia Medical Society, 475
– provincial health survey, 187
nurses, 21, 49, 82, 99, 108, 110, 112, 129, 131, 167, 191, 203, 222–4; air ambulance (flight) nurses, 218–20; psychiatric nurses, 191–2; public health nurses, 110, 117, 184, 195–6, 213, 216, 224; registered nurses, 187, 218, 220
nursing stations (northern), 203, 221–4
nutritionists, 99, 184
Nystrom, Lorne, 463, 628n46

Old Age Security, 415
Ono, Yoko, 458
Ontario, 34–5, 125, 190, 198, 437, 463; CCF-NDP in, 127, 129, 131, 249–51, 254, 324, 345–7, 371–2, 414,

436, 456–7, 465, 470; Dominion-Provincial Reconstruction Conference, 8, 125, 129, 133, 135, 138–9, 141, 176–7, 239; hospital insurance, 242–55, 257, 260, 264–5, 568n49, 569n81; Ontario Dental Association, 407; Ontario Hospital Association, 249; Ontario Medical Association (OMA), 18, 187, 297; provincial health survey, 187; Robartscare and medical care insurance, 417, 421–2, 429, 432, 440–1, 444, 448, 476

On-to-Ottawa Trek. *See* Regina Riot

optical services, coverage of 22, 274, 319, 335, 346, 360, 364, 419, 443, 447

oral health care, 108, 203, 215, 224–8

organized farm groups (Canada), 39; relationship with CCF-NDP, 40, 46, 51, 168, 290, 307–9, 336, 342; support for Medicare, 109, 114, 117, 131, 452; tensions with organized labour, 306–8, 342

organized labour (Canada): support for Medicare, 287–8, 325–8, 330, 341, 428, 484; relationship with CCF-NDP, 39, 59, 306–10, 332, 341, 349, 354, 372, 482

organized medicine, 9, 12, 15, 17–18, 117; Canada, 187, 232, 252, 265–6, 268, 360; cooperation (CPS, OMA, CMA, AMA) during 1960 Saskatchewan election, 197; influence of physicians who left NHS, 273; in New Zealand, 147; regulatory college subsumed into provincial medical associations, 94, 391, 499n9, 524n33; Saskatchewan, 172, 189, 205, 228, 270, 273, 277, 281, 287, 301, 325, 333, 339, 352–3 (*see also* College of Physicians and Surgeons of Saskatchewan); in the United States, 156

Osmond, Dr. Humphrey, 193–5, 198

osteomyelitis, 26–8, 77

Ottawa, ON, 58, 60, 71, 95; Beechwood Cemetery, 487

*Ottawa Citizen*, 368, 408, 419, 446, 488

Oxford, University of, 285, 549n122

Palliser Triangle. *See* Great Depression

Patterson, William J., 84, 125–6, 128

Peacock, Dr. George W., 269, 377

Pearson, Lester B. (Mike), 5, 285, 307, 310, 345, 348, 403–4, 413–19, 421–2, 435, 456, 461, 479–80, 552n40; changing health ministers, 438; election of 1962, 358, 365, 403; election of 1963, 414–16; and legislation for national medicare 439–47, 452–4; merger discussions with NDP, 415–16; national medicare, 425–34, 438–47, 452–4

Pederson, Martin, 284

Pelican Narrows, SK, 223

Pelletier, Gérard, 435

Perth, Scotland, 25

pharmaceuticals. *See* prescription drugs

Phelps, Joe, 88, 92

physicians: chief medical officers, 99, 107, 110, 117, 156, 215; general practitioners (GPs), 99, 145, 147, 152, 379, 388; minimum ratio of GPs to general population, 112; physician payment, 93; physician-sponsored health insurance companies (*see* Group Medical Services and Medical Services Incorporated); psychiatrists, 176, 192–7; public health doctors, 99;

radiologists in hospitals, 149, 214; specialists, 17, 66, 85, 99, 112, 117, 147, 149, 152, 172, 182, 329, 379–82, 388, 431, 472–3, 475

Poland, 27, 75

polio, 168

polyclinics, 9, 99, 106, 108, 152, 155, 172, 207, 274, 382, 528nn84–5; definition of, 106

Popular Front, 48, 53, 74

population health, 46, 106–7, 117, 181, 494; determinants of health, 494–5; health outcomes, 112, 203, 478

Portage la Prairie, MB, 33

Prairie provinces, 34, 125; Dry Belt, 35, 533n151; Palliser Triangle, 35, 72; prairie populism, 306, 403

Presbyterian Church, 25, 33, 36, 156

prescription drugs, 66, 94, 99, 143; excluded from universal health coverage, 274; as part of comprehensive health insurance, 79, 84, 136, 147, 319, 346, 360, 365, 413, 419, 431, 443

preventive care (prevention). *See* public health

primary health care, 112, 117, 213–14, 478; GP-based primary care, 136, 145, 155, 214; group practice, 66, 155, 280, 381, 383, 400, 483; primary care clinics (and centres), 9, 94, 106, 152, 155, 172, 382; primary mental health care, 198

Prince Albert, SK, 35, 104, 110, 135, 183, 199, 211, 362, 383, 534n155

Prince Edward Island, 125, 134–5; hospital insurance, 245, 263, 265; medical care insurance, 432

private health insurance, 13–15, 21, 232–3, 249, 265, 271, 283, 288, 473, 491; administrative costs, 279–80, 344; critiques of, 295, 335; Hall Commission and, 408, 419

Progressive Conservative Party (PC): of British Columbia, 168, 230; of Canada, 19, 64, 129, 260–3, 283, 358–9, 364–5, 367, 371–2, 402–3, 405–6, 410–11, 414, 435–7, 445, 460, 463, 475, 481–2, 491; of Manitoba, 432; of Nova Scotia, 475; of Ontario, 129, 244, 250, 422, 432; of Saskatchewan, 18, 49, 84, 263, 284, 298, 300, 407, 424, 510n152, 523n25

Progressive Party, 61

prosthetics, 419

psychedelic, 194

psychiatric (mental) hospitals, 189

psychiatry, 190, 197–201; community psychiatry, 192, 197–201

public health, 46, 65, 93, 97, 99, 101, 107, 110, 122, 130, 151, 156, 159, 175, 213, 215, 220, 378, 491–2
- communicable disease control: measles, 224; smallpox, 224; syphilis, 109; typhoid, 224; tuberculosis (*see* tuberculosis (TB) control). *See also* sexually transmitted disease control
- disease surveillance, 215–16, 560n34
- health promotion, 99, 110, 213, 215, 226, 327
- illness prevention and preventive medicine, 46, 82, 94, 99, 105–7, 107, 110, 117, 122, 130, 213, 215, 224–6, 227, 274, 280, 290, 326–7, 351, 478, 483, 494
- immunization, 21, 117, 224
- infant mortality, 217
- National Health Grants, public health and research, 175, 181, 184
- nutrition, 131, 262

- public health and safety inspection, 110, 213
- public health education, 21, 45, 106–7, 131, 226
- public health regions. *See* health regions

Quebec City, QC, 80
Quebec (province), 125, 177, 244, 371, 406, 438, 470
- CCF-NDP in, 319, 323, 416, 435, 462–3, 486, 488, 631n85
- Créditistes. *See* Social Credit Party of Canada
- Dominion-Provincial Reconstruction Conference, 133–6, 138–9, 141, 176–7, 239
- Federation of Medical Specialists (Fédération des Médecins spécialistes du Québec), 472–3
- hospital insurance, 168, 242, 245, 247, 254, 264–5
- medical care insurance, 429, 432, 444, 448, 484, 618n138; doctors' (specialists) strike (1970) and, 472–3, 475
- Padlock Act, 136
- provincial health survey, 187
- Quebec Chamber of Commerce, 472–3
- Quebec Manufacturers Association, 472–3
- Quiet Revolution (Révolution tranquille), 323
Quiring, David, 221–2; *CCF Colonialism in Northern Saskatchewan*, 221

Rands, Stan, 381–3, 589n91
Reagan, Ronald, 361
recall (defined), 63
Reconstruction Party, 76
Redgrave, Vanessa, 467
Regier, Erhart, 376, 601n6
Regina, SK, 35, 41, 45–7, 58–62, 70–1, 92–5, 103–4, 110, 112, 114, 154, 158–60, 168, 199, 210, 359–65, 369–73, 384–5. 408–9, 485, 504n75; City of Regina tax assessor, 165; Hotel Saskatchewan, 93; Hungarian Centre, 298; Lakeview United Church, 375–6; mayor of, 164; Regina City Hall, 164; Regina Little Theatre, 467; Regina Voice of Women, 359; Trianon ballroom, 336
Regina Cancer Clinic, 104
Regina General Hospital, 60, 101, 111, 165, 190, 195; psychiatric wing, 111
Regina Labor Council, 288
*Regina Leader-Post*, 48, 60, 69, 84, 104, 158, 168–9, 313, 318, 320–1, 323, 336, 343–4, 353, 362, 366, 370, 373, 388, 409, 425
Regina Manifesto, 45–6, 48–9, 66, 126, 307, 470, 485
Regina Riot, 58–62
regional health authorities. *See* health regions
regionalization. *See* health regions
regions. *See* health regions
Registers Nurses' Association of Saskatchewan, 187
Reiman, Oral, 342–4
relief. *See* Great Depression
relief camps. *See* Great Depression
Rhodes, Cecil, 6
Rhodes scholars (Oxford University), 245, 285, 412
Robarts, John P., 422, 429, 432, 446
Robartscare. *See* Ontario
Robbins, Arthur, 164–5
Robertson, Stuart, 383

Robichaud, Louis, 430, 432, 450, 617n136
Roemer, Dr. Milton I., 159–60, 546n73; Roemer's Law, 160
Roman Catholic Church, 48, 75, 89, 104, 167, 220, 222–3, 297, 376, 404, 406
Romanow, Roy, xiii
Roosevelt, Franklin (F.D.R.), 9, 64, 67, 72, 97, 157; as role model for T.C., 516n88
Rorem, Rufus, 530n113
Rosenfeld, Dr. Leonard Sidney (Len), 157–61, 166, 170, 182, 543n42, 545n65
Rosetown, SK, 69
Ross, Dr. Donovan, 439
Rotberg, Robert, 6
Roth, F. Burns, 198, 206–7, 211, 213, 227–8, 236, 251–2, 254–5, 271, 289, 291, 383, 556n104, 558n4, 558n8
Rowell-Sirois Commission, 125–7, 139
Royal Canadian Air Force (RCAF), 218, 513n32; RCAF Norsemen aircraft, 218
Royal Canadian Military Corps, 108
Royal Canadian Mounted Police (RCMP), 39, 58, 60–1; Security Service's surveillance of T.C., 469, 630n76
Royal Commission on Agriculture and Rural Life, 278, 530n119
Royal Commission on Dominion-Provincial Relations. *See* Rowell–Sirois Commission
Royal Commission on Health Services. *See* Hall Commission
Royal Flying Doctor Service, Australia, 218, 220
rural health centres. *See* health centres

Saint John, NB, 25
Saltcoats, SK, 119
Sandy Bay (Snake Lake), SK, 223
sanitary officers. *See* public health
Saskatchewan:
– CCF-NDP in, 8, 11–19, 46–54, 80–95, 113, 125–6, 168–73, 283–8, 296–300, 459, 463, 475; change of leadership (1961), 336–8
– elections: 1934, 47–52, 68; 1944, 37, 81–6; 1948, 168–74, 204; 1952, 173; 1956, 356, 592n39; 1960, 272, 296–300; 1961 Weyburn by-election, 342–5; 1964, 277, 424
– impact of drought: and depression, 34–7; on oral health, 224
– natural resources, 81, 88, 204, 208–9, 220–1, 335
– "next-year country," 204
– northern areas, 218, 220–4; health policies in, 218, 221–2; historical debate concerning CCF's policies in, 221–2; nursing stations, 223
– population of, 110, 211
– provincial health survey, 176, 181, 186–9, 211, 553n55
– rural nature of, 35, 105, 110, 112–13, 120, 148, 203, 208, 217–25, 275; lack of access to dentists, 224–5; rural electrification, 208–10
– wheat economy, 35, 64, 173, 204–5, 208, 224, 231, 285; King Wheat, 35; Saskatchewan Wheat Pool, 40, 51, 205
Saskatchewan, government of:
– Adult Education Division, 118–20, 382
– Bill of Rights, 86, 335
– Budget Bureau, 164, 351
– cancer clinics. *See* cancer
– Department of Cooperation and Cooperative Development, 205

- Department of Public Health, 36, 107–8, 145, 147, 153, 182, 184, 190, 192, 205, 211, 213, 215, 217–18, 222–8, 270, 280, 291, 293, 326–7, 329, 331, 339, 341, 381, 396; Division of Dental Health, 225–7; Psychiatric Services Branch (PSB), 192–4, 196–9, 339, 381–2
- Department of Social Welfare, 91, 195, 205, 291; Economic Advisory and Planning Board (EAPB), 137, 164, 173, 199, 228, 242, 271, 275, 358, 477
- Health Services Act, 111, 121, 529n103
- Health Services Planning Commission (HSPC), 107, 110–12, 114–23, 146–58, 161–7, 181–2, 186–7, 210–13, 217, 248, 250, 268, 351–3, 381, 532n138
- innovations (policy and administrative), 22, 86, 168, 181, 230, 492
- Public Assistance Medical Plan, 110–11, 143, 146, 224
- Saskatchewan Legislative Assembly, 11–12, 16
- social welfare, 86, 91, 111, 205, 327
- Trade Union Act (1944), 86

Saskatchewan Air Ambulance Service, 168, 203, 218–20, 389, 490, 561n46

Saskatchewan Association of Rural Municipalities (SARM). *See* municipalities

Saskatchewan Urban Municipalities Association (SUMA). *See* municipalities

Saskatchewan Chamber of Commerce, 304, 325

Saskatchewan doctors' strike (1962), 375–400; CPS versus community clinics (*see* community clinics); end of strike (*see* Saskatoon Agreement); media attention, 380–1, 368; mediator (*see* Stephen Taylor); miscalculations by government and CPS, 379–80; recruitment of doctors outside province, 368, 378–81; social consequences, 417; strike strategy committee, 395–6; Lloyd's desire to end strike, 386, 392

Saskatchewan Federation of Labour (SFL), 287, 296, 325, 339, 341

Saskatchewan Hospital Association (SHA), 101, 149, 162–3, 212, 352–3, 391

Saskatchewan Hospital Services Plan (SHSP), 142–74, 158, 164–74; administrative costs compared to private hospital insurance plans, 279–80; billing system, 165; collection of hospital premiums (taxes) (*see* municipal governments); compared to Alberta's original hospital plan, 235–7; compulsory versus voluntary, 150, 235–6; differences with national health system design, 157; financing of, 145, 149–50, 154, 173–5; hospital expansion under, 166–8; hospital tax (premium), 149–50, 160, 162, 164; launch of, 164–6; national influence of, 156, 230, 421, 491–3; payment of hospitals, 154, 163, 211–12; preparing for implementation, 160–4; reason preceded medical services insurance plan, 145–6; registration, 150, 160, 162; risk pooling, 155; staff, 166; single-payer design, 152, 189, 236; standardized forms

(hospital administration and discharge), 161; time devoted to, 211; utilization of, 166–8
Saskatchewan Hospitalization Act (1946), 151–3, 160–1
Saskatchewan Medical Association. *See* College of Physicians and Surgeons of Saskatchewan
Saskatchewan Medical Care Insurance Act, 12, 23, 335, 376; agency clause amendments of April 1962, 355–6; consultation on original bill (1961), 329, 331–4; Diefenbaker on T.C.'s political use of, 407; legislative debate on original 1961 bill, 11–23, 334–5; preparation and passage of original 1961 bill, 328, 335–6; proposed amendments to avert doctors' strike in June 1962, 376–7
Saskatchewan Medical Care Plan:
– continuation after CCF-NDP election loss in 1964, 427
– doctor-patient relationship and, 346–7, 357, 382
– election of 1960 as referendum on medical care plan, 277, 283, 286–6
– financing of, 295, 330–1
– Medical Care Insurance Commission (MCIC), 331, 355, 361, 377–8, 380, 383, 386, 391, 396–400, 430, 480; establishment and appointment of, 350–2
– operating principles: acceptability to public and physicians, 281, 329; government as single payer, 280–1; high-quality services, 280; public administration, 280, 301; universality, 279
– physician payment, 329, 331, 370
– single-payer nature of, 398

*Saskatchewan Medical Quarterly*, 116, 532n132
Saskatchewan Plan. *See* mental health reform
Saskatchewan Power Corporation (SaskPower), 208, 210
Saskatchewan Psychiatric Nurses Association, 258
Saskatoon, SK, 15, 104, 110, 112, 154, 183–4, 192, 199, 210, 225, 363–4, 370, 376, 388–400, 504n75; Bessborough Hotel, 389, 394, 396; Medical Arts Building, 392–4
Saskatoon Agreement, 375, 392–400, 424; choice of payment system for physicians, 396–8, 400; community clinics, 399–400; drafting of, 396; extra-billing of patients, 397–8; negotiations, 393–6; rights of physicians, 398–9; as template for other provinces, 400; threat of two-tier care, 398
*Saskatoon Star Phoenix*, 69, 324, 363–4, 369, 406, 411
schizophrenia, 193–4
Schreyer, Edward Richard (Ed), 465–6, 471
Scotland, 8, 24–5, 29–31, 231, 323
Scott, Frank (F.R.), 45, 62, 65, 73, 92, 127, 129, 132, 136–7, 306, 403, 488, 630n77
Scottish Co-operative Wholesale Society, 25, 28
Scotton, Cliff, 358, 370, 436, 612n44
Seberg, Jean, 467
Second World War, 5, 73, 119, 129, 378, 411; atomic bomb, Hiroshima, 135; Pearl Harbor, attack on, 156; threat of, 73–8
secular society, rise of, 404–5
sexually transmitted disease control, 43, 99, 107–9, 168, 181

Sharp, Mitchell, 439, 446–7, 450–1, 623n61, 623n66; and delay in implementation of national medicare, 445–6; desire for postponement of national medicare, 451–4

Shaunavon, SK, 104, 122, 214

Sheps, Cecil G., 108–9, 150–3, 158, 160, 213, 218, 280

Sheps, Mindel Cherniak, 102–11, 153, 158, 213–14, 225, 274, 280, 382; appointment and background, 102–3; secretary, Health Services Planning Commission, 111–23; secretary, Sigerist Commission, 103–8; work on hospital insurance, 139, 148–50

Shoyama, Thomas K. (Tommy), 199, 201, 403, 434, 480, 567n48, 633n120, 634n122; advisor to T.C. for 1962 election campaign, 358, 360, 367, 548n117; and hospital insurance, 242–3, 252, 254–5; and medical care insurance, 271, 367, 385; move to federal government, 403, 436, 477; role in Established Programs Financing, 477, 480; and Saskatchewan doctors' strike, 385, 394–6, 399

Sicks, Timothy E., 468

Sifton, Sir Clifford, 69

Sifton press, 69, 154, 158, 277, 344, 363, 370, 392, 424, 515n66, 544n43

Sigerist, Henry E., 85, 93–110, 117–19, 151, 155, 157, 160, 214, 224, 274, 280, 382, 524n26; founder of *American Review of Soviet Medicine*, 99; Sigerist Commission, 101–5; Sigerist Report, 105–11, 214; *Socialized Medicine in the Soviet Union* (1937), 97, 103

Skelton, Douglas Alexander (Alex), 138–40

Smallwood, Joseph Roberts (Joey), 232, 247, 255, 432

Smishek, Walter, 296, 312; dissent, Thompson Committee report, 325–8, 330–1, 339

Smith, Dr. Stanley, 27

social care. *See* home care; long-term care

Social Credit Party: of Alberta, 44, 55, 67–70, 134, 190, 232–3, 298; of British Columbia, 231, 254, 298, 413, 422–3, 432; of Canada, 19, 66–70, 291, 359, 371, 414, 424, 434, 443, 448, 573n128, 599n182, 611n41; of Saskatchewan, 284, 298, 300, 515n68, 522n13

social credit theory, 68

social gospel, 32–3, 56

social health insurance system, Bismarckian, 65–6, 98, 146, 149, 526n53, 547n102

social justice, 221, 336, 446, 506n89

social workers in health care, 99, 108, 196, 381–2, 467

socialized health services (socialized medicine), 41, 46, 49, 62, 66, 81–2, 84, 93–103

sociology, discipline of, 37, 42, 65, 197

SOS Medicare conference, 482–4

South African War, 25, 28

South Saskatchewan Regiment, 77

Soviet Union (USSR), 39, 48, 73–4, 78, 95–100, 104–7, 347, 378

Spanish Civil War, 73–5, 99–100, 285; Spanish Hospital and Medical Aid Committee, 285

Spencer, Henry, 66

Spry, Graham, 65, 384, 399, 403, 516n89; advising T.C. on medicare

as election issue (1960), 286–7; as agent general for Saskatchewan in London, UK, 285–6, 378, 574n139; background, 285–6; recruitment of doctors in UK during doctors' strike, 378–81
Stalinism, 97
Standard Oil, 285
Stanfield, Robert, 460–2, 475, 480
State Hospital and Medical League (SHML), 62, 82, 93–4, 104, 107, 110, 114, 382, 524n31
Staveley, J.H. (Jun), 342–5, 352, 592n39
Stevens, H.H., 76
St-Laurent, Louis, 139–40, 174, 186, 234, 262, 264, 425, 456, 463, 466, 492; National Health Grants Program, 175, 177, 179–80, 186; national hospital insurance, 229–30, 232, 237–48, 251–60, 264
Stony Rapids, SK, 223
Strachan, Dr. C.L. (Leslie), 407, 409
Strachan, Robert, 423, 616n107
Strasbourg, SK, 104
Strathcona Baptist Church, Edmonton, 55
Strum, Gladys, 84
Sturgis, SK, 119
Supreme Court of Canada, 407, 427, 490
Sutherland, Donald, 467–8
Sutherland, Irene, 220
Sutherland, Kiefer, 467
Sutherland, Rachel, 467
Sweden, 65, 67
Swift Current, SK, 120–3, 199, 205, 214–15; Swift Current Health Region (No. 1) (*see* health regions); Swift Current Union Hospital District, 167, 214
Switzerland, 96
Sydney, NS, 359

Talnicoff, Mark, 31, 34, 504n64
Tansley, Donald D., 430, 480, 635n133; Medical Care Insurance Commission, chair of, 351–2, 378, 383, 395–6
tariffs, 72
Task Force on the Structure of Canadian Industry. *See* Watkins Report
Tawney, R.H., 5
tax-rental agreements. *See* federalism
Taylor, Charles, 464, 631n85
Taylor, E.P., 412
Taylor, Elizabeth, 467
Taylor, George, 383
Taylor, Malcolm G., 164, 427, 444, 481, 484; as health administrator in Saskatchewan, 181–2, 186–9, 570n86; *Health Insurance and Canadian Public Policy* (1978), 164, 250, 259; health policy consultant, Ontario government, 248–51, 254–5
Taylor, Stephen (Lord), 375, 380, 384–8, 392–9; initial recruitment and arrival in Canada, 384–5; negotiating the Saskatoon Agreement, 392–9
tertiary care (hospitals), 99, 106, 110, 112, 213–14
Tetley, William, 472
Thatcher, Ross, 283–4, 324, 331–2, 342–4, 350, 398, 424–5, 430; on deterrent fees (1968), 459, 463, 475; opposition to Saskatchewan Medical Care Insurance Plan, 17–20, 336, 339, 352, 361, 387–8; position on national medical care plan, 432, 440, 453; retention of Saskatchewan Medical Care Insurance Plan, as premier, 427–8; role in defection of Hazen Argue, 347–8

Thompson Committee, xiii, 16, 272, 282, 288, 299; appointment of chair, 288–90; appointment of members, 290–1, 296; chair's threatened resignation, 303–5; final report, 314; interim report, 296, 314, 325–32; relationship with organized medicine, 290–6, 302–6; T.C.'s objectives for, 289; timeline and timing, 291, 296, 301, 303, 314–15, 352
Thompson, Walter P., 288–90; public attack on, 312–14
Thomson, Watson, 119–20, 381–2
*Time* magazine, 95
Tisdale, SK, 199
*Titanic*, 25
Titmuss, Richard, 380, 602n17
Toronto, ON, 53, 73, 181, 243, 261, 300, 311, 316, 348, 364, 372, 376, 378–9, 384, 412, 459; Maple Leaf Gardens, 437; Toronto Psychiatric Hospital, 190
trade unions. *See* organized labour
Trew, Beatrice, 89–90, 522n18
Trudeau, Pierre E., 435, 455–6, 458–63, 480–2, 624n4; changing mechanism for federal health transfers, 476–80; T.C.'s dislike of, 480
Trudeaumania (1968), 455–6, 463, 465
tuberculosis (TB) control, 22, 93, 99, 113, 175, 181, 218, 224, 256, 261, 294; tuberculosis sanitoriums, 104, 105, 130, 256
Tucker, Walter, 78, 170, 184
Tulchinsky, Dr. Theodore (Ted), 379
Turnbull, Olaf, 337–8, 590n14

Ukraine, 27
Ukrainian (ethnicity), 48

Underhill, Frank, 45, 65, 403, 516n89; *In Search of Canadian Liberalism* (1960), 403
unemployment, 29, 58, 64, 72, 132, 367, 588n82
unemployment insurance, 36, 46, 97, 124, 128, 140, 147, 186, 244
United Church, 34, 36, 376, 485, 505n84, 518n106
United Farmers of Canada (Saskatchewan Section), 40–1, 46–7
United Kingdom, 5, 24, 29, 65, 75, 77–8, 86, 106, 127, 130, 163, 170, 231, 229, 278, 285, 306–7, 324, 375, 380, 384, 386, 412, 415, 490; British Labour Party, 5, 30, 130, 285, 306, 324; National Health Service (NHS), 14, 21, 142, 146, 163, 299, 302, 361, 378–80, 384, 494; Royal Academy of Dramatic Art, London, 467; St. George's Hospital, London, 193
United Mine Workers of America's Memorial Hospital Association, 206
United Nations (UN), 86
Universal Declaration of Human Rights (UN), 86
universal health coverage (UHC), 4–5, 98; centralized versus decentralized administration, 161, 217, 236–7, 268, 274–7, 560n40; comprehensive health insurance, 12, 21–2, 65, 79, 121–4, 128, 130, 132, 141–4, 154, 171, 175–6, 178, 180, 186, 188–9, 207, 224, 229–30, 232, 238–40, 254, 331, 335, 346, 413, 420, 435, 443, 456; means test as inimical to, 14, 21, 235–6, 246, 271, 335, 414; single-payer design, 4, 189, 213, 236–7, 246, 258, 265, 268, 273, 280–1, 287–8, 302, 304, 325,

355, 405, 408, 419, 421, 483, 489, 490–3; single-tier services, 4, 265, 268, 325, 398, 421, 483–4, 489–92; staging in phases, 136, 253, 255, 266, 268, 274, 278
Université de Montréal, 481
University of Alberta, 55
University of California at Berkeley, 167, 181, 521n6, 551n30
University of California at Los Angeles (UCLA), 120, 147, 533n148, 546n73
University of Chicago, 37, 42, 54–5
University of Manitoba, 42, 108, 285, 534n155, 592n31
University of Toronto, 45, 61, 177, 181–2, 190, 198, 206, 215, 250, 378, 436, 470
University of Saskatchewan, 63, 107–8, 135, 137, 192–3, 197–8, 215, 272, 288, 290, 296, 312–13, 338, 351, 378; dentistry college, 108; medical college, 94, 98, 107–8, 282
Uranium City, SK, 223
user fees, 14, 215, 217, 231–2, 235–7, 256, 265, 290, 326, 330–1, 355, 377, 397–8, 448, 455, 459, 475–6, 481–6
US Public Health Service, 106, 157, 159–60

Vancouver, BC, 58, 316, 370, 413, 436–7, 446, 457
*Vancouver Sun*, 414
Van Wart, Dr. Arthur, 407, 409–10
venereal disease control. *See* sexually transmitted disease control
Vietnam War, 402, 405, 469
Vipond, Reverend Reid, 376
Voice of Women, 359
voluntary health insurance. *See* private health insurance
Vulcan Iron Works, Winnipeg, 26

Wadena, SK, 104, 199
Waffle, 458, 469–72; Waffle manifesto, 469–71
wait lists, 490
Wakabayashi, Art, 430
War Measures Act, T.C.'s opposition to, 473–4
Wartime Tax Rental Agreement, 139. *See also* federalism
Washington, DC, 9, 157–8, 160, 206
Watkins, Mel, 469–71, 474, 627n31
Watkins Report, 470, 627(n31)
welfare state, 5, 65, 78–80, 95, 124, 126, 128, 132–4, 136, 138, 141, 234–5, 243, 262, 265, 307, 380, 402–5, 420, 433, 447
*Western Labor News*, 29
Weyburn Independent Labour Association, 39–40
Weyburn Independent Labour Party, 40
Weyburn mental hospital. *See* hospitals
*Weyburn Review*, 36, 38–9, 47
Weyburn, SK, 8, 11, 35–40, 49, 66–7, 77, 171, 342
Whiting, Cliff, 290–1
Wigle, Dr. William, 389
Williams, Charles, 168–9
Williams, George H., 39–40, 46, 50–1, 59, 62, 69, 80–1, 88–9, 129
Winnipeg, MB, 25–32, 34, 52–3, 71, 102–3, 108, 154, 210, 470; North End, 26, 29–31, 37, 274; Winnipeg City Council, 428
Winnipeg Community Welfare Planning Council, 426
Winnipeg Declaration, CCF (1956), 307, 319, 470–1, 485
*Winnipeg Free Press*, 69, 285, 412, 544n43
Winnipeg General Strike, 29

Winnipeg Grenadiers, 77
Winters, Robert, 456
Wiseman, Nelson, 48
Wolfe, Dr. Samuel (Sam), 351, 378–9, 382–3, 484, 602n13, 608n89
Woodsworth, J.S., 26–7, 29, 32, 37, 40–1, 46, 53–4, 60–1, 65, 75–7
World Health Organization (WHO), 182, 278
World Youth Congress, 73

X-ray. *See* diagnostic services

Yale University, 94–5, 98–9, 105, 150–1, 158
Yorkton, SK, 70, 199, 340
Young Communist League, 59
Young Men's Christian Association (YMCA), 156
Young, E.J., 66–7, 70

Zedong, Mao, 285